Clinical
Neurology

a LANGE medical book

Clinical
Neurology

second edition

David A. Greenberg, MD, PhD
Associate Professor of Neurology
and Attending Physician
University of California, San Francisco

Michael J. Aminoff, MD, FRCP
Professor of Neurology
and Attending Physician
University of California, San Francisco

Roger P. Simon, MD
Professor of Neurology
University of California, San Francisco
Chief of Neurology
San Francisco General Hospital

APPLETON & LANGE
Norwalk, Connecticut

0-8385-1311-5

Copyright © 1993 by Appleton & Lange
Simon & Schuster Business and Professional Group
First Edition Copyright © 1989 by Appleton & Lange
A Publishing Division of Prentice Hall

93 94 95 96 97 / 10 9 8 7 6 5 4 3 2 1

Prentice Hall International (UK) Limited, *London*
Prentice Hall of Australia Pty. Limited, *Sydney*
Prentice Hall Canada, Inc., *Toronto*
Prentice Hall Hispanoamericana, S.A., *Mexico*
Prentice Hall of India Private Limited, *New Delhi*
Prentice Hall of Japan, Inc., *Tokyo*
Simon & Schuster Asia Pte. Ltd., *Singapore*
Editora Prentice Hall do Brasil Ltda., *Rio de Janeiro*
Prentice Hall, *Englewood Cliffs, New Jersey*

PRINTED IN THE UNITED STATES OF AMERICA

Table of Contents

Preface

Clinical Neurology is designed to provide medical students, house officers, and non-neurologist practitioners with an organized clinical approach to the evaluation and treatment of neurological complaints.

Chapters 1 through 11 are organized according to the major problems with which neurological disorders commonly present. Within each chapter, we develop an approach to diagnosis, drawing upon basic neuroanatomical principles, clinical history-taking, general physical and neurological examinations, and laboratory data. We then review the various diseases that can lead to the problem under consideration, emphasizing relevant aspects of epidemiology, basic neuroscience, pathophysiology and pathology, differential diagnosis, laboratory investigations, treatment, and prognosis. This format offers the student a guided approach to the analysis of individual patients' presenting complaints, while still enabling the busy practitioner to review a specific disorder quickly. A new chapter on *Neurological Investigations*—Chapter 12—covers the use of lumbar puncture, electrophysiological studies, cranial and spinal imaging, ultrasonography, and biopsies in neurological diagnosis. Appendices provide methods for obtaining and recording a detailed neurological history and examination, performing a briefer screening examination, and examining the functions of selected peripheral nerves.

The second edition of *Clinical Neurology* has been thoroughly revised and updated. In preparing and revising this book, we have been guided by our clinical experience and teaching of neurology at the University of California Medical Center and San Francisco General Hospital. We have chosen approaches and illustrative material that have been helpful to students taking their first neurology clerkship, to more advanced students, and to house officers. The book contains 225 illustrations and tables—most of them original—to clarify neuroanatomical concepts and examination techniques and to provide organized schemes for analyzing clinical findings, formulating differential diagnoses, and treating neurological emergencies. References to selected reviews and other timely articles in the neurological literature follow each chapter; they have been chosen for their likely value to readers of this book.

We have tried to make *Clinical Neurology* useful; we hope that we have succeeded, and we continue to welcome suggestions from readers. The present edition reflects the enormously helpful suggestions of medical students, house officers, and faculty members at the University of California who have used this book since its initial publication. In this respect, we are especially grateful to Megan Burns, Cathleen Miller, Lydia Bayne, Robert Messing, Donna Ferriero, Daniel Lowenstein, Philip Gutin, and Mark Rosenblum. We thank Ken and Cathleen Miller for preparing the new illustrations, Muriel Solar for editing the text, and Alisa Gean for providing CT and MR scans. Finally, we wish to thank the past and present staff at Appleton & Lange for their support at all steps in the production of this book.

David A. Greenberg
Michael J. Aminoff
Roger P. Simon

San Francisco
May, 1992

Disorders of Cognitive Function: Approach to Diagnosis & Acute Confusional States

1

Disorders of cognitive function can impair the level of consciousness (arousal or wakefulness) or the content of consciousness. Disturbances of the **level** of consciousness range in severity from mild confusional states to coma; disturbances of the **content** include both global cognitive disorders (dementia) and more restricted defects in memory, language, or other functions.

Confusional states are discussed in this chapter. Dementia and memory disorders are discussed in detail in Chapter 2, and coma in Chapter 11; these conditions are mentioned more briefly here.

Disturbances of the Level of Consciousness

Abnormalities of the level of consciousness occur when the ascending reticular activating system (Figure 1–1) or both cerebral hemispheres are anatomically or functionally disrupted.

Severe dysfunction produces **coma,** in which the

Table 1–1. Differences between acute confusional states and dementia.

	Acute Confusional State	Dementia
Level of consciousness	Impaired	Not impaired, except occasionally late in course
Course	Acute to subacute; fluctuating	Chronic; steadily progressive
Autonomic hyperactivity	Often present	Absent
Prognosis	Usually reversible	Usually irreversible

patient is unresponsive and unarousable. Less severe dysfunction results in **acute confusional states,** in which the patient responds to at least some stimuli in a purposeful manner but is sleepy, disoriented, and inattentive.

In some instances, agitation rather than drowsiness may predominate. This is the syndrome of **delirium,** which is often characterized by autonomic disturbances (fever, tachycardia, hypertension, sweating, pallor, or flushing), hallucinations, and motor abnormalities (tremor, asterixis, myoclonus). Delirium frequently alternates with drowsiness.

Disturbances of the Content of Consciousness

Many pathological conditions can impair the content of consciousness without altering the level of consciousness. Focal involvement of the brain by structural lesions or selective regional vulnerability to more diffuse processes can lead to isolated disorders of such functions as language or memory.

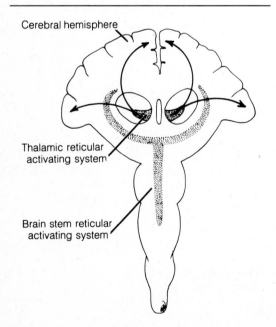

Cerebral hemisphere

Thalamic reticular activating system

Brain stem reticular activating system

Figure 1–1. Brain stem recticular activating system and its ascending projections to the thalamus and cerebral hemispheres.

Certain diffuse, chronic pathological processes can lead to widespread deterioration of mental function, or dementia. Dementia differs from acute confusional states in several respects (see Table 1–1).

I. APPROACH TO DIAGNOSIS

Evaluation of the patient with a suspected cognitive disorder is aimed at determining the following:

(1) Whether such a disorder is present.

(2) Whether impairment of function is global or circumscribed.

(3) Whether the picture is that of a confusional state or dementia.

(4) Whether a treatable pathological process exists.

The approach to diagnosis outlined below, which is designed to answer these questions, applies to any patient with a cognitive disorder. Once the nature of the cognitive disorder is established, the specific cause of an acute confusional state (discussed later in this chapter), dementia, or amnestic syndrome (see Chapter 2) can be investigated.

HISTORY

History of Present Illness

The history should establish the temporal course of the disorder and provide clues to its cause. When dementia is suspected, it is crucial to have a source of information other than the patient—usually a close relative—who can furnish details about the patient's previous level of functioning, the time when dysfunction became evident, and the nature of any changes in personality, behavior, mood, intellect, judgment, memory, or facility with language. Associated problems such as gait disorders, incontinence, and headaches should also be explored. If the patient appears to be in an acute confusional state, the observations of police officers or ambulance attendants may be the only historical information available.

Prior Medical History

A. Cardiovascular System: A history of stroke, hypertension, vasculitis, or cardiac disease may suggest a vascular cause of a confusional state or multi-infarct dementia.

B. Diabetes: Cognitive disturbance in diabetic patients may relate to a hyperosmolar nonketotic state or to insulin-induced hypoglycemia.

C. Seizure Disorder: A history of epilepsy should suggest the possibility of a postictal state or head trauma in a confused patient.

D. Head Trauma: Recent head trauma suggests intracranial hemorrhage. Remote head trauma may produce amnestic syndrome or chronic subdural hematoma with dementia.

E. Alcoholism: Alcoholism predisposes patients to conditions that may present as an acute confusional state; these include intoxication, withdrawal, postictal state, head trauma, hepatic encephalopathy, and Wernicke's encephalopathy. Chronic memory disturbance in an alcoholic is likely to be the result of Korsakoff's syndrome.

F. Drug History: Information about the patient's medications is invaluable. A confusional state can result from intentional or accidental overdose with insulin, sedative-hypnotics, opioids, antidepressants, antipsychotic agents, or hallucinogens. The patient's tolerance to such drugs often declines with age, and cognitive disturbances may be the result of adverse reactions to doses that are well accepted by younger patients. It should be noted that sedative drug withdrawal can also lead to a confusional state.

G. Psychiatric History: A history of psychiatric illness may suggest an accidental or intentional overdose with benzodiazepines, antidepressants, or antipsychotic agents; a previously undiagnosed medical disorder capable of producing organic psychosis (hypothyroidism, vitamin B_{12} deficiency); or a functional disorder masquerading as an acute confusional state or dementia.

H. Other: Homosexual or bisexual men, intravenous drug users and their sexual partners, and recipients of blood or clotting factor transfusions are at particular risk for developing confusional states or dementia related to acquired immunodeficiency syndrome (AIDS).

Family History

The family history is most useful when a heredodegenerative disorder is being considered as the cause of dementia.

GENERAL PHYSICAL EXAMINATION

A general physical examination helps to classify the disorder as either an acute confusional state or dementia and may suggest a systemic disease as its cause (Tables 1–2 and 1–3).

Vital Signs & General Appearance

Fever, tachycardia, hypertension, and sweating occur in many confusional states and should suggest such a state rather than dementia. Meningitis or systemic infection must receive early consideration in the febrile patient. Hypertension should alert the physician to the possibility of hypertensive encephalopathy, intracranial hemorrhage, renal disease, or Cushing's syndrome. Hypothermia occurs with exposure to cold, ethanol or sedative drug intoxication, hypoglycemia, hepatic encephalopathy, Wernicke's encephalopathy, hypothyroidism, or shock. In most dementias, the patient does not appear acutely ill unless a systemic disorder is also present.

Skin & Mucous Membranes

Jaundice suggests hepatic disease, and lemon-yellow coloration of the skin may occur in vitamin B_{12} deficiency. Coarse dry skin, dry brittle hair, and subcutaneous edema are characteristic of hypothyroidism. Petechiae are seen in meningococcemia, and petechiae or ecchymoses may reflect coagulopathy caused by liver disease, disseminated intravascular coagulation, or thrombotic thrombocytopenia purpura. Hot, dry skin is characteristic of intoxication with anticholinergic drugs. Cushing's syndrome may be associated with acne. Hyperpigmentation of the skin may be evidence of Addison's disease. Needle tracks associated with intravenous drug use suggest drug overdose or infective endocarditis.

Head & Neck

Examination of the head may reveal evidence of recent trauma, such as scalp lacerations or contusions, postauricular hematoma (Battle's sign), periorbital hematoma (raccoon eyes), hemotympanum, or cerebrospinal fluid (CSF) otorrhea or rhinorrhea. Percussion of the skull over a subdural hematoma may cause pain or may be associated with a sound described as stony dullness.

Meningeal signs, such as neck stiffness on passive flexion, thigh flexion upon flexion of the neck (Brudzinski's sign), or resistance to passive extension of the knee with the hip flexed (Kernig's sign), are seen in meningitis and subarachnoid hemorrhage.

Chest & Abdomen

Cardiac murmurs may be associated with infective endocarditis and its neurological sequelae. Abdominal examination may reveal a source of systemic infection or suggest liver disease. Rectal examination may provide evidence of gastrointestinal bleeding, which is often the precipitating factor in hepatic encephalopathy.

Table 1–2. Clinical features helpful in the differential diagnosis of acute confusional states.

Feature	Most Suggestive of	Feature	Most Suggestive of
Headache	Head trauma, meningitis, subarachnoid hemorrhage	Tetany	Hypocalcemia
Vital signs		**Cranial nerves**	
Fever	Infectious meningitis, anticholinergic intoxication, withdrawal from ethanol or sedative drugs	Papilledema	Hypertensive encephalopathy, intracranial mass
Hypothermia	Intoxication with ethanol or sedative drugs, hepatic encephalopathy, hypoglycemia, hypothyroidism	Dilated pupils	Head trauma, anticholinergic intoxication, withdrawal from ethanol or sedative drugs, sympathomimetic intoxication
Hypertension	Anticholinergic intoxication, withdrawal from ethanol or sedative drugs, hypertensive encephalopathy, subarachnoid hemorrhage, sympathomimetic intoxication	Constricted pupils	Opioid intoxication
Tachycardia	Anticholinergic intoxication, withdrawal from ethanol or sedative drugs, thyrotoxicosis	Nystagmus/ophthalmoplegia	Intoxication with ethanol or sedative drugs, vertebrobasilar ischemia, Wernicke's encephalopathy
Bradycardia	Hypothyroidism	**Motor**	
Hyperventilation	Hepatic encephalopathy, hyperglycemia, pulmonary encephalopathy	Tremor	Withdrawal from ethanol or sedative drugs, sympathomimetic intoxication, thyrotoxicosis
Hypoventilation	Intoxication with ethanol or sedative drugs, opioid intoxication	Asterixis	Metabolic encephalopathy
General examination		Hemiparesis	Cerebral infarction, head trauma, hyperglycemia, hypoglycemia
Meningismus	Meningitis, subarachnoid hemorrhage	**Other**	
		Seizures	Withdrawal from ethanol or sedative drugs, head trauma, hyperglycemia, hypoglycemia
Skin rash	Meningococcal meningitis	Ataxia	Intoxication with ethanol or sedative drugs, Wernicke's encephalopathy

NEUROLOGICAL EXAMINATION

Mental Status Examination

Evaluation of mental status (see box, p 5) helps to classify a cognitive disorder as a confusional state, dementia, a circumscribed cognitive disturbance (aphasia, amnesia), or a psychiatric illness. The mental status examination is most useful if performed in a standardized fashion—and with the understanding that complex functions can be adequately evaluated only when the basic processes upon which they depend are preserved. Functions such as memory, language, calculation, or abstraction cannot be reliably assessed in the patient who is barely arousable or extremely inattentive.

In performing the mental status examination, the level of consciousness and attention are evaluated first. If these are impaired, an acute confusional state exists, and it may be difficult or impossible to conduct the remainder of the mental status examination. If the level of consciousness and attention are adequate, more complex cortical functions are examined next to determine whether there is global cortical dysfunction, which indicates dementia.

A. Level of Consciousness: The level of consciousness is described in terms of the patient's apparent state of wakefulness and response to stimuli. Impairment of the level of consciousness should always be documented by a written description of the patient's responses to specific stimuli rather than by the use of such nonspecific and imprecise terms as "lethargy," "stupor," or "semicoma."

1. Normal–The patient with a normal level of consciousness appears awake and alert, with eyes open at rest. Unless there is deafness or a language disorder, verbal stimulation results in appropriate verbal responses.

2. Impaired–Mild impairment of consciousness may be manifested by sleepiness from which the patient is easily aroused when spoken to. As consciousness is further impaired, the intensity of stimulation required for arousal increases, the duration of arousal declines, and the responses elicited become less purposeful.

B. Attention: Attention is the ability to focus on a particular sensory stimulus to the exclusion of others; **concentration** is sustained attention. These processes are grossly impaired in acute confusional states, usually less impaired in dementia, and unaffected by focal brain lesions. Attention can be tested by asking the patient to repeat a series of digits or to indicate when a given letter appears in a random series. A normal person can repeat five to seven digits correctly and identify a letter in a series without error.

C. Language and Speech: The essential elements of language are comprehension, repetition, flu-

Table 1–3. Clinical features helpful in the differential diagnosis of dementia.

Feature	Most Suggestive of
History	
(Male) homosexuality, intravenous drug abuse, hemophilia, or blood transfusion	AIDS dementia complex
Family history	Huntington's disease, Wilson's disease
Headache	Brain tumor, chronic subdural hematoma
Vital signs	
Hypothermia	Hypothyroidism
Hypertension	Multi-infarct dementia
Hypotension	Hypothyroidism
Bradycardia	Hypothyroidism
General examination	
Meningismus	Chronic meningitis
Jaundice	Acquired hepatocerebral degeneration
Kayser-Fleischer rings	Wilson's disease
Cranial nerves	
Papilledema	Brain tumor, chronic subdural hematoma
Argyll Robertson pupils	Neurosyphilis
Ophthalmoplegia	Progressive supranuclear palsy
Pseudobulbar palsy	Multi-infarct dementia, progressive supranuclear palsy
Motor	
Tremor	Acquired hepatocerebral degeneration, Wilson's disease, AIDS dementia complex
Asterixis	Acquired hepatocerebral degeneration
Myoclonus	Creutzfeldt-Jakob disease, AIDS dementia complex
Rigidity	Acquired hepatocerebral degeneration, Creutzfeldt-Jakob disease, progressive supranuclear palsy, Wilson's disease
Chorea	Huntington's disease, Wilson's disease
Other	
Gait apraxia	Normal pressure hydrocephalus
Polyneuropathy with hyporeflexia	Neurosyphilis, vitamin B_{12} deficiency, AIDS dementia complex

---

MENTAL STATUS EXAMINATION

Level of consciousness
Attention and concentration
Language and speech
  Comprehension
  Repetition
  Fluency
  Naming
  Reading
  Writing
  Calculation
  Speech
Mood and behavior
Content of thought
  Hallucinations
  Delusions
  Abstraction
  Judgment
Memory
  Immediate recall
  Recent memory
  Remote memory
Integrative sensory function
  Astereognosis
  Agraphesthesia
  Two-point discrimination
  Allesthesia
  Extinction
  Unilateral neglect and anosognosia
  Disorders of spatial thought
Integrative motor function
  Apraxia

---

ency, naming, reading, and writing, all of which should be tested when a language disorder (**aphasia**) is suspected. Calculation disorders (**acalculia**) are probably closely related to aphasia. Speech, the motor activity that is the final step in the expression of language, is mediated by the lower cranial nerves and their supranuclear connections. **Dysarthria,** a disorder of articulation, is sometimes difficult to distinguish from aphasia but it always spares oral and written language comprehension and written expression.

Aphasia may be a feature of diffuse cortical disease, as it is in certain dementias, but language impairment with otherwise normal cognitive function should suggest a focal lesion in the dominant hemisphere. A disorder of comprehension (**receptive,** or **Wernicke's, aphasia**) commonly leads to a false impression of a confusional state or psychiatric disturbance.

There are a variety of aphasic syndromes, each characterized by a particular pattern of language impairment; several have fairly precise pathoanatomical correlations (Figure 1–2).

D. Mood and Behavior: Demented patients may be apathetic, inappropriately elated, or depressed, and their moods can fluctuate. If the examination is otherwise normal, early dementia can easily be confused with depression. Delirious patients are agitated, noisy, and easily provoked to anger.

E. Content of Thought: Abnormalities of thought content may can help to distinguish between

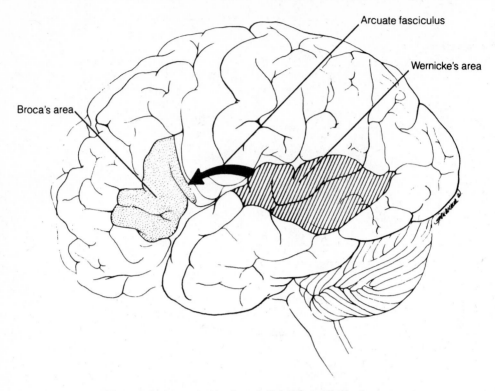

Figure 1–2. Anatomical basis and clinical features of aphasias.

Pathological Site	Type of Aphasia	Language Functions Preserved		
		Comprehension	Repetition	Fluency
Wernick's area	Receptive	−	−	+
Arcuate fasciculus	Conductive	+	−	+
Broca's area	Expressive	+	−	−

organic and psychiatric disease. **Visual hallucinations** are common in acute confusional states, while **auditory hallucinations** and **fixed delusions** are most common with psychiatric disorders. **Impairment of abstraction** may be revealed by the patient's concrete (literal) interpretation of proverbs or inability to recognize conceptual differences and similarities. **Judgment** is commonly tested by asking what the patient would do in a hypothetical situation, such as finding a stamped, addressed letter on the sidewalk.

F. Memory:

1. Functional components of memory–Memory is the ability to register, store, and ultimately retrieve information. Storage and retrieval of memories can be impaired by either diffuse cortical disease or focal bilateral dysfunction of the medial temporal lobes or their connections.

a. Registration–The ability to receive information through the various sensory modalities is largely a function of attention.

b. Storage–The process whereby selected new information is learned, or memorized, may be mediated by limbic structures, including the hippocampus. Stored memories are reinforced by repetition and by emotional significance; they are thought to be diffusely distributed in association areas of the cerebral cortex.

c. Retrieval–This is the ability to access previously learned information.

2. Amnesia–Memory disorder (amnesia) may be an isolated deficit or one feature of global cognitive dysfunction. If the dysfunction is due to an acute confusional state, impairment of attention will result in defective registration and an inability to learn new material. Problems with recent and—to a lesser extent—remote memory are more likely to be present in dementia.

In **psychogenic amnesia,** subjective and emotionally charged memories are more affected than is retention of objective facts and events; in **organic amnesia,** the reverse is true. Isolated loss of memory for personal identity (the inability to remember one's own name) in an awake and alert patient is virtually pathognomonic of a psychogenic disorder.

Additional terms sometimes used to denote aspects of acute-onset amnesia (eg, following head trauma) include **retrograde amnesia,** loss of memory for events immediately prior to the onset of the disorder, and **anterograde** or **posttraumatic amnesia,** impairment of memory in the period following the insult.

3. Testing of memory–Memory is assessed clinically by testing **immediate recall, recent memory,** and **remote memory,** which correspond roughly to registration, storage, and retrieval, respectively.

a. Immediate recall–Tests of immediate recall are similar to tests of attention and include having the patient repeat a random series of numbers or other information that has not been previously learned. The ability to repeat implies that the material has been registered. Most normal adults can repeat a series of seven numbers forward and five backward without difficulty.

b. Recent memory–Tests of recent memory assess the ability to learn new material. Typically, the patient is given three or four items to remember and asked to recall them three minutes later. Nonverbal tests requiring that an object previously shown to the patient be selected from a group of objects may be useful, especially for patients with expressive aphasia. Orientation to place and time, which represents newly learned information, is another important test of recent memory.

c. Remote memory–The practical distinction between recent and remote memory is that only the former requires an ongoing ability to learn new information. Remote memory is tested by asking the patient to recall material that someone of comparable cultural and educational background can be assumed to know. Common examples are personal, historical, or geographic data, but the questions selected must be appropriate for the patient, and personal items must be verifiable.

G. Integrative Sensory Function: Sensory integration disorders from parietal lobe lesions are manifested by misperception of or inattention to sensory stimuli on the contralateral side of the body, when the primary sensory modalities are intact.

Patients with parietal lesions may exhibit the following signs:

1. Astereognosis–The patient cannot identify, by touch, an object placed in the hand.

2. Agraphesthesia–The patient is unable to identify a number written on the hand.

3. Absence of two-point discrimination–This is an inability to differentiate between a single stimulus and two simultaneously applied adjacent, but separated, stimuli that can be distinguished by a normal person.

4. Allesthesia–This is misplaced localization of a tactile stimulus.

5. Extinction–A visual or tactile stimulus is perceived when applied alone to the side contralateral to the lesion but not when stimuli are applied bilaterally.

6. Unilateral neglect and anosognosia–Body image disorders caused by parietal lobe lesions take the form of unilateral neglect. The patient tends not to use the contralateral limbs, may deny that there is anything wrong with them (anosognosia), and may even fail to recognize them.

7. Disorders of spatial thought–These include **constructional apraxia, right/left disorientation, and neglect of external space** on the side opposite the affected parietal lobe. Tests for constructional apraxia include having the patient fill in the numbers on a clock face, copy geometric figures, or build figures with blocks.

H. Integrative Motor Function: Apraxia is the inability to perform previously learned tasks, such as finger snapping or clapping the hands together, despite intact motor and sensory function. Unilateral apraxias are commonly caused by contralateral premotor frontal cortex lesions. Bilateral apraxias, such as gait apraxia, may be seen with bifrontal or diffuse cerebral lesions.

Gait & Station

It is useful to observe the patient standing and walking early in the neurological examination, since these activities may reveal additional neurological abnormalities associated with disturbed cognitive function.

Cranial Nerves

In patients with impaired cognitive function, abnormalities associated with cranial nerves may suggest the underlying cause.

A. Lesions of the Eyes and Ears:

1. Papilledema suggests an intracranial mass, hypertensive encephalopathy, or other process that increases intracranial pressure.

2. In the confused patient, **pupillary constriction** suggests opiate ingestion; **dilated pupils** are characteristic of anticholinergic intoxication but may also be a manifestation of generalized sympathetic hyperactivity. **Small, irregular pupils** that react poorly to light—but better to accommodation—can be seen in neurosyphilis.

3. Sedative drugs and Wernicke's encephalopathy produce **nystagmus** or **ophthalmoplegia.** Selective **impairment of vertical gaze (especially downward)** occurs early in progressive supranuclear palsy.

B. Pseudobulbar Palsy: This syndrome is characterized by dysarthria, dysphagia, hyperactive jaw jerk and gag reflexes, and uncontrollable laughing or crying unrelated to emotional state (**pseudobulbar affect**). It results from bilateral interruption of the corticobulbar and corticospinal tracts. Dementing processes that produce this syndrome include progressive supranuclear palsy and multi-infarct dementia.

C. Multiple Cranial Neuropathies: These can accompany infectious or noninfectious meningitis or AIDS dementia complex.

Motor Findings

A. Acute Confusional State: In the acutely confused patient, a variety of motor abnormalities may suggest the cause.

1. Hemiparesis is most apt to be due to an intracranial structural lesion, although focal neurological signs may be present in such metabolic disorders as hypoglycemia and nonketotic hyperglycemia.

2. Tremor is common in sedative drug or ethanol withdrawal and other states accompanied by autonomic hyperactivity.

3. Asterixis, a flapping tremor of the outstretched hands or feet, is seen in hepatic, renal, and pulmonary encephalopathy and in drug intoxication.

4. Myoclonus, which consists of rapid shocklike muscle contractions, can occur with uremia, cerebral hypoxia, or hyperosmolar nonketotic states.

5. Cerebellar signs such as broad-based ataxic gait and, often, dysmetria on heel-knee-shin maneuver accompany Wernicke's encephalopathy and sedative drug intoxication.

B. Dementia: Motor signs are useful in the differential diagnosis of dementia.

1. Chorea–Huntington's disease, Wilson's disease.

2. Tremor, rigidity, or bradykinesia–Wilson's disease, acquired hepatocerebral degeneration.

3. Myoclonus–Creutzfeldt-Jakob disease, AIDS dementia complex.

4. Ataxia–Spinocerebellar degenerations, Wilson's disease, paraneoplastic syndromes, Creutzfeldt-Jakob disease, AIDS dementia complex.

5. Paraparesis–Vitamin B_{12} deficiency, hydrocephalus, AIDS dementia complex.

Abnormalities of Sensation & Tendon Reflexes

Dementias associated with prominent sensory abnormalities and loss of tendon reflexes include vitamin B_{12} deficiency, neurosyphilis, and AIDS dementia complex.

Primitive Reflexes

A number of reflexes that are present in infancy and subsequently disappear may be released by frontal lobe dysfunction in later life. It is presumed that such release results from loss of cortical inhibition of these primitive reflexes (frontal release signs), which include palmar and plantar grasps as well as palmomental, suck, snout, rooting, and glabellar reflexes. Although these responses are often seen in both acute confusional states and dementia, many can also occur in normal elderly adults. Their presence alone does not constitute evidence of cognitive dysfunction.

1. The **palmar grasp** reflex is elicited by stroking the skin of the patient's palm with the examiner's fingers. If the reflex is present, the patient's fingers close around those of the examiner. The force of the patient's grasp may increase when the examiner attempts to withdraw the fingers, and the patient may be unable to voluntarily release the grasp.

2. The **plantar grasp** reflex consists of flexion and adduction of the toes in response to stimulation of the sole of the foot.

3. The **palmomental reflex** is elicited by scratching along the length of the palm of the hand and results in contraction of ipsilateral chin (mentalis) and perioral (orbicularis oris) muscles.

4. The **suck reflex** consists of involuntary sucking movements following the stimulation of the lips.

5. The **snout reflex** is elicited by gently tapping the lips and results in their protrusion.

6. In the **rooting reflex,** stimulation of the lips causes their deviation toward the stimulus.

7. The **glabellar reflex** is elicited by repetitive tapping on the forehead. Normal subjects blink only in response to the first several taps; persistent blinking is an abnormal response (**Myerson's sign**).

LABORATORY INVESTIGATIONS

Laboratory studies are critical in diagnosing disorders of cognitive function. Useful investigations are listed in Tables 1–4 and 1–5; those most likely to establish or support a diagnosis in acute confusional states are complete blood count, arterial blood gases and pH, serum sodium, serum glucose, serum urea nitrogen and creatinine, liver function tests, drug screens, stool test for occult blood, lumbar puncture, brain CT scan or MRI, and electroencephalogram.

Some of these studies can yield a specific diagnosis. Abnormal arterial blood gas or CSF profiles, for example, narrow the differential diagnosis to one or a few possibilities (Tables 1–6 and 1–7).

Reversible dementia may be diagnosed on the basis of laboratory studies (see Table 1–5). The most common reversible dementias are those due to intracranial masses, normal pressure hydrocephalus, thyroid dysfunction, and vitamin B_{12} deficiency.

II. ACUTE CONFUSIONAL STATES

The common causes of acute confusional states are listed in Table 1–8.

Table 1–4. Laboratory studies in acute confusional states.

Test	Most Useful in Diagnosis of
Blood	
WBC	Meningitis
PT and PTT	Hepatic encephalopathy
Arterial blood gas	Hepatic encephalopathy, pulmonary encephalopathy, uremia
Sodium	Hyponatremia
Serum urea nitrogen and creatinine	Uremia
Glucose	Hyperglycemia, hypoglycemia
Osmolality	Alcohol intoxication, hyperglycemia
Liver function tests, ammonia	Hepatic encephalopathy, Reye's syndrome
Thyroid function tests	Hyperthyroidism, hypothyroidism
Calcium	Hypercalcemia, hypocalcemia
Drug screen	Drug intoxications
Cultures	Meningitis
FTA or MHA-TP	Syphilitic meningitis
HIV antibody titer	Acquired immunodeficiency syndrome and related disorders
Urine, gastric aspirate	
Drug screen	Drug intoxication
Stool	
Guaiac	Hepatic encephalopathy
ECG	Anticholinergic intoxication, vascular disorders
Cerebrospinal fluid	
WBC, RBC	Meningitis, encephalitis, subarachnoid hemorrhage
Gram's stain	Bacterial meningitis
AFB stain	Tuberculous meningitis
India ink preparation	Cryptococcal meningitis
Cultures	Infectious meningitis
Cytology	Neoplastic meningitis
Glutamine	Hepatic encephalopathy
VDRL	Syphilitic meningitis
Cryptococcal antigen	Cryptococcal meningitis
CT brain scan or MRI	Cerebral infarction, intracranial hemorrhage, head trauma, Toxoplasmosis, herpes simplex encephalitis, subarachnoid hemorrhage
EEG	Complex partial seizures, herpes simplex encephalitis, nonconvulsive seizures

Table 1–5. Laboratory studies in dementia.

Test	Most Useful in Diagnosis of
Blood	
Hematocrit, mean corpuscular volume (MCV), peripheral blood smear, vitamin B_{12} level	Vitamin B_{12} deficiency
Thyroid function tests	Hypothyroidism
Liver function tests	Acquired hepatocerebral degeneration, Wilson's disease
Ceruloplasmin, copper	Wilson's disease
FTA or MHA-TP	Neurosyphilis
HIV antibody titer	AIDS dementia complex
Cerebrospinal fluid	
VDRL	Neurosyphilis
Cytology	Neoplastic meningitis
CT scan or MRI	Brain tumor, chronic subdural hematoma, multi-infarct dementia, normal pressure hydrocephalus
EEG	Creutzfeldt-Jakob disease

DRUGS

Many drugs can cause acute confusional states, especially when taken in greater than customary doses, in combination with other drugs, by patients with altered drug metabolism from hepatic or renal failure, or in the setting of preexisting cognitive impairment. A partial list of drugs that can produce acute confusional states is provided in Table 1–9. Classes of drugs that are most commonly abused or employed in suicide attempts are discussed individually below.

Table 1–6. Arterial blood gases in acute confusional states.

Pattern	Differential Diagnosis
Metabolic acidosis (with increased anion gap)	Diabetic ketoacidosis, lactic acidosis (postictal, shock, sepsis), toxins (methanol, ethylene glycol, salicylates,[1] paraldehyde), uremia
Respiratory alkalosis	Hepatic encephalopathy, pulmonary insufficiency, salicylates[1], sepsis
Respiratory acidosis	Pulmonary insufficiency, sedative drug overdose

[1]Salicylates produce a combined acid-base disorder.

Table 1–7. Cerebrospinal fluid profiles in acute confusional states.

	Appearance	Opening Pressure	Red Blood Cells	White Blood Cells	Glucose	Protein	Glutamine	Smears	Cultures
Normal	Clear, color-less	70–200 mm H_2O	0/μL	≤ 5 mono-nuclear/μL	≥ 45 mg/dL	≤ 45[1] mg/dL	< 25 μg/dL	–	–
Bacterial meningtitis	Cloudy	↑	Normal	↑↑ (PMN)[2]	↓↓	↑↑	Normal	Gram's stain +	+
Tuberculous meningitis	Normal or cloudy	↑	Normal	↑ (MN)[3,5]	↓	↑	Normal	AFB stain +	±
Fungal meningitis	Normal or cloudy	Normal or ↑	Normal	↑ (MN)	↓	↑	Normal	India ink prep + (Cryptococ-cus)	±
Viral meningitis/ encephalitis	Normal	Normal or ↑	Normal[4]	↑ (MN)[5]	Normal[6]	Normal or ↑	Normal	–	–
Parasitic meningitis/ encephalitis	Normal or cloudy	Normal or ↑	Normal	↑ (MN,E)[7]	Normal	Normal or ↑	Normal	Amebas may be seen on wet mount	±
Carcinomatous meningitis	Normal or cloudy	Normal or ↑	Normal	Normal or ↑ (MN)	↓↓	Normal or ↑	Normal	Cytology +	-
Subarachnoid hemorrhage	Pink-red (su-pernatant yellow)	↑	↑	Normal or ↑ (PMN)[8]	Normal or ↓[8]	↑	Normal	–	–
Hepatic encepha-lopathy	Normal	Normal	Normal	Normal	Normal	Normal	↑	–	–

[1]Lumbar cerebrospinal fluid.
[2]PMN = polymorphonuclear predominance.
[3]MN = mononuclear (lymphocytic or monocytic) predominance.
[4]Red blood cell count may be elevated in herpes simplex encephalitis.
[5]PMN predominance may be seen early in course.
[6]Glucose may be decreased in herpes or mumps infections.
[7]E = eosinophils often present.
[8]Pleocytosis and low glucose, sometimes seen several days after hemorrhage, reflect chemical meningitis caused by subarachnoid blood.
+ = Positive; – = Negative; ± = Can be positive or negative.

ETHANOL INTOXICATION

Clinical Findings

Ethanol intoxication produces a confusional state that may be associated with nystagmus, dysarthria, and limb and gait ataxia. In nonalcoholics, although the severity and clinical features of encephalopathy correlate roughly with blood ethanol levels, clinical manifestations decline over hours despite a stable blood ethanol level. Chronic alcoholics, who have developed a tolerance to ethanol, may have very high levels without appearing intoxicated. Laboratory studies useful in confirming the diagnosis include blood alcohol levels and serum osmolality. In alcohol intoxication, serum osmolality determined by direct measurement exceeds the calculated osmolality (2 × serum sodium + 1/20 serum glucose + 1/3 serum urea nitrogen) by 22 mosm/L for every 100 mg/dL of ethanol present.

The clinical picture of ethanol intoxication is mim-icked by intoxication with any sedative drug but can often be differentiated by the history, the odor of alcohol on the breath, or toxicological blood and urine analysis. Moreover, sedative drugs do not increase serum osmolality.

Complications

Intoxicated patients are at high risk for head trauma and hemostatic disorders. Alcohol ingestion may cause life-threatening hypoglycemia, and chronic alcoholism is associated with an increased incidence of bacterial meningitis. These possibilities must be investigated.

Treatment

Treatment is generally not required unless a withdrawal syndrome ensues (see below). Alcoholic patients should, however, receive thiamine to prevent Wernicke's encephalopathy (see below).

Table 1–8. Common causes of acute confusional states.

Metabolic Disorders

Drugs[1]
Ethanol intoxication
Ethanol withdrawal
Sedative drug intoxication
Sedative drug withdrawal
Opioids
Anticholinergics
Sympathomimetics
Hallucinogens
Endocrine disorders
Hypothyroidism
Hyperthyroidism
Hypoglycemia
Hyperglycemia
Electrolyte disorders
Hyponatremia
Hypocalcemia
Hypercalcemia
Nutritional disorders
Wernicke's encephalopathy
Vitamin B_{12} deficiency
Organ system failure
Hepatic encephalopathy
Reye's syndrome
Uremia
Dialysis disequilibrium
Pulmonary encephalopathy

Infectious and Noninfectious Meningitis/Encephalitis

Bacterial meningitis
Tuberculous meningitis
Syphilitic meningitis
Viral meningoencephalitis
Herpes simplex virus encephalitis
Acquired immunodeficiency syndrome
Fungal meningitis
Parasitic infections
Neoplastic meningitis

Vascular Disorders

Hypertensive encephalopathy
Subarachnoid hemorrhage
Vertebrobasilar ischemia
Right (nondominant) hemisphere infarction
Systemic lupus erythematosus
Disseminated intravascular coagulation
Thrombotic thrombocytopenic purpura

Head Trauma

Concussion
Intracranial hemorrhage

Seizures

Postictal state
Complex partial seizure

[1]See also Table 1–9.

Table 1–9. Drugs associated with acute confusional states.

Acyclovir	Cycloserine
Aminocaproic acid	Cyclosporine
Amphetamines	Digitalis glycosides
Anticholinergics	Disulfiram
Anticonvulsants	Ethanol
Antidepressants	Hallucinogens
Antihistamines	Isoniazid
(H_1 and H_2)	Levodopa
Antipsychotics	Lidocaine
L-Asparaginase	Methylxanthines
Baclofen	Nonsteroidal anti-
Barbiturates	inflammatory
Benzodiazepines	drugs
Beta-adrenergic	Opioids
receptor antagonists	Penicillin
Bromocriptine	Quinacrine
Chloroquine	Quinidine
Clonidine	Quinine
Cocaine	Thyroid hormones
Corticosteroids	

1. TREMULOUSNESS & HALLUCINATIONS

This benign, self-limited condition occurs within two days after cessation of drinking. It is characterized by tremulousness, agitation, anorexia, nausea, insomnia, tachycardia, and hypertension. Confusion, if present, is mild. Illusions and hallucinations, usually visual in character, occur in about 25% of patients.

Treatment with diazepam, 5–20 mg, or chlordiazepoxide, 25–50 mg, orally every four hours, will terminate the syndrome and prevent more serious consequences of withdrawal.

ETHANOL WITHDRAWAL

Three common withdrawal syndromes are recognized (Figure 1–3). Because of the associated risk of Wernicke's encephalopathy (discussed later), patients presenting with these syndromes should be given thiamine, 100 mg/d, intravenously or intramuscularly, until a normal diet can be ensured.

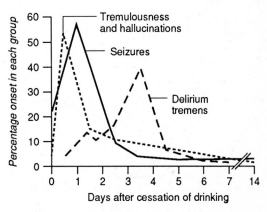

Figure 1–3. Ethanol withdrawal syndromes in relation to the time since cessation of drinking. (Data from Victor M, Adams RD: The effect of alcohol on the nervous system. *Res Publ Assoc Res Nerv Ment Dis* 1952;32:526—573.)

2. SEIZURES

Ethanol withdrawal seizures occur within 48 hours after the beginning of abstinence; in about two-thirds of cases they occur within 7 to 24 hours. Roughly 40% of patients who experience seizures have a single seizure; more than 90% have between one and six. In 85% of the cases, the interval between the first and last seizures is six hours or less. Anticonvulsant treatment is usually not required, since seizures cease spontaneously in most cases. Unusual features such as focal seizures, prolonged duration of seizures (> 6–12 hours), more than six seizures, status epilepticus, or a prolonged postictal state should prompt a search for other causes. The patient should be observed for 6–12 hours to make certain that atypical features are not present.

Because about one-third of patients with withdrawal seizures develop delirium tremens, prophylactic doses of diazepam or chlordiazepoxide are sometimes administered.

3. DELIRIUM TREMENS

This most serious of ethanol withdrawal syndromes typically begins three to five days after cessation of drinking and lasts for up to 72 hours. It is characterized by confusion, agitation, fever, sweating, tachycardia, hypertension, and hallucinations. The mortality rate (up to 15%) is usually due to concomitant infection, pancreatitis, cardiovascular collapse, or trauma. Treatment consists of diazepam, 10–20 mg intravenously, repeated every five minutes as needed until the patient is calm, and correction of fluid and electrolyte abnormalities and hypoglycemia. The total requirement for diazepam may exceed 100 mg/h. Concomitant β-adrenergic receptor blockade with atenolol, 50–100 mg/d, has also been recommended.

SEDATIVE DRUG INTOXICATION

Clinical Findings

The classic signs of sedative drug overdose are confusional state or coma, respiratory depression, hypotension, hypothermia, reactive pupils, nystagmus or absence of ocular movements, ataxia, dysarthria, and hyporeflexia. (Commonly used sedative-hypnotic drugs are listed in Table 1–10.) Glutethimide or very high doses of barbiturates may produce large, fixed pupils. Decerebrate and decorticate posturing can occur in coma that is caused by sedative drug overdose.

The diagnosis can be confirmed by toxicological analysis of blood, urine, or gastric aspirate; blood levels of short-acting agents, however, do not correlate with clinical severity.

Table 1–10. Sedative-hypnotic drugs causing confusional states or coma.[1]

Drug	Half-Life (hrs)	Hypnotic Dose (mg)
Barbiturates		
Phenobarbital (Luminal)	80–120	100–320
Amobarbital (Amytal)	8–42	65–200
Pentobarbital (Nembutal)	15–48	100
Secobarbital (Seconal)	15–40	100–200
Benzodiazepines		
Diazepam (Valium)	30–60	5–10
Chlordiazepoxide (Librium)	5–15	50–100
Flurazepam (Dalmane)	50–100	15–30
Clorazepate (Tranxene)	50–80	15–30
Lorazepam (Ativan)	10–20	2–4
Oxazepam (Serax)	5–10	15–30
Temazepam (Restoril)	10–17	15–30
Triazolam (Halcion)	1.5–3	0.25–0.5
Other		
Meprobamate Miltown)	6–17	800
Ethchlorvynol (Placidyl)	10–25	500–1000
Methaqualone (Quaalude)	10–42	150–300
Glutethimide (Doriden)	5–22	250–500
Chloral hydrate (Noctec)	4–9.5	500–1000

[1]Data from Harvey SC: Hypnotics and sedatives. In Gilman AG, Goodman LS, Rall TW, Murad F: The Pharmacological Basis of Therapeutics, 7th ed. Macmillan, 1985.

Treatment

Management is directed at supporting the patient's respiratory and circulatory function. Morbidity is most often the result of aspiration pneumonia (with or without systemic sepsis) or iatrogenic pulmonary edema caused by fluid overload. Early gastric lavage may reduce further absorption of the drugs, but it carries the risk of aspiration. Forced diuresis with alkalinization of the urine increases the clearance of phenobarbital; it is ineffective for short-acting barbiturates, however, and may lead to fluid overload. Hemodialysis may be indicated when barbiturate overdose is complicated by clinical deterioration despite conservative therapy or when drug elimination is impaired by renal failure.

Prognosis

Barring the development of infections or cardiovascular complications, patients who arrive at the hospital with adequate cardiopulmonary function should survive without sequelae.

SEDATIVE DRUG WITHDRAWAL

Clinical Findings

Like ethanol, sedative drugs can produce confusional states or seizures when stopped abruptly. The frequency and severity of withdrawal syndromes depend upon the duration of drug intake and the dose and half-life of the drug. The syndromes can be associated with any sedative drug; they occur most often in patients who have been taking the drug in large doses for at least several weeks. Intermediate- or short-acting agents are those most likely to produce withdrawal symptoms when discontinued.

Withdrawal syndromes commonly develop one to three days after the use of short-acting agents has ceased but may not appear until a week or more after longer-acting drugs have been discontinued. The symptoms are identical to those of ethanol withdrawal and are similarly self-limited. Myoclonus and seizures may appear after three to eight days, however, and require treatment. Seizures usually occur only when the average daily drug intake is several times the usual hypnotic dose (see Table 1–10). For example, at least 800 mg/d of secobarbital must be ingested for withdrawal seizures to occur. A syndrome indistinguishable from delirium tremens may also appear at this time; this also tends to be restricted to patients taking several times the drug's daily sedative dose.

Test of Tolerance

Pharmacologic confirmation of sedative drug withdrawal syndrome is provided by the **pentobarbital challenge test,** in which the patient is given pentobarbital, 200 mg orally or intramuscularly, and evaluated about one hour later. The absence of signs of sedative drug intoxication (sedation, nystagmus, dysarthria, or ataxia) establishes that tolerance is present and requires special treatment.

Treatment

When tolerance has been demonstrated, phenobarbital, a long-acting barbiturate, is administered orally to maintain a calm state without signs of intoxication. The recommended dosage is 30 mg for each hypnotic dose customarily taken per day (Table 1–10), giving up to 500 mg/d of phenobarbital in three divided doses. A starting dose of 120 mg of phenobarbital three times daily can be used instead and adjusted if withdrawal symptoms recur or toxicity becomes evident. The maintenance dose of phenobarbital is continued for two days and then tapered at a rate of 30 mg/d. For most patients, it should be possible to discontinue the drug within two weeks.

OPIOIDS

Clinical Findings

Numerous naturally occurring and synthetic opioids exist, all exhibiting similar actions. These agents can produce analgesia, mood changes (euphoria or dysphoria), confusional states, coma, respiratory depression, pulmonary edema, nausea and vomiting, pupillary constriction, hypotension, urinary retention, and reduced gastrointestinal motility. Their chronic use is associated with tolerance and physical dependence.

Confusional states and coma are seen with accidental overdose in opioid addicts, iatrogenic overdose, or suicide attempts. While physical examination may reveal needle tracks or any of the above-mentioned systemic signs, the cardinal features of opioid overdose are pinpoint pupils—which usually constrict in bright light—and respiratory depression. These features can also result from pontine hemorrhage. Opioid overdose is distinguished by the patient's response to the opioid antagonist **naloxone.** After administration of naloxone, pupillary dilation and full recovery of consciousness occur promptly. When large doses of opioids or multiple drug ingestions are involved, a slight dilation of the pupils may be the only observable effect.

Treatment

Treatment of opioid overdose may necessitate ventilatory support and reversal of the opiate's effects by the intravenous administration of naloxone, 0.4–0.8 mg, as required. Because naloxone's action may be as short as one hour—and many opioids are longer-acting—it should be readministered as the patient's condition dictates.

Complications & Prognosis

Because opioid overdose and its complications must be recognized and treated promptly, patients with confusional states or coma of uncertain cause should receive 0.8 mg of naloxone intravenously, immediately upon arrival in the emergency room. Systemic complications—pulmonary edema, hypotension, and infection—require specific courses of management. With appropriate treatment, patients should recover uneventfully.

ANTICHOLINERGIC DRUGS

Parasympatholytic anticholinergic agents block muscarinic acetylcholine receptors in both autonomic end organs and the brain. These drugs are commonly used in the treatment of gastrointestinal disturbances, parkinsonism, motion sickness, and insomnia. Antipsychotic drugs, tricyclic antidepressants, and antihistamines also exhibit prominent anticholinergic activity.

Clinical Findings

Overdose with any of these agents can produce a confusional state with characteristic features related to autonomic dysfunction: an agitated delirium with hallucinations, fixed and dilated pupils, blurred vision, dryness of the skin and mucous membranes, flushing, fever, urinary retention, and tachycardia.

In the case of antipsychotic or antidepressant ingestion the diagnosis can be confirmed by toxicological analysis of blood or urine. Symptoms usually resolve spontaneously.

Treatment

Treatment is rarely required unless life-threatening cardiac arrhythmias occur. The cholinesterase inhibitor **physostigmine** can reverse the abnormality by interfering with the breakdown of released acetylcholine. Physostigmine may produce severe bradycardia, seizures, or increased salivary secretion, however—with the attendant hazards of aspiration or respiratory compromise—and so is rarely used.

SYMPATHOMIMETIC DRUGS

The sympathomimetics include common drugs of abuse, such as cocaine and amphetamines, as well as methylphenidate, antidepressants, and monoamine oxidase inhibitors. The clinical effects of antidepressant overdose are largely related to their anticholinergic effects (discussed above).

Cocaine inhibits synaptic uptake of the catecholamine neurotransmitters norepinephrine and dopamine. Amphetamines also inhibit uptake and—in addition—promote catecholamine release. These actions produce central stimulant and peripheral sympathomimetic effects.

Clinical Findings

Sympathomimetic intoxication can produce a confusional state characterized by hallucinations, hyperactivity, stereotyped behavior, and schizophreniform paranoid psychosis. Physical examination typically shows tachycardia, hypertension, and dilated pupils. Hyperthermia, tremors, and seizures may occur, and cardiac arrhythmias are a source of serious morbidity. Cocaine and amphetamine abuse have been associated with thrombotic, embolic, and hemorrhagic strokes (see Chapter 10).

Treatment

Because the actions of amphetamines last longer than do those of cocaine, amphetamine intoxication is more likely to require treatment. Haloperidol, 2 mg intramuscularly every hour or 5 mg every four hours, can be used to offset the central dopaminergic effects and thus the psychotic manifestations of overdose. Alpha-adrenergic blocking agents may be useful in the treatment of life-threatening hypertension.

HALLUCINOGENIC DRUGS

Hallucinogenic agents can produce confusional states severe enough to require medical attention. While lysergic acid diethylamide (LSD) and related drugs (eg, 2,5-dimethoxy-4-methylamphetamine [DOM]; N,N-dimethyltryptamine [DMT]; 3,4-methylenedioxyamphetamine [MDA]; mescaline; psilocybin) almost never cause life-threatening emergencies, phencyclidine (PCP) may produce seizures, coma, and death.

1. LSD

LSD intoxication may be manifested by nystagmus, ataxia, hypertonia, hyperreflexia, insomnia, and signs of sympathetic overactivity (dilated pupils, mild tachycardia, hypertension, and hyperthermia). Seizures are rare, and changes in mental status are usually the most striking feature. Alterations of affect or mood may be prominent. Cognitive changes include thought disorder, distortion of time sense, and feelings of detachment. Visual and somatosensory illusions or hallucinations are a hallmark of the syndrome.

A bad trip may result when the dysphoric effects of LSD predominate. Treatment usually involves verbal calming and reassurance; benzodiazepines may be of benefit if these palliative measures are ineffective.

2. PCP

PCP intoxication can be a medical emergency. The patient may be drowsy or agitated, with disorientation, amnesia, hallucinations, paranoia, and violent behavior. Neurological examination may show large or small pupils, horizontal and vertical nystagmus, ataxia, hypertonicity, hyperreflexia, and myoclonus. There may be analgesia to a surprising degree. Hypertension, malignant hyperthermia, status epilepticus, coma, and death can result from intoxication with large doses of PCP.

Patients who have taken PCP tend to be less amenable to talking down than are those who have ingested LSD or other hallucinogens. Benzodiazepines may be useful for both sedation and treating muscle spasms. Phenothiazines should probably be avoided because they tend to lower the seizure threshold and induce hypotension; butyrophenones (eg, haloperidol) are preferred if an antipsychotic agent is required. Specific treatment with antihypertensives, anticonvulsants, and dantrolene (for malignant hyperthermia) may be required. Symptoms and signs usually resolve within 24 hours but occasionally last for days or weeks.

ENDOCRINE DISTURBANCES

HYPOTHYROIDISM

Clinical Findings

Profound hypothyroidism (myxedema) may produce a confusional state, coma, or dementia in addition to its systemic effects. The mechanisms responsible for these effects are unknown but may involve disruption of neuronal metabolism and autonomic function. Cognitive dysfunction is usually manifested by flat affect and psychomotor retardation, agitation, or a florid psychosis. The neurological examination may show dysarthria, deafness, or cerebellar signs; the most characteristic abnormality is a delayed relaxation phase of tendon reflexes. Untreated, the condition can progress to seizures and coma.

Laboratory abnormalities include low T_3 and T_4 levels and elevated TSH and serum cholesterol. Hypoglycemia and hyponatremia may occur, and arterial blood gases may reveal respiratory acidosis. CSF protein is typically elevated; CSF pressure is occasionally increased.

Treatment

Treatment is of the underlying thyroid disorder. In severe myxedema madness or coma, however, rapid thyroid replacement is indicated, since the disorder may otherwise be fatal. **Levothyroxine** (T_4) should be given intravenously as an initial dose of 200–500 μg over five to ten minutes, followed by 100 μg intravenously every 24 hours. **Hydrocortisone sodium succinate,** 100 mg intravenously every eight hours, should also be administered: adrenal insufficiency may coexist with hypothyroidism or be precipitated by its treatment.

HYPERTHYROIDISM

Clinical Findings

While minor neuropsychiatric symptoms, including euphoria, anxiety, fatigue, emotional lability, and insomnia, are not uncommon in untreated hyperthyroidism, acute exacerbation of the disorder (**thyrotoxic crisis**) may be associated with a confusional state that can progress to coma and death. Precipitating factors include infection, trauma, and metabolic disorders, with systemic manifestations of hyperthyroidism usually present.

In younger patients, thyrotoxic confusional states are characterized by an agitated delirium that may be accompanied by hallucinations or psychosis (**activated crisis**). Patients more than 50 years of age tend to be apathetic and depressed (**apathetic crisis**); cardiovascular disorders are prominent in this group. Seizures may occur, especially in patients with preexisting epilepsy. The general neurological examination shows an exaggerated physiological (action) tremor and hyperreflexia; ankle clonus and extensor plantar responses are rare.

The diagnosis of hyperthyroidism is confirmed by assay of thyroid hormones (T_3 and T_4) in the blood.

Differential Diagnosis

Because many of the symptoms of thyrotoxicosis are manifestations of a hyperadrenergic state, the syndrome may be closely mimicked by sympathomimetic drug intoxication.

Treatment

Treatment of thyrotoxic crisis includes administration of propranolol, beginning with 10–20 mg orally every six hours and increasing the dose as needed to control tachycardia. Hyperthermia, fluid and electrolyte disorders, cardiac arrhythmias, and congestive heart failure should be corrected. Because hyperthyroidism tends to enhance the metabolism of endogenous steroid hormones, dexamethasone, 2 mg orally or intravenously every six hours, should be administered. In more severe cases, patients should receive antithyroid drugs (propylthiouracil, 300–400 mg orally, followed by 200 mg every four hours) and iodine (SSKI, 5 drops orally every eight hours, or sodium iodide, 1 g intravenously every 24 hours). The underlying disorder that precipitated thyrotoxic crisis should be sought.

Prognosis

Even with treatment, thyrotoxic crisis is associated with mortality rates as high as 30%.

HYPOGLYCEMIA

Of all the disorders that produce metabolic encephalopathy, hypoglycemia imposes the most urgent demand for immediate attention. Prompt treatment is essential because hypoglycemic encephalopathy may progress rapidly from a reversible to an irreversible stage, and definitive therapy can be quickly and easily administered.

Severe hypoglycemia is most often the result of exogenous insulin administration in diabetic patients. It is less commonly caused by alcoholism, malnutrition, hepatic failure, insulinoma, and non-insulin-secreting tumors (especially retroperitoneal, thoracic, or pelvic fibromas, sarcomas, and fibrosarcomas).

The brain relies on glucose almost exclusively for energy metabolism. Brain glucose reserves at any given time are sufficient to support brain function for only a few minutes. In the usual clinical setting of hypoglycemia, where some glucose continues to be supplied to the brain and the delivery of blood and oxygen is unimpaired, neurological symptoms usually develop over the course of a few minutes to several hours. While no strict correlation between blood glucose levels and the severity of neurological dysfunction can be demonstrated, prolonged hypoglycemia at levels of 30 mg/dL or lower invariably leads to irreversible brain damage.

Clinical Findings

The early signs of hypoglycemic encephalopathy (Table 1–11) include manifestations of sympathetic nervous system hyperactivity (tachycardia, sweating, and pupillary dilation), followed by a confusional state characterized either by somnolence or by agitated delirium. The autonomic warning signs of hunger, sweating, and tachycardia may be absent in patients with autonomic neuropathy or pharmacological β-adrenergic blockade. Neurological dysfunction progresses in a rostral-caudal fashion (see Chapter 11), much as might be produced by a mass lesion causing transtentorial herniation. Coma ensues, with spasticity, extensor plantar responses, and decorticate or decerebrate posturing. Signs of brain stem dysfunction subsequently appear, including abnormal ocular movements and loss of pupillary reflexes. Respiratory depression, bradycardia, hypotonia, and hyporeflexia ultimately supervene, at which point irreversible brain damage is imminent.

Hypoglycemic coma is often associated with focal neurological signs and focal or generalized seizures.

The diagnosis is confirmed by measuring blood glucose levels. The tragic consequences of failure to treat such a condition early can be avoided only if blood glucose determination is performed promptly and glucose given to *every* patient presenting with encephalopathy or coma.

Treatment

Glucose—50 mL of 50% dextrose intravenously—should be administered *immediately,* before the blood glucose level is known (a normal blood glucose level indicated by dipstick methods should not be relied upon). Improvement in the level of consciousness is evident within minutes after glucose administration in patients with reversible hypoglycemic encephalopathy. The consequences of inadvertently worsening what later proves to be hyperglycemic encephalopathy are never as serious as those of a failure to treat hypoglycemia.

HYPERGLYCEMIA

Two distinct hyperglycemic syndromes in diabetic patients, **diabetic ketoacidosis** and **hyperosmolar nonketotic hyperglycemia,** are associated with encephalopathy that can progress to coma. Either syndrome, distinguished by a variety of clinical and laboratory features (Table 1–12), may be the presenting manifestation of diabetes.

Impaired cerebral metabolism, intravascular coagulation from hyperviscosity, and brain edema resulting from rapid correction of hyperglycemia are important factors in the genesis of neurological symptoms in hyperglycemic encephalopathies. While the severity of hyperosmolarity correlates well with depression of consciousness, the degree of systemic acidosis does not.

Clinical Findings

A. Symptoms and Signs: Symptoms of developing hyperglycemic encephalopathies include blurred vision, dry skin, anorexia, polyuria, and polydipsia. Physical examination may show hypotension and other signs of dehydration, especially in hyperosmolar nonketotic hyperglycemia. Deep, rapid (Kussmaul) respiration characterizes diabetic ketoacidosis. Depending upon the severity of the encepha-

Table 1–11. Signs and symptoms of hypoglycemia after insulin administration.

Time after Insulin Administration	Symptoms and Signs
30 minutes	Perspiration, salivation, somnolence, excitement and restlessness, tachycardia (if stimulated), bradycardia (if somnolent)
2–3 hours	Loss of contact with environment; myoclonus; primitive reflexes (grasping, sucking); reactive, dilated pupils
4–5 hours	Coma, depressed responses to pain, roving eye movements, tonic and torsional muscular spasms, extensor plantar responses
5–6 hours	Decerebrate rigidity
6–7 hours	Small pupils, bradycardia, flaccid muscle tone, depressed reflexes

Table 1–12. Features of hyperglycemic encephalopathies.

	Diabetic Ketoacidosis	Hyperosmolar Nonketotic State
Patient age	Young	Middle-aged to elderly
Type of diabetes	Juvenile-onset or insulin-dependent	Adult-onset
Blood glucose (mg/dL)	300–600	> 800
Serum osmolality (mosm/L)	< 350	> 350
Ketosis	+	−
Metabolic acidosis	+	−
Coma	Uncommon	Common
Focal neurologic signs	−	+
Seizures	−	+

+ = Present; − = Absent.

lopathy, impairment of consciousness varies from mild confusion to coma. Focal neurological signs and generalized or focal seizures are common in hyperosmolar nonketotic hyperglycemia but not in diabetic ketoacidosis.

B. Laboratory Findings: Important laboratory findings in diabetic ketoacidosis and hyperosmolar nonketotic hyperglycemia are shown in Table 1–12. Associated abnormalities may include hypokalemia (although serum potassium may be initially elevated in the face of intracellular potassium depletion), hypophosphatemia, and hypomagnesemia. A white blood cell count, microscopic examination of the urine, a chest x-ray, and blood and urine cultures should be obtained to search for an underlying infection as the precipitating cause of hyperglycemia. An ECG may reveal abnormalities related to hypokalemia.

C. Diagnostic Pitfalls: Three common pitfalls may prevent the correct diagnosis of diabetic ketoacidosis or hyperosmolar nonketotic hyperglycemia.

1. Failure to consider the diagnoses in patients without a history of diabetes–Up to 15% of patients with diabetic ketoacidosis and 40% of those with hyperosmolar nonketotic hyperglycemia have no such history.

2. Incorrect differentiation between hypoglycemia and hyperglycemia as the cause of encephalopathy or coma in a patient known to be diabetic–Early hypoglycemia is characterized by such signs of sympathetic nervous system overactivity as clammy skin. These signs are absent in hyperglycemic states, where dehydration produces dry skin and decreased tissue turgor. Determining blood glucose levels easily distinguishes these conditions.

3. The erroneous assumption that focal neurological signs must be due to a structural brain lesion–A patient with either hypoglycemia or hyperosmolar nonketotic hyperglycemia may present with a strokelike syndrome and go untreated when a vascular cause is assumed. Blood glucose concentrations should therefore be determined promptly in all patients presenting stroke or focal or generalized seizures.

Treatment

A. Diabetic Ketoacidosis: An initial dose of regular insulin, 10–20 units, should be given as an intravenous bolus, followed by continuous intravenous infusion at a rate of 10–15 units/h. The dose should be reduced as serum glucose levels decline. The patient's levels of serum glucose, bicarbonate, ketones, potassium, and phosphate should be carefully monitored. Fluids are given as normal saline until the glucose level drops to 250 mg/dL, at which time 5% dextrose is substituted.

A number of hazards attend therapy. Rapid correction of hyperglycemia may be associated with brain edema. Severe hypokalemia can be induced by rapid

redistribution of potassium into the intracellular compartment following insulin administration, even in patients with hyperkalemia at presentation, who are likely to have profound intracellular potassium depletion. Administering bicarbonate to correct systemic acidosis may worsen CSF acidosis, since CO_2 readily diffuses from blood to CSF and is converted to bicarbonate, which exits less readily. Treatment with bicarbonate may also exacerbate hypokalemia and should be reserved for special situations, including coma with an arterial pH of less than 7.00, hypotension that fails to respond to intravenous fluid administration, cardiac arrhythmias related to hyperkalemia, and hypoventilation.

B. Hyperosmolar Nonketotic Hyperglycemia: This disorder is typically treated with an initial dose of 20 units of regular insulin intravenously followed by 5–15 units/h by continuous intravenous infusion until the serum glucose level declines to about 250 mg/dL. Insulin can then be given subcutaneously.

Fluid replacement is most important in treating patients with hyperglycemic nonketotic coma. These patients are dehydrated and markedly hyperosmolar; 0.5 N saline should be administered. Patients who are also in circulatory collapse should begin normal saline. Care is required to ensure proper replacement of water and sodium.

Prognosis

The mortality rate in diabetic ketoacidosis is reported to be 6–9%. Most deaths are related to associated sepsis, cardiovascular or cerebrovascular complications, or renal failure. Mortality rates as high as 40–70% are reported for hyperosmolar nonketotic hyperglycemia; they are largely due to failure to recognize the condition in elderly patients with no history of diabetes or who present with stroke or seizures.

HYPOADRENALISM

Primary adrenocortical insufficiency (**Addison's disease**) results from inadequate production of glucocorticoids by the adrenal glands as a result of autoimmune disease, infection (eg, tuberculosis), hemorrhage, or acute withdrawal from corticosteroid therapy. Secondary adrenocortical insufficiency is due to impaired secretion of corticotropin (ACTH), usually caused by pituitary or hypothalamic tumors. Neurological involvement may result from the hypoadrenalism itself or from such complications as hyponatremia, hypoglycemia, or hypotension.

Clinical Findings

A. Symptoms and Signs: Clinical features include fatigue, weakness, weight loss, anorexia, hyperpigmentation of the skin, hypotension, nausea and vomiting, abdominal pain, and diarrhea or constipation. Neurological involvement is manifested by confusional states, seizures, or coma.

B. Laboratory Findings: Abnormal laboratory findings include decreased serum sodium, glucose, and bicarbonate; decreased plasma cortisol; increased serum potassium; and eosinophilia. The diagnosis of primary adrenocortical insufficiency is confirmed by a defective response to ACTH administration (ACTH stimulation test).

Treatment

Acute adrenocortical insufficiency (**Addisonian crisis**) is treated with hydrocortisone, 100 mg intravenously every 6 hours for 24 hours with subsequent tapering, and correction of hypovolemia, hypoglycemia, electrolyte disturbances, and precipitating illnesses (eg, infections). The crisis can be prevented by supplemental administration of glucocorticoids to patients with chronic adrenocortical insufficiency who develop severe medical illnesses or undergo surgery.

HYPERADRENALISM

Hyperadrenalism (**Cushing's syndrome**) results from hypersecretion of glucocorticoids by the adrenal glands, hypersecretion of ACTH by the pituitary gland (Cushing's disease) or from other sites, or the administration of exogenous glucocorticoids or ACTH.

Clinical Findings

A. Symptoms and Signs: Clinical features include truncal obesity, facial flushing, hirsutism, menstrual irregularities, hypertension, weakness, cutaneous striae, acne, and ecchymoses. Neuropsychiatric disturbances are common and include depression or euphoria, anxiety, irritability, memory impairment, psychosis, delusions, and hallucinations; fully developed acute confusional states are rare, however. Mild polycythemia and leukocytosis may occur. Hypokalemia, which is uncommon, suggests ectopic ACTH secretion or adrenal carcinoma.

B. Laboratory Findings: The diagnosis of hyperadrenalism is confirmed by an elevated 24-hour-urine free cortisol level or a defective response to a low-dose dexamethasone-suppression test. The cause of hyperadrenalism can then be determined by measuring basal plasma ACTH levels and by a high-dose dexamethasone-suppression test.

Treatment

Treatment of pituitary tumors is with transsphenoidal hypophysectomy; adrenal or ectopic ACTH-secreting tumors are also treated surgically. Drugs that suppress ACTH secretion (eg, bromocriptine) or glucocorticoid secretion (eg, mitotane) are used as adjuncts to surgery or with patients for whom surgery is impossible or unsuccessful.

ELECTROLYTE DISORDERS

HYPONATREMIA

Clinical Findings

A. Symptoms and Signs: Hyponatremia, particularly when acute in onset, leads to cerebral dysfunction by means of brain cell swelling that results from hypo-osmolality of extracellular fluid. Symptoms of severe hyponatremia include headache, lethargy, confusion, weakness, muscle cramps, nausea, and vomiting. The general examination may suggest dehydration, euhydration, or edema. Neurological signs include a confusional state or coma, papilledema, tremor, asterixis, rigidity, extensor plantar responses, and focal or generalized seizures. Hyponatremia may produce focal signs by unmasking preexisting structural brain lesions, such as infarcts.

B. Laboratory Findings: Neurological disorders caused by hyponatremia are usually associated with serum sodium levels less than 120 meq/L (Figure 1-4), but abnormalities may be seen following a rapid fall to 130 meq/L—while chronic hyponatremia with levels as low as 110 meq/L may be asymptomatic.

Treatment

Treatment of hyponatremia is most effective when the underlying abnormality is corrected. Immediate management includes water restriction or, for severe symptoms, infusion of hypertonic saline with or without intravenous furosemide.

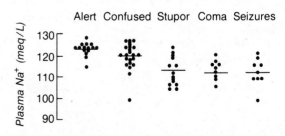

Figure 1–4. Relationship between plasma sodium concentration and neurological manifestations of hyponatremia. (Reproduced, with permission, from Arieff AI, Llach F, Massry SG: Neurological manifestations and morbidity of hyponatremia: Correlation with brain water and electrolytes. *Medicine* 1976;55:121—129.)

The most important complication of treatment is **central pontine myelinolysis,** a disorder of white matter most common in alcoholics and other malnourished patients who undergo overcorrection or excessively rapid correction of hyponatremia. Clinical features include a confusional state, paraparesis or quadriparesis, dysarthria, dysphagia, hyper- or hyporeflexia, and extensor plantar responses. Severe cases can result in the locked-in syndrome (see Chapter 11), coma, or death. MRI may show pontine and extrapontine white matter lesions.

Since no treatment is available for central pontine myelinolysis, prevention assumes special importance. There is widespread, but not unanimous, agreement that this may best be achieved by restricting water intake and using small amounts of hypertonic saline to raise the serum sodium concentration to 120–130 mmol/L at a rate not exceeding 12 mmol/L/d.

Prognosis

Untreated hyponatremic encephalopathy can produce irreversible brain damage or death.

HYPERCALCEMIA

Neurological symptoms of hypercalcemia result from a calcium-induced increase in the depolarization threshold of nerve and muscle, with consequent underexcitability.

Clinical Findings

A. Symptoms and Signs: Symptoms of hypercalcemia include thirst, polyuria, constipation, nausea and vomiting, abdominal pain, anorexia, and flank pain from nephrolithiasis. Neurological symptoms are universally present with serum calcium levels higher than 17 mg/dL (8.5 meq/L) and include headache, weakness, and lethargy.

Physical examination may show dehydration, abdominal distention, focal neurological signs, myopathic weakness, and a confusional state that can progress to coma. Seizures occur rarely. The myopathy spares bulbar muscles and tendon reflexes are usually normal.

B. Laboratory Findings: The diagnosis is confirmed by an elevated serum calcium level. The ECG may show a shortened QT interval. The hematocrit and serum urea nitrogen can help to quantify the extent of dehydration. Elevated parathyroid hormone levels may be detected by radioimmunoassay. Abdominal x-rays may demonstrate intestinal ileus or metastatic calcification. Patients presenting with hypercalcemia should be fully evaluated for the presence of occult cancers.

Treatment

Severe hypercalcemia is initially treated with vigorous intravenous hydration using 0.5-N or normal saline and usually requires central venous pressure monitoring. Fluid replacement promotes both rehydration and calciuresis. Intravenous furosemide (20–40 mg every two hours) enhances calciuresis and is useful in preventing overhydration.

HYPOCALCEMIA

Neurological symptoms of hypocalcemia are produced by neuronal hyperexcitability resulting from a lowered depolarization threshold.

Clinical Findings

A. Symptoms and Signs: Symptoms include irritability, delirium, psychosis with hallucinations, depression, nausea, vomiting, abdominal pain, and paresthesias of the circumoral region and distal extremities. The most characteristic physical signs are those of overt or latent tetany. Neural hyperexcitability is exhibited by contraction of facial muscles in response to percussion of the facial (VII) nerve anterior to the ear (**Chvostek's sign**). **Carpopedal spasm** may occur spontaneously or following tourniquet-induced limb ischemia (**Trousseau's sign**). Cataracts and papilledema are sometimes present, and chorea has been reported as well. Seizures or laryngospasm can be life-threatening.

B. Laboratory Findings: Serum calcium levels are below the normal range (9–11 mg/dL or 4.5–5.5 meq/L) in symptomatic hypocalcemia, but their interpretation requires consideration of other factors. Protein-bound (and thus total) calcium is decreased by hypoalbuminemia (0.8 mg/dL for each 1 g/L decrease in albumin) without affecting the ionized calcium concentration. Hypocalcemia with normal ionized calcium is asymptomatic. Serum potassium should be determined, because hyperkalemia exacerbates the adverse cardiac effects of hypocalcemia. Serum magnesium should be assayed also, since hypomagnesemia may be the cause of the hypocalcemia; in this case it is correctable by magnesium administration alone. Alkalosis (revealed by arterial blood gases) may be a contributing factor. Parathormone levels can be determined by radioimmunoassay, and the ECG may show a prolonged QT interval.

Treatment

Treatment of severe hypocalcemia requires administration of intravenous calcium gluconate, 100–200 mg calcium over 10–15 minutes, followed by intravenous drip infusion. The same regimen is effective in treating intoxication with calcium channel antagonist drugs. Maintenance with oral calcium preparations and a low-phosphorus diet can be initiated later. Vitamin D preparations are useful adjunctive therapy for chronic hypocalcemia that is refractory to calcium replacement alone. Seizures are treated with phenytoin or phenobarbital, both of which inhibit tetany.

NUTRITIONAL DISORDERS

WERNICKE'S ENCEPHALOPATHY

Wernicke's encephalopathy usually occurs as a complication of chronic alcoholism, but it occurs also in a variety of disorders associated with malnutrition. It is produced by deficiency of **thiamine** (vitamin B_1), which, as the pyrophosphate, is a required cofactor for decarboxylation of pyruvic acid and ketoglutaric acid and for transferring glycolaldehyde groups in the hexose monophosphate shunt.

Pathology
Pathologically, Wernicke's encephalopathy is characterized by neuronal loss, demyelination, and gliosis in periventricular gray matter regions. Proliferation of small blood vessels and petechial hemorrhages may be seen. The areas most commonly involved are the medial thalamus, mammillary bodies, periaqueductal gray matter, the cerebellar vermis, and the oculomotor, abducens, and vestibular nuclei. How thiamine deficiency produces these effects is unclear.

Clinical Findings
A. Symptoms and Signs: The classic syndrome comprises the triad of **ophthalmoplegia, ataxia,** and a **confusional state.** The most common ocular abnormalities are nystagmus, abducens (VI) nerve palsy, and horizontal or combined horizontal-vertical gaze palsy. Ataxia affects gait primarily; ataxia of the arms is uncommon, as is dysarthria. The mental status examination reveals global confusion with a prominent disorder of immediate recall and recent memory. The confusional state progresses to coma in a small percentage of patients. Most patients have associated neuropathy with absent ankle jerks. Hypothermia and hypotension may occur, presumably as a result of hypothalamic involvement. Pupillary abnormalities, including mild anisocoria, or a sluggish reaction to light, are occasionally seen.

B. Laboratory Findings: The peripheral blood smear may show macrocytic anemia. The CSF is usually normal, although protein may be mildly elevated (< 90 mg/dL). Elevated CSF pressure, decreased glucose, or pleocytosis should prompt a search for other or additional disease. MRI may show atrophy of the mammillary bodies.

Treatment
Treatment requires prompt administration of thia-mine. An initial dose of 100 mg intravenously is given, always before or simultaneously with the infusion of dextrose; administration of dextrose without thiamine can precipitate or exacerbate the syndrome. Parenteral thiamine is continued for several days to ensure repletion of tissue stores. The maintenance requirement for thiamine—about 1 mg/d—is usually available in the diet, although enteric absorption of thiamine is impaired in alcoholics.

Prognosis
Following treatment, ocular abnormalities usually begin to improve within one day, ataxia and confusion within a week. Ophthalmoplegia, vertical nystagmus, and acute confusion should be entirely reversible, usually within one month. Horizontal nystagmus and ataxia, however, resolve completely in only about 40% of cases. The major long-term complication of Wernicke's encephalopathy is Korsakoff's syndrome (see Chapter 2).

VITAMIN B_{12} DEFICIENCY

A deficiency of vitamin B_{12} **(cyanocobalamin)** can produce many neurological disorders, including peripheral neuropathy, subacute combined degeneration of the spinal cord, nutritional amblyopia (visual loss), and cognitive dysfunction that ranges from a mild confusional state to dementia or psychosis (megaloblastic madness). Neurological abnormalities may precede the development of macrocytic anemia. The most frequent cause of vitamin B_{12} deficiency is **pernicious anemia,** a defective production of intrinsic factor associated with gastric atrophy and achlorhydria, that is most common in persons of northern European ancestry.

Clinical Findings
A. Symptoms and Signs: The presenting symptoms are most commonly due to anemia or orthostatic lightheadedness. Associated leukopenia and thrombocytopenia occasionally lead to infection or bleeding diathesis. The initial symptoms of vitamin B_{12} deficiency may also be neurological, however. Distal paresthesias, gait ataxia, a bandlike sensation of tightness around the trunk or limbs, and Lhermitte's sign (an electric-shocklike sensation along the spine precipitated by neck flexion) may be present. When cerebral involvement predominates, the major clinical feature is mood disorder, confusional state, or psychosis.

On general physical examination, diagnostic clues include low-grade fever, glossitis, lemon-yellow discoloration of the skin, and cutaneous hyperpigmentation. Spinal cord involvement (when present) is manifested by prominent impairment of vibratory and joint position sense, sensory gait ataxia, spastic paraparesis with extensor plantar responses, loss of tendon reflexes in the legs (from associated peripheral nerve involvement), and urinary retention. Cerebral involvement can produce confusion, depression, agitation, or psychosis with hallucinations.

B. Laboratory Findings: Hematological abnormalities include macrocytic anemia, bone marrow megaloblastosis, leukopenia with hypersegmented neutrophils, and thrombocytopenia with giant platelets. Because folate deficiency may produce identical hematological changes, the diagnosis must be confirmed by the serum vitamin B_{12} level. When this level is low, **Schilling's test** determines whether defective intestinal absorption of vitamin B_{12} (such as that produced by pernicious anemia) is the cause.

Liver function tests may show mild abnormalities. The CSF is usually normal, but a slight increase in protein is sometimes found.

Differential Diagnosis

The greatest difficulty in differential diagnosis arises when cerebral symptoms occur without anemia or spinal cord disease. In this situation, a psychiatric disorder can easily be diagnosed erroneously unless the serum vitamin B_{12} level is determined. Diagnosis of this deficiency while its neurological manifestations are still reversible is possible only if a vitamin B_{12}-level determination is routinely included in the evaluation of cognitive disorders, myelopathy, and peripheral neuropathy, whether or not anemia is present.

Treatment

When neurological manifestations are present, treatment is by prompt intramuscular administration of cyanocobalamin after blood is drawn to determine the serum vitamin B_{12} level. Daily injections are continued for one week, and Schilling's test is performed to determine the cause of deficiency. If, as in pernicious anemia, the deficiency state is not correctable by dietary supplementation or by treatment of a malabsorption syndrome, intramuscular doses of vitamin B_{12} are given at weekly intervals for several months and monthly thereafter. The optimal dose has not been determined. While the daily maintenance requirement is only about 2–5 μg, doses of at least 30 μg should be given to ensure repletion of body stores, and doses as high as 1000 μg are often advocated.

Prognosis

The extent to which the neurological consequences of vitamin B_{12} deficiency are reversible depends upon their duration. Abnormalities present for more than one year are less likely to be corrected with treatment. Encephalopathy may begin to clear within 24 hours after the first vitamin B_{12} dose, but full neurological recovery, when it occurs, may take several months. Reversal of hematopoietic suppression is heralded by reticulocytosis within the first week of treatment.

ORGAN SYSTEM FAILURE

HEPATIC ENCEPHALOPATHY

Hepatic encephalopathy occurs as a complication of cirrhosis, portosystemic shunting, chronic active hepatitis, or of fulminant hepatic necrosis following viral hepatitis. Alcoholism is the most common underlying disorder. The syndrome may be chronic and progressive or acute in onset; in the latter case, gastrointestinal hemorrhage is a frequent precipitating cause.

Pathophysiology

Liver disease produces cerebral symptoms by impairing the hepatocellular detoxifying mechanisms or by the portosystemic shunting of venous blood. As a result, ammonia and other toxins accumulate in the blood and diffuse into the brain. Increased activity of γ-aminobutric acid (GABA)-containing neuronal pathways in the brain associated with elevated levels of endogenous benzodiazepine receptor agonists may be involved in the pathogenesis of cerebral symptoms.

Clinical Findings

A. Symptoms and Signs: Symptoms of hepatic encephalopathy may precede systemic symptoms of liver failure, such as nausea, anorexia, and weight loss. A history of recent gastrointestinal bleeding, overindulgence in high-protein foods, the use of sedatives or diuretics, or systemic infection may provide a clue to the cause of clinical decompensation.

General physical examination may reveal signs of liver disease. Cognitive disturbances include somnolence or an agitated delirium, which fluctuates in severity and may progress to coma. Ocular reflexes are usually brisk. Nystagmus, tonic downward ocular deviation, and disconjugate eye movements may be seen. The most helpful neurological sign in suggesting liver disease (or other metabolic disturbances) as the cause of encephalopathy is **asterixis**—a flapping tremor of the outstretched hands or feet that results from impaired postural control. Motor abnormalities other than asterixis are often prominent and include tremor, myoclonus, paratonic rigidity, spasticity, decorticate or decerebrate posturing, and extensor plantar responses. Focal neurological signs and focal or generalized seizures may occur.

B. Laboratory Findings: Laboratory studies may show elevated serum bilirubin, transaminases, ammonia, PT, and PTT. Respiratory alkalosis is usually present. Common complications of hepatic failure that must be identified because they require specific therapy include hypoglycemia and gastrointestinal bleeding. Elevated CSF pressure and protein and a mild pleocytosis occasionally occur, and xanthochromia may be seen with serum bilirubin concentrations above 10 mg/dL. The most specific CSF abnormality is elevated **glutamine,** a major intermediary in brain ammonia metabolism (Figure 1–5). The EEG may be diffusely slowed, with triphasic waves.

Differential Diagnosis

In cases of encephalopathy with asterixis, liver disease must be distinguished from other metabolic causes. Focal neurological signs, posturing, and extensor plantar responses may suggest a mass lesion, but in hepatic encephalopathy these signs are not associated with pupillary abnormalities or absent ocular reflexes. The clinical picture of hepatic encephalopathy may be mimicked by Reye's syndrome (see below), and a liver biopsy may be necessary to distinguish between Reye's syndrome and other causes of hepatic failure in the pediatric age group.

Treatment

Treatment involves restricting dietary protein, reversing electrolyte disturbances and hyperglycemia, discontinuing drugs that may have caused decompensation, providing effective antibiotics for infections, and correcting coagulopathy with fresh-frozen plasma or vitamin K. Oral or rectal administration of lactulose, 20–30 g three or four times daily, decreases colonic pH and thus ammonia absorption. Neomycin, 1–3 g orally four times daily, may reduce ammonia-forming bacteria in the colon. Although levodopa has been reported to be useful in treating acute hepatic encephalopathy, it has not been widely employed for that purpose. Some success has also been reported with the experimental benzodiazepine receptor antagonist flumazenil.

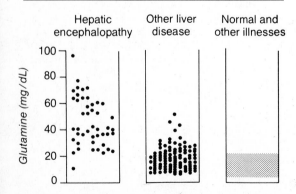

Figure 1–5. Range of CSF glutamine concentrations in hepatic encephalopathy. (Reproduced, with permission, from Plum F: The CSF in hepatic encephalopathy. *Exp Biol Med* 1971;4:34—41.)

Prognosis

Prognosis in hepatic encephalopathy is most closely correlated with the severity of hepatocellular rather than neurological dysfunction.

REYE'S SYNDROME

Reye's syndrome is an idiopathic disorder characterized by encephalopathy or coma with laboratory evidence of hepatic dysfunction. It can occur at any time from infancy to early adulthood, although children 6–11 years of age are most commonly affected.

The syndrome typically has its onset several days after a viral illness, especially varicella or influenza B. Administration of salicylates appears to be an additional risk factor. Reye's syndrome is characterized pathologically by cerebral edema and fatty degeneration of the liver, kidneys, heart, and pancreas. The mechanism through which visceral disorders produce cerebral involvement is unclear.

Reye's syndrome typically begins with the development over a period of hours to days of an encephalopathy that is characterized by lethargy and vomiting and may progress to agitated delirium and coma. Signs of coma evolve in a rostral-caudal fashion (see Chapter 11).

Typical laboratory findings include hypoglycemia, hypophosphatemia, and evidence of hepatic dysfunction (elevated ammonia, transaminases, PT, and PTT). Jaundice is uncommon. Lumbar puncture reveals elevated pressure, elevated CSF glutamine, normal or elevated protein, normal or decreased glucose, and no pleocytosis. The EEG shows diffuse slowing.

Complications of Reye's syndrome, including death, are related to increased intracranial pressure, hypoglycemia, electrolyte abnormalities, and coagulopathy.

Treatment includes administration of glucose (1–2 mL/kg of 50% dextrose intravenously followed by continuous intravenous infusion as needed), intracranial pressure monitoring, intubation, hyperventilation, and mannitol (0.25–2 g/kg intravenously). If these measures fail, induction of barbiturate coma may be useful. Pentobarbital is administered as an initial dose of 3–5 mg/kg intravenously, followed by continuous intravenous infusion at a rate of 1–2 mg/kg/h. Overall mortality rates of up to 40% have been cited, with higher rates in cases complicated by coma, decerebrate posturing, respiratory arrest, or seizures.

UREMIA

Renal failure, particularly when acute in onset or rapidly progressive, is commonly associated with encephalopathy. The severity of measured biochemical abnormalities correlates poorly with symptoms; CSF acidosis is rare, and cerebral edema is not a factor.

Uremic encephalopathy is characterized clinically by a quiet or delirious confusional state that may progress to coma, with hyperventilation and prominent motor manifestations. The motor signs include tremor, asterixis, myoclonus, and tetany. Focal or generalized seizures and focal neurological signs are common. Meningeal signs are sometimes seen, and decorticate and decerebrate posturing may occur.

Laboratory abnormalities include elevated serum urea nitrogen and creatinine and metabolic acidosis. Hyperkalemia from renal failure can be life-threatening. The CSF may exhibit elevated pressure, mild mononuclear or polymorphonuclear pleocytosis, and increased protein. The EEG is diffusely slowed and may show triphasic complexes and sometimes paroxysmal activity that includes spikes or sharp waves.

In patients with confusional states and asterixis, uremia must be distinguished from hepatic encephalopathy, pulmonary encephalopathy, hyponatremia, and drug intoxication or withdrawal. Disorders other than uremia that can produce metabolic acidosis include drug intoxications, diabetic ketoacidosis, sepsis, seizures, and hypoperfusion.

Immediate management of uremic encephalopathy includes appropriate hydration, protein and salt restriction, and treating such complications as hypernatremia, hypertension, and seizures. Definitive long-term management requires dialysis or reversal of the inciting cause (eg, urinary tract obstruction). While dialysis reverses the encephalopathy, clinical improvement still often lags behind normalization of serum urea nitrogen and creatinine.

DIALYSIS DISEQUILIBRIUM

While dialysis can reverse uremic encephalopathy, it can also produce an encephalopathy known as **dialysis disequilibrium syndrome.** Symptoms are thought to result from rapid removal of urea and other molecules from the blood, leading to relative hypoosmolality of extracellular fluid, with a shift of water into the brain. A rapid correction of systemic acidosis may also exacerbate CSF acidosis as CO_2 diffuses into the CSF. Symptoms resolve upon reequilibration of the brain with plasma osmolality. Dialysis disequilibrium is most common with a patient's first hemodialysis and may begin during treatment or as long as 24 hours after treatment. It is rarely a complication of maintenance hemodialysis in patients with chronic, stable renal failure.

Symptoms include headache, irritability, obtundation, delirium, nausea, and muscle cramps. More severe abnormalities—asterixis, myoclonus, seizures, and coma—occur in a small proportion of patients. The syndrome, which can last for several days, should be suspected when a patient deteriorates during or following dialysis despite improvement in the biochemical indices of renal function. The EEG may deteriorate during or after dialysis—sometimes before any clinical change has occurred—showing increased paroxysmal activity with spikes and sharp waves.

Dialysis disequilibrium syndrome can be prevented by correcting uremia more gradually or using briefer periods of dialysis at reduced rates of blood flow. Specific treatment is not generally required unless seizures occur.

PULMONARY ENCEPHALOPATHY

Patients with chronic lung disease or with brain stem or neuromuscular disorders that affect respiratory function may develop encephalopathy related to hypoventilation. While several potential pathophysiological mechanisms are present in this condition, the abruptness of its onset and the degree of hypercapnia are most directly related to neurological dysfunction. Carbon dioxide diffuses readily from blood into the CSF, resulting in CSF acidosis. This probably accounts for the more marked neurological impairment seen in respiratory acidosis than in metabolic acidosis of equal severity. Such factors as hypoxia and cerebral edema may also contribute to the clinical syndrome.

Symptoms of pulmonary encephalopathy include headache, confusion, and somnolence. Examination shows papilledema, asterixis or myoclonus, and an alteration in the level of consciousness ranging from mild confusion to coma. Tendon reflexes are often decreased, but pyramidal signs may be present, and seizures occur occasionally. Focal neurological signs are characteristically absent.

Arterial blood gases demonstrate the respiratory acidosis, and a chest x-ray may show emphysema, pulmonary congestion, or cardiac enlargement.

While the diagnosis is easily made when the full clinical syndrome is present, partial manifestations call for investigation of other conditions. Headache and papilledema, for example, can be produced by intracranial mass lesions; asterixis is a prominent manifestation of other metabolic or toxic encephalopathies.

Untreated pulmonary encephalopathy may lead to coma and death. Treatment involves ventilatory support with intubation, if necessary, to decrease hypercapnia and maintain adequate oxygenation. Administration of high concentrations of oxygen to the unintubated patient (intended to correct hypoxia) may cause the loss of the hypoxia-stimulated respiratory drive in patients whose response to hypercapnia is already compromised. Naloxone should be given when opiates might be responsible for the decompensation of respiratory function. Bicarbonate administration increases in PCO_2 with subsequent diffusion of

CO_2 across the blood-brain barrier and worsened CSF acidosis, leading to paradoxical clinical deterioration while systemic acidosis is improving.

INFECTIOUS & NONINFECTIOUS MENINGITIS & ENCEPHALITIS

BACTERIAL MENINGITIS

Bacterial meningitis is a leading cause of acute confusional states and one in which early diagnosis greatly improves the outcome. Conditions that predispose patients to its development include systemic (especially respiratory) or parameningeal infection, head trauma, anatomical meningeal defects, previous neurosurgical procedures, cancer, alcoholism, and other immunodeficiency states. The etiologic organism varies with age and with the presence of predisposing conditions (Tables 1–13 and 1–14).

Pathogenesis

Bacteria typically gain access to the central nervous system by colonizing the mucous membranes of the nasopharynx, leading to local tissue invasion, bacteremia, and hematogenous seeding of the subarachnoid space. Bacteria can also spread to the meninges directly, through anatomical defects in the skull or from parameningeal sites such as the paranasal sinuses or middle ear. Polysaccharide bacterial capsules, lipopolysaccharides, and outer membrane proteins may contribute to the bacterial invasion and virulence. Low levels of antibody and complement in the subarachnoid space are inadequate to contain the infection. The resulting inflammatory response is associated with the release of humoral factors, including interleukin-1, tumor necrosis factor, and arachidonic acid metabolites, which pro-

Table 1–13. Common etiological agents in bacterial meningitis, based on age.

Age	
Birth to 1 month	*Escherichia coli*, group B streptococci, *Listeria monocytogenes*
1–3 months	*Escherichia coli*, group B streptococci, *Listeria monocytogenes*, *Haemophilus influenzae*, *Streptococcus pneumoniae*
3 months to 18 years	*Haemophilus influenzae*, *Neisseria meningitidis*, *Streptococcus pneumoniae*
18–50 years	*Streptococcus pneumoniae*, *Neisseria meningitidis*
Older than 50 years	*Streptococcus pneumoniae*, *Neisseria meningitidis*, gram-negative bacilli

Table 1–14. Common etiological agents in bacterial meningitis, based on predisposing condition.

Predisposing Condition	
Chronic otitis media	*Streptococcus pneumoniae*, other *Streptococcus* species, *Bacteroides fragilis*, gram-negative bacilli
Malignant external otitis (diabetics)	*Pseudomonas* species
Head trauma or neurosurgical procedures	*Streptococcus pneumoniae*, other *Streptococcus* species, *Bacteroides fragilis*, gram-negative bacilli, *Staphylococcus aureus*
CSF shunt infection	*Staphylococcus epidermidis*, *Staphylococcus aureus*
Splenectomy	*Streptococcus pneumoniae*, *Haemophilus influenzae*
Neutropenia	*Pseudomonas aeruginosa*, *Escherichia coli*, *Listeria monocytogenes*, *Streptococcus pneumoniae*, *Klebsiella* species, gram-negative bacilli, *Staphylococcus aureus*

mote blood-brain barrier permeability, vasogenic cerebral edema, changes in cerebral blood flow, and perhaps direct neuronal toxicity.

Pathologically, bacterial meningitis is characterized by leptomeningeal and perivascular infiltration with polymorphonuclear leukocytes and an inflammatory exudate. These changes tend to be most prominent over the cerebral convexities in *Streptococcus pneumoniae* and *Haemophilus* infection and over the base of the brain when *Neisseria meningitidis* is the causative organism. Brain edema, hydrocephalus, and cerebral infarction may occur, although actual bacterial invasion of the brain is rare.

Clinical Findings

A. Symptoms and Signs: At the time of presentation, most patients have experienced symptoms of meningitis for one to seven days. The symptoms include fever, confusion, vomiting, headache, and neck stiffness, but the full syndrome is often not present.

Physical examination may show fever and signs of systemic or parameningeal infection, such as skin abscess or otitis. A petechial rash is seen in 50–60% of patients with *N meningitidis* meningitis. Signs of meningeal irritation (see p 3) are seen in about 80% of cases; they are often absent at the extremes of age or with profoundly impaired consciousness. The level of consciousness, when altered, ranges from mild confusion to coma. Focal neurological signs, seizures, and cranial nerve palsies may occur.

B. Laboratory Findings: Blood counts may reveal polymorphonuclear leukocytosis related to systemic infection or leukopenia reflecting immunosuppression. In associated bacteremia, the causative organism can be cultured from the blood in 40–90% of cases. X-rays of the chest, sinuses, or mastoid bones may indicate a primary site of infection. A brain CT scan may show contrast enhancement of the cerebral convexities, the base of the brain, or the ventricular ependyma. The EEG is usually diffusely slowed, and focal abnormalities suggest the possibility of focal cerebritis, abscess formation, or scarring.

While these studies are helpful in some cases, the essential investigation in all cases of suspected meningitis is prompt lumbar puncture and CSF examination. CSF pressure is elevated in about 90% of cases, and the appearance of the fluid ranges from slightly turbid to grossly purulent. CSF white cell counts of 1000–10,000/μL are usually seen, consisting chiefly of polymorphonuclear leukocytes, although mononuclear cells may predominate in *Listeria monocytogenes* meningitis. Protein concentrations of 100–500 mg/dL are most common. The CSF glucose level is lower than 40 mg/dL in about 80% of cases; it may be immeasurably low. Gram-stained smears of CSF identify the causative organism in 70–80% of cases. CSF culture, which is positive in about 80% of cases, provides a definitive diagnosis and allows determination of antibiotic sensitivity. Other techniques, such as countercurrent immunoelectrophoresis (CIE) and latex agglutination tests, can be useful in identifying the causative organism in patients with partially treated bacterial meningitis.

Differential Diagnosis

The signs of meningeal irritation may also be seen with subarachnoid hemorrhage, but the distinction is easily made when lumbar puncture shows bloody CSF. Early viral meningitis can produce polymorphonuclear pleocytosis, and symptoms identical to those of bacterial meningitis, but a repeat lumbar puncture after 6–12 hours should demonstrate a shift to lymphocytic predominance, and the CSF glucose level is normal.

Prevention

Children should be routinely immunized against *H influenzae* by vaccination. A vaccine is also available for some strains of *N meningitidis* and is recommended for travelers to areas of ongoing epidemics. The risk of contracting *H influenzae* or *N meningitidis* meningitis can be reduced in household and other close contacts of affected patients by the prophylactic administration of rifampin, 20 mg/kg/d orally, given as a single daily dose for four days (*H influenzae*) or as two divided doses for two days (*N meningitidis*).

Treatment

Unless the physical examination shows focal neurological abnormalities or papilledema, lumbar puncture should be performed immediately; if the CSF is not clear and colorless, antibiotic treatment (see below) is started without delay. When focal signs or papilledema are present, blood and urine should be taken for culture, antibiotics begun, and a brain CT scan obtained. If the scan shows no focal lesion that would contraindicate lumbar puncture, the puncture is then performed. The initial choice of antibiotics is empirical, based upon the patient's age (Table 1–13) and the predisposing factors (Table 1–14). Neonates in the first week of life should receive ampicillin, 100 mg/kg, and gentamicin, 2.5 mg/kg, intravenously twice daily, to cover *E coli, Streptococcus,* and *L monocytogenes*. Beyond the first week and up to three months of age, ampicillin is given in the same manner, but the gentamicin is increased to three times per day; cefotaxime, 50 mg/kg intravenously every six hours, can be substituted for gentamicin. Older infants and children are also treated with cefotaxime, 50 mg/kg intravenously every six hours; cephtriaxone, 50 mg/kg intravenously every 12 hours; or a combination of ampicillin, 100 mg/kg, and chloramphenicol, 25 mg/kg, intravenously four times per day, to cover *H influenzae* and *N meningitidis*. Adults, in whom *S pneumoniae* is the most likely organism, are given penicillin G, 2 million units intravenously every two hours, or ampicillin, 2 g intravenously every four hours. A combination of ampicillin, 2 g intravenously every four hours, and either cefotaxime, 2 g intravenously every four hours, or ceftriaxone, 2–3 g intravenously every 12 hours, is recommended for patients over 50 years of age.

Patients with head trauma or those who have had recent neurosurgical procedures require coverage for *Staphylococcus* (nafcillin or oxacillin, 3 g intravenously every six hours) and gram-negative bacilli (gentamicin, 1.7 mg/kg intravenously every eight hours). With immunosuppression, a combination of ticarcillin, 50 mg/kg intravenously, and gentamicin, 1.7 mg/kg intravenously, every eight hours, is recommended. Therapy is adjusted as indicated when the Gram's stain or culture and sensitivity results become available (Tables 1–15 and 1–16). Lumbar puncture should be repeated to assess the response to therapy. CSF should be sterile after 24 hours, and a decrease in pleocytosis and the proportion of polymorphonuclear leukocytes should be apparent within three days. Antibiotic treatment is continued for 10–14 days in most cases, although seven days may be adequate for meningitis caused by *N meningitidis* and that from *H influenzae* in children. Gram-negative bacillary meningitis should be treated for three weeks.

The use of corticosteroids as an adjunct to antibiotic treatment of bacterial meningitis is controversial. Nonetheless, dexamethasone, 0.6 mg/kg intravenously every six hours for the first four days of antibiotic therapy, may reduce the incidence of hearing loss following meningitis in children.

Table 1–15. Treatment of bacterial meningitis of known cause.

Organism	Drug(s) of Choice	Alternative(s)
Gram-positive		
Streptococcus pneumoniae	Penicillin G or ampicillin	Cefotaxime, ceftriaxone, or chloramphenicol
Streptococci groups A, B	Penicillin G	Erythromycin, cefotaxime, or ceftriaxone
Streptococcus group D	Penicillin G + gentamicin	Cefotaxime, ceftriaxone, or vancomycin
Staphylococcus sp.		
Methicillin-sensitive	Nafcillin or oxacillin	Vancomycin
Methicillin-resistant	Vancomycin	Trimethoprim-sulfamethoxazole
Listeria monocytogenes	Ampicillin + gentamicin	Trimethoprim-sulfamethoxazole
Gram-negative		
Neisseria meningitidis	Penicillin G	Cefotaxime, ceftriaxone, or chloramphenicol
Haemophilus influenzae		
Beta-lactamase-negative	Ampicillin	Cefotaxime, ceftriaxone, or chloramphenicol
Beta-lactamase-positive	Cefotaxime or ceftriaxone	Chloramphenicol
Escherichia coli	Cefotaxime or ceftriaxone	Ampicillin + gentamicin
Pseudomonas aeruginosa	Ceftazidime + gentamicin	Piperacillin + gentamicin

Prognosis

Complications of bacterial meningitis include headache, seizures, hydrocephalus, inappropriate secretion of antidiuretic hormone, residual neurological deficits (including cognitive disturbances and cranial—especially VIII—nerve abnormalities), and death. A CT scan will confirm suspected hydrocephalus. Fluid and electrolyte status should be carefully monitored in patients with meningitis. *N meningitidis* infections may be complicated by adrenal hemorrhage related to meningococcemia, resulting in hypotension and often death (**Waterhouse-Friderichsen syndrome**).

The morbidity and mortality rates of bacterial meningitis are high. Fatalities occur in about 25% of patients with *S pneumoniae,* 10% with *N meningitidis,* and 5% with *H influenzae* meningitis. Factors that worsen prognosis include extremes of age, delays in diagnosis and treatment, a complicating illness, stupor or coma, seizures, and focal neurological signs.

Table 1–16. Antibiotic dosage in adult meningitis.

Antibiotic	Intravenous Dose	Dose Interval
Ampicillin[1]	2 g	q4h
Cefotaxime[1]	2 g	q4h
Ceftazidime[1]	2–4 g	q8h
Ceftriaxone	2–3 g	q12h
Chloramphenicol	1–1.5 g	q6h
Erythromycin	1–2 g	q6h
Gentamicin[1,2]	1.7 mg/kg	q8h
Nafcillin	1.5–2 g	q4h
Oxacillin	1.5–2 g	q4h
Penicillin G[1]	2×10^6 units	q2h
Piperacillin[1]	2–3 g	q4h
Trimethoprim-sulfamethoxazole[1]	500 mg trimethoprim	q8h
Vancomycin[1]	1 g	q12h

[1]Reduce dose in patients with renal failure
[2]Plus 10 mg intrathecally q24h

TUBERCULOUS MENINGITIS

Tuberculous meningitis is an important diagnostic consideration in patients who present with a confusional state, especially if there is a history of pulmonary tuberculosis, alcoholism, corticosteroid treatment, HIV infection, or other conditions associated with impaired immune responses. It should also be considered if patients are from areas (eg, Asia, Africa) or groups (eg, the homeless and inner-city drug users) with a high incidence of tuberculosis.

Tuberculous meningitis usually results from reactivation of latent infection with *Mycobacterium tuberculosis.* Primary infection, typically acquired by inhaling bacillus-containing droplets, may be associated with metastatic dissemination of blood-borne bacilli from the lungs to the meninges and the surface of the brain. Here the organisms remain in a dormant state in tubercles that can rupture into the subarachnoid space at a later time, resulting in tuberculous meningitis.

Pathology

The principal neuropathological finding is a basal meningeal exudate containing mainly mononuclear cells. Tubercles may be seen on the meninges and surface of the brain. The ventricles may be enlarged as a result of hydrocephalus, and their surfaces may show ependymal exudate or granular ependymitis. Arteritis can result in cerebral infarction, and basal inflammation and fibrosis can compress cranial nerves.

Clinical Findings

A. Symptoms and Signs: Symptoms have usually been present for less than four weeks at the time of presentation and include fever, lethargy or confusion, and headache. Weight loss, vomiting, neck stiffness, visual impairment, diplopia, focal weakness, and seizures may also be noted. A history of contact with known cases of tuberculosis is usually absent.

Fever, signs of meningeal irritation, and a confusional state are the most common findings on physical examination, but all may be absent. Papilledema, ocular palsies, and hemiparesis are sometimes seen. Complications include spinal subarachnoid block, hydrocephalus, brain edema, cranial nerve palsies, and stroke caused by vasculitis or compression of blood vessels at the base of the brain.

B. Laboratory Findings: Only about one-half to two-thirds of patients show a positive skin test or evidence of active or healed tubercular infection on chest x-ray. The only investigation that can establish the diagnosis is CSF analysis. CSF pressure is usually increased, and the fluid is typically clear and colorless but may form a clot upon standing. Lymphocytic and mononuclear cell pleocytosis of 50–500 cells/µL is most often seen, but polymorphonuclear pleocytosis can occur early and may give an erroneous impression of bacterial meningitis. CSF protein is usually more than 100 mg/dL and may exceed 500 mg/dL, particularly in patients with spinal subarachnoid block. The glucose level is usually decreased and may be less than 20 mg/dL. A decreased chloride level, formerly thought to be specifically associated with tuberculous meningitis, is no longer considered diagnostically useful. Acid-fast smears of spinal fluid should be performed in all cases of suspected tuberculous meningitis, but they are positive in only a minority of cases. Definitive diagnosis is most often made by culturing *M tuberculosis* from the CSF, a process that usually takes several weeks and requires large quantities of spinal fluid for maximum yield. Finally, the CT scan may show contrast enhancement of the basal cisterns and cortical meninges, or hydrocephalus.

Differential Diagnosis

Many other conditions can cause a subacute confusional state associated with mononuclear cell pleocytosis, including syphilitic, fungal, neoplastic, and partially treated bacterial meningitis. These can be diagnosed by appropriate smears, cultures, and serological and cytological examinations.

Treatment

Treatment should be started as early as possible; it should not be withheld while awaiting culture results. The decision to treat is based on the CSF findings described above; lymphocytic pleocytosis and decreased glucose are particularly suggestive, even if acid-fast smears are negative. Triple therapy is indicated, consisting of isoniazid, 300 mg/d; rifampin, 600 mg/d; and pyrazinamide, 10–15 mg/kg twice daily. Each of these drugs is given orally. Triple therapy is continued for two months, followed by seven months of treatment with isoniazid and rifampin alone. If a drug-resistant strain of *M tuberculosis* is suspected, a fourth drug (streptomycin, 500 mg orally twice daily, or ethambutol, 15 mg/kg/d orally) should be added—and treatment for 18–24 months may be required. When streptomycin is used, it should be discontinued after three months because of its ototoxicity. Corticosteroids (eg, prednisone, 60 mg/d orally in adults or 1–3 mg/kg/d orally in children, tapered gradually over 3–4 weeks) are indicated as adjunctive therapy in patients with spinal subarachnoid block. They may also be indicated in seriously ill patients with focal neurological signs or with increased intracranial pressure from cerebral edema. The risk of using corticosteroids may be high, however, especially if tuberculous meningitis has been mistakenly diagnosed in a patient with fungal meningitis. Therefore, if fungal meningitis has not been excluded, antifungal therapy (see below) should be added together with corticosteroids. Pyridoxine, 50 mg/d, can be used to decrease the likelihood of isoniazid-induced polyneuropathy. Complications of therapy include hepatic dysfunction (isoniazid, rifampin, and pyrazinamide), polyneuropathy (isoniazid), optic neuritis (ethambutol), seizures (isoniazid), and ototoxicity (streptomycin).

Prognosis

Even with appropriate treatment, about one-third of patients with tuberculous meningitis succumb. Coma at the time of presentation is the most significant predictor of a poor prognosis.

SYPHILITIC MENINGITIS

Acute or subacute syphilitic meningitis usually occurs within two years after primary syphilitic infection. It is most common in young adults, affects men more often than women, and requires prompt treatment to prevent the irreversible manifestations of tertiary neurosyphilis.

In about one-fourth of patients with *Treponema pallidum* infection, treponemes gain access to the central nervous system, where they produce a meningitis that is usually asymptomatic (**asymptomatic neurosyphilis**). Asymptomatic invasion of the central nervous system is associated with CSF pleocytosis, elevated protein, and positive serological tests for syphilis.

Clinical Findings

A. Symptoms and Signs: In a few patients, syphilitic meningitis is a clinically apparent acute or subacute disorder. At the time of presentation, symptoms such as headache, nausea, vomiting, stiff neck, mental disturbances, focal weakness, seizures, deafness, and visual impairment have usually been present for up to two months.

Physical examination may show signs of meningeal irritation, confusion or delirium, papilledema, hemiparesis, and aphasia. The cranial nerves most frequently affected are (in order) the facial (VII), acoustic (VIII), oculomotor (III), trigeminal (V), abducens (VI), and optic (II) nerves, but other nerves may be involved as well. Fever is typically absent.

B. Laboratory Findings: The diagnosis is established by CSF findings. Opening pressure is normal or slightly elevated. Pleocytosis is lymphocytic or mononuclear in character, with white cell counts usually in the range of 100–1000/μL. Protein may be mildly or moderately elevated (< 200 mg/dL) and glucose mildly decreased. CSF VDRL and serum FTA or MHA-TP tests are usually positive. Protein electrophoretograms of CSF may show discrete gamma globulin bands (oligoclonal bands) not visible in normal CSF.

Treatment

Acute syphilitic meningitis is usually a self-limited disorder with no or minimal sequelae. Subsequent development of more advanced manifestations of neurosyphilis, including vascular and parenchymatous disease (eg, tabes dorsalis, general paresis, optic neuritis, myelitis), can be prevented by adequate treatment of the early syphilitic infection.

Syphilitic meningitis is treated with aqueous penicillin G, $2–4 \times 10^6$ units intravenously every four hours for ten days. For penicillin-allergic patients, tetracycline or erythromycin, 500 mg orally every six hours for 20 days, can be substituted. The CSF should be examined every six months until all findings are normal. Another course of therapy must be given if the CSF cell count or protein remains elevated.

LYME DISEASE

Lyme disease is a tick-borne disorder that results from systemic infection with the spirochete *Borrelia burgdorferi*. The disease occurs in Europe, the northeastern and western United States, and Australia; most cases occur during the summer months. Primary infection may be manifested by an expanding erythematous annular skin lesion (**erythema chronicum migrans**) that usually appears over the thigh, groin, or axilla. Less distinctive symptoms include fatigue, headache, fever, neck stiffness, joint or muscle pain, anorexia, sore throat, and nausea. Neurological involvement may be delayed for up to ten weeks and is characterized by meningitis or meningoencephalitis and disorders of the cranial or peripheral nerves or nerve roots. Cardiac abnormalities (conduction defects, myocarditis, pericarditis, cardiomegaly, or heart failure) can also occur at this stage. Lyme meningitis usually produces prominent headache that may be accompanied by signs of meningeal irritation, photophobia, pain when moving the eyes, nausea, and vomiting. When encephalitis is present, it is usually mild and characterized by insomnia, emotional lability, or impaired concentration and memory. The

CSF usually shows a lymphocytic pleocytosis with 100–200 cells/μL, slightly elevated protein, and normal glucose. Oligoclonal IgG bands may be detected. Definitive diagnosis is made by serological testing for *B burgdorferi*. Treatment is with intravenous penicillin (as described above for syphilitic meningitis) or with ceftriaxone, 1 g intravenously twice daily for 14 days. Symptoms typically resolve within ten days in treated cases. Untreated or inadequately treated infections may lead to recurrent oligoarthritis, and chronic neurological disorders including memory, language, and other cognitive disturbances; focal weakness; and ataxia. In such cases, a CT scan or MRI may show hydrocephalus, lesions in white matter resembling those seen in multiple sclerosis, or abnormalities suggestive of cerebral infarction. Subtle chronic cognitive or behavioral symptoms should not be attributed to Lyme encephalitis in the absence of serological evidence of *B burgdorferi* exposure, CSF abnormalities, or focal neurological signs. The peripheral neurological manifestations of Lyme disease are discussed in Chapter 7.

VIRAL MENINGITIS & ENCEPHALITIS

Viral infections of the meninges (**meningitis**) or brain parenchyma (**encephalitis**) often present as acute confusional states. Children and young adults are frequently affected. Viral meningitis is most often caused by enteric viruses (Table 1–17). Although the etiological agent is not identified in most cases of viral encephalitis, childhood exanthems, arthropod-borne agents, and herpes simplex type 1 are the more commonly recognized causes (Table 1–18).

Pathology

Viral infections can involve the central nervous system in three ways, through **hematogenous** dissemination of systemic viral infection (eg, arthropod-borne viruses); the **neuronal** spread of the virus (eg, herpes simplex, rabies) by axonal transport; and **autoimmune** responses causing postinfectious demyelination (eg, varicella, influenza).

Pathological changes in viral meningitis consist of an inflammatory meningeal reaction mediated by lymphocytes. Encephalitis is characterized by perivascular cuffing, lymphocytic infiltration, and microglial proliferation mainly involving subcortical gray matter regions. Intranuclear or intracytoplasmic inclusions are often seen.

Clinical Findings

A. Symptoms and Signs: Clinical manifestations of viral meningitis include fever, headache, neck stiffness, photophobia, pain with eye movement, and mild impairment of consciousness. Patients usually do not appear as ill as those with bacterial meningitis. Systemic viral infection may be

Table 1–17. Etiological agents in viral meningitis.

Virus	Incidence	Seasonal Variation	Source	Susceptible Population	Systemic Involvement	Laboratory Findings
Echoviruses	30%	Summer, fall	Fecal-oral	Children, members of affected families	Maculopapular, vesicular, or petechial skin rash; gastroenteritis	...
Coxsackie A	10%	Summer, fall	Fecal-oral	Children, members of affected families	Maculopapular, vesicular, or petechial skin rash; herpangina; gastroenteritis	...
Coxsackie B	40%	Summer, fall	Fecal-oral	Children, members of affected families	Maculopapular, vesicular, or petechial skin rash; pleuritis, pericarditis, myocarditis, orchitis; gastroenteritis	...
Mumps	15%	Late winter, spring	Inhalation	Children, male more than female	Parotitis, orchitis, oophoritis, pancreatitis	Amylase ↑; CSF glucose may be ↓
Herpes simplex (type 2)	Uncommon	...	Genital infection	Neonates with affected mothers	Vesicular genital lesions	...
Adenovirus	Uncommon	...	Inhalation	Infants, children	Pharyngitis, pneumonitis	...
Lymphocytic choriomeningitis	Uncommon	Late fall, winter	Mouse	Laboratory workers	Pharyngitis, pneumonitis	Marked CSF pleocytosis (1000–10,000 WBC/μL)
Hepatitis viruses	Uncommon	...	Fecal-oral, venereal, transfusion	IV drug users, male homosexuals, blood recipients	Jaundice, arthritis	Liver function abnormalities
Epstein-Barr virus (infectious mononucleosis)	Uncommon	...	Oral contact	Teenagers, young adults	Lymphadenopathy, pharyngitis, maculopapular skin rash, palatal petechiae, splenomegaly	Atypical lymphocytes, positive heterophil, liver function abnormalities

reflected by skin rash, pharyngitis, lymphadenopathy, pleuritis, carditis, jaundice, organomegaly, diarrhea, or orchitis. Such associations often suggest a particular etiologic agent. Because viral encephalitis involves the brain directly, marked alterations of consciousness, seizures, and focal neurological signs can occur. When signs of meningeal irritation and brain dysfunction coexist, the condition is termed **meningoencephalitis.**

B. Laboratory Findings: CSF analysis is the most important laboratory investigation. CSF pressure is normal or increased, and a lymphocytic or monocytic pleocytosis is present, with cell counts usually less than 1000/μL. (Higher counts can be seen in lymphocytic choriomeningitis or herpes simplex encephalitis.) A polymorphonuclear pleocytosis can occur early in viral meningitis, while red blood cells may be seen with herpes simplex encephalitis. Protein is normal or slightly increased (usually 80–200 mg/dL). Glucose is usually normal; it may be de-

creased in mumps, herpes zoster, or herpes simplex encephalitis. Gram's stains and bacterial, fungal, and acid-fast bacilli (AFB) cultures are negative. Oligoclonal bands and CSF protein electrophoresis abnormalities may be present. An etiologic diagnosis can often be made by virus isolation or by acute and convalescent CSF antibody titers.

Blood counts may show a normal white cell count, leukopenia, or mild leukocytosis. Atypical lymphocytes in blood smears and a positive heterophil (Monospot) test suggest infectious mononucleosis. Serum amylase is frequently elevated in mumps; abnormal liver function tests are associated with both hepatitis viruses and infectious mononucleosis. The EEG is diffusely slowed, especially if there is direct cerebral involvement; more characteristic findings can be found in encephalitis caused by herpes simplex infection (see below).

Table 1–18. Etiological agents in viral encephalitis

Type of Encephalitis	Vector	Geographic Distribution	Comments
Childhood exanthems			
Measles, varicella, mumps, rubella	Human	Worldwide.	Measles and mumps uncommon in USA because of vaccination.
Arthropod-borne (Arbo) viruses			
Alphaviruses			
Eastern equine	Mosquito	USA (Atlantic and Gulf coasts), Caribbean, South America.	Children usually affected; mortality 50–75%; neurological sequelae common.
Western equine	Mosquito	Western and central USA, South America.	Infants and adults >50 years usually affected; mortality 5–15%; neurological sequelae uncommon except in infants.
Venezuelan equine	Mosquito	Florida, southwestern USA, Central and South America.	Adults usually affected; mortality 1%; neurological sequelae rare.
Flaviviruses			
Japanese B	Mosquito	China, Southeast Asia, India.	Vaccine available.
St. Louis	Mosquito	USA (rural west and midwest, New Jersey, Florida, Texas), Caribbean, Central and South America.	Adults >50 years most often affected; mortality 2–20%; neurological sequelae in about 20%.
Murray Valley	Mosquito	Australia, New Guinea.	
West Nile	Mosquito	Middle East, Africa.	
Rocio	Mosquito	Brazil.	
Kyasanur Forest	Tick	India.	
Powassan	Tick	New York, Ontario.	
Russian spring-summer	Tick	Northern Europe, Siberia.	
Louping-ill	Tick	United Kingdom.	
Bunyaviruses			
California (including LaCrosse)	Mosquito	North America.	Children usually affected; mortality <1%; neurological sequelae uncommon.
Rift Valley	Mosquito	Africa.	
Orbiviruses			
Colorado tick fever	Tick	Western and Rocky Mountain states of USA.	
Other			
Herpes simplex (type 1)	Human	Worldwide.	Focal neurological signs common; responds to treatment with acyclovir.
Herpes simplex (type 2)	Human	Worldwide.	Encephalitis usually affects neonates; causes meningitis in older children and adults.
Rabies	Foxes, bats, dogs, skunks, cattle	Worldwide.	Invariably fatal unless vaccine and antiserum administered before symptoms occur following bite by affected animal.

Differential Diagnosis

The differential diagnosis of meningitis with mononuclear cell pleocytosis includes partially treated bacterial meningitis as well as syphilitic, tuberculous, fungal, parasitic, neoplastic, and other meningitides. Evidence of systemic viral infection and CSF wet mounts, stained smears, cultures, and cytological examination can distinguish among these possibilities. When presumed early viral meningitis is associated with a polymorphonuclear pleocytosis of less than 1000 white blood cells/μL and normal CSF glucose, one of two strategies can be used. The patient can be treated for bacterial meningitis until the results of CSF cultures are known, or treatment can be withheld and lumbar puncture repeated in 6–12 hours. If the meningitis is viral in origin, the second sample should show a mononuclear cell pleocytosis. The syndrome of viral encephalitis may clinically resemble that from metabolic disorders, but it can be distinguished by spinal fluid findings.

A disorder that may be clinically indistinguishable from viral encephalitis is the **immune-mediated encephalomyelitis** that may follow viral infections such as influenza, measles, or chickenpox. Progressive neurological dysfunction typically begins a few days after the viral illness but can also occur either simultaneously or up to several weeks later. Neurological abnormalities result from perivenous demyelination, which often severely affects the brain stem. The CSF shows a lymphocytic pleocytosis, usually with cell counts of 50–150/μL, and mild protein elevation.

Treatment

Except for herpes simplex encephalitis, which is discussed separately (see below), no specific therapy for viral meningitis and encephalitis is available. Corticosteroids are of no benefit except in immune-mediated postinfectious syndromes. Headache and severe hyperthermia can be treated with aspirin or acetaminophen; mild fever requires no treatment and may even contribute to the host response to the virus. Seizures usually respond to phenytoin or phenobarbital. Supportive measures in comatose patients include mechanical ventilation and intravenous or nasogastric feeding.

Prognosis

Symptoms of viral meningitis usually resolve spontaneously within two weeks regardless of the causative agent, although residual deficits may be seen. The outcome of viral encephalitis varies with the specific virus, however; eastern equine and herpes simplex virus infections are associated with severe morbidity and high mortality rates. Mortality rates as high as 20% have also been reported in immune-mediated encephalomyelitis following measles infections.

HERPES SIMPLEX VIRUS (HSV) ENCEPHALITIS

Specific antiviral therapy is available for this disorder, which is the most common type of sporadic fatal encephalitis in the United States. About two-thirds of cases involve patients over 40 years of age. Primary herpes infections most often present as stomatitis (HSV type 1) or a venereally transmitted genital eruption (HSV type 2). The virus migrates along nerve axons to sensory ganglia, where it persists in a latent form—and may be subsequently reactivated. It is not clear whether HSV type 1 encephalitis, the most common type in adults, represents a primary infection or a reactivation of latent infection. Neonatal HSV encephalitis usually results from acquisition of type 2 virus during passage through the birth canal of a mother with active genital lesions. Central nervous system involvement by HSV type 2 in adults usually causes meningitis, rather than encephalitis.

Pathology

The pathological picture of HSV type 1 encephalitis is that of an acute, necrotizing, asymmetrical hemorrhagic process with lymphocytic and plasma cell reaction, which usually involves the medial temporal and inferior frontal lobes. Intranuclear inclusions may be seen in the neurons and glia. In patients who recover, the chronic state is characterized by cystic necrosis of the involved regions.

Clinical Findings

A. Symptoms and Signs: The clinical syndrome may include headache, stiff neck, vomiting, behavioral disorders, memory loss, anosmia, aphasia, hemiparesis, and focal or generalized seizures. Active herpes labialis is seen occasionally, but its presence does not increase the likelihood that the encephalitis is due to HSV. The encephalitis is usually rapidly progressive over several days and may result in coma or death. The most common sequelae in patients who survive HSV encephalitis are memory and behavior disturbances, reflecting the predilection of the process for limbic structures.

B. Laboratory Findings: The CSF in HSV type 1 encephalitis most often shows increased pressure, lymphocytic or mixed lymphocytic and polymorphonuclear pleocytosis (50–100 white blood cells/μL), mild protein elevation, and normal glucose. Red blood cells, xanthochromia, and decreased glucose are seen in some cases. The virus generally cannot be isolated from the CSF. The EEG may show periodic slow-wave complexes arising from one or both temporal lobes, and CT scans and MRI may show abnormalities in one or both temporal lobes. These can extend to frontal or parietal regions and are sometimes enhanced with the infusion of contrast material (Figure 1–6). It should be noted that imaging studies may also be normal. Definitive diagnosis is possible only by biopsy of affected brain areas, with the choice of biopsy site guided by the EEG, CT, or MRI findings.

Differential Diagnosis

The symptoms and signs are not specific for herpes infection. The greatest diagnostic difficulty is distinguishing between HSV encephalitis and brain abscess. The latter is suggested by systemic bacterial infection, a slower progression of deficits, less-marked CSF pleocytosis, a continuous polymorphic slow-wave disturbance in the EEG, and symmetrical contrast enhancement of the rim of the lesion seen on CT scan. The two disorders often cannot be differentiated on clinical grounds alone, however. Final diagnoses in patients undergoing brain biopsy for suspected HSV encephalitis have included vasculitis, other viral infections, bacterial abscess, fungal infections, tumor, Reye's syndrome, parasitic infections, and tuberculosis. Because many of these conditions require specific therapy and none are favorably affected by the treatment used for HSV encephalitis, some clini-

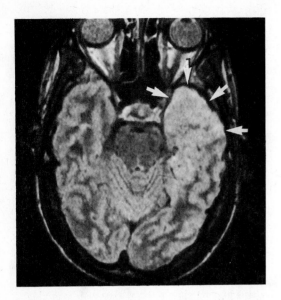

Figure 1–6. T2-weighted MRI in herpes simplex encephalitis. Note the lack of differentiation between gray and white matter, because of edema, in the left anterior temporal lobe (arrows) compared to the right. (Courtesy of A Gean.)

cians argue that all patients with suspected HSV encephalitis should undergo brain biopsy to establish a definitive diagnosis. The most commonly accepted approach, however, is to treat patients with probable HSV encephalitis as described below and to reserve biopsies for those who fail to improve.

Treatment

The most effective drug is **acyclovir,** given intravenously at a dosage of 30 mg/kg/d, divided into three daily doses, each given over one hour. Treatment is continued for ten days. Complications reported include erythema at the intravenous infusion site. **Vidarabine,** 15 mg/kg/d intravenously, administered over 12 hours each day for ten days, is less effective. Complications of this therapy include overhydration, skin rash, diarrhea, decreased leukocyte and platelet counts, and increased hepatic enzymes. For both drugs, treatment is started as early as possible, since outcome is greatly influenced by the severity of dysfunction at the time treatment is initiated. Treatment is discontinued if a subsequent brain biopsy establishes another diagnosis.

Prognosis

Prognosis is influenced by the patient's age and level of consciousness at presentation and the treatment. Patients under the age of 30 years and those who are only lethargic at the onset of treatment are more likely to survive than are older or comatose patients. Reported mortality rates are 44% at six months

in vidarabine-treated patients and 28% at 18 months in patients given acyclovir. Acyclovir also increases the fraction of patients with no or only minor neurological sequelae from 5% to 38%, compared with vidarabine. It is not known whether a combination of acyclovir and vidarabine has greater efficacy than either drug used alone.

ACQUIRED IMMUNODEFICIENCY SYNDROME (AIDS)

AIDS is a disorder caused by systemic infection with human immunodeficiency virus-1 (HIV-1) and characterized by opportunistic infections, malignant neoplasms (typically non-Hodgkins lymphoma or Kaposi's sarcoma), and a variety of neurological disturbances. Transmission occurs through sexual activity or by transfer of virus-contaminated blood or blood products. Individuals at particular risk of infection include homosexual and bisexual men, intravenous drug users who share needles, hemophiliacs who have received factor VIII transfusions, and the sexual partners of all the foregoing. AIDS can also be transmitted through heterosexual intercourse, by blood transfusions, or, in medical personnel, by accidental puncture with contaminated needles.

Neurological complications of AIDS include dementia (see Chapter 2), myelopathy (see Chapter 6), neuropathy (see Chapter 7), myopathy (see Chapter 6), and stroke (see Chapter 10). Patients with AIDS can also develop acute confusional states related to any of the disorders (discussed later in this chapter) that produce such states in persons without AIDS. In addition, patients with AIDS are at increased risk for developing acute confusional states resulting from direct viral involvement of the nervous system, opportunistic infections, and tumors associated with AIDS (Table 1–19). Treatment of AIDS is discussed in the section on AIDS dementia complex in Chapter 2.

1. HIV-1 MENINGITIS

Patients infected with HIV-1 can develop a syndrome characterized by headache, fever, signs of meningeal irritation, cranial nerve (especially VII) palsies, other focal neurological abnormalities, or seizures. This usually occurs at about the time of HIV-1 seroconversion. An acute confusional state may occasionally also be present. HIV-1 meningitis is associated with mononuclear pleocytosis of up to about 200 cells/μL and may represent the initial immunologic response of the nervous system to HIV-1 infection. A similar CSF profile has been found in some asymptomatic patients undergoing lumbar puncture shortly after HIV-1 seroconversion. Symptoms usually resolve spontaneously within about one month. Other causes of pleocytosis associated with

Table 1–19. Causes of acute confusional states in patients with AIDS.

Meningitis
  HIV-1 meningitis
  Cryptococcal meningitis
Encephalitis
  Herpes simplex encephalitis
  Varicella-zoster encephalitis
  Cytomegalovirus encephalitis
Intracerebral mass lesions
  Cerebral toxoplasmosis
  Primary central nervous system lymphoma
Metabolic encephalopathies
  Pulmonary encephalopathy (related to *Pneumocystis carinii*
    pneumonia)
  Drug toxicity
Stroke
Seizures

AIDS, including cryptococcal meningitis, herpes-simplex encephalitis, and cerebral toxoplasmosis, must be excluded; specific treatments exist for these conditions.

2. CRYPTOCOCCAL MENINGITIS

Cryptococcal meningitis occurs in 5–10% of patients with AIDS. Clinical features include headache, confusion, stiff neck, fever, nausea and vomiting, seizures, and cranial nerve palsies. Because the CSF is otherwise normal in about 20% of patients with AIDS and cryptococcal meningitis, CSF cryptococcal antigen titers should always be obtained. Laboratory abnormalities and recommended treatment are discussed in the section on fungal meningitis (below).

3. HERPES SIMPLEX & VARICELLA-ZOSTER ENCEPHALITIS

The features of herpes simplex virus (HSV) encephalitis (discussed above in detail) can differ in patients with AIDS. While HSV encephalitis in immunocompetent adults is almost always due to type 1 virus, either type 1 or type 2 HSV can produce the disorder in patients with AIDS. The focal neurological signs and CSF abnormalities usually associated with HSV encephalitis may be absent in AIDS, and the disorder may follow a more indolent course. Varicella-zoster virus, a herpesvirus that rarely causes encephalitis in immunocompetent individuals, may do so in patients with AIDS. Treatment is as described above for HSV encephalitis.

4. CYTOMEGALOVIRUS ENCEPHALITIS

Cytomegalovirus, another herpesvirus, has been implicated as a cause of retinitis and polyradiculomyelitis (see Chapter 6) in patients with AIDS. Cytomegalovirus can also be identified in CSF and biopsy specimens from patients with AIDS who are neurologically asymptomatic, acutely confused, or demented. The extent to which cytomegalovirus contributes to the pathogenesis of the last two syndromes is uncertain.

5. CEREBRAL TOXOPLASMOSIS

Cerebral toxoplasmosis is the most common cause of intracerebral mass lesions in patients with AIDS. A confusional state lasting days to weeks exists at the time of presentation in about 30% of patients. Other clinical features include fever, focal neurological abnormalities such as cranial nerve palsies or hemiparesis, seizures, headache, and signs of meningeal irritation. Serological tests for toxoplasmosis are unreliable in patients with AIDS. CT scanning typically reveals one or more lesions, which often show a contrast enhancement of the rim and are commonly located in the basal ganglia; MRI is more sensitive than CT in revealing the lesions.

Because toxoplasmosis is so often the cause of intracerebral mass lesions in AIDS and is readily treatable, patients with such lesions that are not obviously due to stroke should be treated for presumed toxoplasmosis (Figure 1–7), as described in the section on parasitic infections (below). Up to 90% of patients respond favorably to therapy within the first few weeks and the majority survive longer than six months.

6. PRIMARY CENTRAL NERVOUS SYSTEM LYMPHOMA

Primary central nervous system lymphoma, an otherwise rare tumor, is the most common brain tumor associated with AIDS and, after toxoplasmosis, the second most common cause of intracerebral mass lesions in AIDS. Systemic non-Hodgkin's lymphoma also occurs with increased frequency in patients with AIDS; in contrast to primary CNS lymphoma, however, it usually produces lymphomatous meningitis (see section on neoplastic meningitis below) rather than intracerebral masses.

Clinical features of primary CNS lymphoma usually evolve over several weeks, which is slower than the typical course of developing cerebral toxoplasmosis. Most patients have a confusional state at the time of presentation. Other symptoms and signs include hemiparesis, aphasia, seizures, cranial nerve palsies and headache. Signs of meningeal irritation are exceptional and suggest another cause of neuro-

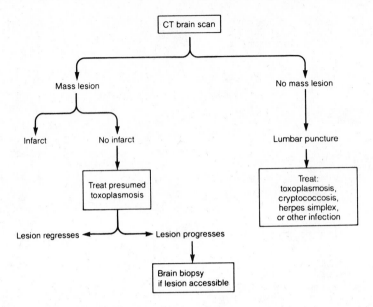

Figure 1–7. Diagnostic evaluation of central nervous system dysfunction in patients with HIV infection.

logical involvement. CSF commonly shows elevated protein and mild mononuclear pleocytosis, and glucose may be low; cytology is rarely positive. CT scanning shows single or multiple contrast-enhanced lesions, which cannot be distinguished definitively by appearance or location from those seen with toxoplasmosis. Here, too, MRI is more sensitive than CT.

Patients with AIDS and one or more intracerebral mass lesions that fail to respond to treatment for toxoplasmosis within three weeks should undergo brain biopsy for histologic diagnosis of lymphoma. Although corticosteroid treatment and radiation therapy may prolong survival, most patients die within a few months.

7. PULMONARY ENCEPHALOPATHY

Pneumocystis carinii pneumonia develops eventually in more than 80% of patients with AIDS. While this opportunistic protozoan does not affect the nervous system directly, pulmonary involvement may lead to hypoxia and a resulting confusional state. Pulmonary encephalopathy is discussed above in the section on organ system failure.

8. DRUG TOXICITY

Patients with AIDS, especially those with AIDS dementia complex or CNS infections or tumors, may be especially sensitive to drug-induced and other metabolic disturbances that produce acute confusional states. Antidepressants may be of particular concern as causative agents.

9. STROKE

As described below in the section on vascular disorders, stroke can cause acute confusional states, especially when it affects the brain stem or right cerebral hemisphere. Ischemic strokes may occur in patients with AIDS, especially when the disorder is complicated by cryptococcal meningitis.

10. SEIZURES

A confusional state typically follows generalized tonic-clonic seizures, and confusion may be a major manifestation of complex partial seizures. Seizures are common in patients with AIDS, especially those with AIDS dementia complex, cerebral toxoplasmosis, or cryptococcal meningitis.

FUNGAL MENINGITIS

In a small fraction of patients with systemic fungal infections (**mycoses**), fungi invade the central nervous system to produce meningitis or focal intraparenchymal lesions (Table 1–20). Several of these fungi are opportunistic organisms that cause infection in patients with cancer, patients receiving corticosteroids or other immunosuppressive drugs, and other debilitated hosts. Intravenous drug abuse is a potential route for infection with *Candida* and *Aspergillus*. Diabetic acidosis is strongly correlated with rhinocerebral mucormycosis. In contrast, meningeal infections with *Coccidioides, Blastomyces,* and *actinomyces* usually occur in previously healthy individ-

Table 1–20. Etiological agents in fungal meningitis.

Name	Geographic Distribution	Opportunistic Infection	Systemic Involvement	Distinctive CSF Findings	Treatment
Cryptococcus neoformans	Nonspecific	Sometimes (including AIDS)	Lungs, skin, bones, joints	Viscous fluid, positive India ink prep, positive cryptococcal antigen	Amphotericin B + Flucytosine (amphotericin B or amphotericin B + Fluconazole for AIDS patients)
Coccidioides immitis	Southwestern USA	No	Lungs, skin, bones	Positive complement fixation	Amphotericin B (intravenous and intrathecal)
Candida species	Nonspecific	Yes	Mucous membranes, skin, esophagus, GU tract, heart	Positive Gram's stain	Amphotericin B
Aspergillus species	Nonspecific	Yes	Lungs, skin	Polymorphonuclear pleocytosis	Amphotericin B
Mucor species	Nonspecific	Yes, diabetics	Orbits, paranasal sinuses		Amphotericin B + correction of hyperglycemia and acidosis
Histoplasma capsulatum	Eastern and mid-western USA	Sometimes	Lungs, skin, mucous membranes, heart, viscera		Amphotericin B
Blastomyces dermatitidis	Mississippi River Valley	No	Lungs, skin, bones, joints, viscera		Amphotericin B
Actinomyces israelii[1]	Nonspecific	No	Jaw, lungs, abdomen, orbits, sinuses, skin	Sulfur granules, positive Gram's stain, AFB smear	Penicillin G or tetracycline
Nocardia species[1]	Nonspecific	Yes	Lungs, skin	Positive Gram's stain, AFB smear	Sulfonamides

[1] Actinomyces and Nocardia are filamentous bacteria that are traditionally considered together with fungi.

uals. *Cryptococcus* (the most common cause of fungal meningitis in the United States) and *Histoplasma* infection can occur in either healthy or immunosuppressed patients. Cryptococcal meningitis is the most common fungal infection of the nervous system in AIDS, but *Coccidioides* and *Histoplasma* infections can also occur in this setting. Geographic factors are also important in the epidemiology of certain mycoses (see Table 1–20).

Pathogenesis

Organisms reach the central nervous system by hematogenous spread from the lungs, heart, gastrointestinal or genitourinary tract, or skin or by direct extension from parameningeal sites such as the orbits or paranasal sinuses. Invasion of the meninges from a contiguous focus of infection is particularly common in mucormycosis but may also occur in aspergillosis and actinomycosis.

Pathology

Pathological findings in fungal infections of the nervous system include a primarily mononuclear meningeal exudative reaction, focal abscesses or granulomas in the brain or spinal epidural space, cerebral infarction related to vasculitis, and ventricular enlargement caused by communicating hydrocephalus.

Clinical Findings

Fungal meningitis is usually a subacute illness that clinically resembles tuberculous meningitis. A history of such predisposing conditions as carcinoma, hematological cancer, AIDS, diabetes, organ transplantation, treatment with corticosteroids or cytotoxic agents, prolonged antibiotic therapy, or intravenous drug use increases the suspicion of opportunistic infection. Questions should be asked about recent travel through areas where certain fungi are endemic.

A. Symptoms and Signs: Common symptoms include headache and lethargy or confusion. Nausea, vomiting, visual loss, seizures, or focal weakness may be noted, while fever may be absent. In a diabetic patient with acidosis, complaints of facial or eye pain, nasal discharge, proptosis, or visual loss should urgently alert the physician to the likelihood of *Mucor* infection.

Careful examination of the skin, orbits, sinuses, and chest may reveal evidence of systemic fungal infection. Neurological examination may show signs of meningeal irritation, a confusional state, papilledema, visual loss, ptosis, exophthalmos, ocular or other cranial nerve palsies, and focal neurological abnormalities such as hemiparesis. Because some fungi (most commonly *Cryptococcus*) can cause spinal cord compression, there may be evidence of spine

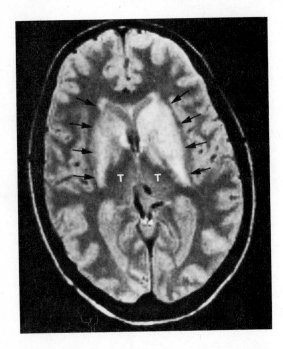

Figure 1–8. T2-weighted MRI in cryptococcal meningitis. Note the bilateral increase in signal in the basal ganglia (arrows) with relative sparing of the thalami (T). This is due to the presence of gelatinous fungal pseudocysts in the territory of the lenticulostriate arteries. (Courtesy of A Gean.)

tenderness, paraparesis, pyramidal signs in the legs, and loss of sensation over the legs and trunk.

B. Laboratory Findings: Blood cultures should be obtained. Serum glucose and arterial blood gas levels should be determined in diabetic patients. The urine should be examined for *Candida.* Chest x-ray may show hilar lymphadenopathy, patchy or miliary infiltrates, cavitation, or pleural effusion. The CT scan or MRI may demonstrate intracerebral mass lesions associated with *Cryptococcus* (Figure 1–8) or other organisms, a contiguous infectious source in the orbit or paranasal sinuses, or hydrocephalus.

CSF pressure may be normal or elevated, and the fluid is usually clear. It may be viscous in the presence of numerous cryptococci, but the presence of alcohol (once considered indicative of cryptococcal infection) is not a reliable finding. Lymphocytic pleocytosis of up to 1000 cells/μL is common, but a normal cell count or polymorphonuclear pleocytosis can be seen in early fungal meningitis and normal cell counts are common in immunosuppressed patients. *Aspergillus* infection typically produces a polymorphonuclear pleocytosis. CSF protein, which may be normal initially, subsequently rises, usually to levels not exceeding 200 mg/dL. Higher levels (< 1 g/dL) suggest possible subarachnoid block. Glucose is normal or decreased but rarely below 10 mg/dL. Micro-

scopic examination of Gram-stained and acid-fast smears and India ink preparations may reveal the infecting organism (Table 1–20). Fungal cultures of CSF and other body fluids and tissues should be obtained, but they are often negative. In suspected **mucormycosis,** biopsy of the affected tissue (usually nasal mucosa) is essential. Useful CSF serological studies include cryptococcal antigen and *Coccidioides* complement-fixing antibody. Cryptococcal antigen is more sensitive than India ink for detecting *Cryptococcus,* and should always be looked for in both CSF and serum when that organism is suspected (in patients with AIDS, for example).

Differential Diagnosis

Fungal meningitis may mimic brain abscess and other subacute or chronic meningitides, such as those due to tuberculosis or syphilis. CSF findings and contrast CT scans are useful in differential diagnosis.

Treatment & Prognosis

For most organisms causing fungal meningitis, treatment is begun with **amphotericin B,** 1 mg intravenously as a test dose given over 20–30 minutes, followed the next day by 0.25 mg/kg intravenously given over two to six hours. The dose is then increased daily in 5- to 10-mg increments until a maximal dose of 0.5–0.6 mg/kg/d is reached. Treatment is usually continued for 12 weeks. Nephrotoxicity is common with amphotericin B and may force interruption of therapy for two to five days.

In patients with *Coccidioides* meningitis or those not responding to intravenous therapy, intrathecal amphotericin B (usually administered via an Ommaya reservoir) is added. The drug is given as a 0.1-mg test dose diluted in 10 mL of CSF, with or without added corticosteroids, and increased to 0.25-0.5 mg every other day.

In cryptococcal meningitis, **flucytosine,** 150 mg/kg/d orally, added to amphotericin B and given in four divided doses, reduces the duration of therapy from 12 to 6 weeks. The dose of flucytosine must be reduced in renal failure; the major side effect is bone marrow suppression, which is usually reversible. Because of this toxicity, flucytosine is usually omitted when treating cryptococcal meningitis in patients with AIDS. For patients with AIDS and cryptococcal meningitis who do not respond to amphotericin B alone, **fluconazole** can be added at an initial dose of 400 mg, followed by 200 mg/d, orally or intravenously, for at least 10–12 weeks after CSF cultures are negative. Long-term maintenance therapy with fluconazole, 100–200 mg/d orally, may also reduce the likelihood of recurrence following successful treatment of cryptococcal meningitis in patients with AIDS.

Rapid correction of hyperglycemia and acidosis must be combined with amphotericin B treatment and surgical debridement of necrotic tissue in diabetics with mucormycosis.

Mortality rates remain high in fungal meningitis. The complications of therapy are frequent, and neurological residua are common.

PARASITIC INFECTIONS

Protozoal and helminthic infections are important causes of central nervous system disease, particularly in immunosuppressed patients (including those with AIDS), and in certain regions of the world (Table 1–21). Rickettsia, the parasitic bacteria that cause Rocky Mountain spotted fever, rarely affect the nervous system.

1. MALARIA

Malaria is caused by the protozoan *plasmodium falciparum* or another *Plasmodium* species that is transferred to humans by the female *Anopheles* mosquito. Clinical features include fever, chills, myalgia, nausea and vomiting, anemia, renal failure, and pulmonary edema. Although malaria is, worldwide, the most common parasitic infection of humans, cerebral involvement is rare. Plasmodia reach the central nervous system in infected red blood cells and cause occlusion of cerebral capillaries. Neurological involvement becomes apparent weeks after infection. In addition to acute confusional states, cerebral malaria can produce seizures and, rarely, focal neurological abnormalities. The diagnosis is made by finding plasmodia in red blood cells of peripheral blood smears.

Table 1–21. Parasitic infections of the central nervous system.

Parasite	Epidemiological and Geographic Factors	Clinical Syndrome	Laboratory Findings	Treatment
Protozoa				
Plasmodium falciparum (malaria)	Africa, South America, Southeast Asia, Oceania.	Acute confusional state, coma, seizures.	Anemia, organisms within red blood cells on peripheral blood smear.	Chloroquine phosphate (chloroquine-sensitive) or quinine sulfate and pyrimethamine-sulfadioxine (chloroquine-resistant).
Toxoplasma gondii	Malignancy or immunosuppression (including AIDS).	Single or multiple focal mass lesions; meningoencephalitis; encephalopathy ± asterixis, myoclonus, or seizures.	Positive CT/MRI brain scan; positive Sabin-Feldman dye test; positive IgM antibody; CSF: normal or lymphocytic pleocytosis, organism on wet mount.	Pyrimethamine and either trisulfapyrimidines or sulfadiazine.
Naegleria fowleri (primary amebic meningoencephalitis)	Freshwater swimming in southeastern USA.	Acute fulminant meningoencephalitis with prominent headache and meningeal signs.	CSF: polymorphonuclear pleocytosis, motile organisms on wet mount.	Amphotericin B.
Acanthamoeba or *Hartmanella* species (granulomatous amebic encephalitis)	Chronic illness or immunosuppression.	Subacute-chronic meningoencephalitis, often with seizures and focal neurological signs.	CSF: lymphocytic or polymorphonuclear pleocytosis, sluggish organisms on wet mount.	None proven.
Helminths				
Taenia solium (cysticercosis)	Latin America.	Mass lesion or meningoencephalitis, often presenting with headache or seizures.	CSF: lymphocytic pleocytosis, eosinophilia, positive complement fixation or hemagglutination; calcifications on soft tissue x-rays or brain CT scan.	Praziquantel or albendazole, corticosteroids, surgical excision of solitary lesion, shunting for hydrocephalus.
Angiostrongylus cantonensis (eosinophilic meningitis)	Hawaii, Asia.	Acute-subacute meningitis with headache; stiff neck, vomiting, fever, and paresthesias in about half of patients; self-limited course of 1–2 weeks.	Peripheral blood eossinophilia; CSF: eosinophilic and lymphocytic pleocytosis.	None (self-limited) or mebendazole (investigational).
Rickettsia				
Rickettsia rickettsii (Rocky Mountain spotted fever)	Southeastern USA.	Acute fever, headache, rash; confusion uncommon.	Positive Weil-Felix reaction.	Tetracycline or chloramphenicol.

The CSF may show increased pressure, xanthochromia, mononuclear pleocytosis, or mildly elevated protein.

Prophylaxis

Malaria prophylaxis is recommended for travelers to endemic areas and consists of chloroquine phosphate, 500 mg orally, weekly. If exposure to chloroquine-resistant strains is expected, mefloquine (250 mg orally weekly for four weeks, then every other week for four weeks) should be given instead. Both regimens are started one week before the initial exposure and continued for four weeks after exposure ends.

Treatment

Treatment of **chloroquine-sensitive malaria** consists of chloroquine phosphate, 1 gram orally upon diagnosis, followed by 500 mg orally 6, 24, and 48 hours later. **Chloroquine-resistant malaria** is treated with quinine sulfate (650 mg orally every eight hours for three days) and pyrimethamine-sulfadoxine (3 tablets orally immediately). Parenteral treatment of malaria, which is not widely available, consists of quinine dihydrochloride, 600 mg intravenously over two to four hours every eight hours, up to a maximum of three doses; or quinine gluconate, 10 mg/kg intravenously over one hour followed by constant infusion at 0.02 mg/kg/min for up to three days. Oral therapy is then instituted as described above. Exchange transfusion is a useful adjunctive therapy.

Cerebral edema is not a consistent finding in cerebral malaria and corticosteroids are *not* helpful and may, in fact, be deleterious. The mortality rate in cerebral malaria is 20–50% and reaches 80% in cases complicated by coma and seizures.

2. TOXOPLASMOSIS

Acquired (as opposed to congenital) toxoplasmosis results from ingestion of *Toxoplasma gondii* cysts in raw meat or cat excrement and it is usually asymptomatic. Symptomatic infection is associated with underlying malignant disease (especially Hodgkin's disease), immunosuppressive therapy, or AIDS. Systemic manifestations include skin rash, lymphadenopathy, myalgias, arthralgias, carditis, pneumonitis, and splenomegaly. CNS involvement can take several forms (Table 1–21).

Clinical Findings

The CSF may be normal, or it may show mild mononuclear cell pleocytosis or slight protein elevation. A CT scan may show one or more ring-enhancing lesions, especially if a double dose of contrast material is used. Lesions revealed by CT scan may fail to enhance, however, and autopsy-proved lesions may not be detected by CT. MRI is superior to CT scanning for demonstrating cerebral toxoplasmosis (Figure 1–9).

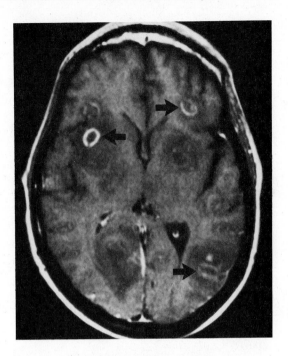

Figure 1–9. T1-weighted, gadolinium-enhanced MRI in cerebral toxoplasmosis complicating HIV infection. Note the multiple ring-enhanced lesions (arrows) with surrounding edema. (Courtesy of A Gean.)

The diagnosis is made by blood tests demonstrating a high (≥ 1:32,000) or rising Sabin-Feldman dye test titer or IgM antibodies to *Toxoplasma* by indirect immunofluorescent techniques. Accurate diagnosis requires appropriate serological studies in the immunosuppressed patient who develops neurological symptoms.

Treatment

Treatment with pyrimethamine, 25 mg/d orally, and either trisulfapyrimidines or sulfadiazine, 100 mg/kg/d orally in four divided doses, should be continued for at least one month. Clindamycin, 600 mg orally four times a day, may be substituted for sulfonamides in patients who develop drug sensitivity rashes. Folinic acid (leucovorin), 10 mg orally daily, is added to prevent pyrimethamine-induced leukopenia and thrombocytopenia. In patients with AIDS, treatment for at least three to six months is required; even then, relapses are common, and some clinicians advocate lifelong treatment.

3. PRIMARY AMEBIC MENINGOENCEPHALITIS

The free-living ameba *Naegleria fowleri* causes primary amebic meningoencephalitis in previously healthy young patients exposed to polluted water.

Amebas gain entry to the central nervous system through the cribriform plate, producing a diffuse meningoencephalitis that affects the base of the frontal lobes and posterior fossa. It is characterized by headache, fever, nausea and vomiting, signs of meningeal irritation, and disordered mental status. Seizures and focal neurological signs are rare. The CSF shows a polymorphonuclear pleocytosis with elevated protein and low glucose; highly motile, refractile trophozoites can be seen on wet mounts of centrifuged CSF.

The disease is usually fatal within one week, although treatment with amphotericin B, 1 mg/kg/d intravenously, may be effective, as may a combination of amphotericin B, miconazole, and rifampin.

4. GRANULOMATOUS AMEBIC ENCEPHALITIS

Granulomatous amebic encephalitis results from infection with the *Acanthamoeba/Hartmanella* species and commonly occurs in the setting of chronic illness or immunosuppression. The disorder typically lasts for periods from one week to two or three months and is characterized by subacute or chronic meningitis and granulomatous encephalitis. The cerebellum, brain stem, basal ganglia, and cerebral hemispheres are affected. An acute confusional state is the most common clinical finding. Although fever, headache, and meningeal signs are less common than in primary amebic meningoencephalitis (each occurring in only about half of patients), seizures and hemiparesis are more common. Cranial nerve palsies, cerebellar ataxia, and aphasia may occur. Pleocytosis may be primarily lymphocytic or polymorphonuclear; protein is elevated, and glucose is low or normal. Sluggishly motile trophozoites may be seen on wet mounts. Successful treatment has not been reported.

5. CYSTICERCOSIS

Cysticercosis is common in Mexico, Central and South America, and certain regions of Africa, Asia, and Europe. The disease follows ingestion of larvae of the pork tapeworm *(Taenia solium)* and affects the brain in 60–90% of cases. Larvae undergo hematogenous dissemination, forming cysts in the brain, ventricles, and subarachnoid space. Neurological manifestations of cysticercosis result from the mass effect of intraparenchymal cysts, obstruction of CSF flow by intraventricular cysts, or inflammation that causes basilar meningitis. They include seizures, headache, focal neurological signs, hydrocephalus, myelopathy, and subacute meningitis. Peripheral blood eosinophilia, soft tissue calcifications on x-ray, or the presence of parasites in the stool suggests the diagnosis. The CSF typically shows a lymphocytic pleocytosis

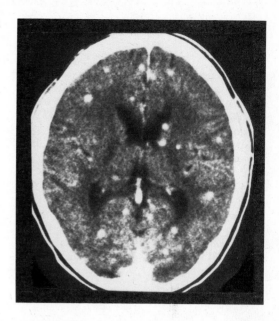

Figure 1–10. Contrast-enhanced CT scan in cerebral cysticercosis. Note the multiple bilateral, small, rounded areas of high density, which represent intraparenchymal cysts. (Courtesy of A Gean.)

(< 100 cells/μL), with eosinophils usually but not always present. Opening pressure is often increased but may be decreased with spinal subarachnoid block. Protein is increased to 50–100 mg/dL, and glucose is 20–50 mg/dL in most cases. Complement fixation and hemagglutination studies can assist in the diagnosis. The CT scan (Figure 1–10) may show contrast-enhanced mass lesions with surrounding edema, intracerebral calcifications, or ventricular enlargement. Myelography should be performed in suspected spinal subarachnoid block.

The indications for treatment of cerebral cysticercosis are controversial. However, patients with symptomatic neurological involvement (usually seizures) and either meningitis or one or more noncalcified intraparenchymal cysts should probably receive praziquantel, 50 mg/kg/d in three divided doses, for 14 days, or albendazole, 15 mg/kg/d in three divided doses, for 30 days. Patients with seizures should also receive anticonvulsants. Corticosteroids are indicated for increased intracranial pressure or lesions near the cerebral aqueduct or intraventricular foramina; these may progress to cause obstructive hydrocephalus. Single accessible intraparenchymal lesions can be removed surgically, and shunting is required for intraventricular lesions causing hydrocephalus, which are unlikely to respond to drugs.

6. *ANGIOSTRONGYLUS CANTONENSIS* MENINGITIS

Angiostrongylus cantonensis is endemic to Southeast Asia and to Hawaii and other Pacific islands. Infection is transmitted by ingestion of infected raw mollusks and produces meningitis with CSF eosinophilia (Table 1–22). Most patients complain of headache, and about half report stiff neck, vomiting, fever, and paresthesias. Most patients have a CSF leukocytosis of 150–1500/μL, mild elevation of protein, and normal glucose. The acute illness usually resolves spontaneously in one to two weeks, although paresthesias may persist longer.

Mebendazole, 100 mg orally twice daily for five doses, is an experimental drug for treating *Angiostrongylus* infections, but its efficacy is unproved in humans. Analgesics, corticosteroids, and reduction of CSF pressure by repeated lumbar punctures may be of value.

7. ROCKY MOUNTAIN SPOTTED FEVER

Rocky Mountain spotted fever is caused by *Rickettsia rickettsii*, an intracellular parasite transmitted to humans by tick bites. *R rickettsii* damages endothelial cells, leading to vasculitis, microinfarcts, and petechial hemorrhage. Initial symptoms include fever, headache, and a characteristic rash that involves the palms and soles and spreads centrally. Neurological involvement, which is uncommon, produces a confusional state and, less often, coma or focal neurological abnormalities. The CSF is normal or shows a mild mononuclear pleocytosis. Treatment is with tetracycline, 25–50 mg/kg/d orally, or chloramphenicol, 50 mg/kg/d orally, in four daily doses. Neurological residua are rare and mortality is less than 5%.

Table 1–22. Causes of cerebrospinal fluid eosinophilia.

Common causes
  Taenia solium (cysticercosis)
  Angiostrongylus cantonensis (eosinophilic meningitis)
Uncommon causes
  Other helminthic infections
  Coccidioides immitis meningitis
  Hematologic malignancies with meningeal infiltration
  Foreign matter (including myelography dye) in subarachnoid space
Possible causes (less well documented)
  Neurosyphilis
  Tuberculous meningitis
  Nonhematologic malignancies with meningeal infiltration
  Lymphocytic choriomeningitis
  Polyarteritis nodosa
  Allergic reactions

NEOPLASTIC MENINGITIS

Diffuse metastatic seeding of the leptomeninges may complicate systemic cancers (especially carcinoma of the breast or lung, lymphoma, melanoma, and acute lymphocytic leukemia), producing neurological syndromes with prominent cognitive dysfunction. Primary brain tumors may be associated with meningeal gliomatosis, and medulloblastomas and pineal tumors have a particular propensity for meningeal dissemination.

Neoplastic meningitis usually occurs from three months to five years after the diagnosis of cancer. It may, however, be the presenting manifestation of the cancer, or it may occur only after many years of illness—sometimes in apparently cured patients. Its most frequent symptoms are headache and cognitive disorders, including lethargy, confusion, and memory impairment. Nausea, vomiting, seizures, and gait abnormalities are also common.

Clinical Findings

A. Symptoms and Signs: Abnormal neurological signs are often more striking than the symptoms and usually suggest involvement at multiple levels of the neuraxis. Cognitive dysfunction may take the form of confusion, lethargy, or dementia. Cranial nerve abnormalities most often affect the optic (II), oculomotor (III), trochlear (IV), abducens (VI), facial (VII), and acoustic (VIII) nerves. Other common findings include focal weakness, isolated or asymmetrical areflexia, extensor plantar responses, focal sensory loss, gait disorders, and dysarthria. Signs of meningeal irritation, however, are frequently absent.

B. Laboratory Findings: The most useful diagnostic procedure is lumbar puncture, which may show increased opening pressure, pleocytosis and elevated protein, and markedly decreased or even immeasurably low glucose. Neoplastic meningitis is diagnosed by finding malignant cells in the CSF; large volumes of fluid and repeated lumbar punctures increase the yield of cytological studies. The diagnosis should not be abandoned because of one or two negative cytological tests. CSF β_2-microglobulin can be a useful marker for leptomeningeal leukemia and lymphoma, and elevated β-glucuronidase and carcinoembryonic antigen may aid the diagnosis of carcinomatous meningitis from melanoma or lung or breast carcinoma. Where clinically indicated, a CT brain scan, an MRI or a metrizamide CT study of the spine, or myelography is performed to exclude the possibility of intraparenchymal metastasis or spinal cord compression by epidural metastasis.

Differential Diagnosis

Neoplastic meningitis can simulate infectious meningitis, metabolic encephalopathy, intraparenchymal or spinal epidural metastasis, remote effects of carcinoma, or chemotherapeutic drug toxicity and may coexist with any of these conditions. CSF cytological tests and cultures, blood studies, and appropriate radiological investigations may be required to distinguish among these possibilities.

Treatment & Prognosis

Treatment of neoplastic meningitis involves irradiation of symptomatic regions of the neuraxis and, in some cases, intrathecal chemotherapy. Treatment frequently leads to symptomatic improvement; it can also enhance the quality of life and prolong survival by several months. The prognosis is best in patients with leptomeningeal metastasis from lymphoma or carcinoma of the breast.

VASCULAR DISORDERS

HYPERTENSIVE ENCEPHALOPATHY

A sudden increase in blood pressure, with or without preexisting chronic hypertension, may result in encephalopathy and headache, which develop over a period of several hours to days. Vomiting, visual disturbances, focal neurological deficits, and focal or generalized seizures can also occur. Blood pressure in excess of 250/150 mm Hg is usually required to precipitate the syndrome in patients with chronic hypertension, while previously normotensive patients may be affected at lower pressures. Coexisting renal failure appears to increase the risk of hypertensive encephalopathy.

Cerebrovascular spasm, impaired autoregulation of cerebral blood flow, and intravascular coagulation have all been proposed as causes. These processes can lead to small infarcts and petechial hemorrhages that affect the brain stem most prominently and other subcortical gray and white matter regions to a lesser extent. Cerebral edema appears unlikely as an important pathogenetic factor in hypertensive encephalopathy.

Clinical Findings

A. Symptoms and Signs: The physical findings most useful in confirming the diagnosis are those seen on ophthalmoscopy. Retinal arteriolar spasm is almost invariably present. Papilledema, retinal hemorrhages, and exudates are usually present.

B. Laboratory Findings: Lumbar puncture may show normal or elevated CSF pressure and protein. Low-density areas in white matter have been seen on CT scan. Blood studies are important to determine whether uremia is present, since hypertensive encephalopathy and uremia can occur together.

Differential Diagnosis

Hypertensive encephalopathy is a diagnosis of exclusion. Stroke and subarachnoid hemorrhage also produce encephalopathy with acutely elevated blood pressure, and when focal neurological abnormalities are present, stroke is by far the most likely diagnosis. Elevated blood pressure, headache, papilledema, and altered consciousness are also seen with intracranial hemorrhage; where this is a consideration, it can be excluded by CT scan or MRI.

Prevention

Hypertensive encephalopathy is best prevented by early treatment of uncomplicated hypertension and by prompt recognition of elevated blood pressure in settings—such as acute glomerulonephritis or eclampsia—in which it tends to occur in previously normotensive patients.

Treatment

The diagnosis of hypertensive encephalopathy is established when it is shown that rapid resolution of symptoms occurs when the blood pressure is lowered. This is accomplished by administration of sodium nitroprusside by continuous intravenous infusion, beginning at a rate of 0.5 µg/kg/min, which is increased to as much as 3–10 µg/kg/min as required. Alternative approaches include diazoxide, 50–100 mg by intravenous bolus every 5–10 minutes (to a maximum of 600 mg) or 10–30 mg/min by constant intravenous infusion, or labetalol, 20–80 mg by intravenous bolus every 5-10 minutes (to a maximum of 600 mg) or 0.5–2 mg/min by constant intravenous infusion. The patient must be carefully monitored and the infusion rate adjusted to maintain a therapeutic effect *without producing hypotension.* In the first hour of treatment, mean arterial blood pressure should be reduced by no more than 20–25% and diastolic pressure should not be allowed to fall below 100 mm Hg. Treatment should be terminated immediately if neurological function worsens.

Prognosis

Untreated hypertensive encephalopathy can result in stroke, coma, and death. Prompt treatment is usually associated with full clinical recovery.

SUBARACHNOID HEMORRHAGE

Subarachnoid hemorrhage must receive early consideration in the differential diagnosis of an acute confusional state. This disorder is discussed in Chapter 3.

VERTEBROBASILAR ISCHEMIA

Transient ischemia or stroke in the distribution of the posterior cerebral circulation can produce an acute confusional state. Vertebrobasilar ischemia is discussed in Chapter 9.

RIGHT (NONDOMINANT) HEMISPHERIC INFARCTION

Agitated confusional states with sudden onset can result from infarction (usually embolic) in the areas served by the inferior division of the nondominant (usually right) middle cerebral artery. If the superior division is spared, there is no hemiparesis. The agitation is often so pronounced as to suggest the diagnosis of an alcohol withdrawal syndrome; autonomic hyperactivity is not present, however. The diagnosis is suggested by the sudden (strokelike) onset of an agitated confusional state and confirmed by CT brain scan or MRI. Rarely, isolated anterior cerebral artery infarcts or posterior cerebral artery infarcts cause acute confusion.

SYSTEMIC LUPUS ERYTHEMATOSUS

Among the disorders associated with systemic vasculitis, systemic lupus erythematosus (SLE) is the most common cause of encephalopathy. SLE is nine times more common in women than in men and usually has its onset between the ages of 10 and 40 years. Neurological involvement is reported in 37–75% of patients. The clinical features that correlate best with nervous system involvement are active mucocutaneous or visceral vasculitis and thrombocytopenia, but clinically active systemic disease need not be present for neurological symptoms to occur.

Neuropathologic findings in patients who die with SLE involving the central nervous system include fibrinoid degeneration of arterioles and capillaries, microinfarcts, and intracerebral hemorrhages. True vasculitis affecting cerebral blood vessels is rare.

Clinical Findings

A. Symptoms and Signs: The most common neurological features are seizures and an altered mental status. Disorders of cognitive function may take the form of a quiet confusional state, agitated delirium, or schizophreniform psychosis with hallucinations, paranoia, or autistic behavior. Alternatively, patients may present with affective disorders characterized by depression or mania. Seizures are usually generalized but may be focal. Less common neurological manifestations include visual impairment, ptosis, diplopia, focal weakness (hemiparesis or paraparesis), tremor, chorea, cerebellar ataxia, and polyneuropathy.

B. Laboratory Findings: Although a variety of laboratory abnormalities can be found in SLE with or without neurological involvement, no laboratory finding is diagnostic of nervous system involvement. The CSF shows mild elevation of protein or a modest—usually mononuclear—pleocytosis in about one-third of cases. The EEG frequently shows diffuse slowing or focal abnormalities. Antibodies to ribosomal P proteins have been reported in serum from patients with lupus psychosis.

Differential Diagnosis

Even in patients with known SLE, encephalopathy can be caused by a variety of factors other than cerebral lupus per se. Coagulopathy, concurrent infection, uremia from nephritis, and multiple emboli related to endocarditis must be excluded. A common dilemma is the need to distinguish cerebral lupus from steroid-induced psychosis in patients receiving corticosteroid therapy. Cerebral lupus is by far the more frequent problem, particularly in patients receiving low or tapering doses of steroids.

Treatment

Cerebral lupus is treated with corticosteroids, which are begun at a dosage equivalent to 60 mg/d of prednisone or increased by 5–10 mg of prednisone per day in patients already receiving steroids. Dosages as high as 2 mg/kg/d may be required. After symptoms resolve, steroids should be tapered to a low maintenance dose. Seizures are treated with anticonvulsants.

Prognosis

Neurological symptoms caused by SLE improve in more than 80% of the patients treated with corticosteroids. Symptoms may also resolve without treatment, however, and cerebral involvement has not been shown to adversely affect the overall prognosis.

DISSEMINATED INTRAVASCULAR COAGULATION

Disseminated intravascular coagulation (DIC) results from pathological activation of the coagulation and fibrinolytic systems, usually in the setting of a severe underlying systemic disease. The principal manifestation is hemorrhage. Neurological symptoms are common and may precede the abnormalities that provide a definitive hematological diagnosis (see below).

DIC tends to occur at the extremes of age, but patients of any age can be affected. The syndrome is most often seen as a complication of severe systemic illness. Common findings in the brain include small multifocal infarctions and petechial hemorrhages involving both gray and white matter. Subdural hematoma, subarachnoid hemorrhage, and hemorrhagic infarction in the distribution of large vessels may occur.

Clinical Findings

Systemic symptoms of DIC most often relate to hemorrhage. Bleeding can affect the skin, mucous membranes, or gastrointestinal or genitourinary tract and can result in hypotension or oliguria. Neurological involvement is commonly manifested by a confusional state that takes the form of lethargy or agitated delirium and can progress to coma. Focal neurological signs and seizures also occur; the focal signs can be transient.

Definitive diagnosis of DIC requires evidence of disordered coagulation and fibrinolysis. The coagulation defect is associated with thrombocytopenia and usually with prolonged PT and PTT, although the latter tests may be normal. The most useful finding is decreased plasma fibrinogen. Accelerated fibrinolysis is documented by elevated serum fibrinogen-fibrin degradation products (FDP-fdp). Additional laboratory studies may show prolonged whole-blood clot formation, rapid clot lysis, and anemia with fragmented red blood cells.

Differential Diagnosis

Because neurological involvement in DIC most often presents as encephalopathy in a patient with a severe underlying disease, a variety of conditions related to the primary disorder must be excluded. These include metabolic encephalopathy, meningoencephalitis, metastatic involvement of the brain or meninges, or stroke caused by nonbacterial thrombotic (marantic) endocarditis. Thrombotic thrombocytopenic purpura (TTP) is distinguished by its tendency to occur in previously healthy patients and by its association with normal plasma fibrinogen and normal or only slightly elevated FDP-fdp.

Treatment

Treatment of DIC is directed at the underlying disease. Transfusion of red blood cells, platelets, and coagulation factors from fresh-frozen plasma may be indicated. Transfused platelets are often rapidly destroyed, however, and transfused coagulation factors may be converted to anticoagulant FDP-fdp and thus worsen the hemorrhagic tendency. Heparin has sometimes been advocated because of its ability to inhibit the coagulation cascade, but its utility is uncertain.

Prognosis

The prognosis is probably related to the severity of the underlying disease, which itself is the usual cause of death. Mild, unrecognized transient DIC probably occurs frequently in hospitalized patients who recover fully.

THROMBOTIC THROMBOCYTOPENIC PURPURA

Thrombotic thrombocytopenic purpura (TTP) is a rare multisystem disorder of unknown cause, classically defined by the clinical pentad of thrombocytopenic purpura, microangiopathic hemolytic anemia, neurological dysfunction, fever, and renal disease. Both injury to vascular endothelial cells and increased platelet aggregation have been proposed as primary pathogenetic mechanisms. The result in either case is platelet-fibrin thrombus formation leading to occlusion of small blood vessels, especially at arteriolar-capillary junctions. Pathological findings in the brain include disseminated microinfarctions and, less frequently, petechial hemorrhages that are present mainly in gray matter.

Clinical Findings

A. Symptoms and Signs: Patients most often present with such neurological symptoms as altered consciousness, headache, focal neurological signs, or seizures or with cutaneous hemorrhages in the form of purpura, ecchymoses, or petechiae. Other common symptoms include malaise, fatigue, generalized weakness, nausea, vomiting, diarrhea, fever, and abdominal pain. Bleeding from sites other than the skin may occur. The physical examination is most helpful in documenting the presence of fever, cutaneous hemorrhage, and neurological dysfunction.

TTP usually follows an acute, fulminant course but can be a chronic progressive or remitting and relapsing disorder lasting from months to years. Neurological symptoms in particular may be fleeting and recurrent. Recent studies report survival of about half the patients.

B. Laboratory Findings: Hematologic studies show a Coombs-negative hemolytic anemia with hemoglobin levels usually less than 10 g/dL, normochromic red blood cell indices, fragmented and misshapen erythrocytes, and often nucleated red cells. Platelet counts are less than 20,000/μL in about half the cases and less than 60,000/μL in almost all; the white blood cell count is normal or elevated. Coagulation studies are normal or slightly abnormal in most patients: PT and PTT are normal in about 90% of cases and fibrinogen is normal in 80%. Fibrinogen-fibrin degradation products (FDP-fdp) are normal in about half the cases and slightly elevated in one-fourth. Renal involvement may cause gross or microscopic hematuria, proteinuria, or azotemia. Spinal fluid is usually normal, though protein may be elevated. Antemortem pathological diagnosis may be made by gingival biopsy or splenectomy.

Differential Diagnosis

DIC is also associated with hemolytic anemia or thrombocytopenia. Idiopathic thrombocytopenic purpura (ITP) is not accompanied by microangiopathic hemolytic anemia or by evidence of multisystem disease. The hemolytic anemias of SLE, autoimmune hemolytic anemia (AIHA), and Evans syndrome (both ITP and AIHA) are Coombs-positive.

Treatment

Recommended therapy includes plasma exchange or fresh-frozen plasma, 2 units intravenously every six hours; aspirin, 325 mg/d orally; dipyridamole, 75 mg orally every six hours; and methylprednisolone, 1 mg/kg/d intravenously.

HEAD TRAUMA

Blunt head trauma can cause a confusional state or coma. Acceleration or deceleration forces and physical deformation of the skull can produce disruption of white matter by shearing forces; contusion from contact between the inner surface of the skull and the polar regions of the cerebral hemispheres; torn blood vessels; vasomotor changes; brain edema; and increased intracranial pressure.

CONCUSSION

Concussion is characterized by transient (lasting seconds to minutes) loss of consciousness without structural pathological features. Its pathophysiological mechanism is unknown. Unconsciousness is associated with normal pupillary and ocular reflexes, flaccidity, and extensor plantar responses. As consciousness returns, the patient is left with a confusional state that usually lasts from minutes to hours. A prominent feature of the posttraumatic confusional state is both retrograde and anterograde amnesia. These aspects are considered further in Chapter 2. Patients with simple concussion usually recover uneventfully, although the posttraumatic syndrome of headache, dizziness, or mild cognitive impairment may persist for weeks.

When unconsciousness is prolonged—or delayed in onset following a lucid interval—the possibility of posttraumatic intracranial hemorrhage should be considered. The presence of focal neurological abnormalities following concussion should arouse a similar concern.

INTRACRANIAL HEMORRHAGE

Traumatic intracranial hemorrhage can be epidural, subdural, or intracerebral in location. **Epidural hematoma** most often results from a lateral skull fracture that lacerates the middle meningeal artery or vein. Patients may or may not lose consciousness initially, but in either event a lucid interval of from several hours to one or two days is followed by the rapid evolution—over hours—of headache, progressive obtundation, hemiparesis, and finally ipsilateral pupillary dilatation from uncal herniation. Death may follow if treatment is delayed.

The course of **subdural hematoma** following head injury can be acute, subacute, or chronic, and in each case headache and altered consciousness are its principal manifestations. Delay in diagnosis and treatment may lead to a fatal outcome. In contrast to epidural hematoma, the time between trauma and the onset of symptoms is typically longer, the hemorrhage tends to be located over the cerebral convexities, and associated skull fractures are uncommon. Subdural hematoma in the posterior fossa is rare.

Intracerebral contusion (bruising) or **hemorrhage** related to head injury is usually located at the frontal or temporal poles. Because of the superficial location of traumatic intracerebral hemorrhage, blood typically enters the CSF, resulting in signs of meningeal irritation and—sometimes—hydrocephalus. As with epidural and subdural hematoma, focal neurological signs are usually absent or subtle.

The diagnosis of posttraumatic intracranial hemorrhage is made by CT scan. Epidural hematoma tends to appear as a biconvex, lens-shaped, extra-axial mass that may cross the midline or the tentorium, but not the cranial sutures. Subdural hematoma, in contrast, is typically crescent-shaped and may cross the cranial sutures, but not the midline or tentorium. The density relative to the adjacent brain is variable. Intracerebral hemorrhage or contusion is typically a radiodense collection that may be surrounded by an area of edema. Midline structures may be displaced contralaterally by the space-consuming hematoma.

Epidural and subdural hematomas are treated by surgical evacuation. The decision to use surgery to treat intracerebral hematoma depends upon the clinical course and location. Evacuation, decompression, or shunting for hydrocephalus may be indicated.

SEIZURES

POSTICTAL STATE

Generalized tonic-clonic (grand mal) seizures are typically followed by a transient confusional state (postictal state) that resolves within one to two hours. If there are no witnesses to the seizure itself, patients may present with a confusional state or agitated delirium with no apparent cause. Disturbances of recent memory and of attention are prominent.

When postictal coma and confusion do not clear rapidly, an explanation must be sought for the prolonged postictal state. This occurs in three settings: status epilepticus, an underlying structural brain abnormality (eg, stroke, tumor, intracranial hemorrhage), and an underlying diffuse cerebral disorder (eg, dementia, meningitis or encephalitis, metabolic encephalopathy).

Patients with an unexplained prolonged postictal state should be evaluated by means of blood chemistry studies, lumbar puncture, EEG, and (when indicated) CT scan.

COMPLEX PARTIAL SEIZURES

Complex partial (formerly called **temporal lobe** or **psychomotor**) seizures produce alterations in consciousness characterized by confusion alone or, more commonly, by cognitive, affective, psychomotor, or psychosensory symptoms. Complex partial seizures rarely cause diagnostic problems in the patient presenting with an acute confusional state, because spells are typically brief and stereotypical, psychomotor manifestations are often obvious to the observer, and patients themselves may describe classic cognitive, affective, or psychosensory symptoms (as discussed in Chapter 9).

Impaired consciousness in complex partial seizures takes the form of a confusional state that may be characterized by a withdrawn or unresponsive state or by agitated behavior. Automatisms such as staring, repetitive chewing, swallowing, lip-smacking, or picking at clothing are most helpful in suggesting the diagnosis of complex partial seizures in an apparently confused patient.

Complex partial status epilepticus, which is rare, lasts for hours to days. In some cases it results in bilateral hippocampal lesions with a postictal inability to acquire new memories, at least for several months. Periods of unresponsiveness, staring, and automatisms alternate with a twilight state characterized by confusion, amnesia, partial responsiveness, and semi-purposeful behavior.

An acute confusional state caused by complex partial seizures may need to be distinguished from the postictal state following generalized tonic-clonic seizures, metabolic encephalopathy, or acute psychosis. The EEG is useful in making the distinction.

PSYCHIATRIC DISORDERS

Symptoms similar to those associated with acute confusional states—incoherence, agitation, distractibility, hypervigilance, delusions, and hallucinations—can also be seen in a variety of psychiatric disorders. These include schizophrenia, delusional (paranoid) disorder, other psychotic disorders (brief reactive psychosis, schizophreniform disorder, schizoaffective disorder, atypical psychosis), mood (bipolar and depressive) disorders, anxiety disorders (posttraumatic stress disorder), and factitious disorder with psychological symptoms. Such diagnoses may be mistakenly assigned to patients with acute confusional states; conversely, patients with psychiatric disturbances may be thought—incorrectly—to have organic disease.

Unlike acute confusional states, psychiatric disorders are rarely acute in onset but typically develop over a period of at least several weeks. The history may reveal previous psychiatric disease or hospitalization or a precipitating psychological stress.

Physical examination may show abnormalities related to autonomic overactivity, including tachycardia, tachypnea, and hyperreflexia but no definitive signs of neurological dysfunction.

While the mental status examination in acute confusional states of metabolic origin is characterized by a fluctuating level of consciousness and disorientation, patients with psychiatric disorders tend to maintain a consistent degree of cognitive impairment and to be oriented to person, place, and time. Disorientation as to person, especially in the face of preserved orientation in other spheres, is virtually diagnostic of psychiatric disease. Patients with psychiatric disorders exhibit a normal level of consciousness, usually appearing awake and alert, and memory is intact. Disturbances in the content and form of thought (eg, persecutory delusions, delusions of reference, loosening of associations), perceptual abnormalities (eg, auditory hallucinations), and flat or inappropriate affect are common, however.

Routine laboratory studies are normal in acute functional psychosis; they should be performed in any case to exclude organic disorders. Initial treatment of functional psychoses or manic episodes consists of intramuscular administration of phenothiazines or butyrophenones. Psychiatric consultation should be sought concerning the long-term management of any psychiatric disorder.

REFERENCES

General

Plum F, Posner JB: *The Diagnosis of Stupor and Coma,* 3rd ed. Vol 19 of: *Contemporary Neurology Series.* Davis, 1980.

Strub RL, Black FW: *The Mental Status Examination in Neurology.* Davis, 1977.

Drug Intoxication & Withdrawal

Charness ME, Simon RP, Greenberg DA: Ethanol and the nervous system. *N Engl J Med* 1989;321:442–454.

Khantzian EJ, McKenna GJ: Acute toxic and withdrawal reactions associated with drug use and abuse. *Ann Intern Med* 1979;90:361–372.

Larson EB et al: Adverse drug reactions associated with global cognitive impairment in elderly persons. *Ann Intern Med* 1987;107:169–173.

Logan WJ: Neurological aspects of hallucinogenic drugs. Pages 47–78 in: *Current Reviews.* Vol 13 of: *Advances in Neurology.* Friedlander WJ (editor). Raven Press, 1975.

Lowenstein DH et al: Acute neurological and psychiatric complications associated with cocaine abuse. *Am J Med* 1987;83:841–846.

Pearlson GD: Psychiatric and medical syndromes associated with phencyclidine (PCP) abuse. *Johns Hopkins Med J* 1981;148:25–33.

Roy-Byrne PP, Hommer D: Benzodiazepine withdrawal: Overview and implications for the treatment of anxiety. *Am J Med* 1988;84:1041–1052.

Hypo- & Hyperglycemia

Guisado R, Arieff AI: Neurological manifestation of diabetic comas: Correlation with biochemical alterations in the brain. *Metabolism* 1975;24:665–679.

Malouf R, Brust JC: Hypoglycemia: Causes, neurological manifestations, and outcome. *Ann Neurol* 1985;17:421–430.

Hyponatremia

Brunner JE et al: Central pontine myelinolysis and pontine lesions after rapid correction of hyponatremia: A prospective magnetic resonance imaging study. *Ann Neurol* 1990;27:61–66.

Wernicke's Encephalopathy

Charness ME, Simon RP, Greenberg DA: Ethanol and the nervous system. *N Engl J Med* 1989;321:442–454.

Victor M, Adams RD, Collins GH: *The Wernicke-Korsakoff Syndrome.* Vol 30 of: *Contemporary Neurology Series.* Davis, 1989.

Vitamin B$_{12}$ Deficiency

Lindenbaum J et al: Neuropsychiatric disorders caused by cobalamin deficiency in the absence of anemia or macrocytosis. *N Engl J Med* 1988;318:1720–1728.

Uremia & Dialysis Disequilibrium

Fraser CL, Arieff AI: Nervous system complications in uremia. *Ann Intern Med* 1988;109:143–153.

Harris CP, Townsend JJ: Dialysis disequilibrium syndrome. *West J Med* 1989;151:52–55.

Raskin NH, Fishman RA: Neurological disorders in renal failure. (2 parts.) *N Engl J Med* 1976;294:143–148 and 204–210.

Bacterial Meningitis

Lukes SA et al: Bacterial infections of the CNS in neutropenic patients. *Neurology* 1984;34:269–275.

Tunkel AR, Wispelwey B, Scheld WM: Bacterial meningitis: Recent advances in pathophysiology and treatment. *Ann Intern Med* 1990;112:610–623.

Lyme Disease

Steere AC: Lyme disease. *N Engl J Med* 1989;321:586–596.

Viral Meningitis & Encephalitis

Whitley RJ: Viral encephalitis. *N Engl J Med* 1990;323:242–250.

Herpes Simplex Virus Encephalitis

Whitley RJ: Herpes simplex virus infections of the central nervous system: A review. *Am J Med* 1988;85(Suppl 2A):61–67.

AIDS

Chuck SL, Sande MA: Infections with cryptococcus neoformans in the acquired immunodeficiency syndrome. *N Engl J Med* 1989;321:794–799.

Glatt AE, Chirgwin K, Landesman SH: Treatment of infections associated with human immunodeficiency virus. *N Engl J Med* 1988;318:1439–1448.

McArthur JC: Neurological manifestations of AIDS. *Medicine* 1987;66:407–437.

Remick SC et al: Primary central nervous system lymphoma in patients with and without the acquired immune deficiency syndrome: A retrospective analysis and review of the literature. *Medicine* 1990;69:345–360.

Rosenblum ML, Levy RM, Bredesen DE: *AIDS and the Nervous System.* Raven Press, 1988.

Tuberculous Meningitis

Ogawa SK et al: Tuberculous meningitis in an urban medical center. *Medicine* 1987;66:317–326.

Roberts FJ: Problems in the diagnosis of tuberculous meningitis. *Arch Neurol* 1981;38:319–320.

Syphilitic Meningitis

Jordan KG: Modern neurosyphilis: A critical analysis. *West J Med* 1988;149:47–57.

Musher DM, Hamill RJ, Baughn RE: Effect of human immunodeficiency virus (HIV) infection on the course of syphilis and on the response to treatment. *Ann Intern Med* 1990;113:872–881.

Simon RP: Neurosyphilis. *Arch Neurol* 1985;42:606–613.

Fungal Meningitis

Bozette SA et al: A placebo-controlled trial of maintenance therapy with fluconazole after treatment of cryptococcal meningitis in the acquired immunodeficiency syndrome. *N Engl J Med* 1991;324:580–584.

Drugs for treatment of fungal infections. *Med Lett* 1992;34:14–16.

Walsh TJ, Hier DB, Caplan LR: Fungal infections of the central nervous system: Comparative analysis of risk factors and clinical signs in 57 patients. *Neurology* 1985;35:1654–1657.

Parasitic Infections

Drugs for parasitic infections. *Med Lett Drugs Ther* 1992;34:17–26.

Nash TE, Neva FA: Recent advances in the diagnosis and treatment of cerebral cysticercosis. *N Engl J Med* 1984;311:1492–1495.

Navia BA et al: Cerebral toxoplasmosis complicating the acquired immune deficiency syndrome: Clinical and neuropathological findings in 27 patients. *Ann Neurol* 1986;19:224–238.

Salata RA, King CH, Mahmoud AAF: Parasitic infection of the central nervous system. Pages 643–672 in: *Neurology and General Medicine.* Aminoff MJ (editor). Churchill Livingstone, 1989.

Neoplastic Meningitis

Olson ME, Chernik NL, Posner JB: Infiltration of the leptomeninges by systemic cancer: A clinical and pathologic study. *Arch Neurol* 1974;30:122–137.

Hypertensive Encephalopathy

Calhoun DA, Oparil S: Treatment of hypertensive crisis. *N Engl J Med* 1990;323:1177–1183.

Systemic Lupus Erythematosus

Adelman DC, Saltiel E, Klinenberg JR: The neuropsychiatric manifestations of systemic lupus erythematosus: An overview. *Semin Arthritis Rheum* 1986;15:185–199.

O'Connor P: Diagnosis of central nervous system lupus. *Can J Neurol Sci* 1988;15:257–260.

Disseminated Intravascular Coagulation

Collins RC et al: Neurological manifestations of intravascular coagulation in patients with cancer: A clinicopathologic analysis of 12 cases. *Neurology* 1975;25:795–806.

Thrombotic Thrombocytopenic Purpura

Schmidt JL: Thrombotic thrombocytopenic purpura: Successful treatment unlocks etiologic secrets. *Mayo Clinic Proc* 1989;64:956–961.

Psychiatric Disorders

Anderson WH, Kuehnle JC: Diagnosis and early management of acute psychosis. *N Engl J Med* 1981;305:1128–1130.

2

Disorders of Cognitive Function: Dementia & Amnestic Syndromes

I. DEMENTIA

Dementia refers to an acquired, generalized, and often progressive impairment of cognitive function that affects the content, but not the level, of consciousness. Although its incidence increases with advancing age (it has been estimated to affect 5–20% of individuals over age 65), dementia is not an invariable accompaniment of aging. It reflects instead an underlying pathology that affects the cerebral cortex, its subcortical connections, or both.

Minor changes in neurological function, including alterations in memory and other cognitive spheres, are associated with normal aging (Table 2–1). Enlargement of ventricles and cerebral cortical sulci seen on CT or MRI scans (Figure 2–1) is also common with normal aging. These findings should not by themselves be considered indicative of dementia.

Table 2–1. Neurological changes in normal aging.

Cognitive
  Memory loss (benign senescent forgetfulness)
Neuro-ophthalmologic
  Small, sluggishly reactive pupils
  Impaired upgaze
  Impaired convergence
Motor
  Muscular atrophy (intrinsic hand and foot muscles)
  Increased muscle tone
  Flexion (stooped) posture
  Gait disorders (small-stepped or broad-based gait)
Sensory
  Impaired vision
  Impaired hearing
  Impaired taste
  Impaired olfaction
  Decreased vibration sense
Reflexes
  Primitive reflexes
  Absent abdominal reflexes
  Absent ankle jerks

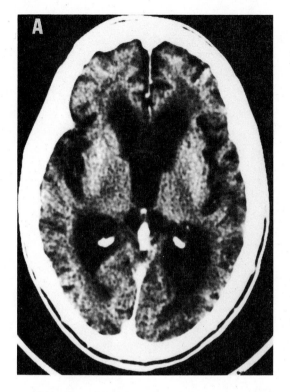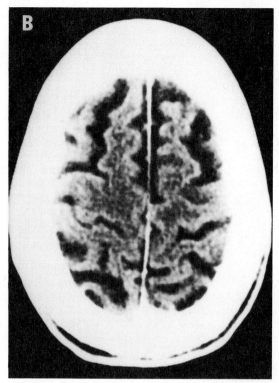

Figure 2–1. CT scan in cerebrocortical atrophy, showing ventricular dilation (A) and prominent cortical sulci (B).

The first step in evaluating a patient with a disorder of cognitive function is to classify the disorder as either a disturbance of the level of consciousness (wakefulness or arousal), such as an acute confusional state or coma, or a disturbance of the content of consciousness, in which wakefulness is preserved. The latter category includes both global cognitive disorders (dementia) and more circumscribed deficits, such as aphasia and amnestic syndromes. This distinction is important because the initial classification of the disorder determines the subsequent diagnostic approach. The most common problem in this area is distinguishing dementia from an acute confusional state, such as that produced by drug intoxication. The clinical features presented in Table 1–1 may be useful in making this distinction.

Another common problem is differentiating between dementia and so-called pseudodementia, such as that produced by depression. (The pseudodementia of depression is discussed later in this chapter.)

APPROACH TO DIAGNOSIS

The goal in clinical evaluation of patients with suspected dementia is to find a treatable cause. Although only about 10% of dementias are reversible, the possibility of reversing or arresting the disorder through appropriate treatment and dramatically improving the quality and duration of life justifies a thorough diagnostic investigation. A diagnosis is important in other cases for purposes of genetic counseling or for alerting family members and medical personnel to the risk of a transmissible disease.

The approach to diagnosis in patients with disorders of cognitive function, including dementia, is considered in detail in Chapter 1; it is reviewed here only briefly.

History

Since dementia implies deterioration in cognitive ability, it is important to establish that the patient's previous level of functioning has declined. Additional data can help to establish the cause of dementia, including the time course of deterioration; associated symptoms such as headache, gait disturbance, or incontinence; family history of a similar condition; concurrent medical illnesses that can produce dementia; the use of alcohol and prescribed or unprescribed drugs; and sexual preference.

General Physical Examination

The general physical examination can contribute to the etiological diagnosis when it reveals signs of a systemic disease responsible for the dementia. Particularly helpful signs are listed in Table 1–3.

Mental Status Examination

The mental status examination (see Chapter 1) helps to determine whether it is the level or the content of consciousness that is impaired and whether the cognitive dysfunction is global or circumscribed.

A disorder of the level of consciousness is suggested by sleepiness, inattention, impairment of immediate recall, or disorientation as to place or time. Abnormalities in these areas are unusual in dementia until the disorder is far advanced.

To determine the scope of the cognitive dysfunction (global or circumscribed), various spheres of cognition are tested in turn. These include memory, language, parietal lobe functions (pictorial construction, right-left discrimination, localization of objects in space), and frontal lobe or diffuse cerebral cortical functions (judgement, abstraction, thought content, the ability to perform previously learned acts). Multiple areas of cognitive function are impaired in dementia.

Neurological Examination

Certain disorders that produce dementia also affect vision, coordination, or motor or sensory function. Detecting such associated neurological abnormalities can help to establish an etiological diagnosis. Neurological signs suggesting causes of dementia are listed in Table 1–3.

Laboratory Investigations

Laboratory studies that can help to identify the cause of dementia are listed in Table 1–5.

DIFFERENTIAL DIAGNOSIS

Common Causes of Dementia

Although a wide variety of diseases can produce dementia (Table 2–2), it is generally agreed that Alzheimer's disease is by far the most common cause. Multi-infarct dementia is the next most common; other causes of dementia, including all reversible dementias, are comparatively rare.

Treatable Causes of Dementia

Treatable causes of dementia—such as normal pressure hydrocephalus, intracranial mass lesions, vitamin B_{12} deficiency, hypothyroidism, and neurosyphilis—are rare. They are the most important disorders to diagnose promptly, however, because treatment can arrest or reverse the intellectual decline.

Table 2–2. Causes of cognitive dysfunction in patients referred for evaluation of dementia.[1]

Cause	Percentage
Dementia	
Alzheimer's disease	57
Multi-infarct dementia	13
Alcohol-related	4
Normal pressure hydrocephalus	2
Metabolic[2]	2
Neoplasm	2
Parkinson's disease	1
Huntington's disease	1
Infection[3]	<1
Subdural hematoma	<1
Other	7
Pseudodementia	
Depression	5
Drug-induced encephalopathy	2
Other	4

[1]Data are from 32 clinical series published between 1966 and 1987, as compiled by Clarfield AM. The reversible dementias: Do they reverse? *Ann Intern Med* 1988;109:476.
[2]Includes hypothyroidism, vitamin B_{12} deficiency, and hepatocerebral degeneration.
[3]Includes neurosyphilis.

Other Important Causes of Dementia

Recognizing that the dementia is caused by Huntington's disease allows patients with this disorder (and their families) to benefit from genetic counseling. If Creutzfeldt-Jakob disease or AIDS dementia complex is diagnosed, precautions can be instituted against transmission; the course of AIDS dementia complex may also be modified by antiviral treatment. Progressive multifocal encephalopathy may indicate underlying immunosuppression that is due to human immunodeficiency virus (HIV) infection, lymphoma, leukemia, or another disorder.

Controversial Causes of Dementia

Some disorders to which dementia is often attributed may not directly cause the disorder. For example, the existence of a primary alcoholic dementia is questionable, since dementia in alcoholic patients may be the result of such related problems as head trauma or nutritional deficiency. Dementia in patients with Parkinson's disease sometimes represents coexisting Alzheimer's disease.

Pseudodementias

About 15% of patients referred for evaluation of possible dementia instead have other disorders (pseudodementias), such as depression. Drug intoxication, commonly cited as a cause of dementia in the elderly, actually produces an acute confusional state, rather than dementia.

IDIOPATHIC DEGENERATIONS

ALZHEIMER'S DISEASE

General Considerations

Alzheimer's disease, by far the single most common cause of dementia, becomes increasingly common with advancing age and has an equal incidence in both sexes. A slowly progressive disorder of unknown cause that cannot be diagnosed with certainty on clinical grounds, it is characterized by typical histopathological features: neurofibrillary tangles, neuritic plaques, and granulovacuolar degeneration. Pick's disease, a closely related dementing process in which atrophy is most conspicuous in the frontal and temporal lobes, may be clinically indistinguishable from Alzheimer's disease. Although a distinction was formerly made between presenile Alzheimer's disease and senile dementia of the Alzheimer type, these conditions appear to be clinically and pathologically identical.

Pathogenesis

A. Genetic: Alzheimer's disease usually occurs sporadically; it is genetically based in certain settings, however. These include both **trisomy 21 (Down's syndrome),** which is associated with a high incidence of Alzheimer's disease beginning in the fourth decade, and **familial Alzheimer's disease,** an autosomal dominant disorder. Although familial Alzheimer's disease is genetically heterogeneous, the gene defect has been localized to the amyloid precursor protein gene on chromosome 21 in some kindreds, and to a nearby site in other kindreds. It is not known whether the apparently sporadic cases of Alzheimer's disease also represent genetic disorders that are masked by incomplete penetrance or by the age-dependent nature of the disease.

B. Infectious: No infectious agent has been identified in Alzheimer's disease.

C. Toxic: A role has been proposed for aluminum toxicity in the pathogenesis of Alzheimer's disease. This is based on findings that the concentration of aluminum in the brain increases with age, and aluminum is present in the neurofibrillary tangles and neuritic plaques of brains from patients with Alzheimer's disease. In addition, aluminum-containing dialysates may be responsible for a dementia associated with chronic hemodialysis (see *Dialysis Dementia,* below). It is, however, unlikely that exposure to aluminum in antacids, drinking water, or cooking utensils increases the risk of developing Alzheimer's disease.

Endogenous excitotoxins, eg, the amino acid neurotransmitters glutamate and aspartate, may contribute to neuronal death in Alzheimer's disease, but this hypothesis is unproven.

D. Neurochemical: Changes in several neurotransmitter and neuromodulator systems have been found in the brains of patients dying of Alzheimer's disease; whatever the underlying cause of the disorder, these changes may contribute to its clinical expression. The acetylcholine-synthesizing enzyme **choline acetyltransferase** is markedly depleted in the cerebral cortex and hippocampus of patients with Alzheimer's disease. Degeneration of the nucleus basalis of Meynert (the principal origin of cortical cholinergic innervation) and of the cholinergic septal-hippocampal tract may underlie this abnormality. Several neurotransmitters (acetylcholine, somatostatin, vasopressin, β-endorphin, corticotropin, substance P) are depleted in the brains of patients with Alzheimer's disease, perhaps as a result of the selective loss of certain neuronal populations.

Clinical Findings

A. Early Manifestations: Impairment of recent memory is typically the first sign of Alzheimer's disease—often noticed only by family members. As the memory disorder progresses, the patient becomes disoriented to time and then to place. Aphasia, anomia, and acalculia may develop, forcing the patient to leave work or give up the management of family finances. The depression apparent in the earlier stages of the disorder may give way to an agitated, restless state. Apraxias and visuospatial disorientation ensue, causing the patient to become lost easily. Primitive reflexes (see Chapter 1) are commonly found. A frontal lobe gait disorder may become apparent, with short, slow, shuffling steps, flexed posture, wide base, and difficulty in initiating walking.

B. Late Manifestations: In the late stages, previously preserved social graces are lost, and psychiatric symptoms, including psychosis with paranoia, hallucinations, or delusions, may be prominent. Seizures occur in some cases. Examination at this stage may show extrapyramidal rigidity and bradykinesia. Rare and usually late features of the disease include myoclonus, incontinence, spasticity, extensor plantar responses, and hemiparesis. Mutism, incontinence, and a bedridden state are terminal manifestations, and death typically occurs from five to ten years after the onset of symptoms.

Investigative Studies

Laboratory investigations do not assist in the diagnosis—except to exclude other disorders. The CT scan or MRI often shows cortical atrophy and enlarged ventricles, but such changes may also be seen in elderly nondemented patients.

Differential Diagnosis

A. Early Dementia: Alzheimer's disease must be distinguished from depression and from such pure disorders of memory as the Korsakoff amnestic syndrome associated with chronic alcoholism.

B. More Advanced Dementia: Multi-infarct dementia and Creutzfeldt-Jakob disease must often be considered.

1. Multi-infarct dementia is suggested by a step-wise progression of deficits, pseudobulbar palsy, or focal sensorimotor abnormalities.

2. Creutzfeldt-Jakob disease is characterized by a shorter course than Alzheimer's disease (often leading to death within one year), prominent myoclonus, cerebellar dysfunction, more frequent pyramidal and extrapyramidal signs, visual disturbances, and a characteristic electroencephalographic pattern of periodic complexes.

Treatment

No treatment is currently available to reverse the existing deficits or arrest the disease's progression. Several pharmacological treatments have been proposed, including cerebral vasodilators (papaverine, dihydroergotoxine), central nervous system stimulants (amphetamines, pentylenetetrazol, procainamide), opioid antagonists (naloxone), and neuropeptides (vasopressin), but none has proved helpful. Because cholinergic neuronal pathways degenerate and choline acetyltransferase is depleted in the brains of patients with Alzheimer's disease, cholinergic replacement therapy might be of value. Experimental drugs that might be useful in this form of therapy include acetylcholine precursors (choline, lecithin), drugs that stimulate acetylcholine release (piracetam, 4-aminopyridine), acetylcholinesterase inhibitors (physostigmine, tacrine), and muscarinic cholinergic receptor agonists (arecholine). Some of these agents are under investigation, but none has yet been shown to be beneficial.

Prognosis

Early in the course of the disease, patients can usually remain at home and continue social, recreational, and limited professional activities. Early diagnosis can allow patients time to plan orderly retirement from work, to arrange for management of their finances, and to discuss with the physician and family members the management of future medical problems. Patients in advanced stages of the disease may require care in a nursing facility and the use of psychoactive medications. These patients must be protected and prevented from injuring themselves and their families by injudicious actions or decisions. Death from inanition or infection generally occurs five to ten years after the first symptoms.

HUNTINGTON'S DISEASE

Huntington's disease is an autosomal dominant heredodegenerative condition characterized by a movement disorder, psychiatric symptoms, and dementia.

Dementia, which usually becomes apparent after chorea and psychiatric symptoms have been present for a few years, precedes chorea in about one-fourth of cases. A memory disturbance affecting all aspects of memory is an early and prominent feature; aphasia, apraxia, agnosia, and global cognitive dysfunction tend to occur later. Huntington's disease is discussed further in Chapter 8.

PROGRESSIVE SUPRANUCLEAR PALSY

Progressive supranuclear palsy is an idiopathic degenerative disorder that primarily affects subcortical gray matter regions of the brain. The classic clinical features are supranuclear ophthalmoplegia, pseudobulbar palsy, axial dystonia with or without extrapyramidal rigidity of the limbs, and dementia. The disorder of movement is a conspicuous feature of this syndrome, which is discussed further in Chapter 8.

SPINOCEREBELLAR DEGENERATIONS

Many idiopathic degenerative disorders that affect the cerebellum and its connections can be associated with dementia. These include **Friedreich's ataxia** and other **spinocerebellar, cerebellar parenchymal,** and **cerebellar outflow tract degenerations.**

These disorders can be combined with extrapyramidal manifestations (**multiple systems atrophy**) or autonomic insufficiency (**Shy-Drager syndrome**). They can be sporadic or familial in occurrence. In the latter case, dementia may be present in family members otherwise unaffected by the disease. The distinguishing features of the spinocerebellar degenerations are discussed in Chapter 4.

Among the spinocerebellar degenerations, cognitive disorders are most often described in Friedreich's ataxia and include mental retardation, dementia, and psychiatric disturbances. (Most patients with Friedreich's ataxia, however, do not exhibit these abnormalities.) Dementia also occurs in a substantial fraction of patients with the Ramsay Hunt syndrome of myoclonic cerebellar dyssynergia. It is a less common feature of idiopathic spinocerebellar degenerations of adult onset.

VASCULAR DISORDERS

MULTI-INFARCT DEMENTIA

Multi-infarct dementia is second only to Alzheimer's disease as a cause of dementia. It can result from bilateral cortical infarctions in the distribution of major cerebral vessels or from widespread small (lacunar) infarcts (see Chapter 10) producing a **lacunar state.**

Patients with multi-infarct dementia typically have a history of hypertension, a stepwise progression of deficits, a more or less abrupt onset of dementia, and focal neurological symptoms or signs. Despite extensive pathological changes, they may remain functionally well compensated until a new and perhaps otherwise innocuous infarct tips the balance.

Clinical Findings

The neurological examination commonly shows pseudobulbar palsy with dysarthria, dysphagia, and pathological emotionality (**pseudobulbar affect**), focal motor and sensory deficits, ataxia, gait apraxia, hyperreflexia, and extensor plantar responses. Multi-infarct dementia may be associated with a memory disorder caused by bilateral infarction in the distribution of the posterior cerebral arteries, but aphasia, apraxia, and agnosia are uncommon.

Investigative Studies

The MRI (Figure 2–2) may show multiple small subcortical lucencies, though these are often too small to be seen. Extensive areas of low density in subcortical white matter are seen in **Binswanger's disease (subcortical arteriosclerotic encephalopa-**

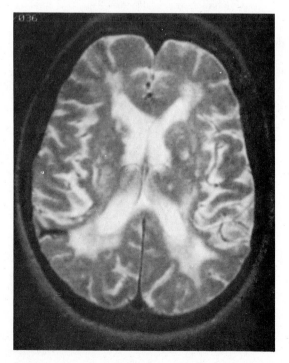

Figure 2–2. T2-weighted MRI in multi-infarct dementia, showing foci of abnormal high signal intensity adjacent to the lateral ventricles and within the basal ganglia.

thy), which may be a related condition. (MRI is more sensitive than CT for detecting these abnormalities.)

Additional laboratory studies should be performed to exclude cardiac emboli, polycythemia, thrombocytosis, cerebral vasculitis, and meningovascular syphilis as causes of multiple infarctions, particularly in younger patients or those without a history of hypertension.

Treatment

Hypertension, when present, should be treated to reduce the incidence of subsequent infarction and to prevent other end-organ diseases.

CHRONIC SUBDURAL HEMATOMA

Chronic subdural hematoma is the most readily treatable intracranial mass lesion causing dementia. Patients aged 50–70 years are most commonly affected. The most frequently identified precipitating factor is head trauma, which is often minor. Other factors that increase the risk of head trauma or the severity of the resulting hemorrhage include alcoholism, cerebral atrophy, epilepsy, the use of anticoagulants, ventricular shunts, and long-term hemodialysis. The onset of symptoms may be delayed for months, and medical attention may not be sought for some time after the symptoms are first noted. Hematomas are bilateral in about one-sixth of cases.

Clinical Findings

Headache is the initial symptom in most patients. Alterations in mental status, ranging from a confusional state to dementia, hemiparesis, and vomiting, may ensue. Cognitive dysfunction and hemiparesis are the most frequent findings, followed by papilledema and extensor plantar responses. Although aphasia, visual field defects, and seizures are uncommon, they can occur.

Investigative Studies

The hematoma can usually be seen on CT scan (Figure 2–3) as an extra-axial crescent-shaped area of decreased density, with ipsilateral obliteration of cortical sulci and often ventricular compression. The scan should be carefully reviewed for evidence of bilateral subdural collections. Isodense collections may become more apparent after contrast infusion. In a few cases, demonstration of the hematoma may require cerebral arteriography, which should always be undertaken bilaterally.

Treatment

Unless contraindicated by medical problems or evidence of spontaneous improvement, symptomatic hematomas should be surgically evacuated.

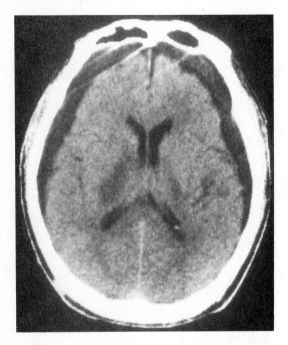

Figure 2–3. CT scan in chronic subdural hematoma, showing bilateral low-density collections between the inner table of the skull and the cerebral hemispheres.

NORMAL-PRESSURE HYDROCEPHALUS

Normal-pressure hydrocephalus, a potentially reversible cause of dementia, is characterized by the clinical triad of dementia, gait apraxia, and incontinence. It may be idiopathic or secondary to conditions that interfere with cerebrospinal fluid absorption, such as meningitis or subarachnoid hemorrhage. The dementia is often mild and insidious in onset. It is characterized initially by mental slowness and apathy and subsequently by global cognitive dysfunction. Deterioration of memory is common, but focal cognitive disorders such as aphasia and agnosia are rare.

Pathophysiology

Normal-pressure hydrocephalus is sometimes called **communicating** (because the ventricles remain in communication) or **nonobstructive hydrocephalus** (because the flow of CSF between the ventricles is not obstructed). It is presumed to be due to impaired CSF absorption from arachnoid granulations in the subarachnoid space over the convexity of the hemispheres (Figure 2–4), eg, from meningeal fibrosis and adhesions following meningitis or subarachnoid hemorrhage. In contrast, **noncommunicating** or **obstructive hydrocephalus** is caused by a blockade of CSF circulation *within* the ventricular system (eg, by an intraventricular cyst or tumor) and is associated with increased CSF pressure and often with headache and papilledema.

Clinical Findings

Normal-pressure hydrocephalus usually develops over a period of weeks to months; a gait disorder is often the initial manifestation. This typically takes the form of **gait apraxia,** characterized by unsteadiness on standing and difficulty in initiating walking even though there is no weakness or ataxia. The patient can perform the leg movements associated with walking, bicycling, or kicking a ball and can trace figures with the feet while lying or sitting but is unable to do so when the legs are bearing weight. The patient typically appears to be glued to the floor, and walking, once under way, is slow and shuffling. Pyramidal signs, including spasticity, hyperreflexia, and extensor plantar responses, are sometimes present. Motor perseveration (the inappropriate repetition of motor activity) and grasp reflexes in the hands and feet may occur. Urinary incontinence is a later development, and patients may be unaware of it; fecal incontinence is uncommon.

Investigative Studies

Lumbar puncture reveals normal or low opening pressure. The CT scan or MRI typically shows enlarged lateral ventricles without increased prominence of cortical sulci (Figure 2–5) and is the most useful investigative procedure in predicting the response to treatment. Radionuclide cisternography classically shows isotope accumulation in the ventricles, delayed clearance, and failure of ascent over the cerebral convexities. This pattern is not necessarily present in patients who respond to shunting, however.

Differential Diagnosis

A variety of conditions that produce dementia must be considered in the differential diagnosis. Alzheimer's disease tends to follow a longer course, often with prominent focal cortical dysfunction and enlarged cortical sulci shown in a CT scan or MRI. Parkinsonism may be simulated by the gait disorder but can be distinguished by extrapyramidal rigidity, tremor, and response to antiparkinsonian medications. Multi-infarct dementia should be suspected if the disorder follows a stepwise course, or pseudobulbar palsy, focal sensorimotor signs, or a history of stroke are encountered.

Treatment

Some patients, especially those with hydrocephalus from meningitis or subarachnoid hemorrhage, re-

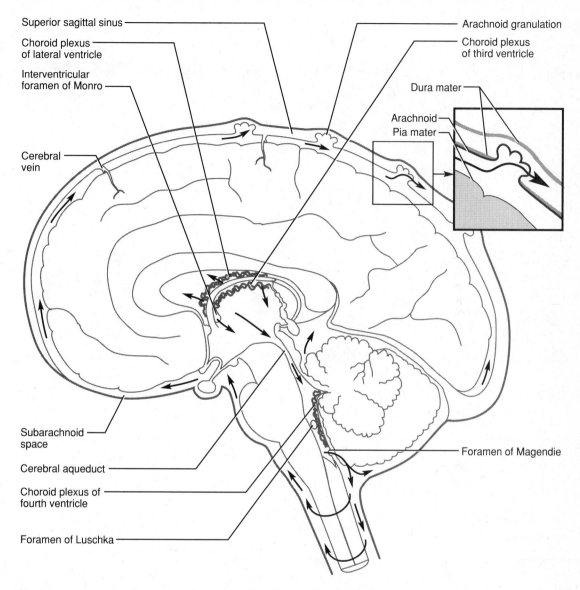

Figure 2–4. Circulation of cerebrospinal fluid (CSF). CSF is produced by the choroid plexus, which consists of specialized secretory tissue located within the cerebral ventricles. It flows from the lateral and third ventricles through the cerebral aqueduct and fourth ventricle and exits the ventricular system through two laterally situated foramina of Luschka and a single, medially located formen of Magendie. CSF then enters and circulates through the subarachnoid space surrounding the brain and spinal cord. It is ultimately absorbed through arachnoid granulations into the venous circulation.

cover or improve following ventriculoatrial, ventriculoperitoneal or lumboperitoneal shunting. In idiopathic normal-pressure hydrocephalus, about one-half of patients have sustained improvement, and about one-third have a good or excellent response (ie return to work) after shunting (Table 2–3). Predictors of a favorable response to shunting are arguable, but they probably include prominent gait disorder, ventricular enlargement without cortical atrophy on CT scan or MRI, and perhaps also transient gait improvement following lumbar puncture (see Table 2–4). Complications of shunting occur in about one-third of patients and include shunt infection, subdural hematoma, and shunt malfunction that necessitates replacement.

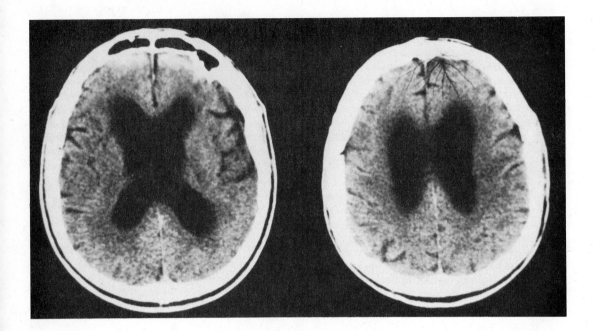

Figure 2–5. CT scan (at two levels) in normal pressure hydrocephalus, showing enlarged lateral ventricles without enlargement of the cortical sulci.

NEOPLASTIC DISEASES

BRAIN TUMOR

Cognitive dysfunction is a common presenting manifestation of brain tumor. Brain tumors produce dementia and related syndromes by a combination of local and diffuse effects, including edema, compression of adjacent brain structures, increased intracranial pressure, and impairment of cerebral blood flow. The tumors most likely to produce generalized cerebral syndromes are gliomas arising in the frontal or temporal lobes or the corpus callosum. Although such lesions tend to infiltrate subcortical white matter extensively, they initially give rise to few focal neurological signs.

Clinical Findings

The dementia associated with brain tumor is characterized by prominent mental slowness, apathy, impaired concentration, and subtle alterations in personality. Depending on the areas of involvement, memory disorder, aphasia, or agnosia may be seen early. Brain tumors ultimately produce headache, seizures, or focal sensorimotor disturbances, often after cognitive disturbances have been present for weeks or months and have been attributed to depression or aging.

Investigative Studies

Tumors and associated edema are best seen with CT scan or MRI, which may suggest the nature of the tumor. If the CT or MRI picture is not sufficiently characteristic to suggest appropriate therapy, brain biopsy may be required for diagnosis. If a metastatic lesion is suspected, screening, with careful examination of the skin and breasts, chest x-ray, stool test for occult blood, and urinalysis, should be undertaken to detect a primary site of occult systemic malignant disease.

Treatment & Prognosis

Treatment of brain tumor consists of surgical excision of benign neoplasms, such as meningioma, and sometimes of solitary metastases. Malignant tumors are treated with cranial irradiation, and corticosteroids are given to treat the associated brain edema. Chemotherapeutic regimens for primary brain tumors are under investigation, but thus far none have been clearly shown to improve results in patients receiving irradiation and steroids.

Primary supratentorial malignant brain tumors eventually cause death from brain herniation; death

Table 2–3. Outcome of CSF shunting for idiopathic normal-pressure hydrocephalus at 3 months.[1]

Outcome	Percentage
Improvement	
Excellent	8
Good	25
Fair	19
Transient	11
No improvement	
Unchanged	27
Worsened	3
Died	6
Complications	
Subdural hematoma	28
Seizure	8
Shunt infection	3

[1]Data from Black PMcL: CSF shunts for dementia, incontinence, and gait disturbance. *Clin Neurosurg* 1985;32:632.

in patients with metastatic brain tumor is usually related to the extracerebral disease.

NEOPLASTIC MENINGITIS

Neoplastic meningitis, discussed in Chapter 1 as a cause of confusional states, may also produce dementia that is commonly associated with headache as well as symptoms and signs of dysfunction at multiple sites in the nervous system. The diagnosis is established by cytological studies of the CSF, and irradiation of involved areas of the nervous system is the mainstay of therapy.

Table 2–4. Predictors of improvement after CSF shunting for idiopathic normal-pressure hydrocephalus.[1]

Predictor	Percentage Improved[2]
Clinical pattern	
Gait disorder, dementia, incontinence	69
Gait disorder and dementia	67
Gait disorder and incontinence	71
Gait disorder alone	50
Dementia alone	0
Primary disturbance	
Gait disorder	77
Dementia or incontinence	42
CT scan	
Only ventricles enlarged	81
Ventricles and cortical sulci enlarged	58
Radionuclide cisternography	
Abnormal	71
Normal	67

[1]Data from Black PMcL: CSF shunts for dementia, incontinence, and gait disturbance. *Clin Neurosurg* 1985;32:632.
[2]Includes excellent, good, fair, and transient improvement.

CENTRAL NERVOUS SYSTEM INFECTIONS

NEUROSYPHILIS

Neurosyphilis, a rare cause of dementia and organic psychosis since the widespread use of penicillin, is reemerging as an important problem in HIV-infected patients. **Parenchymatous neurosyphilis** produces the syndromes of general paresis and tabes dorsalis, which can occur both together and in association with optic atrophy.

Clinical Findings

A. General Paresis: The usual cause of dementia and psychiatric disorders related to neurosyphilis, general paresis was responsible for about 20% of cases of symptomatic neurosyphilis in the pre-penicillin era. It developed in about 5% of patients with untreated syphilis, most commonly 10–15 years after the primary infection. A chronic meningoencephalitis caused by active spirochetal infection, its onset may be characterized by gradual deterioration of memory or alterations in affect, personality, or behavior. Global intellectual deterioration ensues, and grandiosity, depression, psychosis, and focal weakness may be prominent features of the clinical picture. The terminal stages can include incontinence, frequent seizures, or recurrent strokes. Neurological examination may show tremors of the face and tongue, paucity of facial expressions, dysarthria, and pyramidal signs.

B. Taboparesis: Where tabes dorsalis (see Chapter 7) coexists with general paresis (taboparesis), signs and symptoms include Argyll Robertson pupils (see Chapter 5), lancinating pains, areflexia, posterior column sensory deficits with sensory ataxia and Romberg's sign, incontinence, impotence, Charcot (hypertrophic) joints, and genu recurvatum (hyperextended knees). Optic atrophy may also be present.

Investigative Studies

Serological studies are essential for diagnosis. Treponemal blood tests (FTA-ABS or MHA-TP) are reactive in almost all patients with active neurosyphilis, but nontreponemal blood tests (VDRL or RPR) can be negative. A treponemal blood test should therefore be obtained in all suspected cases. If this is nonreactive, neurosyphilis is effectively excluded; if it is reactive, lumbar puncture should be performed to confirm the diagnosis of neurosyphilis and to provide a baseline CSF profile against which to gauge the efficacy of future treatment. The CSF in active neurosyphilis always shows a lymphocytic pleocytosis and reactive nontreponemal CSF serology; CSF protein elevation, increased gamma globulin, and oligoclonal bands may also be present.

Treatment

Neurosyphilis is treated with a ten-day course of aqueous penicillin G, $2–4 \times 10^6$ units intravenously every four hours. Tetracycline or erythromycin can be used for patients allergic to penicillin. Fever and leukocytosis may occur shortly after therapy is started (**Herxheimer's reaction**) but are transient. Failure of the CSF to return to normal within six months requires retreatment.

Prognosis

After penicillin (or other antibiotic) treatment for general paresis, the clinical condition may improve or stabilize; in some cases it continues to deteriorate. Patients with persistent CSF abnormalities or symptomatic progression despite therapy should be retreated. Patients with reactive CSF serological tests but no pleocytosis are unlikely to respond to penicillin therapy but are usually treated nevertheless.

CREUTZFELDT-JAKOB DISEASE

Creutzfeldt-Jakob disease is an invariably fatal transmissible disorder of the central nervous system and is characterized by rapidly progressive dementia and variable focal involvement of the cerebral cortex, basal ganglia, cerebellum, brain stem, and spinal cord. A proteinaceous infectious particle (**prion**) has been proposed as the etiological agent, and prion proteins can be demonstrated by immunohistological methods in the brains of patients with Creutzfeldt-Jakob disease. Prions have also been implicated in two other rare dementing disorders—**kuru,** a disease of Fore-speaking tribes of New Guinea (apparently spread by cannibalism), and **Gerstmann-Straussler syndrome,** a familial disorder characterized by dementia and ataxia. Creutzfeldt-Jakob disease may have an incubation period of decades; the route of infection is unknown.

While transmission from humans to animals has been demonstrated experimentally, documented human-to-human transmission (by corneal transplantation, cortical electrode implantation, or administration of human growth hormone) is rare. The infectious agent is present in the CSF of humans and in the blood of experimental animals but not in nasopharyngeal secretions, semen, urine, or feces. Conjugal cases are rare and do not necessarily imply spouse-to-spouse transmission.

The annual incidence of Creutzfeldt-Jakob disease is about 1:1,000,000 population. The naturally acquired disease occurs in patients 20–80 years of age, with a peak incidence between 50 and 75 years and an equal sex incidence. More than one member of a family is affected in 4–8% of cases.

Clinical Findings

The clinical picture may be that of a diffuse central nervous system disorder or of a more localized dysfunction (Table 2–5). Dementia is present in virtually all cases and may begin as a mild global cognitive impairment or a focal cortical disorder such as aphasia, apraxia, or agnosia. Progression to akinetic mutism or coma typically ensues over a period of months. Psychiatric symptoms including anxiety, euphoria, depression, labile affect, delusions, hallucinations, and changes in personality or behavior may be prominent.

Aside from cognitive abnormalities, the most frequent clinical manifestations are myoclonus (often induced by a startle), extrapyramidal signs (rigidity, bradykinesia, tremor, dystonia, chorea, or athetosis), cerebellar signs, and extrapyramidal signs. Visual field defects, cranial nerve palsies, and seizures occur less often.

Investigative Studies

The most helpful noninvasive laboratory test is the EEG (Figure 2–6), which may show a typical but nonspecific pattern of periodic sharp waves or spikes. CSF protein may be mildly elevated (<100 mg/dL). Definitive diagnosis is by brain biopsy.

Differential Diagnosis

A variety of other disorders must be distinguished from Creutzfeld-Jakob disease. Alzheimer's disease is often a consideration, especially in patients with a less fulminant course and a paucity of cerebellar and extrapyramidal signs. Where subcortical involvement is prominent, Parkinson's disease, cerebellar degeneration, or progressive supranuclear palsy may be suspected. Striking focal signs raise the possibility of an intracerebral mass lesion. Acute metabolic disor-

Table 2–5. Clinical features of Creutzfeldt-Jakob Disease.[1]

Cortical	
Dementia	96%
Behavioral abnormalities	49%
Other	47%
Motor	
Myoclonus	88%
Extrapyramidal signs	67%
Cerebellar disorder	61%
Pyramidal signs	43%
Lower motor neuron signs	11%
Sensory	
Visual disturbances	31%
Cranial nerve palsy	16%
EEG	
Periodic complexes	80%

[1]After Brown P et al: Creutzfeldt-Jakob disease: Clinical analysis of a consecutive series of 230 neuropathologically verified cases. *Ann Neurol* 1986;20:597.

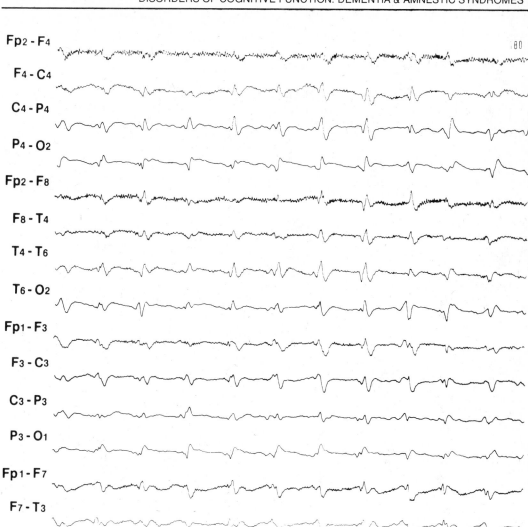

Figure 2–6. Electroencephalogram of a patient with Creutzfeldt-Jakob disease, showing triphasic waves with sharpened outlines; these occur repetitively about once every second.

ders that produce altered mentation and myoclonus (eg, sedative drug withdrawal) can mimic Creutzfeldt-Jakob disease.

Prognosis

No treatment is currently available. The disease is usually relentlessly progressive and, although transient improvement may occur, invariably fatal. In most cases, death occurs within one year after the onset of symptoms.

PROGRESSIVE MULTIFOCAL LEUKOENCEPHALOPATHY

Progressive multifocal leukoencephalopathy is thought to be due to infection with a papovavirus called **JC virus.** While antibodies to this virus are present in most of the adult population, symptomatic infection is rare. The disease is most common in patients with AIDS, lymphoma or leukemia, carcinoma, sarcoidosis, tuberculosis, or pharmacological immunosuppression following renal transplantation. It is rare in patients with normal immune function. The virus infects oligodendrocytes, leading to diffuse and patchy demyelination that most prominently affects white matter of the cerebral hemispheres but also involves the brain stem and cerebellum. Gray matter involvement and inflammatory changes are minimal.

Clinical Findings

The disorder is a subacute infection that runs a progressive course, usually leading to death in three to six months. Fever and systemic manifestations are absent. The clinical picture is dominated by cognitive disturbances, usually dementia, and focal cortical dysfunction. Hemiparesis, visual deficits, aphasia, dysarthria, sensory impairment, and dysphagia are also common. Ataxia is seen less frequently; headache is uncommon, and seizures do not occur.

Investigative Studies

The CSF is usually normal but may show a mild increase in pressure, white cell count, or protein. The CT scan is characterized by low-density areas within the subcortical white matter. Multifocal white matter abnormalities may also be seen on MRI (Figure 2–7). When the diagnosis is in doubt, it can be established by brain biopsy.

Treatment & Prognosis

The disorder has been almost uniformly fatal, and treatment with such antiviral agents as cytosine

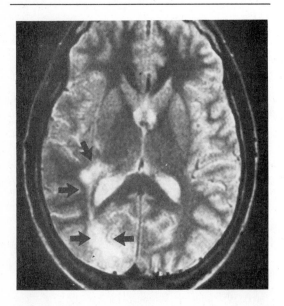

Figure 2–7. T2-weighted MRI in progressive multifocal leukoencephalopathy, showing abnormally high signal intensity (arrows) in white matter of the right parietal and occipital lobes. (Courtesy of A Gean.)

arabinoside, adenine arabinoside, or amantadine has generally been unsuccessful.

AIDS DEMENTIA COMPLEX

AIDS dementia complex (also called subacute encephalitis, AIDS encephalopathy, or AIDS-related dementia) is the most common neurological complication of AIDS, occurring in up to 70% of patients. While especially common in severely immunosuppressed patients late in the course of the disease, it can also be an early or presenting manifestation.

Pathogenesis

AIDS dementia complex results from direct invasion of the brain by a retrovirus, **human immunodeficiency virus-1 (HIV-1).** The virus and viral DNA and RNA can be isolated from the brain and CSF of affected patients, and antibodies against HIV-1 are produced within the central nervous system. The virus appears to reach the central nervous system early in the course of systemic HIV-1 infection, although the manner in which it does so is disputed. Monocytes, macrophages, and microglia are the principal cell types affected, but whether these cells are infected before or after entering the brain is uncertain. Neurological involvement at this stage may be asymptomatic, or it can produce transient symptomatic HIV-1 meningitis (see Chapter 1). The infection then seems to be contained until progressive immunosuppression impairs the normal host defense mechanisms, leading to increased HIV-1 production in the brain and, perhaps, the emergence of neurotropic strains. Productive viral infection within the brain seems to be associated with multinucleated cells (see below).

HIV-1 does not appear to replicate within neurons, astrocytes, or oligodendrocytes in vivo, and the loss of these cell types is not prominent in brains of patients with AIDS dementia complex. It has therefore been suggested that neuronal function is impaired by an indirect neurotoxic mechanism. This might involve viral products (such as the HIV-1 envelope protein **gp120,** which blocks the action of the neurotrophic factor **neuroleukin**) or the release from infected macrophages of cytokines or molecules that mimic the effects of excitotoxic amino acids.

Pathology

The earliest histopathological sign of AIDS dementia complex is pallor of subcortical and periventricular cerebral white matter associated with reactive astrocytosis but few inflammatory changes. More advanced cases are associated with parenchymal and perivascular infiltration by macrophages, microglia, lymphocytes, and multinucleated cells; the last are thought to result from the virus-induced fusion of macrophages. These changes affect the white matter, basal ganglia, thalamus, and pons and are accompanied by reactive astrocytosis. Spongy vacuolation of white matter occurs infrequently. Neuronal loss has been reported. The spinal cord may also be affected by a vacuolar myelopathy (see Chapter 6) resembling that caused by vitamin B_{12} deficiency.

Clinical Findings

The onset of AIDS dementia complex is usually insidious and is associated with cognitive and behavioral symptoms, such as forgetfulness, apathy, social withdrawal, impaired balance, leg weakness, and deterioration of handwriting (Table 2–6). Examination at this early stage may also show cerebellar ataxia,

pyramidal signs such as hyperreflexia and extensor plantar responses, weakness in one or both legs, postural tremor, and dysarthria. As the disease progresses, hypertonia, fecal and urinary incontinence, primitive reflexes, myoclonus, seizures, quadriparesis, and organic psychosis with delusions and visual hallucinations can occur.

Investigative Studies

Antibodies to HIV are detectable in the blood. The CSF is usually abnormal and may show a mild to moderate elevation of protein (<200 mg/dL); a modest, usually mononuclear pleocytosis (<50 cells/μL); and oligoclonal bands. CT scans and MRI usually demonstrate cerebrocortical atrophy with ventricular dilation and may also show diffuse involvement of subcortical white matter (Figure 2–8).

Treatment

Treatment with **zidovudine** (also known as **azidothymidine,** or **AZT),** 100 mg orally five times daily, is recommended for patients with symptomatic HIV-1 infection or with asymptomatic infection and CD4+ lymphocyte counts lower than 500/μL. Zidovudine is not curative in such patients but it can decrease the frequency of opportunistic infections and prolong survival. Zidovudine has also been reported to improve cognitive function in AIDS pa-

Table 2–6. Clinical features of AIDS dementia complex.[1]

Feature	Percentage of Patients	
	Early Stage	Late Stage
Symptoms		
Memory loss	80	74
Behavioral changes (eg, social withdrawal)	30	11
Depression	30	16
Motor symptoms (eg, imbalance, weakness, deteriorated handwriting)	20	21
Apathy	15	58
Confusion	15	42
Hallucinations	5	11
Signs		
Cognitive		
Psychomotor retardation	61	84
Dementia	39	100
Psychosis	5	16
Mutism	0	40
Motor		
Ataxia	34	71
Hypertonia	22	44
Tremor	16	45
Paraparesis or quadriparesis	13	33
Monoparesis or hemiparesis	5	2
Myoclonus	0	20
Other		
Hyperreflexia	36	78
Primitive reflexes	22	38
Seizures	7	20
Incontinence	0	47
Investigative studies[2]		
CSF		
Mononuclear pleocytosis	19	
Increased protein	66	
Decreased glucose	1	
Oligoclonal IgG bands	25	
Imaging		
Cerebral cortical atrophy (CT)	79	
Cerebral cortical atrophy (MRI)	55	
White matter lesions (CT)	11	
White matter lesions (MRI)	35	

[1]Adapted from Navia BA et al: The AIDS dementia complex. 1. Clinical features. 2. Neuropathology. *Ann Neurol* 1986; 19:517–524 and 525–535. and McArthur JC: Neurologic manifestations of AIDS. *Medicine* 1987;66:407–437.
[2]All stages.

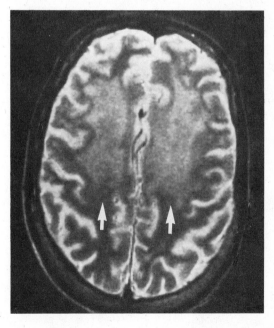

Figure 2–8. T2-weighted MRI in AIDS dementia complex, showing extensive, bilaterally symmetrical increases in signal intensity (arrows) in white matter (centrum semiovale) of the frontal lobes. (Courtesy of A Gean.)

tients without frank dementia, and in some patients with AIDS dementia complex. The drug's side effects include generalized weakness and malaise, gastrointestinal disturbances (anorexia, nausea, vomiting), insomnia, dizziness, headache, and myalgia. More serious adverse effects include anemia, which can sometimes be controlled by blood transfusions or administration of epoetin, and neutropenia. Zidovudine may also produce a mitochondrial myopathy (see Chapter 6) that responds to nonsteroidal anti-inflammatory drugs, prednisone, or discontinuing the drug.

Bone marrow toxicity limits the use of zidovudine in many patients, and resistance to the drug may develop after several months of treatment. In such cases, and depending on availability, it may be possible to substitute one of the investigational antiviral agents. These also have serious side effects: Didanosine (dideoxyinosine) can produce pancreatitis, thrombocytopenia, and painful polyneuropathy; dideoxycytidine is associated with stomatitis and painful polyneuropathy; and foscarnet is nephrotoxic and can cause leukopenia.

Prognosis

The course may be steadily progressive, or it can be acutely exacerbated by concurrent pulmonary infection. Patients usually die from one to nine months after the onset of dementia from aspiration or opportunistic infection.

METABOLIC DISORDERS

HYPOTHYROIDISM

Hypothyroidism (myxedema), which is discussed in Chapter 1 as a cause of acute confusional states, can also produce a reversible dementia or chronic organic psychosis. The dementia is a global disorder characterized by mental slowness, memory loss, and irritability. Focal cortical deficits do not occur. Psychiatric manifestations are typically prominent and include depression, paranoia, visual and auditory hallucinations, mania, and suicidal behavior.

Associated neurological symptoms and signs may be helpful in pointing to hypothyroidism as the cause of dementia. The most suggestive finding in this regard is delayed relaxation of the tendon reflexes. Patients with myxedema may complain of headache, hearing loss, tinnitus, vertigo, weakness, or paresthesia. Examination may show deafness, dysarthria, or cerebellar ataxia.

The diagnosis of myxedema is based upon the laboratory finding of decreased blood levels of T_4 and T_3, usually associated with increased TSH. Treatment consists of levothyroxine administration and corticosteroids as described in Chapter 10. Cognitive dysfunction is usually reversible with treatment.

VITAMIN B_{12} DEFICIENCY

Vitamin B_{12} deficiency is a rare cause of reversible dementia and organic psychosis. Like the acute confusional state associated with vitamin B_{12} deficiency (see Chapter 1), such syndromes can occur with or without hematological and other neurological manifestations.

The dementia consists of global cognitive dysfunction with mental slowness, impaired concentration, and memory disturbance; aphasia and other focal cortical disorders do not occur. Psychiatric manifestations are often prominent and include depression, mania, and paranoid psychosis with visual and auditory hallucinations. Laboratory findings and treatment are discussed in Chapter 1.

WILSON'S DISEASE

Wilson's disease (hepatolenticular degeneration), a rare but treatable hereditary disorder that produces dementia and extrapyramidal symptoms, is discussed in Chapter 8.

ACQUIRED HEPATOCEREBRAL DEGENERATION

Acquired (non-Wilsonian) hepatocerebral degeneration is an uncommon complication of chronic hepatic cirrhosis with spontaneous or surgical portosystemic shunting. The mechanisms underlying cerebral symptoms are unclear but may be related to failure of the liver to detoxify ammonia. Neurological symptoms precede hepatic symptoms in about one-sixth of patients.

Clinical Findings

Systemic manifestations of chronic liver disease are usually present. The neurological syndrome is characterized by a fluctuating but generally progressive course over one to nine years, often punctuated by bouts of acute hepatic encephalopathy (see Chapter 1). Dementia, dysarthria, and a variety of cerebellar, extrapyramidal, and pyramidal signs are the most common manifestations. Dementia is marked by mental slowness, apathy, impaired attention and concentration, and memory disturbance. The patient appears alert, in contrast to the somnolence or delirium seen in acute hepatic encephalopathy.

Cerebellar signs include gait and limb ataxia and dysarthria; nystagmus is rare. Extrapyramidal involvement may produce rigidity, resting tremor, dystonia, chorea, or athetosis. Adventitious movements tend to be most marked in the head, face, and neck. Asterixis, intention or action myoclonus, hyperreflexia, and extensor plantar responses are common findings; paraparesis occurs rarely.

Because episodes of acute hepatic encephalopathy may be superimposed on the chronic neurological disorder, it may be difficult to determine the relative contributions of acute and chronic syndromes to the clinical state of the patient. The diagnosis of acute hepatic encephalopathy is suggested by somnolence or agitated delirium, acute neurological deterioration, or ongoing gastrointestinal bleeding.

Investigative Studies

Laboratory studies show abnormal hepatic blood chemistries and elevated blood ammonia, but the degree of abnormality bears no direct relationship to the severity of neurological symptoms. The CSF is normal, except for increased glutamine and an occasional mild elevation of protein.

Differential Diagnosis

Several disorders resemble acquired hepatocerebral degeneration, but they can be distinguished by clinical or laboratory features. In Wilson's disease, the onset is typically earlier, and neurological involvement often precedes hepatic involvement. Kayser-Fleischer rings and laboratory evidence of abnormal copper metabolism are present, but there is no episodic encephalopathy. The ataxia of alcoholic cerebellar degeneration primarily affects gait rather than causing limb ataxia and dysarthria.

Treatment & Prognosis

Patients may benefit from a low-protein diet, lactulose, neomycin, or portosystemic shunting. Shunting may also precipitate or worsen neurological symptoms, however. Improvement following levodopa or bromocriptine therapy has been described. Death ultimately results from progressive hepatic failure or variceal bleeding.

ALCOHOLISM

Several complications of alcoholism are known to cause dementia. These include acquired hepatocerebral degeneration as a result of alcoholic liver disease, chronic subdural hematoma from head trauma (discussed above), and certain rare disorders resulting from nutritional deficiency.

Pellagra, caused by deficiency of nicotinic acid (niacin), affects neurons in the cerebral cortex, basal ganglia, brain stem, cerebellum, and anterior horns of the spinal cord. Systemic involvement is manifested by diarrhea, glossitis, anemia, and erythematous skin lesions. Neurological involvement may produce de-

mentia; psychosis; confusional states; pyramidal, extrapyramidal, and cerebellar signs; polyneuropathy; and optic neuropathy. Treatment is with nicotinamide, but the neurological deficits may persist despite treatment.

Marchiafava Bignami syndrome is characterized by necrosis of the corpus callosum and subcortical white matter and occurs most often in malnourished alcoholics. The course can be acute, subacute, or chronic. Clinical features include dementia, spasticity, dysarthria, gait disorder, and coma. The diagnosis can sometimes be made by CT scan or MRI. No specific treatment is available, but cessation of drinking and improvement of nutrition are advised. The outcome is variable: patients may die, survive with dementia, or recover.

The **Korsakoff amnestic syndrome** is a common and well-recognized cause of cognitive dysfunction in malnourished alcoholic patients. Because this disorder produces selective impairment of memory rather than global cognitive dysfunction, it is discussed in the section on amnestic syndromes (below).

It has been proposed that dementia can occur as a direct result of the toxic effects of ethanol on the brain, but this is disputed, and no distinctive corresponding abnormalities have been identified in the brains of demented alcoholics. Therefore, alcoholism should not be considered an adequate explanation for dementia, at least until other causes—especially those that are treatable—have been investigated and excluded.

DIALYSIS DEMENTIA

A subacute progressive—and ultimately fatal—dementia is an uncommon accompaniment of chronic hemodialysis; the mean duration of hemodialysis at the onset of the symptom is 39 months. The neurological symptoms are prominent dysarthria (often the earliest feature), multifocal myoclonus, and generalized or occasionally partial motor seizures. The symptoms are initially intermittent, being maximal following dialysis; they later become permanent, and dementia supervenes. The mean survival time in established cases is six months.

The interictal EEG is invariably abnormal, showing paroxysmal high-voltage slowing with intermixed spikes and slow waves. The CSF examination is normal. Brain CT studies show diffuse atrophy.

The ability of diazepam to reverse the clinical electroencephalographic features of dialysis dementia suggests an epileptic component to the disorder. Aluminum in the dialysate is a major etiological suspect, since elevated aluminum levels have been found in the brains of patients with dialysis dementia, and removing trace metals from the dialysate has markedly decreased the syndrome's incidence. Reports of the therapeutic effectiveness of renal transplantation have been conflicting.

HEAD TRAUMA

Severe open or closed head injury, particularly when followed by a prolonged period of unconsciousness, may cause posttraumatic syndromes with impaired memory and concentration, personality changes, headache, focal neurological disorders, or seizures. Cognitive impairment is nonprogressive, and the cause is usually obvious.

A syndrome of delayed and progressive posttraumatic dementia following repeated head injury (**dementia pugilistica**) has been described in boxers. It may begin—and typically continues to progress—years after the episodes of trauma have ceased. Dementia is characterized by cheerful or labile affect, mental slowness, memory deficit, and irritability. Associated neurological abnormalities include tremor, rigidity, bradykinesia, dysarthria, cerebellar ataxia, pyramidal signs, and seizures. Neuroradiological investigations may show cortical atrophy and cavum septi pellucidi.

PSEUDODEMENTIA OF DEPRESSION

Depression is the disorder most commonly mistaken for dementia. Because depression is common and usually treatable, distinguishing between the two conditions is of obvious clinical importance.

Both dementia and the pseudodementia of depression can be characterized by mental slowness, apathy, self-neglect, withdrawal, irritability, difficulty with memory and concentration, and changes in behavior and personality. In addition, depression can be a feature of most dementing illnesses, and the two disorders frequently coexist. Clinical features of help in the differentiation are listed in Table 2–7.

If depression is identified as a significant problem and is not correctable by treatment of an underlying disease or by a change in medication, it should be treated directly. Modes of treatment include psychotherapy, tricyclic and related antidepressants, monoamine oxidase inhibitors, and electroconvulsive therapy.

II. AMNESTIC SYNDROMES

A disorder of memory (**amnestic syndrome**) may occur as one feature of an acute confusional state or dementia or as an isolated abnormality (Table 2–8). The latter condition is discussed in this section.

Memory

Memory is a complex function that can be viewed as comprising phases of **registration, storage,** and **retrieval** (see Chapter 1). Autopsy and MRI studies of the brains of patients with memory disorders suggest that the hippocampus and related structures, such as the dorsomedial nucleus of the thalamus, are important in memory processing. Bilateral damage to these regions results in impairment of **short-term memory,** which is manifested clinically by the inability to form new memories. **Long-term memory,** which involves retrieval of previously learned information, is relatively preserved, perhaps because well-established memories are stored in diffuse regions of the cerebral cortex. Some patients with amnestic syndromes may attempt to fill in gaps in memory with false recollections (**confabulation**), which can take the form of elaborate contrivances or of genuine memories misplaced in time. The longest-standing and most deeply ingrained memories, however, such

Table 2–7. Dementia and the pseudodementia of depression: distinguishing features.

Dementia	Depression
Insidious onset	Abrupt onset
Progressive deterioration	Plateau of dysfunction
No prior history of depression	Prior history of depression may exist
Patient typically unaware of extent of deficits, does not complain of memory loss	Patient aware of and may exaggerate deficits, frequently complains of memory loss
Somatic complaints uncommon	Somatic complaints or hypochondriasis common
Variable affect	Depressed affect
Few vegetative symptoms	Prominent vegetative symptoms
Impairment often worse at night	Impairment usually not worse at night
Neurological examination and laboratory studies may be abnormal	Neurological examination and laboratory studies normal

Table 2–6. Causes of amnestic syndromes.

Acute
  Accompanying acute confusional states
  Head trauma
  Hypoxia or ischemia
  Bilateral posterior cerebral artery infarction
  Transient global amnesia
  Alcoholic blackouts
  Wernicke's encephalopathy
  Psychogenic amnesia
Chronic
  Accompanying dementias
  Alcoholic Korsakoff amnestic syndrome
  Postencephalitic amnesia
  Brain tumor
  Paraneoplastic limbic encephalitis

as one's own name, are almost always spared in organic memory disturbances. In contrast, such personal memories may be prominently or exclusively impaired in **psychogenic amnesia.**

The cellular basis of memory is poorly understood, but repetitive neuronal firing produces lasting pre- and postsynaptic changes that facilitate neurotransmission at hippocampal synapses (**long-term potentiation**). These changes appear to result from the release of glutamate, which stimulates the entry of calcium into postsynaptic neurons and the production of a retrograde chemical messenger (perhaps nitric oxide) that acts on presynaptic nerve terminals to increase transmitter release upon subsequent firing.

ACUTE AMNESIA

HEAD TRAUMA

Head injuries resulting in loss of consciousness are invariably associated with an amnestic syndrome. Patients seen shortly after such an injury exhibit a confusional state in which they are unable to incorporate new memories (**anterograde,** or **posttraumatic amnesia;** see Figure 2–9), although they may behave in an apparently normal automatic fashion. In addition, **retrograde amnesia** is present, covering a variable period prior to the trauma. Features characteristic of **transient global amnesia** (see below) may be seen.

As full consciousness returns, the ability to form new memories is restored. Events occurring in the confusional interval tend to be permanently lost to memory, however. Exceptions are islands of memory, for a lucid interval between trauma and unconsciousness, or for periods of lesser impairment in the course of a fluctuating posttraumatic confusional state. The period of retrograde amnesia begins to shrink, with the most remote memories the first to return. The severity of the injury tends to correlate with the duration of confusion and with the extent of permanent retrograde and posttraumatic amnesia.

HYPOXIA OR ISCHEMIA

Because of the selective vulnerability of pyramidal neurons in the Sommer sector (h1 sector of Scholz) of the hippocampus, conditions resulting in cerebral hypoxia or ischemia (eg, cardiac arrest, carbon monoxide poisoning) can produce amnestic syndromes. Amnesia tends to occur in patients in whom coma has lasted at least 12 hours. There is severe impairment of the ability to incorporate new memories, with relative preservation of registration and remote memory; patients typically appear to have an isolated disorder of short-term memory. A period of retrograde amnesia preceding the insult may occur. Patients exhibit a lack of concern about their impairment and sometimes confabulate. Amnesia following cardiac arrest may be the sole manifestation of neurological dysfunction, or it may coexist with other cerebral watershed syndromes, such as bibrachial paresis, cortical blindness, or visual agnosia (see Chapter 10). Recovery often occurs within several days, although deficits may persist.

Amnestic syndromes from **carbon monoxide poisoning** are frequently associated with affective disturbances. Other associated abnormalities include focal cortical and extrapyramidal dysfunction. Acute carbon monoxide poisoning is suggested by cherry-red coloration of the skin and mucous membranes, elevated carboxyhemoglobin levels, or cardiac arrhythmia. The CT brain scan may show lucencies in the basal ganglia and dentate nuclei.

BILATERAL POSTERIOR CEREBRAL ARTERY INFARCTION

The posterior cerebral artery supplies the medial temporal lobe, thalamus, posterior internal capsule, and occipital cortex (Figure 2–10). Ischemia or infarction in this territory, typically when bilateral, may produce a transient or permanent amnestic syndrome. Emboli in the vertebrobasilar system (see Chapter 10) are frequent causes of such disorders.

The amnestic syndrome is usually associated with unilateral or bilateral hemianopia and sometimes with visual agnosia, alexia without agraphia, anomia, sensory disturbances, or signs of upper midbrain dysfunction (especially impaired pupillary light reflex). Recent memory tends to be selectively impaired, with relative preservation of remote memory and registration.

The CT scan shows lucencies—which may or may not be enhanced by use of contrast material—in any combination of the above-mentioned regions. Evaluation and treatment are described in Chapter 10.

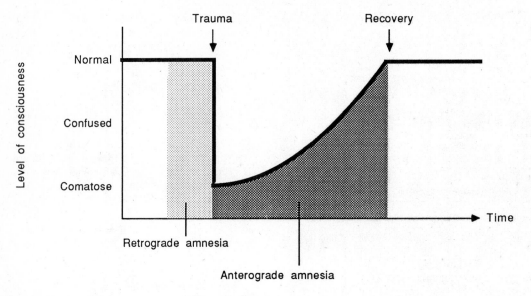

Figure 2–9. Retrograde and anterograde amnesia in posttraumatic memory disorders. Head trauma may produce transient coma, followed by a confusional state during which the patient is unable to form new memories. With recovery, this ability is restored, but there is persistent amnesia for the period of coma and confusion **(anterograde amnesia)** and for a variable period preceding the trauma **(retrograde amnesia)**; the latter deficit may improve with time.

TRANSIENT GLOBAL AMNESIA

Transient global amnesia is a syndrome of acute memory loss that tends to occur in middle-aged or elderly patients with risk factors for atherosclerotic disease, especially a prior ischemic event in the posterior cerebral circulation. While the cause may be vascular in origin, it is often not determined. The disorder is recurrent in fewer than 10% of patients.

A primary disorder of short-term memory that can last for minutes or days, it typically lasts for hours. Patients appear agitated and perplexed and may repeatedly inquire about their whereabouts, the time, and the nature of what they are experiencing. Knowledge of personal identity is preserved, as are remote memories and registration. New memories cannot be formed, however, which accounts for the patient's repetitive questions. Retrograde amnesia for a variable period preceding the episode may be present, but this period shrinks as the episode resolves.

The patient's obvious concern about the condition distinguishes transient global amnesia from most other organically based amnestic syndromes and may give rise to the suspicion that amnesia is psychogenic. A CT scan or MRI may demonstrate focal thalamic or temporal lobe abnormalities.

ALCOHOLIC BLACKOUTS

Short-term consumption of large amounts of ethanol by alcoholic or nonalcoholic individuals may lead to "blackouts"—transient amnestic episodes that are not due to global confusion, seizures, head trauma, or the Wernicke-Korsakoff syndrome. These spells are characterized by an inability to form new memories, without impairment of long-term memory or immediate recall. Although the cause is unknown, alcoholic blackouts may result from ethanol-induced depression of synaptic (especially serotonin- or glutamate-mediated) neurotransmission. The disorder is self-limited and no specific treatment is required, but reduction of the ethanol intake should be counseled, and thiamine should be given to treat possible Wernicke's encephalopathy (see Chapter 1).

WERNICKE'S ENCEPHALOPATHY

Wernicke's encephalopathy is caused by thiamine deficiency and classically produces an acute confusional state, ataxia, and ophthalmoplegia. Amnesia may be the major or sole cognitive disturbance, however, especially after thiamine treatment is begun and other cognitive abnormalities improve. Since patients with Wernicke's encephalopathy usually present with global confusion rather than isolated amnesia, the disorder is discussed more fully in Chapter 1.

PSYCHOGENIC AMNESIA

Amnesia may be a manifestation of a dissociative disorder (psychogenic amnesia) or of malingering. In such patients a prior psychiatric history, additional

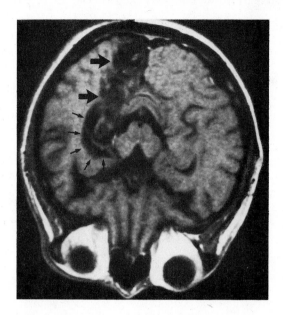

Figure 2–10. T1-weighted MRI in a patient with an old left posterior cerebral artery occlusion, showing tissue loss in the medial temporal (small arrows) and occipital (large arrows) lobes and associated dilation of the temporal and occipital horns of the lateral ventricle. (Courtesy of A Gean.)

psychiatric symptoms, or a precipitating emotional stress can often be identified.

Psychogenic amnesia is characterized by an isolated or a disproportionate loss of personal memories. The patient may be unable to remember his own name—an exceedingly rare finding in organic amnesia. Despite such disorientation to person, orientation to place and time may be preserved. In addition, recent memories may be less affected than remote memories—the reverse of the pattern customarily seen in amnesia caused by organic disease.

Examination under hypnosis or after administration of amobarbital sodium may be helpful in establishing that amnesia is of psychogenic origin.

CHRONIC AMNESIA

ALCOHOLIC KORSAKOFF AMNESTIC SYNDROME

The Korsakoff amnestic syndrome, which occurs in chronic alcoholism and other malnourished states, is thought to be caused by thiamine deficiency. It is usually preceded by one or more episodes of

Wernicke's encephalopathy (see Chapter 1), but such a history may be lacking. The memory disorder may be related to bilateral degeneration of the dorsomedial thalamic nuclei.

An amnestic syndrome of variable severity follows recovery from Wernicke's encephalopathy in about three-fourths of cases and is often associated with polyneuropathy and other residua such as nystagmus or gait ataxia. The essential defect is an inability to form new memories, resulting in significant impairment of short-term memory. Long-term memory is also frequently affected, although to a lesser extent. Registration is intact. Patients are typically apathetic and lack insight into their disorder. They may attempt to reassure the physician that no impairment exists and try to explain away their obvious inability to remember. Confabulation is often, but not invariably, a feature.

Korsakoff's syndrome can be prevented or its severity decreased by prompt administration of thiamine to patients with Wernicke's encephalopathy. Patients with established Korsakoff's syndrome should also receive thiamine to prevent the progression of deficits, although existing deficits are unlikely to be reversed.

POSTENCEPHALITIC AMNESIA

Patients who recover from acute viral encephalitis—particularly that caused by **herpes simplex** (see Chapter 1)—may be left with a permanent and static amnestic syndrome. The syndrome is similar to that produced by chronic alcoholism in that an inability to form new memories is its outstanding feature. Remote memories are affected to a lesser extent than are recent ones, and registration is intact. Confabulation may occur. Often there is total amnesia for the period of the acute encephalitis.

Patients may also exhibit other symptoms of limbic system disease. These include docility, indifference, flatness of mood and affect, inappropriate jocularity and sexual allusions, hyperphagia, impotence, repetitive stereotyped motor activity, and the absence of goal-oriented activity. Complex partial seizures, with or without secondary generalization, may occur.

BRAIN TUMOR

Brain tumor is a rare cause of amnestic syndrome. Tumors that can present in this manner include those that are located in the third ventricle or that compress its floor or walls from without. The amnestic syndrome closely resembles that of Korsakoff's syndrome. In addition, patients with deep midline tumors often exhibit marked lethargy, headache, endocrine disturbances, visual field deficits, or papilledema.

The diagnosis of brain tumor is made by CT scan

or MRI. Treatment consists of surgery or irradiation or both, depending upon the type of tumor and its location.

PARANEOPLASTIC LIMBIC ENCEPHALITIS

An inflammatory and degenerative disorder of gray matter regions of the central nervous system can occur as a rare effect of systemic cancer. When limbic structures are primarily affected, the clinical picture is that of an amnestic syndrome. The cause is not known, but (by analogy to other paraneoplastic neurological syndromes) antineuronal autoantibodies may be involved.

Paraneoplastic limbic encephalitis is most often associated with small cell cancer of the lung, and symptoms typically precede diagnosis of the underlying cancer. Histopathological findings include neuronal loss, reactive gliosis, microglial proliferation, and perivascular lymphocytic cuffing. Gray matter of the hippocampus, cingulum, piriform cortex, inferior frontal lobes, insula, and amygdala is characteristically affected. Symptoms develop over several weeks. The disorder is characterized by profound impairment of recent memory, corresponding to the inability to learn new material. Remote memory is less impaired, and registration is unaffected; confabulation occurs in some cases. Affective symptoms, either anxiety or depression, are common early features. Hallucinations and complex partial or generalized seizures may occur. In many instances, the amnestic syndrome progresses to a global dementia.

Depending upon the extent to which gray matter regions outside the limbic system are involved, cerebellar, pyramidal, bulbar, and peripheral nerve disturbances may coexist with the amnestic disorder.

The CSF may show a modest mononuclear pleocytosis and mildly elevated protein. Diffuse slowing or bitemporal slow waves and spikes are sometimes seen on EEG. An MRI may reveal abnormal signal intensity in the medial temporal lobes.

The paraneoplastic amnestic syndrome can be static, it can progress, or it can remit. Because no specific treatment is available, excluding treatable disorders is of primary importance. Korsakoff's syndrome caused by thiamine deficiency should especially be considered, because patients with cancer are susceptible to nutritional deficiency and thiamine administration may prevent these symptoms from worsening.

REFERENCES

Dementia (General)
Clarfield AM: The reversible dementias: Do they reverse? *Ann Intern Med* 1988;109:476–486.

Larson EB et al: Dementia in elderly outpatients: A prospective study. *Ann Intern Med* 1984;100:417–423.

Van Horn G: Dementia. *Am J Med* 1987;83:101–110.

Alzheimer's Disease
Gauthier S et al: Tetrahydroaminoacridine-lecithin combination treatment in patients with intermediate-stage Alzheimer's disease: Results of a Canadian double-blind, crossover, multicenter study. *N Engl J Med* 1990; 322:1272–1276.

Katzman R: Alzheimer's disease. *N Engl J Med* 1986; 314:964–973.

Katzman R, Saitoh T: Advances in Alzheimer's Disease. *FASEB J* 1991;5:278–286.

Kokmen E: Dementia: Alzheimer type. *Mayo Clin Proc* 1984;59:35–42.

Yankner BA, Mesulam M-M: β-amyloid and the pathogenesis of Alzheimer's disease. *N Engl J Med* 1991; 325: 1849–1857.

Multi-infarct Dementia
Fields WS: Multi-infarct dementia. *Neurol Clin* 1986; 4:405–413.

Hachinski VC, Lassen NA, Marshall J: Multi-infarct dementia: A cause of mental deterioration in the elderly. *Lancet* 1974;2:207–210.

Wells CE: Role of stroke in dementia. *Stroke* 1978;9: 1–3.

Chronic Subdural Hematoma
Luxon LM, Harrison MJ: Chronic subdural haematoma. *Q J Med* 1979;48:43–53.

McKissock W, Richardson A, Bloom WH: Subdural hematoma: A review of 389 cases. *Lancet* 1960;1:1365–1369.

Normal-Pressure Hydrocephalus
Black PMcL: CSF shunts for dementia, incontinence, and gait disturbance. *Clin Neurosurg* 1985;32:632–656.

Estanol BV: Gait apraxia in communicating hydrocephalus. *J Neurol Neurosurg Psychiatry* 1981;44:305–308.

Neurosyphilis
Jordan KG: Modern neurosyphilis: A critical analysis. *West J Med* 1988;149:47–57.

Musher DM, Hamill RJ, Baughn RE: Effect of human immunodeficiency virus (HIV) infection on the course of syphilis and on the response to treatment. *Ann Intern Med* 1990;113:872–881.

Creutzfeldt-Jakob Disease
Brown P et al: Creutzfeldt-Jakob disease: Clinical analysis of a consecutive series of 230 neuropathologically verified cases. *Ann Neurol* 1986;20:597–602.

Committee on Health Care Issues, American Neurological Association: Precautions in handling tissues, fluids, and other contaminated materials from patients with documented or suspected Creutzfeldt-Jakob disease. *Ann Neurol* 1986;19:75–77.

Hsaio K, Prusiner SB: Inherited human prion diseases. *Neurology* 1990;40:1820–1827.

Progressive Multifocal Leukoencephalopathy

Krupp LB et al: Progressive multifocal leukoencephalopathy: Clinical and radiographic features. *Ann Neurol* 1985;**17:**344–349.

AIDS Dementia Complex

McArthur JC: Neurological manifestations of AIDS. *Medicine* 1987;66:407–437.

Navia BA, Jordan BD, Price RW: The AIDS dementia complex. 1. Clinical features. 2. Neuropathology. *Ann Neurol* 1986;19:517–524 and 525–535.

Price RW et al: The brain in AIDS: Central nervous system HIV-1 infection and AIDS dementia complex. *Science* 1988;239:586–592.

Schmitt FA et al: Neuropsychological outcome of zidovudine (AZT) treatment of patients with AIDS and AIDS-related complex. *N Engl J Med* 1988; 319:1573–1578.

Yarchoan R et al: Clinical pharmacology of 3'-azido-2',3'- dideoxythymidine (zidovudine) and related dideoxynucleosides. *N Engl J Med* 1989;321:726–738.

Vitamin B$_{12}$ Deficiency

Lindenbaum J et al: Neuropsychiatric disorders caused by cobalamin deficiency in the absence of anemia or macrocytosis. *N Engl J Med* 1988;318:1720–1728.

Wiener JS, Hope JM: Cerebral manifestations of vitamin B$_{12}$ deficiency. *JAMA* 1959;170:1038–1041.

Acquired Hepatocerebral Degeneration

Victor M, Adams RD, Cole M: The acquired (non-Wilsonian) type of chronic hepatocerebral degeneration. *Medicine* 1965;44:345–396.

Alcoholism

Charness ME, Simon RP, Greenberg DA: Ethanol and the nervous system. *N Engl J Med* 1989;321:442–454.

Victor M, Adams RD: The alcoholic dementias. *Handbook Clin Neurol* 1985;46:335–352.

Dialysis Dementia

O'Hare JA, Callaghan NM, Murnaghan DJ: Dialysis encephalopathy: Clinical, electroencephalographic and interventional aspects. *Medicine* 1983;62:129–141.

Pseudodementia of Depression

Finlayson RE, Martin LM: Recognition and management of depression in the elderly. *Mayo Clin Proc* 1982; 57:115–120.

Amnestic Syndromes (General)

Brown TH et al: Long-term synaptic potentiation. *Science* 1988;242:724–728.

Schuman EM, Madison DV: A requirement for the intercellular messenger nitric oxide in long-term potentiation. *Science* 1991;254:1503–1506.

Squire LR: Mechanisms of memory. *Science* 1986; 232:1612–1619.

Head Trauma

Fisher CM: Concussion amnesia. *Neurology* 1966; 16:826–830.

Hypoxia or Ischemia

Caronna JJ: Diagnosis, prognosis, and treatment of hypoxic coma. *Adv Neurol* 1979;26:1–15.

Smith JS, Brandon S: Morbidity from acute carbon monoxide poisoning at three-year follow-up. *Br Med J* 1973;1:318–321.

Transient Global Amnesia

Fisher CM, Adams RD: Transient global amnesia. *Acta Neurol Scand* 1964;40(Suppl 9):1–83.

Miller JW et al: Transient global amnesia: Clinical characteristics and prognosis. *Neurology* 1987;**37:**733–737.

Alcoholic Blackouts, Wernicke's Encephalopathy and Alcoholic Korsakoff Amnestic Syndrome

Charness ME, Simon RP, Greenberg DA: Ethanol and the nervous system. *N Engl J Med* 1989;321:442–454.

Paraneoplastic Limbic Encephalitis

Dropcho EJ: The remote effects of cancer on the nervous system. *Neurol Clin* 1989;**7:**579–603.

3

Headache & Facial Pain

APPROACH TO DIAGNOSIS

PATHOPHYSIOLOGY OF HEADACHE & FACIAL PAIN

Pain-Sensitive Structures

Headache is caused by traction, displacement, inflammation, vascular spasm, or distention of the pain-sensitive structures in the head or neck. Isolated involvement of the bony skull, most of the dura, or most regions of brain parenchyma does not produce pain.

A. Pain-Sensitive Structures Within the Cranial Vault: These include the venous sinuses (eg, sagittal sinus); the anterior and middle meningeal arteries; the dura at the base of the skull; the trigeminal (V), glossopharyngeal (IX), and vagus (X) nerves; the proximal portions of the internal carotid artery and its branches near the circle of Willis; the brain stem periaqueductal gray matter; and the sensory nuclei of the thalamus.

B. Extracranial Pain-Sensitive Structures: These include the periosteum of the skull; the skin; the subcutaneous tissues, muscles, and arteries; the neck muscles; the second and third cervical nerves; the eyes, ears, teeth, sinuses, and oropharynx; and the mucous membranes of the nasal cavity.

Radiation or Projection of Pain

The trigeminal (V) nerve carries sensation from intracranial structures in the anterior and middle fossae of the skull, above the cerebellar tentorium. Discrete intracranial lesions in these locations produce pain that radiates in the trigeminal nerve distribution (Figure 3–1).

The glossopharyngeal (IX) and vagus (X) nerves supply part of the posterior fossa; pain originating in this area may also be referred to the ear or throat (eg, glossopharyngeal neuralgia).

The upper cervical nerves transmit stimuli arising

Headache may be the earliest or the principal manifestation of serious systemic or intracranial disease and therefore requires thorough and systematic evaluation. Headache occurs in all age groups and is the seventh leading reason for medical office visits; the causes are myriad (Table 3–1).

An etiological diagnosis of headache is based on understanding the pathophysiology of head pain; obtaining a history, with characterization of the pain as acute, subacute, or chronic; performing a careful physical examination; and formulating a differential diagnosis.

Table 3–1. Causes of headache and facial pain.

Acute onset
  Common causes
    Subarachnoid hemorrhage
    Other cerebrovascular diseases
    Meningitis or encephalitis
    Ocular disorders (glaucoma, acute iritis)
  Less common causes
    Seizures
    Lumbar puncture
    Hypertensive encephalopathy
    Coitus
Subacute onset
  Giant cell (temporal) arteritis
  Intracranial mass (tumor, subdural hematoma, abscess)
  Pseudotumor cerebri (benign intracranial hypertension)
  Trigeminal neuralgia (tic douloureux)
  Glossopharyngeal neuralgia
  Postherpetic neuralgia
  Hypertension (including pheochromocytoma and the use of
    monoamine oxidase inhibitors plus tyramine)
  Atypical facial pain
Chronic
  Tension headache
  Migraine
  Cluster headache
  Cervical spine disease
  Sinusitis
  Dental disease

from infratentorial and cervical structures; therefore, pain from posterior fossa lesions projects to the second and third cervical dermatomes (Figure 3–1).

HISTORY

Classification & Approach to the Differential Diagnosis

A. Acute Headaches and Facial Pain: Headaches that are new in onset and clearly different from any the patient has experienced previously are commonly a symptom of serious illness and therefore demand prompt evaluation. The sudden onset of "the worst headache I've ever had in my life" (classic subarachnoid hemorrhage), diffuse headache with neck stiffness and fever (meningitis), and head pain centered about one eye (acute glaucoma) are striking examples. Acute headaches may also accompany more benign processes such as viral syndromes or other febrile illnesses.

B. Subacute Headaches and Facial Pain: Subacute headaches occur over a period of weeks to months. Such headaches may also signify serious medical disorders, especially when the pain is progressive or when it develops in elderly patients. Inquiries should be made about recent head trauma (subdural hematoma or postconcussive syndrome); a history of malaise, fever, or neck stiffness (subacute meningitis); other neurological abnormalities or weight loss (primary or metastatic brain tumor);

symptoms of vasculitis, especially giant cell arteritis; and medical conditions (eg, optic neuritis in multiple sclerosis; cutaneous herpes zoster) or medications predisposing to any of the disorders listed in Table 3–1.

C. Chronic Headaches and Facial Pain: Headaches that have occurred for years (eg, migraine or tension headaches) usually have a benign cause, although each acute attack may be profoundly disabling. When treating these patients, it is important to determine whether the present headache is similar to those suffered previously or is new—and thus represents a different process.

Precipitating Factors

Precipitating factors can provide a guide to the cause of headache. Such factors include recent eye or dental surgery; acute exacerbation of chronic sinusitis or hay fever; systemic viral infection; tension, emotional stress, or fatigue; menses; hunger; ice cream; foods containing nitrite (hot dogs, salami, ham, and most sausage), phenylethylamine (chocolate), or tyramine (cheddar cheese); and bright lights. Precipitation of headache by alcohol is especially typical of cluster headache. Chewing and eating commonly trigger glossopharyngeal neuralgia, tic douloureux, and the jaw claudication of giant cell arteritis; these activities also trigger pain in patients with temporomandibular joint dysfunction. The use of oral contraceptive agents or other drugs such as nitrates may precipitate or exacerbate migraine and even lead to stroke. Intense headache can occur in response to coughing in patients with structural lesions in the posterior fossa; in other instances no specific cause for cough headache can be identified.

Prodromal Symptoms

Prodromal symptoms or auras, such as scintillating scotomas or other visual changes, often occur with migraine; they may also occur in patients with a seizure disorder who present with postictal headaches.

Characteristics of Pain

Headache or facial pain is most often described as throbbing; a dull, steady ache; or a jabbing, lancinating pain. **Pulsating, throbbing** pain is frequently ascribed to migraine, but it is equally common in patients with tension headache. A steady sensation of **tightness** or **pressure** is also commonly seen with tension headache. The pain produced by intracranial mass lesions is typically **dull** and **steady. Sharp, lancinating** pain suggests a neuritic cause such as trigeminal neuralgia. **Icepicklike** pain may be described by patients with migraine, cluster headache, or giant cell arteritis.

Headache of virtually any description can occur in patients with migraine or brain tumors, however, so the character of the pain alone does not provide a reliable etiologic guide.

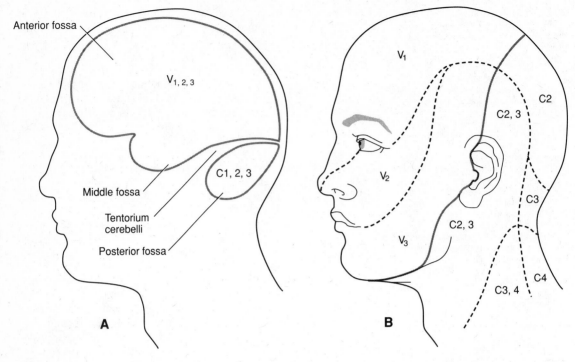

Figure 3–1. Innervation of pain-sensitive intracranial compartments **(A)** and corresponding extracranial sites of pain radiation **(B)**. The trigeminal (V) nerve, especially its ophthalmic (V₁) division, innervates the anterior and middle cranial fossae; lesions in these areas can produce frontal headache. The upper cervical nerve roots (especially C2) innervate the posterior fossa; lesions here can cause occipital headache.

Location of Pain

Unilateral headache is an invariable feature of cluster headache and occurs in the majority of migraine attacks; most patients with tension headache report bilateral pain.

Ocular or **retro-ocular** pain suggests a primary ophthalmologic disorder such as acute iritis or glaucoma, optic (II) nerve disease (eg, optic neuritis), or retro-orbital inflammation (eg, Tolosa-Hunt syndrome). It is also common in migraine or cluster headache.

Paranasal pain localized to one or several of the sinuses, often associated with tenderness in the overlying periosteum and skin, occurs with acute infection or outlet obstruction of these structures.

Headache from intracranial mass lesions may be **focal** ("it hurts right here"), but even in such cases it is replaced by bioccipital and bifrontal pain when the intracranial pressure becomes elevated.

Bandlike or **occipital** discomfort is commonly associated with tension headaches. Occipital localization can also occur with meningeal irritation from infection or hemorrhage and with disorders of the joints, muscles, or ligaments of the upper cervical spine.

Pain within the **first division of the trigeminal nerve** (Figure 3–1B), characteristically described as burning in quality, is a common feature of postherpetic neuralgia.

Lancinating pain localized to the **second** or **third division of the trigeminal nerve** (Figure 3–1B) suggests tic douloureux.

The **pharynx** and **external auditory meatus** are the most frequent sites of pain caused by glossopharyngeal neuralgia.

Associated Symptoms

Manifestations of underlying systemic disease can aid in the etiological diagnosis of headache and should always be sought.

Recent weight loss may accompany cancer, giant cell arteritis, or depression.

Fever or **chills** may indicate systemic infection or meningitis.

Dyspnea or other symptoms of congenital heart disease raise the possibility of subacute infective endocarditis and resultant brain abscess.

Visual disturbances suggest an ocular disorder (eg, glaucoma), migraine, or an intracranial process involving the optic nerve or tract or the central visual pathways.

Nausea and **vomiting** are common in migraine and posttraumatic headache syndromes and can be seen in the course of mass lesions. Some patients with migraine also report that diarrhea accompanies the attacks.

Photophobia may be prominent in migraine and acute meningitis or subarachnoid hemorrhage.

Myalgias often accompany tension headaches, viral syndromes, and giant cell arteritis.

Ipsilateral rhinorrhea and **lacrimation** during attacks typify cluster headache.

Transient loss of consciousness may be a concomitant of both migraine and glossopharyngeal neuralgia.

Other Features of Headache

Temporal pattern of headache. Headaches from mass lesions are commonly maximal on awakening, as are sinus headaches. Headaches from mass lesions, however, increase in severity over time. Cluster headaches frequently awaken patients from sleep; they often recur at the same time each day or night. Tension headaches can develop whenever stressful situations occur and are often maximal at the end of a workday. Migraine headaches are episodic and may be worse during menses (see Figure 3–2).

Conditions relieving headache. Migraine headaches are frequently relieved by darkness, sleep, vomiting, or pressing on the ipsilateral temporal artery, and their frequency is often diminished during pregnancy. Post-lumbar-puncture headaches are typically relieved by recumbency, while headaches caused by intracranial mass lesions may be less severe with the patient standing.

Conditions exacerbating headache. Discomfort exacerbated by rapid changes in head position or by events that transiently raise intracranial pressure, such as coughing and sneezing, is often associated with an intracranial mass but can also occur in migraine. Anger, excitement, or irritation can precipitate or worsen both migraine and tension headaches. Stooping, bending forward, sneezing, or blowing the nose characteristically worsens the pain of sinusitis. Postural headache (maximal when upright, nearly absent when lying down) occurs with low CSF pressure caused by lumbar puncture, head injury, or spinal fluid leak.

Fluctuations in intensity and duration of the headache with no obvious cause, especially when associated with similar fluctuations in mental status, are seen with subdural hematoma.

Past history of headache. The characteristics of the present headache should be compared with those of previous occurrences, since headache with features different from those previously experienced calls for careful investigation.

PHYSICAL EXAMINATION

A general physical examination is mandatory, since headache is a nonspecific accompaniment of many systemic disorders. If possible, the patient should be observed during an episode of headache or facial pain.

Vital Signs

A. Temperature: Although fever suggests a viral syndrome, meningitis, encephalitis, or brain abscess, headache from these causes can occur without fever. Moreover, headache can accompany any systemic infectious illness.

B. Pulse: Tachycardia can occur in a tense, anxious patient with a tension headache or accompany any severe pain. Paroxysmal headache associated with tachycardia and perspiration is characteristic of pheochromocytoma.

C. Blood Pressure: Hypertension per se rarely causes headache unless the blood pressure elevation is acute, as with pheochromocytoma, or very high, as with early hypertensive encephalopathy. Chronic hypertension, however, is the major risk factor for stroke, which can be associated with acute headache. Subarachnoid hemorrhage is commonly followed by marked acute blood pressure elevation.

D. Respiration: Hypercapnia from respiratory insufficiency from any cause can elevate intracranial pressure and produce headache.

General Physical Examination

A. Weight Loss: Weight loss or cachexia in a patient with headache suggests the presence of cancer or chronic infection. Polymyalgia rheumatica-giant

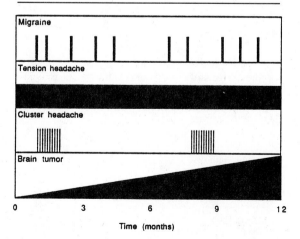

Figure 3–2. Temporal patterns of headache. Migraine headache is episodic and may occur at varying intervals. Tension headache may be present every day. Cluster headache occurs in bouts separated by symptom-free periods. Headache caused by brain tumor often increases in severity with time.

cell arteritis syndromes can also be accompanied by weight loss.

B. Skin: Focal cellulitis of the face or overlying the skull indicates local infection, which may be the source of intracranial abscess or venous sinus thrombosis. Cutaneous abnormalities elsewhere may suggest vasculitis (including that from meningococcemia), endocarditis, or cancer. The neurofibromas or café-au-lait spots of von Recklinghausen's disease (neurofibromatosis) may be associated with benign or malignant intracranial tumors that produce headache. Cutaneous angiomas sometimes accompany arteriovenous malformations (AVMs) of the central nervous system and may be associated with chronic headache—or acute headache if they bleed. Herpes zoster that affects the face and head most often involves the eye and the skin around the periorbital tissue, causing facial pain.

C. Scalp, Face, and Head: Scalp tenderness is characteristic of migraine headache, subdural hematoma, giant cell arteritis, and postherpetic neuralgia. Nodularity, erythema, or tenderness over the temporal artery suggests giant cell arteritis. Localized tenderness of the superficial temporal artery also accompanies acute migraine. Recent head trauma or a mass lesion can cause a localized area of tenderness.

Paget's disease, myeloma, or metastatic cancer of the skull may produce head pain that is boring in quality and associated with skull tenderness. In Paget's disease, arteriovenous shunting within bone may make the scalp feel warm.

Disorders of the eyes, ears, or teeth may cause headache. Tooth percussion may reveal periodontal abscess. Sinus tenderness may indicate sinusitis. A bruit over the orbit or skull suggests an intracranial AVM, a carotid artery-cavernous sinus fistula, an aneurysm, or a meningioma. Lacerations of the tongue raise the possibility of postictal headache. Ipsilateral conjunctival injection, lacrimation, Horner's syndrome, and rhinorrhea occur with cluster headache. Temporomandibular joint disease is accompanied by local tenderness and crepitus.

D. Neck: Cervical muscle spasms occur with tension and migraine headaches, cervical spine injuries, cervical arthritis, or meningitis. Carotid bruits may be associated with cerebrovascular disease.

Meningeal signs must be carefully sought, especially if the headache is of recent onset. Meningeal irritation causes nuchal rigidity mainly in the anteroposterior direction, while cervical spine disorders restrict movement in all directions. Discomfort or hip and knee flexion during neck flexion (Brudzinski's sign) readily indicates meningeal irritation (Figure 3–3).

Meningeal signs may be absent or difficult to demonstrate in the early stages of subacute (eg, tuberculous) meningitis, in the first few hours after subarachnoid hemorrhage, and in comatose patients.

E. Heart and Lung: Brain abscess may be associated with congenital heart disease, which is evi-

denced by murmurs or cyanosis. Lung abscess may also be a source of brain abscess.

NEUROLOGICAL EXAMINATION

Mental Status Examination

During the mental status examination, patients with acute headache may demonstrate confusion, as is commonly seen with subarachnoid hemorrhage and meningitis. Dementia may be the major feature of intracranial tumor, particularly one in the frontal lobe.

Cranial Nerve Examination

Cranial nerve abnormalities may suggest and localize an intracranial tumor or other mass lesion. Papilledema, the hallmark of increased intracranial pressure, may be seen in space-occupying intracranial lesions, carotid artery-cavernous sinus fistula, pseudotumor cerebri, or hypertensive encephalopathy. Superficial retinal (subhyaloid) hemorrhages are characteristic of subarachnoid hemorrhage in adults. Ischemic retinopathy may be found in patients with vasculitis.

Progressive oculomotor nerve palsy, especially when it causes pupillary dilatation, may be the presenting sign of an expanding posterior-communicating-artery aneurysm, or it may reflect increasing intracranial pressure and incipient herniation. Decreased pupillary reactivity occurs in optic neuritis. Extraocular muscle palsies occur in Tolosa-Hunt syndrome. Proptosis suggests an orbital mass lesion or carotid artery-cavernous sinus fistula.

Decreased sensation over the area of pain—most commonly the first division of the trigeminal nerve—is found in postherpetic neuralgia. Trigger areas eliciting pain in and about the face and pharynx suggest trigeminal and glossopharyngeal neuralgia, respectively.

Motor Examination

Asymmetric motor function or gait ataxia in a patient with a history of subacute headache demands complete evaluation to exclude intracranial mass lesions.

Sensory Examination

Focal or segmental sensory impairment or diminished corneal sensation (corneal reflex) is strong evidence against a benign cause of pain.

HEADACHES OF ACUTE ONSET

Sudden onset of new headache may be a symptom of serious intracranial or systemic disease; it must be investigated promptly and thoroughly.

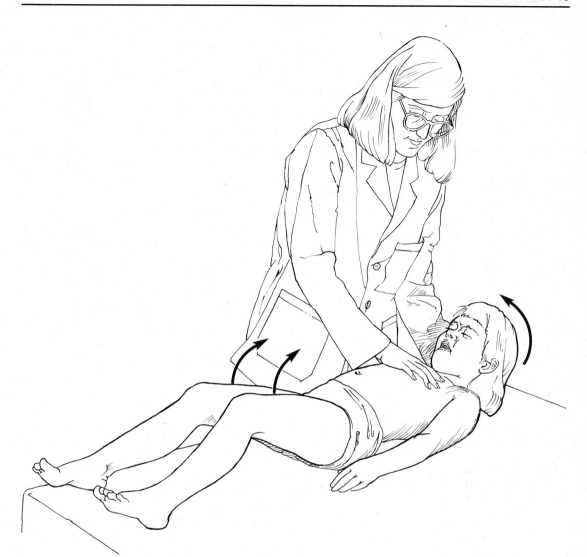

Figure 3–3. Brudzinski's sign. With the patient supine and the examiner's hand on the patient's chest, passive neck flexion (arrow at right) results in flexion at the hips (arrows at left). The sign is present with meningeal irritation from disorders such as infectious meningitis or subarachnoid hemorrhage.

SUBARACHNOID HEMORRHAGE

Spontaneous (nontraumatic) subarachnoid hemorrhage (bleeding into the subarachnoid space), is usually the result of a ruptured cerebral arterial aneurysm or an arteriovenous malformation (AVM). Rupture of a berry aneurysm accounts for about 75% of cases and occurs most often during the fifth and sixth decades, with an approximately equal sex distribution. Hypertension has not been conclusively demonstrated to predispose to the formation of aneurysms but may be responsible for their rupture. Intracranial AVMs, a less frequent cause of subarachnoid hemorrhage (10%), occur twice as often in men and usually bleed in the second to fourth decades, although a significant incidence extends into the 60s. Blood in the subarachnoid space can also result from intracerebral hemorrhage, embolic stroke, and trauma.

Pathology

Cerebral artery aneurysms are most commonly congenital "berry" aneurysms, which result from developmental weakness of the vessel wall, especially at sites of branching. These aneurysmal dilatations arise from intracranial arteries about the circle of Willis at the base of the brain (Figure 3–4) and are multiple in about 20% of cases. Other congenital abnormalities, including polycystic kidney disease and coarctation of the aorta, may be associated with berry aneurysms. Occasionally, systemic infections such as

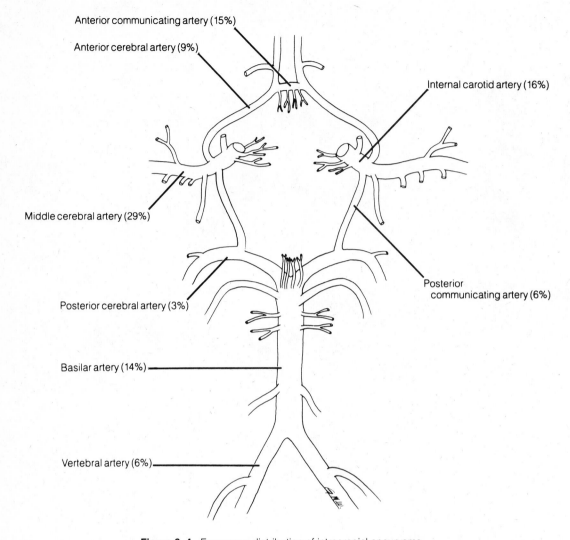

Anterior communicating artery (15%)

Anterior cerebral artery (9%)

Internal carotid artery (16%)

Middle cerebral artery (29%)

Posterior communicating artery (6%)

Posterior cerebral artery (3%)

Basilar artery (14%)

Vertebral artery (6%)

Figure 3–4. Frequency distribution of intracranial aneurysms.

infective endocarditis disseminate to a cerebral artery and cause aneurysm formation; such "mycotic" aneurysms account for 2–3% of aneurysmal ruptures. Mycotic aneurysms are usually more distal (along the course of cerebral arteries) than are berry aneurysms.

Arteriovenous malformations consist of abnormal vascular communications that permit arterial blood to enter the venous system without passing through a capillary bed. They are most common in the middle cerebral artery distribution.

Pathophysiology

Rupture of an intracranial artery elevates intracranial pressure and distorts pain-sensitive structures, producing headache. Intracranial pressure may reach systemic perfusion pressure and acutely decrease cerebral blood flow; together with the concussive effect of the rupture, this is thought to cause the loss of consciousness that occurs at the onset in about 50% of patients. Rapid elevation of intracranial pressure can also produce subhyaloid retinal hemorrhages (Figure 3–5).

Because aneurysmal hemorrhage is usually confined to the subarachnoid space, it does not produce a focal cerebral lesion. Prominent focal findings on neurological examination are accordingly uncommon except with middle cerebral artery aneurysms. Ruptured AVMs, however, produce focal abnormalities that correspond to their parenchymal location.

Clinical Findings

A. Symptoms and Signs: The classic (but not invariable) presentation of subarachnoid hemorrhage is the sudden onset of an unusually severe generalized headache ("the worst headache I ever had in my life"). The absence of headache essentially precludes

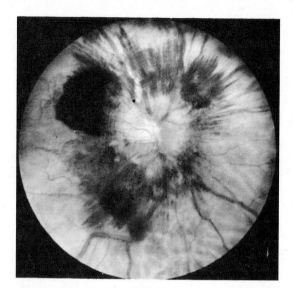

Figure 3–5. Peripapillary intraretinal and preretinal (subhyaloid) hemorrhages associated a sudden increase in intracranial pressure caused by aneurysmal rupture. (Courtesy of WF Hoyt.)

the diagnosis. Loss of consciousness is frequent, as are vomiting and neck stiffness. Symptoms may begin at any time of day and during either rest or exertion.

The most significant feature of the headache is that it is new. Milder but otherwise similar headaches may have occurred in the weeks prior to the acute event. These earlier headaches are probably the result of small prodromal hemorrhages (sentinel, or warning, hemorrhages).

The headache is not always severe, however, especially if the subarachnoid hemorrhage is from a ruptured AVM rather than an aneurysm. Although the duration of the hemorrhage is brief, the intensity of the headache may remain unchanged for several days and subside only slowly over the next two weeks. A recrudescent headache usually signifies recurrent bleeding.

Blood pressure frequently rises precipitously as a result of the hemorrhage. Temperature elevations to as high as 39°C (102.2 °F) may occur during the first two weeks. There is frequently confusion, stupor, or coma. Nuchal rigidity and other evidence of meningeal irritation (Figure 3–3) are common, but these signs may not occur for several hours after the onset of the headache. Preretinal globular subhyaloid hemorrhages (found in 20% of cases) are most suggestive of the diagnosis (Figure 3–5). Because bleeding occurs mainly in the subarachnoid space in patients with aneurysmal rupture, prominent focal signs are uncommon on neurological examination. When present, they may bear no relationship to the site of the

aneurysm. An exception is oculomotor nerve palsy occurring ipsilateral to a posterior communicating artery aneurysm. Bilateral extensor plantar responses are frequent in such cases. Ruptured AVMs may produce focal signs, such as hemiparesis, aphasia, or a defect of the visual fields, that help to localize the intracranial lesion.

B. Laboratory Findings: Patients presenting with subarachnoid hemorrhage are generally investigated first by CT scan, which will usually confirm that hemorrhage has occurred and may help to identify a focal source. CT brain scanning will detect subarachnoid blood in more than 90% of patients with aneurysmal rupture. The test is highly sensitive on the day bleeding occurs; it is most sensitive in patients with altered consciousness. Intracerebral or intraventricular blood, associated hydrocephalus, and infarction can also be identified. Aneurysms may not be evident on the CT scan, but most AVMs can be seen with contrast. MRI is especially useful in detecting small AVMs localized to the brain stem (an area poorly seen on CT scan). If the CT scan fails to confirm the clinical diagnosis, lumbar puncture is performed.

The CSF examination usually reveals markedly elevated pressure, often above the maximum recordable value (600 mm water) using the standard CSF manometer; the fluid is grossly bloody and contains from 100,000 to more than 1 million red cells/μL. As a result of the breakdown of hemoglobin from red cells, the supernatant of the centrifuged CSF becomes yellow (xanthochromic) within several hours (certainly by 12 hours) following the hemorrhage. White cells are initially present in the spinal fluid in the same proportion to red cells as in the peripheral blood. The chemical meningitis caused by blood in the subarachnoid space, however, may produce a pleocytosis of several thousand white blood cells during the first 48 hours and a reduction in CSF glucose between the fourth and eighth days after the hemorrhage. In the absence of pleocytosis, CSF glucose following subarachnoid hemorrhage is normal. The peripheral blood white count is often modestly elevated but rarely exceeds 15,000 cells/μL. The ECG may reveal a host of abnormalities: peaked or deeply inverted T waves, short PR interval, or tall U waves.

Once the diagnosis is confirmed, four-vessel cerebral arteriography is undertaken. Cerebral angiography of both the carotid and vertebral arteries should be performed to visualize the entire cerebral vascular anatomy, since multiple aneurysms occur in 20% of patients and AVMs are frequently supplied from multiple sources. Angiography can be performed at the earliest time convenient for radiology department personnel; emergency studies in the middle of the night are rarely indicated. Angiography is a prerequisite to the rational planning of surgical treatment and is therefore not necessary for patients who are not surgical candidates, eg, those who are deeply comatose.

Differential Diagnosis

The history of a sudden severe headache with confusion or obtundation, nuchal rigidity, a nonfocal neurological examination, and bloody spinal fluid is highly specific for subarachnoid hemorrhage.

Hypertensive intracerebral hemorrhage is also manifested by obtundation and hemorrhagic spinal fluid, but there are prominent focal findings. Bacterial meningitis is excluded by the CSF examination. Ruptured mycotic aneurysm is suggested by other signs of endocarditis. Traumatic spinal puncture can be excluded as the cause of bloody CSF by examination of the centrifuged CSF specimen. Since blood that results from traumatic lumbar puncture does not undergo enzymatic breakdown to bilirubin, centrifugation of the spinal fluid specimen reveals a colorless supernatant.

Complications & Sequelae

A. Recurrence of Hemorrhage: Recurrence of aneurysmal hemorrhage is the major acute complication and roughly doubles the mortality rate. Recurrence of hemorrhage from AVM is less common in the acute period.

B. Intraparenchymal Extension of Hemorrhage: While it is common for hemorrhages from an AVM to involve the cerebral parenchyma, this is far less common with aneurysm. Nevertheless, rupture of an aneurysm of the anterior cerebral or middle cerebral artery may direct a jet of blood into brain parenchyma, producing hemiparesis, aphasia, and sometimes transtentorial herniation.

C. Arterial Vasospasm: Arterial vasospasm at or distant from the site of a ruptured aneurysm occurs in more than one-third of cases. It is most common during the first two weeks following the hemorrhage and often produces focal or diffuse neurological signs that progress over 48–96 hours. The deficits are irreversible in about half the patients; the rest recover over a period of days to months. The diagnosis of spasm is confirmed by angiography, which does not itself increase the risk of spasm. Curiously, vasospasm is not a major complication of ruptured AVMs.

D. Acute or Subacute Hydrocephalus: Acute or subacute hydrocephalus may develop during the first day—or after several weeks—as a result of impaired CSF absorption in the subarachnoid space. Progressive somnolence, nonfocal findings, and impaired upgaze should suggest the diagnosis.

E. Seizures: Seizures occur in fewer than 10% of cases and only following damage to the cerebral hemisphere. Decorticate or decerebrate posturing is common, however, and should not be mistaken for seizures.

F. Other Complications: Although inappropriate secretion of antidiuretic hormone and resultant diabetes insipidus can occur, they are uncommon.

Treatment

A. Medical Treatment: Medical treatment is traditionally directed toward preventing elevation of arterial or intracranial pressure that might rerupture the aneurysm or AVM. Typical measures include absolute bed rest with the head of the bed elevated 15–20 degrees, mild sedation and analgesics for headache, stool softeners to prevent straining during defecation, and antitussive drugs, when indicated, to prevent coughing. Since patients who are hypertensive on admission have an increased mortality risk, reducing the blood pressure (to approximately 160/100 mm Hg) is prudent. Bed rest and mild sedation are often adequate in this regard. Hypotension should be prevented, however, to ensure adequate cerebral perfusion. Intravenous fluids should be administered with care, since overhydration can exacerbate cerebral swelling. Prophylactic use of the calcium channel antagonist drug **nimodipine,** 60 mg orally (or by nasogastric tube) every four hours for 21 days, may reduce the sequelae of cerebral vasospasm in patients with a ruptured aneurysm. The antifibrinolytic agent **aminocaproic acid,** 24–36 g/d by continuous intravenous infusion or divided oral doses, has been shown in some studies to reduce the incidence of rebleeding, but this drug increases ischemic complications such as vasospasm and cerebral infarction.

B. Surgical Treatment:

1. Aneurysm–Definitive surgical therapy consists of clipping or wrapping the aneurysm. The neurological examination is used to grade the patient's clinical state relative to surgical candidacy (Table 3–2). In patients who are fully alert (grades I and II) or only mildly confused (grade III), surgery has been shown to improve the clinical outcome. In contrast, stuporous (grade IV) or comatose (grade V) patients do not appear to benefit from the procedures. Although there is some controversy about the optimal timing of surgery, current evidence supports early intervention, within about two days following the hemorrhage. This approach reduces the period at risk for rebleeding and permits aggressive treatment of vasospasm with volume expansion and pharmacological elevation blood pressure.

2. AVMs–Surgically accessible AVMs may be removed by en-bloc resection or obliterated by ligation of feeding vessels or embolization via local intra-arterial catheter. Because the risk of an early second hemorrhage is much less with AVMs than with aneurysms, surgical treatment can be undertaken electively at a convenient time after the bleeding episode.

Prognosis

The mortality rate from aneurysmal subarachnoid hemorrhage is high. About 20% of patients die before reaching a hospital, 25% die subsequently from the initial hemorrhage or its complications, and 20% die from rebleeding if the aneurysm is not surgically cor-

Table 3–2. Clinical grading of patients with aneurysmal subarachnoid hemorrhage.

Grade	Level of Consciousness	Associated Clinical Features	Surgical Candidate
I	Normal	None or mild headache and stiff neck.	Yes
II	Normal	Moderate headache and stiff neck; minimal neurological deficit (eg, cranial nerve palsy) in some cases.	Yes
III	Confusional state	Focal neurological deficits in some cases.	Yes
IV	Stupor	Focal neurological deficits in some cases.	No
V	Coma	Decerebrate posturing in some cases.	No

rected. Most deaths occur in the first few days after the hemorrhage. The probability of survival following aneurysmal rupture is related to the patient's state of consciousness and the elapsed time since the hemorrhage. On day one, the prognosis for survival for symptom-free and somnolent patients is, respectively, 60% and 30%; such patients still alive at one month have survival probabilities of 90% and 60%, respectively. Recovery from subarachnoid hemorrhage resulting from rupture of intracerebral AVMs occurs in nearly 90% of patients, and although recurrent hemorrhage remains a danger, conservative management compares favorably with surgical therapy.

OTHER CEREBROVASCULAR DISORDERS

Headache may be associated with—or may rarely be the presenting symptom of—**thrombotic** or **embolic stroke.** Compression of pain-sensitive structures is the mechanism of headache in **intracranial hemorrhage,** while pain-sensitive receptors in large cerebral arteries are responsible for headache in thrombotic and embolic stroke. Lacunar strokes, which affect small arterial branches deep in the brain, are not as frequently associated with headache.

Headaches associated with ischemic stroke are typically mild to moderate in intensity, ipsilateral to the involved hemisphere, and nonthrobbing in character. Their location is determined by the pain projection sites of the involved arteries: posterior fossa strokes usually present with occipital headache, whereas carotid lesions usually produce frontal (trigeminal distribution) pain. **Transient ischemic attacks** may be associated with headache in as many as 50% of cases; in perhaps one-third of these, headaches precede the other symptoms.

Headache accompanying **retinal artery embolism** or posterior cerebral artery spasm or occlusion may be erroneously diagnosed as migraine because of the associated visual impairment.

Headache also occurs following **carotid endarterectomy** and may be associated with focal sensory or motor signs of contralateral hemispheric ischemia. This syndrome occurs in the presence of a patent carotid artery on the second or third postoperative day

and typically produces intense throbbing anterior headache that is often associated with nausea.

Headache disorders associated with ischemic or hemorrhagic cerebral infarction require direct treatment of the cerebral lesion combined with the use of analgesics for symptomatic relief.

MENINGITIS OR ENCEPHALITIS

Headache is a prominent feature of inflammation of the brain (encephalitis) or its meningeal coverings (meningitis) caused by bacterial, viral, or other infections; granulomatous processes; neoplasms; or chemical irritants. The pain is caused by inflammation of intracranial pain-sensitive structures, including blood vessels at the base of the brain. The headache syndrome produced is commonly throbbing in character, bilateral, and occipital or nuchal in location. The headache is increased by sitting upright, moving the head, compressng the jugular vein, or performing other maneuvers (eg, sneezing, coughing) that transiently increase intracranial pressure. Photophobia may be prominent. The headache rarely presents suddenly but more commonly develops over hours to days, especially with subacute infections (eg, tuberculous meningitis).

Neck stiffness and other signs of meningeal irritation (Figure 3–3) must be sought with care, since they may not be obvious either early in the course of the illness or when the brain parenchyma, rather than meninges, is the predominant site of involvement. Lethargy or confusion may also be a prominent feature.

The diagnosis is suggested by a CSF examination that shows an increased white blood cell count. Bacterial, syphilitic, tuberculous, viral, fungal, and parasitic infections may be distinguished by CSF VDRL, Gram's stain, acid-fast stain, India ink preparation, and cultures (see Table 1–7). Treatment of meningitis or encephalitis caused by these different organisms is discussed in Chapter 1.

OTHER CAUSES OF ACUTE HEADACHE

1. SEIZURES

Postictal headache that follows generalized tonic-clonic seizures is frequently accompanied by resolving lethargy, diffuse muscle soreness, or tongue laceration. Although this headache requires no specific treatment, it is important to differentiate it from subarachnoid hemorrhage and meningitis. If doubt exists, lumbar puncture should be undertaken.

2. LUMBAR PUNCTURE

Post-lumbar-puncture headache is diagnosed by a history of lumbar puncture—and by the characteristic marked increase in pain in the upright position and relief with recumbency. Headache is caused by persistent spinal subarachnoid leak with resultant traction on pain-sensitive structures at the base of the brain. The risk of this complication can be reduced by using a small-gauge needle for the puncture and removing only as much fluid as needed for the studies to be performed. Low-pressure headache syndromes are usually self-limited. When this is not the case, they may respond to the administration of caffeine sodium benzoate, 500 mg intravenously, which can be repeated after 45 minutes if headache persists or recurs upon standing. In persistent cases, the subarachnoid rent can be sealed by injection of autologous blood into the epidural space at the site of the puncture; this requires an experienced anesthesiologist. Headache similar in character to that caused by lumbar puncture occasionally occurs spontaneously.

3. HYPERTENSIVE ENCEPHALOPATHY

Headache may be due to a sudden elevation in blood pressure such as is caused by pheochromocytoma, sexual intercourse, the combination of monoamine oxidase inhibitors and tyramine-containing foods such as cheddar cheese, or—the most important cause—malignant hypertension. Blood pressures of 250/150 mm Hg or higher—characteristic of malignant hypertension—produce cerebral edema and displace pain-sensitive structures. The pain is described as severe and throbbing. Other signs of diffuse or focal central nervous system dysfunction are present, such as lethargy, hemiparesis, or focal seizures. Treatment is with antihypertensive drugs (see Chapter 1), but care must be taken to avoid hypotension, which can result in cerebral ischemia and stroke.

4. COITUS

Headache during sexual intercourse has been described as the presenting sign of subarachnoid hemorrhage; however, headache in this setting is more often of a benign nature. Men are more often affected than women. The pain may be either a dull, bilateral pain occurring during sexual excitement or a severe, sudden headache occurring at the time of orgasm, presumably caused by a marked increase in systemic blood pressure. Persistent headache following orgasm—worse in the upright posture—has also been described. In the latter case, the symptoms are reminiscent of post-lumbar puncture headache and patients have low opening pressures at lumbar puncture. Each of these headaches—except for those associated with aneurysmal rupture—is benign and subsides over minutes to days.

Patients reporting severe headache in association with orgasm should be evaluated for possible subarachnoid hemorrhage as described on p 77. If no hemorrhage is found, prophylactic treatment with indomethacin, 50 mg orally prior to intercourse, may be effective.

5. OCULAR DISORDERS

Pain about the eye may occur in migraine and cluster headache and is also the presenting feature of iritis and glaucoma. **Acute iritis** produces extreme eye pain that is associated with photophobia. The diagnosis is confirmed by slit lamp examination; acute management involves pharmacological dilatation of the pupil. **Angle-closure glaucoma** produces pain within the globe that radiates to the forehead. When it occurs after middle age, such a pain syndrome should prompt diagnostic tonometry. Acute treatment is with glycerol, 1 mL/kg orally, followed by pilocarpine, 2%, 2 drops every 15 minutes.

HEADACHES OF SUBACUTE ONSET

GIANT CELL ARTERITIS

This disorder, also known as temporal arteritis, is characterized by a subacute granulomatous inflammation (consisting of lymphocytes, neutrophils, and giant cells) that affects the external carotid arterial system, particularly the superficial temporal artery and the vertebral artery. Inflammation of the pain-sensitive arterial wall produces the headache. Thrombosis may occur in the most severely affected arteries.

This syndrome, which affects women twice as frequently as men, is uncommon before age 50 and is frequently associated with nonspecific signs and symptoms, such as malaise, myalgia, weight loss, arthralgia, and fever (the polymyalgia rheumatica complex). The headache can be unilateral or bilateral, fairly severe, and boring in quality. It is characteristically localized to the scalp, especially over the temporal arteries. Scalp tenderness may be especially apparent when lying with the head on a pillow or brushing the hair. Pain or stiffness in the jaw during chewing (jaw claudication) is highly suggestive of giant cell arteritis and is due to arterial ischemia in the muscles of mastication. Involvement of the ophthalmic artery leads to permanent blindness in 50% of untreated patients; in half of these, blindness will become bilateral. The visual loss is most often sudden in onset. Although episodes of transient prodromal blindness have been reported, blindness is unusual as an initial symptom; however, it often occurs within the first month.

The diagnosis is made by biopsy of affected temporal arteries, which are characteristically thickened and nonpulsatile as well as dilated and tender. The temporal arteries may be affected in a patchy manner, and multiple biopsies may be necessary to demonstrate histological vasculitis. The erythrocyte sedimentation rate (ESR) is almost invariably elevated. The mean Westergren ESR is about 100 mm/h in giant cell arteritis (range, 29–144 mm/h) and polymyalgia rheumatica (range, 58–160 mm/h). The normal upper limit of the Westergren ESR in elderly patients is reported to be only as high as 40 mm/h.

Consideration of this diagnosis demands prompt inpatient evaluation if vision is to be preserved. Therapy for giant cell arteritis is prednisone, 40–60 mg/d orally, with decreasing dosage usually after about three months, depending upon the clinical response. The sedimentation rate returns rapidly toward normal with prednisone therapy and must be maintained within normal limits as the drug dose is tapered. Therapy should not be withheld pending biopsy diagnosis and should be continued despite negative biopsy findings if the diagnosis can be made with confidence on clinical grounds. Therapy generally needs to be continued for one to two years. Although dramatic improvement in headache occurs within two to three days after institution of therapy, the blindness is usually irreversible.

INTRACRANIAL MASS

The new onset of headache in middle or later life should always raise concern about a mass lesion. A mass lesion, such as a brain tumor (Table 3–3), subdural hematoma, or abscess (see Chapter 11), may or may not produce headache depending upon whether or not it compresses or distorts pain-sensitive intracranial structures. Only 30% of patients with intracranial tumor present with headache as the first symptom, although 80% have such a complaint at the time of diagnosis. Subdural hematoma (see Chapter 11) frequently presents with conspicuous headache, since its large size increases the likelihood of impinging upon pain-sensitive areas. Headaches associated with brain tumors are most often nonspecific in character, mild to moderate in severity, dull and steady in nature, and intermittent. The pain is characteristically aggravated by a change in position or by maneuvers that increase intracranial pressure, such as coughing, sneezing, and straining at stool. The headache is usually maximal on awakening in the morning and is associated with nausea and vomiting.

An uncommon type of headache that suggests brain tumor is characterized by a sudden onset of severe pain reaching maximal intensity within seconds, persisting for minutes to hours, and subsiding rapidly. Altered consciousness or "drop attacks" may be associated. Although classically associated with third ventricular colloid cysts, these paroxysmal headaches can be associated with tumors at many different intracranial sites.

Suspicion of an intracranial mass lesion demands prompt evaluation, preferably with CT scan or MRI. Lumbar puncture should not be used as a diagnostic screening test, since the results are nonspecific and the procedure may aggravate the symptoms of the intracerebral mass, sometimes with a fatal outcome.

PSEUDOTUMOR CEREBRI

Pseudotumor cerebri (benign intracranial hypertension)is characterized by a diffuse increase in intracranial pressure causing headache, papilledema, and diminished visual acuity. Diplopia may also occur as a result of abducens nerve palsy. Although this condition can accompany many disorders (Table 3–4), most cases are idiopathic. In the idiopathic variety, women are affected much more commonly than men, with a peak incidence in the third decade. Diffuse headache is almost always a presenting symptom, and diplopia and blurred vision occur in 60% of cases. Although visual acuity is normal in 50% of patients at presentation, moderate to severe papilledema is seen in almost 90%. Visual loss from increased intracranial pressure can occur even in the idiopathic form; episodes of clouded vision precede the loss.

The course of the idiopathic disorder is generally self-limited over several months, with no sequelae if intracranial pressure is maintained at a relatively normal level to prevent secondary optic atrophy. Differentiating idiopathic pseudotumor cerebri from intracerebral mass lesions and from the disorders listed in Table 3–4 is critical; evaluation must include MRI or CT brain scanning. These studies typically show small (slitlike) ventricles in pseudotumor cerebri. Elevation of intracranial pressure can be documented by lumbar puncture. If a specific cause is identified, it must be treated appropriately.

Table 3–3. Brain tumors: clinical features.

Tumor Type	Incidence[1] Adults	Incidence[1] Children	Clinical Presentation	Diagnosis	Treatment	Comments
Malignant						
Astroglial tumors Astrocytoma	+++	++++	Headache, focal deficits, seizures.	CT, MRI, biopsy.	Resection, irradiation.	Cerebellar astrocytomas in children may be cured.
Anaplastic astrocytoma	+++	++	Headache, focal deficits, seizures.	CT, MRI, biopsy.	Resection, irradiation, chemotherapy.	Distinguished from astrocytoma by greater hypercellularity and pleomorphism and by vascular proliferation.
Glioblastoma multiforme	++++	+	Headache, focal deficits, seizures.	CT, MRI, biopsy.	Resection, irradiation, chemotherapy, brachytherapy[2].	Distinguished from anaplastic astrocytoma by necrosis.
Oligodendroglioma	+	+	Seizures, headache.	CT, MRI, biopsy.	Resection, irradiation, chemotherapy.	Slow-growing; may calcify. Frontal lobe most common site.
Ependymoma	+	++	Lethargy, vomiting, headache.	CT, MRI.	Resection, irradiation.	Fourth ventricle most common site. Spinal axis irradiation indicated for patients >2 years of age.
Medulloblastoma	+	+++	Lethargy, vomiting, headache.	CT, MRI.	Resection, irradiation (>2 years of age), chemotherapy (<2 years of age).	Cerebellum most common site.
Lymphoma	+	+	Lethargy, confusion, focal deficits, seizures.	CT, MRI, biopsy.	Irradiation, chemotherapy.	May be associated with AIDS; about 50% multifocal.
Pineal region tumors	+	+	Lethargy, vomiting, headache, upgaze paralysis, precocious puberty.	CT, MRI, CSF α-fetoprotein, plasma β-HCG[3] or melatonin, biopsy.	Resection, irradiation.	Germ-cell tumors, pinealoma, pinealoblastoma.
Metastatic tumors	++++	+	Headache, focal deficits, seizures.	CT, MRI, biopsy.	Resection (single metastasis), irradiation.	Common primary sources: lung, melanoma, kidney, colon, breast.
Benign						
Meningioma	+++	+	Seizures, focal deficits, headache.	CT, MRI.	Resection, irradiation (for recurrence).	More common in women, especially those with breast cancer. Common sites: parasagittal cerebral convexity, sphenoid ridge.
Pituitary adenoma	++	+	Amenorrhea, galactorrhea, decreased libido, acromegaly, Cushing's syndrome, hypopituitarism, bitemporal visual field cut, headache.	MRI, serum prolactin, plasma growth hormone after oral glucose, plasma corticotropin (including comparison of levels in right and left petrosal sinuses and superior vena cava), high-dose dexamethasone-suppression test.	Transsphenoidal resection, irradiation, bromocriptine (prolactin-secreting tumors), octreotide (growth hormone-secreting tumors).	Prolactin-secreting, growth hormone-secreting, corticotropin-secreting, and non-secreting tumors.

(continued)

Table 3–3 (cont'd). Brain tumors: clinical features.

Tumor type	Incidence[1] Adults	Incidence[1] Children	Clinical Presentation	Diagnosis	Treatment	Comments
Acoustic neuroma	++	+	Hearing loss, vertigo.	MRI, brain stem-evoked potentials, audiometry.	Resection.	Usually unilateral, but bilateral in neurofibromatosis 2 (autosomal dominant).
Craniopharyngioma	+	++	Impaired growth, decreased libido, bitemporal visual field cut.	CT, MRI.	Resection, irradiation.	Congenital; located in suprasellar region. May calcify.
Epidermoid tumor	+	+	Seizures, cranial nerve palsies, headache.	CT, MRI.	Resection.	Common sites: cerebellopontine angle, suprasellar region, fourth ventricle.
Colloid cyst	+	+	Postural headache, loss of consciousness.	CT, MRI.	Transcallosal or transventricular resection; shunting, aspiration.	Congenital; located in anterior part of third ventricle.
Choroid plexus papilloma	+	+	Headache, lethargy, paraparesis.	CT, MRI.	Resection, shunting.	Lateral and fourth ventricles most common sites.
Hemangioblastoma	+	+	Headache, lethargy, ataxia.	CT, MRI.	Resection.	Usually located in cerebellum; associated with von Hippel-Lindau disease. Hematocrit may be increased with erythropoetin-secreting tumors.

[1]++++ indicates >20% of all brain tumors in age group; +++, 10–20%; ++ 5–10%; + 0–5%.
[2]Radioactive implants.
[3]Human chorionic gonadotropin.

Treatment with acetazolamide, 250 mg orally three times daily, with or without a diuretic (eg, furosemide), may be adequate to control mild intracranial hypertension. In other instances, prednisone, 60–80 mg/d orally, may be necessary. In refractory cases, repeated lumbar punctures or lumboperitoneal shunting procedures protect vision and decrease headache. Transorbital optic nerve sheath fenestration is also used to protect the optic nerve from the pressure injury that is thought to cause blindness.

TRIGEMINAL NEURALGIA

Trigeminal neuralgia (tic douloureux)is a facial-pain syndrome of unknown cause that develops in middle to late life. In many instances, the trigeminal nerve roots are close to some vascular structure, and microvascular compression of the nerve is believed to cause the disorder. Pain is confined mainly to the area supplied by the second and third divisions of the trigeminal nerve (Figure 3–6). Involvement of the first division or bilateral disease occurs in less than

5% of cases. Characteristically, lightninglike momentary jabs of excruciating pain occur and spontaneously abate. Occurrence during sleep is rare. Pain-free intervals may last for minutes to weeks, but long-term spontaneous remission is rare. Sensory stimulation of trigger zones about the cheek, nose, or mouth by touch, cold, wind, talking, or chewing can precipitate the pain. Physical examination discloses no abnormalities. Rarely, similar pain may occur in multiple sclerosis or brain stem tumors, and these possibilities should thus be considered in young patients and in all patients who show neurological abnormalities on examination.

In idiopathic cases, CT scan and MRI fail to show any abnormality, and arteriography is similarly normal. Any vascular structure compressing the nerve roots is generally too small to be seen by these means.

Remission of symptoms with carbamazepine, 400–1200 mg/d orally in three divided doses, occurs within 24 hours in such a high percentage of cases that some believe it to be diagnostic. Rarely, blood dyscrasia occurs as an adverse reaction to carbamazepine. Intravenous administration of pheny-

**Table 3–4. Disorders associated
with pseudotumor cerebri.**

Intracranial venous drainage obstruction (eg, venous sinus
thrombosis, head trauma, polycythemia)
Endocrine dysfunction (eg, obesity, especially with marked
menstrual irregularities; pregnancy; menarche; oral contraceptive therapy; withdrawal from steroid therapy; Cushing's
disease; Addison's disease; hypoparathyroidism)
Vitamin and drug therapy (eg, hypervitaminosis A in children
and adolescents; tetracycline in infants)
Other (eg, chronic hypercapnia, congestive heart failure,
chronic meningitis, hypertensive encephalopathy)
Idiopathic

toin, 250 mg, will abort an acute attack, and
phenytoin, 200–400 mg/d orally, may be effective in
combination with carbamazepine if a second drug is
necessary. Posterior fossa microvascular decompressive surgery has been used in drug-resistant cases.

GLOSSOPHARYNGEAL NEURALGIA

Patients with glossopharyngeal neuralgia, an uncommon pain syndrome, present with either a paroxysmal pain that is identical in quality to that of trigeminal neuralgia, or a continuous burning or aching
discomfort. The pain is localized to the oropharynx,
the tonsillar pillars, the base of the tongue, or the au-

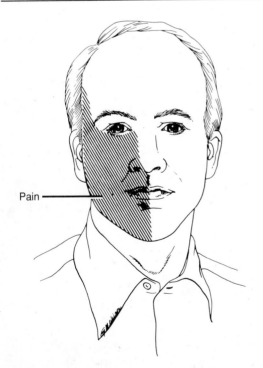

Figure 3–6. Distribution of symptoms in trigeminal
neuralgia.

ditory meatus. The trigger areas are usually around
the tonsillar pillars, so that symptoms are initiated by
swallowing or by talking. Paroxysms of pain can
occur many times daily and may be accompanied by
syncopal episodes caused by transient bradyarrhyth-
mias. Men are affected more often than women, and
symptoms begin at a somewhat younger age than in
trigeminal neuralgia. The diagnosis is established by
the history and by reproducing pain through stimulation of the trigger zones. Examination reveals no abnormal neurological signs. Application of local anesthetics to the trigger area may block the pain
response. Carbamazepine or phenytoin therapy (as
described above for trigeminal neuralgia) usually
produces dramatic relief.

POSTHERPETIC NEURALGIA

Herpes zoster—a vesicular skin eruption in dermatomal distribution, accompanied and followed by
local pain and tenderness—is due to reactivation of
varicella-zoster virus in patients with a history of varicella infection. It becomes increasingly common
with advancing age, in immunocompromised patients, and in patients with certain malignant diseases
(eg, lymphoma). Postherpetic neuralgia is characterized by constant severe stabbing or burning, dyses-
thetic pain that may persist for months or years in a
minority of patients, especially older ones. It occurs
in the same dermatomic distribution as a previous
bout of herpes zoster, conforming to the distribution
of the involved nerve root, where residual scars may
be present. When the head is involved, the first division of the trigeminal nerve is most commonly affected, so that pain is usually localized to the forehead on one side (Figure 3–7). Careful testing of the
painful area reveals decreased cutaneous sensibility
to pinprick. The other major complication of trigeminal herpes is decreased corneal sensation with impaired blink reflex, which can lead to corneal abra-
sion, scarring, and ultimate loss of vision.

The intensity and duration of the cutaneous eruption of herpes zoster are reduced by treatment with
acyclovir, which has not been shown to lessen the
likelihood of postherpetic neuralgia. Corticosteroids
(60 mg/d prednisone, orally for two weeks, with rapid
tapering) taken during the acute herpetic eruption
may reduce the incidence of postherpetic pain, but
their efficacy has been questioned. Once the postherpetic pain syndrome is established, the most useful treatment has been with tricyclic antidepressants
such as amitriptyline, 25–150 mg/d orally, which are
thought to act directly on central nervous system
pain-integration pathways (rather than via an antidepressant effect). Tricyclic antidepressant drugs may
be more effective when combined with a phenothiazine, as in the commercially available preparation
Triavil, which contains perphenazine and amitripty-

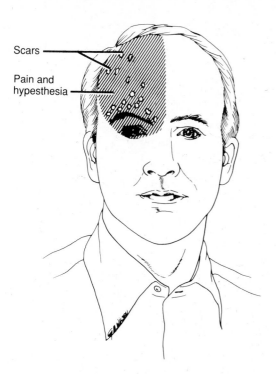

Scars

Pain and hypesthesia

Figure 3–7. Distribution of symptoms and signs in postherpetic neuralgia.

line in combinations of 2 and 10, 4 and 10, 4 and 25, and 4 and 50 mg, respectively. Treatment should be started with a single oral dose at bedtime and the dosage increased as indicated. Relief is often immediate, but treatment may need to be continued indefinitely, since pain often recurs on withdrawal of medication. Patients must be followed cautiously for the development of phenothiazine-induced tardive dyskinesia (see Chapter 8). Fortunately, postherpetic neuralgia subsides within 6–12 months in many patients. Topical application of capsaicin (eg, Zostrix 0.025%) cream, which depletes pain-mediating peptides from peripheral sensory neurons, can also be helpful.

HYPERTENSION

Chronic hypertension is often invoked as a cause of headache, but evidence to support such a connection is sparse. In contrast, headache is a well-established complication of paroxysmal hypertension such as is seen in patients with pheochromocytoma or those ingesting tyramine-rich foods while being treated with monoamine oxidase inhibitors. In pheochromocytoma, headache attacks are brief. They last less than 15 minutes in one-half of patients and are characteristically associated with perspiration and tachycardia. The headache is usually bilateral and may be precipitated by urination if the bladder is involved.

ATYPICAL FACIAL PAIN

Constant, boring, mainly unilateral lower facial pain for which no cause can be found is referred to as atypical facial pain. Unlike trigeminal neuralgia, it is not confined to the trigeminal nerve distribution and is not paroxysmal. This idiopathic disorder must be distinguished from similar pain syndromes related to nasopharyngeal carcinoma, intracranial extension of squamous cell carcinoma of the face, or infection at the site of a tooth extraction. Treatment is with amitriptyline, 20–250 mg/d orally, alone or in combination with phenelzine, 30–75 mg/d orally.

CHRONIC HEADACHES

TENSION HEADACHE

Tension headache is the term used to describe chronic headaches of inapparent cause that lack features characteristic of migraine or cluster headache. The underlying pathophysiological mechanism is unknown, and tension is unlikely to be primarily responsible. Contraction of neck and scalp muscles, which has also been proposed as the cause, is probably a secondary phenomenon. In its classic form (Figure 3–8), tension headache is a chronic disorder that begins after age 20. It is characterized by frequent (often daily) attacks of nonthrobbing, bilateral occipital head pain that is not associated with nausea, vomiting, or prodromal visual disturbance. The pain is sometimes likened to a tight band around the head. Women are more commonly affected than men. Although tension headache and migraine have been traditionally considered distinct disorders, many patients have headaches that exhibit features of both. Thus, some patients who are classified as having tension headaches experience throbbing headaches, unilateral head pain, or vomiting with attacks. In consequence, it may be more accurate to view tension headache and migraine as representing opposite poles of a single clinical spectrum.

Drugs used in the treatment of tension headache include many of the same agents used for migraine (Table 3–5). Acute attacks may respond to aspirin, other nonsteroidal anti-inflammatory drugs, acetaminophen, ergotamine, or dihydroergotamine. For prophylactic treatment, amitriptyline is often effective, and propranolol is useful in some cases. Although many patients respond to benzodiazepines

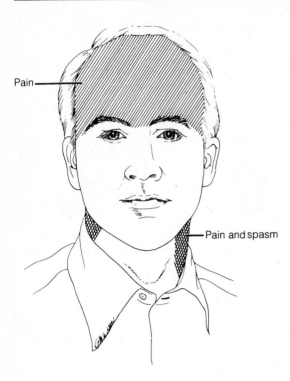

Figure 3–8. Distribution of symptoms and signs in tension headache.

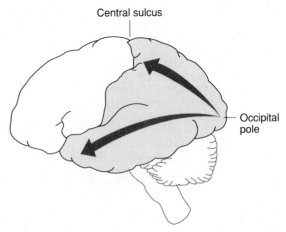

Figure 3–9. Direction of spread (arrows) and maximal extent (stippled region) of depressed cerebral blood flow in classic migraine.

such as diazepam, 5–30 mg/d orally, or chlordiazepoxide, 10–75 mg/d orally, these drugs should be used sparingly because of their addictive potential. Psychotherapy, physical therapy, and relaxation techniques can provide additional benefit in selected cases.

MIGRAINE

Migraine is manifested by headache that is usually unilateral and frequently pulsatile in quality; it is often associated with a visual aura, nausea, vomiting, and photophobia.

Two-thirds to three-fourths of cases of migraine occur in women; the onset is early in life—approximately 25% beginning during the first decade, 55% by 20 years of age, and more than 90% before age 40. A family history of migraine is present in many cases.

Pathogenesis

Intracranial vasoconstriction and extracranial vasodilatation have long been held to be the respective causes of the aura and headache phases of migraine. This theory received support from the efficacy of vasoconstrictive ergot alkaloids (eg, ergotamine) in aborting the acute migraine attack and vasodilators such as amyl nitrite in abolishing the migraine aura. More recent studies of regional cerebral blood flow

during migraine attacks have demonstrated a reduction in regional flow, which begins in the occipital region, during the aura phase of classic migraine. No changes in regional cerebral blood flow occur in common migraine. The reduction in cerebral blood flow, however, spreads according to cytoarchitectural patterns in the cerebral cortex and does not reflect the distribution of major vascular territories (Figure 3–9). In addition, regional cerebral blood flow may remain depressed after focal neurological symptoms have resolved and headache has begun (Figure 3–10). These data imply that vascular abnormalities in migraine may be an epiphenomenon of a primary disturbance in neuronal function.

Serotonergic neurons ramify extensively throughout the brain, and many effective antimigraine drugs act as antagonists or partial agonists at central seroto-

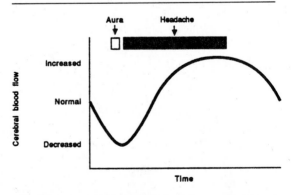

Figure 3–10. Time course of changes in cerebral blood flow in classic migraine. (Adapted from Olesen J et al: Timing and topography of cerebral blood flow, aura, and headache during migraine attacks. *Ann Neurol* 1990;28: 791–798.)

Table 3–5. Drug treatment of migraine headache.

Drug	Route	Strength	Recommended Dose	Comments
Acute treatment				
Simple analgesics				
Aspirin	PO	325 mg.	650–1300 mg.	May cause gastric pain or bleeding.
Naproxen sodium	PO	275, 550 mg.	825–1375 mg.	
Ibuprofen	PO	300, 400, 600, 800 mg.	400–800 mg.	
Acetaminophen[1]	PO	325 mg.	650–1300 mg.	
Ergot preparations				
Ergotamine	Inhaled	0.36 mg per puff.	1–6 puffs; max. 15 per week.	May cause nausea and vomiting; contraindicated by pregnancy or coronary or peripheral vascular disease. Use dihydroergotamine with metoclopramide (see below).
	SL	2 mg.	1–3 tablets; max. 5 per week.	
Ergotamine/caffeine (*Cafergot, Wigraine*)	PO	1/100 mg.	2–6 tablets; max. 10 per week.	
	PR	2/100 mg.	1/4–2 suppositories; max. 5 per week.	
Ergotamine/caffeine, belladonna/pentobarbital (*Cafergot-PB*)	PO	1/100/0.125/30 mg.	2–6 tablets; max. 10 per week.	
	PR	2/100/0.25/60 mg.	1/4–2 suppositories; max. 5 per week.	
Dihydroergotamine	IM, SC, IV	1 mg/mL.	1–2 mg IM or SC. 0.75–1.25 mg IV.	
Narcotic analgesics				
Codeine/aspirin	PO	15, 30, 60/325 mg.	30–120 mg codeine.	
Codeine/acetaminophen	PO	7.5, 15, 30, 60/300 mg.	30–120 mg codeine.	
Meperidine[1]	PO, IM	50, 100 mg.	50–200 mg.	
Other agents				
Sumatriptan	SC	6 mg.	6 mg.	
Isometheptene/dichloralphenazone/acetaminophen (*Midrin*)	PO	65/100/325 mg.	2–5 capsules.	
Caffeine/butalbital/aspirin (*Fiorinal*)	PO	40/50/325 mg.	1–2 tablets or capsules.	
Metoclopramide	PO, IV	5, 10 mg; 5, 10 mg/mL.	10 mg.	Adjunct to treatment; improves enteric drug absorption and reduces nausea.
Prophylactic treatment				
Anti-inflammatory agents				
Aspirin	PO	325 mg.	650 mg bid.	May cause gastric pain or bleeding.
Naproxen sodium	PO	275, 550 mg.	550–825 mg bid.	
Tricyclic antidepressants				
Amitriptyline	PO	10, 25, 50, 75, 100, 150 mg.	10–175 mg hs.	May cause dry mouth, urinary retention, and sedation. Contraindicated in glaucoma or prostatism.
Nortriptyline	PO	10, 25, 50, 75 mg.	10–150 mg hs.	
Doxepin	PO	10, 25, 30, 75, 100, 150 mg.	10–150 mg hs.	
β-receptor antagonists				
Propranolol	PO	10, 20, 40, 60, 80, 90 mg.	20–160 mg bid.	Listed in descending order of efficacy. Symptomatic bradycardia may occur at high doses. Cardioselective agents (atenolol, metoprolol) contraindicated in asthma and congestive heart failure.
	PO (long-acting)	60, 80, 120, 160 mg.	60–320 mg qd.	
Nadolol	PO	40, 80, 120, 160 mg.	40–240 mg qd.	
Atenolol	PO	50, 100 mg.	50–200 mg qd.	
Timolol	PO	10, 20 mg.	10–30 mg bid.	
Metoprolol	PO	50, 100 mg.	50–100 mg bid.	
Ergonovine	PO	0.2 mg.	0.2–0.6 mg tid.	Nausea and vomiting may occur. Contraindicated by pregnancy or coronary or peripheral vascular disease.
Methysergide	PO	2 mg.	2–8 mg qd.	Occurrence of retroperitoneal fibrosis with urethral obstruction and mediastinal fibrosis, although uncommon, should be monitored with creatinine, ultrasound imaging or intravenous urograms, and chest x-rays every six months.

(continued)

Table 3–5 (cont'd). Drug treatment of migraine headache.

Drug	Route	Strength	Recommended Dose	Comments
Cyproheptadine	PO	4 mg.	4–8 mg tid.	Drowsiness common early in treatment.
Calcium channel antagonists				
Verapamil	PO PO (long-acting)	40, 80, 120 mg. 240 mg.	80 mg tid–160 mg qd. 240 mg qd–bid.	Contraindicated by severe left ventricular dysfunction, hypotension, sick sinus syndrome without artificial pacemaker, or second- or third-degree AV nodal heart block. Constipation is most common side effect.
Nimodipine	PO	30 mg.	30 mg qd.	May cause headache, hypotension, edema, flushing.
Nifedipine	PO	10, 20 mg.	10–60 mg tid.	
Diltiazem	PO	30, 60, 90, 120 mg.	60–90 mg qd.	
Other agents				
Ergotamine/phenobarbital/belladonna (*Bellergal-S*)	PO	0.6/40/0.2 mg	1 tablet bid.	May cause nausea and vomiting; contraindicated by pregnancy or coronary or peripheral vascular disease.
Phenelzine	PO	15 mg.	15–90 mg qd.	
Papaverine	PO	100, 150 mg.	150–300 mg bid.	
Phenytoin	PO	30, 50, 100 mg.	200–400 mg qd.	
Valproic acid	PO	125, 250, 500 mg.	250–1,000 mg tid.	

PO = Oral; SL = Sublingual; PR = Rectal; IM = Intramuscular; IV = Intravenous; SC = Subcutaneous.

nin receptors. Serotonin in platelets decreases and urinary serotonin increases during the acute phase of a migraine attack. Depletion of serotonin by reserpine may precipitate migraine. The headache and other manifestations of migraine may thus reflect a disorder of central serotonergic neurotransmission.

Clinical Findings

A. Classic Migraine: Classic migraine headache is preceded by transient neurological symptoms—the aura. The most common auras are visual alterations, particularly hemianopic field defects and scotomas and scintillations that enlarge and spread peripherally (Figure 3–11). A throbbing unilateral headache ensues (Figure 3–12) with or following these prodromal features. The frequency of headache varies, but more than 50% of patients experience no more than one attack per week. The duration of episodes is less than one day in one-half to two-thirds of patients. Remissions are common during pregnancy and after menopause. Occasionally, prodromal symptoms occur without headache (migraine equivalents). Although hemicranial pain is a hallmark of classic migraine, headaches can also be bilateral. Bilateral headache, therefore, does not exclude the diagnosis of migraine, nor does an occipital location—a characteristic commonly attributed to tension headaches. During the headache, prominent associated symptoms include nausea, vomiting, and photophobia. Fluid retention, diarrhea, light-headedness, and fainting also occur, but less often.

B. Common Migraine: The common migraine headache lacks the classic aura, is unilateral less often than the classic type, and is seen more frequently in clinical practice. As in classic migraine, the pain may be described as throbbing. As the pain persists, associated cervical muscle contraction can compound the symptoms. Scalp tenderness is often present during the episode. Vomiting may occasionally terminate the headache.

A useful diagnostic test for both common and classic migraine is reducing headache severity by compressing the ipsilateral carotid or superficial temporal artery.

Precipitating Factors

Migraine attacks can be precipitated by certain foods (tyramine-containing cheeses; meat, such as hot dogs or bacon, with nitrite preservatives; chocolate containing phenylethylamine) and by food additives such as monosodium glutamate, a commonly used flavor enhancer. Fasting, emotion, menses, drugs (especially oral contraceptive agents and vasodilators such as nitroglycerin), and bright lights may also trigger attacks.

Treatment

Acute migraine attacks may respond to simple analgesics (eg, aspirin, acetaminophen). If not, they usually respond to ergot preparations. These drugs (see Table 3–5) must be taken immediately at the onset of symptoms to be maximally effective. Rap-

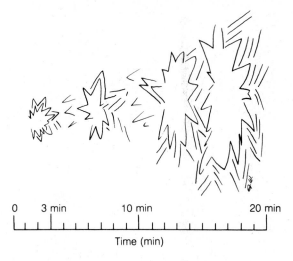

Figure 3–11. Successive maps of scintillating scotoma to show the evolution of fortification figures in a patient with classic migraine.

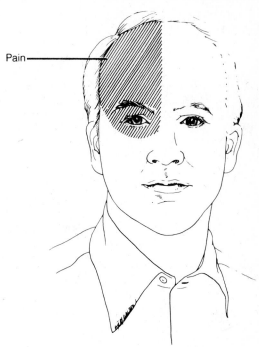

Figure 3–12. Distribution of pain in migraine. Hemicranial pain (the pattern shown) is most common, but the pain can also be holocephalic, bifrontal, or unilateral frontal in distribution or, less commonly, localized to the occiput or the vertex of the skull.

idly absorbed forms (eg, suppository, aerosol) are superior to oral or sublingual preparations. In severe cases, intramuscular or intravenous administration is often most effective. Unfortunately, nausea, which is a prominent feature of migraine, is also a common side effect of the drugs, so that concomitant administration of an antiemetic (eg, metoclopramide, 10 mg orally) may be necessary. Ergot alkaloids are potent vasoconstrictors and are contraindicated in patients with significant hypertension or cardiac disease. Established migraine headaches may respond to dihydroergotamine, sumatriptan, or narcotic analgesics (eg, meperidine, 100 mg intramuscularly).

Several drugs are effective in the prophylactic treatment of migraine (see Table 3–5). Prophylactic treatment is indicated for patients who have frequent attacks—especially more than one per week—and those for whom the ergot alkaloids used for acute treatment are poorly tolerated or contraindicated. Three structurally unrelated agents—propranolol, amitriptyline, and ergonovine—are the mainstays of therapy. Each is effective in a substantial fraction of patients, and patients refractory to one agent may respond to another. The initial choice of medication is usually influenced by consideration of clinical side effects that may be especially troublesome for a particular patient. Propranolol and amitriptyline may be sedating, especially at the onset of treatment. The β-adrenergic-receptor-blocking properties of propranolol often preclude its use in patients with congestive heart failure, asthma, or insulin-dependent diabetes. The anticholinergic actions of amitriptyline may complicate glaucoma and prostatism. Ergonovine may produce gastrointestinal symptoms that could make the drug unacceptable for administration to pa-

tients whose headaches are accompanied by prominent nausea and vomiting.

Calcium channel antagonists such as verapamil and nifedipine are also efficacious in the prophylactic treatment of migraine. Drugs available in other countries or approved in the United States only for other indications include nimodipine and flunarizine; however, both common and classic migraine respond to these drugs. As discussed above, potential side effects should be taken into account in the choice of therapy. Verapamil, which has pronounced effects on cardiac and gastrointestinal calcium channels, may exacerbate atrioventricular nodal heart block and congestive heart failure and frequently causes constipation. Nifedipine and nimodipine, which are more selective for vascular smooth muscle, are associated with a higher incidence of headache, light-headedness, hypotension, and peripheral edema.

CLUSTER HEADACHE

Cluster headache is a common headache syndrome seen much more frequently in men than in women. Cluster headaches characteristically begin at a later age than does migraine, with a mean age at onset of

25 years. There is rarely a family history of such headaches. The syndrome presents as clusters of brief, very severe, unilateral, constant nonthrobbing headaches that last from 10 minutes to a few hours. Unlike migraine headaches, cluster headaches are always unilateral, and usually recur on the same side in any given patient. The headaches commonly occur at night, awakening the patient from sleep, and recur daily, often at nearly the same time of day, for a cluster period of weeks to months. Between clusters, the patient may be free from headaches for months or years.

The headache may begin as a burning sensation over the lateral aspect of the nose or as a pressure behind the eye. Ipsilateral conjunctival injection, lacrimation, nasal stuffiness, and Horner's syndrome are commonly associated with the attack (Figure 3–13). Episodes are often precipitated by the use of alcohol or vasodilating drugs. The response to nitroglycerin challenge, which may be diagnostic, produces a typical headache in 30-60 minutes.

At the onset of a headache cluster, treatment involves measures both to abort the acute attack and to prevent subsequent ones. Acute relief of pain within minutes may be achieved by inhalation of ergotamine tartrate in aerosol form (Table 3–5) or 100% oxygen (8–10 L/min for 10–15 minutes) or by intranasal administration of topical lidocaine (1 mL of 4% solution in the nostril ipsilateral to the pain). Intravenous dihydroergotamine or subcutaneous sumatriptan (Table 3–5) may also be effective.

Several drugs used in the treatment of migraine (see Table 3–5), including ergotamine, dihydroergotamine, methysergide, and calcium channel antagonists are also useful for preventing recurrent symptoms during an active bout of cluster headache. Ergotamine rectal suppositories, inserted at bedtime, may be especially helpful for nocturnal headaches. In addition, dramatic improvement is typically seen with administration of prednisone, 40–80 mg/d orally for one week, discontinued by tapering the dose over the following week. Pain may resolve within hours, and most patients who respond do so within two days. Many neurologists therefore consider prednisone the drug of choice for cluster headache. Alternatively, lithium carbonate or lithium citrate syrup, 300 mg orally three times daily, is highly effective in many cases. Serum lithium levels should be measured at weekly intervals for the first several weeks and should be maintained below 1.2 meq/L to reduce the likelihood of adverse effects. These include disorders of the gastrointestinal (nausea, diarrhea), urinary (polyuria, renal failure), endocrine (hypothyroidism), and nervous (tremor, dysarthria, ataxia, myoclonus, seizures) systems. Chronic rather than episodic cluster headaches may respond dramatically to indomethacin, 25 mg three times daily.

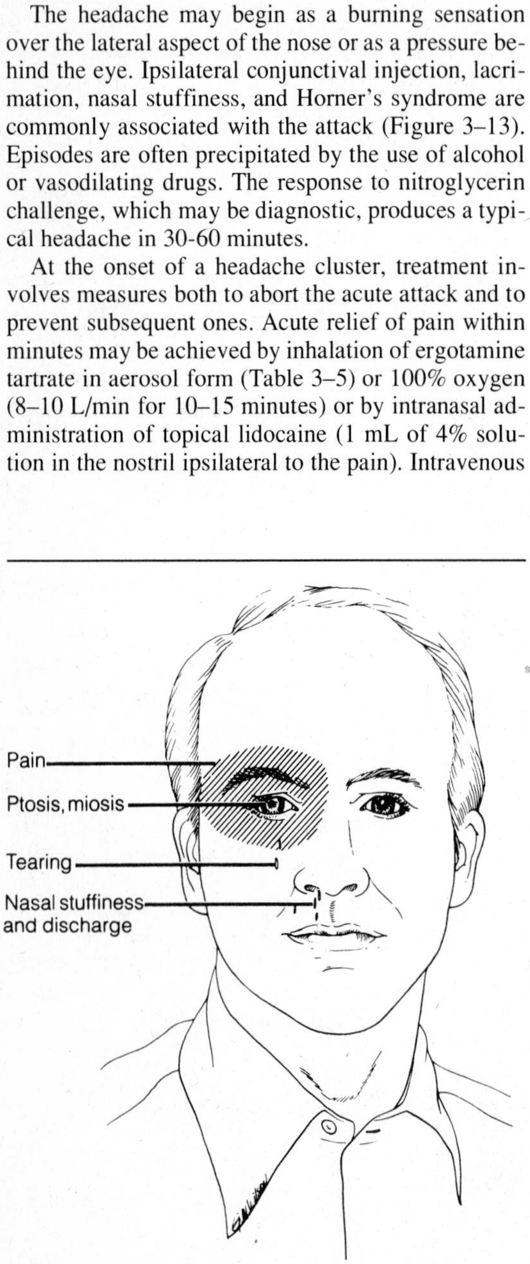

CERVICAL SPINE DISEASE

Injury or degenerative disease processes involving the upper neck can produce pain in the occiput or referred to the orbital regions. The most important source of discomfort is irritation of the second cervical nerve root. In the lower cervical spine, disk disease or abnormalities of the articular processes refer pain to the ipsilateral arm or shoulder, not to the head. Cervical muscle spasm may occur, however.

Acute pain of cervical origin is treated with immobilization of the neck (eg, using a soft collar) and analgesics or anti-inflammatory drugs.

SINUSITIS

Acute sinusitis can produce pain and tenderness localized to the affected frontal or maxillary sinus areas. Inflammation in the ethmoidal or sphenoidal sinuses produces a deep midline pain behind the nose. Sinusitis pain is increased by bending forward and by coughing or sneezing. Tenderness and accentuation of pain on percussion over the frontal or maxillary area are present on examination.

Sinusitis is treated with vasoconstrictor nose drops (eg, phenylephrine, 0.25%, instilled every two to three hours), antihistamines, and antibiotics. In refractory cases, sinus drainage may be necessary.

Figure 3–13. Distribution of symptoms and signs in cluster headache.

Patients who complain of chronic sinus headache rarely have recurrent inflammation of the sinuses; they are much more likely to have migraine or tension headaches.

DENTAL DISEASE

Temporomandibular joint dysfunction is a poorly defined syndrome that is characterized by preauricular facial pain, limitation of jaw movement, tenderness of the muscles of mastication, and "clicking" of the jaw with movement. Symptoms are often associated with malocclusion, bruxism, or clenching of the teeth, and may result from spasm of the masticatory muscles. Some patients benefit from local application of heat, jaw exercises, nocturnal use of a bite guard, or nonsteroidal antiinflammatory drugs.

Infected tooth extraction sites can also give rise to pain, which is characteristically constant, unilateral, and aching or burning in character. Although radiological studies may be normal, injection of a local anesthetic at the extraction site relieves the symptoms. Treatment is with jaw bone curettage and antibiotics.

REFERENCES

Ahlskog JE, O'Neill BP: Pseudotumor cerebri. *Ann Intern Med* 1982;97:249–256.

Black PMcL: Brain tumors. *N Engl J Med* 1991;324:1471–1476,1555-1564.

Goodman BW Jr: Temporal arteritis. *Am J Med* 1979;67:839–852.

Greenberg DA: Calcium channel antagonists and the treatment of migraine. *Clin Neuropharmacol* 1986;9:311–328.

Katusic S et al: Incidence and clinical features of trigeminal neuralgia, Rochester, Minnesota, 1945-1984. *Ann Neurol* 1990;27:89–95.

Lance JW: Headache. *Ann Neurol* 1981;10:1–10.

Lance JW: *Mechanism and Management of Headache,* 4th ed. Butterworths, 1982.

Moskowitz MA: The neurobiology of vascular head pain. *Ann Neurol* 1984;16:157–168.

Olesen J et al: Timing and topography of cerebral blood flow, aura, and headache during migraine attacks. *Ann Neurol* 1990;28:791–798.

Olesen J, Edvinsson L: Migraine: A research field matured for the basic neurosciences. *Trends in Neurosci* 1991;14:3–5.

Portenoy RK, Duma C, Foley KM: Acute herpetic and postherpetic neuralgia: Clinical review and current management. *Ann Neurol* 1986;20:651–664.

Raskin NH: Chemical headaches. *Annu Rev Med* 1981;32:63–71.

Raskin NH: Headaches associated with organic diseases of the nervous system. *Med Clin North Am* 1978;62:459–466.

Raskin NH: *Headache,* 2nd ed. Churchill Livingstone, 1988.

Rushton JG, Stevens JC, Miller RH: Glossopharyngeal (vagoglossopharyngeal) neuralgia: A study of 217 cases. *Arch Neurol* 1981;38:201–205.

The Subcutaneous Sumatriptan International Study Group: Treatment of migraine attacks with sumatriptan. *N Engl J Med* 1991;325:316–321.

The Sumatriptan Cluster Headache Study Group: Treatment of acute cluster headache with sumatriptan. *N Engl J Med* 1991;325:322–326.

4

Disorders of Equilibrium

APPROACH TO DIAGNOSIS

Equilibrium is the ability to maintain orientation of the body and its parts in relation to external space. It depends upon the continuous provision of visual, labyrinthine, and proprioceptive information and its integration in the brain stem and cerebellum.

Disorders of equilibrium result from diseases that affect central or peripheral vestibular pathways, the cerebellum, or the sensory pathways involved in proprioception. Such disorders usually present with one of two clinical problems: **vertigo** or **ataxia**.

1. VERTIGO

Vertigo is the illusion of movement of the body or the environment, sometimes additionally defined as either rotatory or unidirectional. It is often associated with other symptoms, such as **impulsion** (a sensation that the body is being hurled or pulled in space), **oscillopsia** (a visual illusion of moving back and forth), nausea, vomiting, diaphoresis, or gait ataxia.

Distinction Between Vertigo & Other Symptoms

Vertigo must be distinguished from nonvertiginous dizziness, which includes sensations often described by patients as light-headedness, faintness, or giddiness not associated with an illusion of movement. In contrast to vertigo, these sensations are produced by conditions that impair the brain's supply of blood, oxygen, or glucose—eg, excessive vagal stimulation, orthostatic hypotension, cardiac arrhythmias, myocardial ischemia, hypoxia, or hypoglycemia—and may culminate in loss of consciousness (**syncope;** see Chapter 9).

Differential Diagnosis

A. Anatomic Origin: Once vertigo is identified as the problem, the first step in diagnosis is to localize the pathological process in the peripheral or central vestibular pathways (see Figure 4–1).

Peripheral **vestibular lesions** affect the labyrinth of the inner ear or the vestibular division of the acoustic (VIII) nerve. **Central lesions** affect the brain stem vestibular nuclei or their connections. Rarely, vertigo is of **cortical** origin, occurring as a symptom associated with complex partial seizures.

B. Symptomatology: Certain characteristics of vertigo and the associated abnormalities can help differentiate between peripheral and central causes (Table 4–1).

1. Peripheral vertigo tends to occur intermittently, last for briefer periods, and produce more distress than does vertigo of central origin. **Nystagmus** (rhythmic oscillation of the eyeballs) is always associated with peripheral vertigo; it is usually unidirectional and never vertical (see below). Peripheral lesions commonly produce additional symptoms of inner ear or acoustic nerve dysfunction, ie, hearing loss and tinnitus.

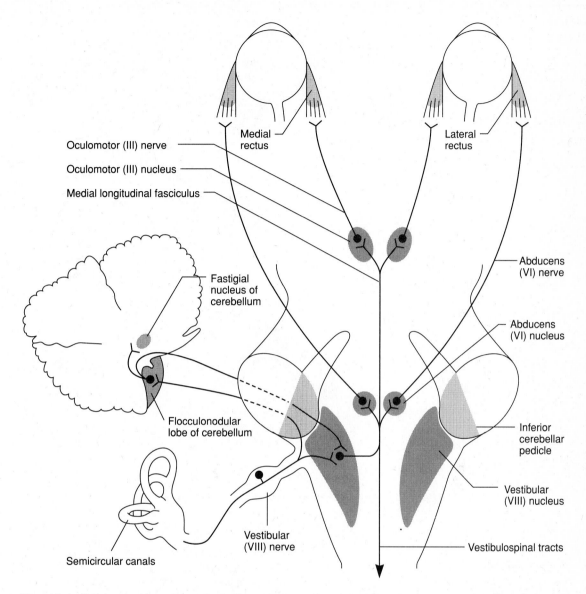

Figure 4–1. Peripheral and central vestibular pathways. The vestibular nerve terminates in the vestibular nucleus of the brain stem and in midline cerebellar structures that also project to the vestibular nucleus. From here, bilateral pathways in the medial longitudinal fasciculus ascend to the abducens and oculomotor nuclei and descend to the spinal cord.

2. Nystagmus may be absent with central vertigo; if present, it can be vertical, unidirectional, or multidirectional, and may differ in character in the two eyes. (Vertical nystagmus is oscillation in a vertical plane; that produced by upgaze or downgaze is not necessarily in the vertical plane.) Central lesions may produce intrinsic brain stem or cerebellar signs, such as motor or sensory deficits, hyperreflexia, extensor plantar responses, dysarthria, or limb ataxia.

2. ATAXIA

Ataxia is incoordination or clumsiness of movement that is not the result of muscular weakness. It is caused by vestibular, cerebellar, or sensory (proprioceptive) disorders. Ataxia can affect eye movement, speech, individual limbs, the trunk, or gait (Table 4–2).

Vestibular Ataxia

Vestibular ataxia results from the same central and peripheral lesions that cause vertigo. Nystagmus is frequently present, typically unilateral, and most pro-

Table 4–1. Characteristics of central and peripheral vertigo.

	Peripheral	Central
Vertigo	Often intermittent; severe.	Often constant; usually less severe.
Nystagmus	Always present; unidirectional, never vertical.	May be absent; uni- or bidirectional, may be vertical.
Associated findings		
Hearing loss or tinnitus	Often present.	Rarely present.
Intrinsic brain stem signs	Absent.	Typically present.

nounced on gaze away from the side of vestibular involvement. Dysarthria does not occur.

Vestibular ataxia is gravity-dependent: Incoordination of limb movements cannot be demonstrated when the patient is examined lying down but becomes apparent when the patient attempts to stand or walk.

Cerebellar Ataxia

Cerebellar ataxia is produced by lesions of the cerebellum itself or its afferent or efferent connections in the cerebellar peduncles, pons, or red nucleus (Figure 4–2). Because of the crossed connection between the frontal cerebral cortex and the cerebellum, unilateral frontal disease can occasionally mimic a disorder of the contralateral cerebellar hemisphere. The clinical manifestations of cerebellar ataxia consist of irregularities in the rate, rhythm, amplitude, and force of voluntary movements.

A. Hypotonia: Cerebellar ataxia is commonly associated with hypotonia, which results in defective posture maintenance. Limbs are easily displaced by a relatively small force and, when shaken by the examiner, exhibit an increased range of excursion. The range of arm swing during walking may be similarly increased. Tendon reflexes take on a pendular quality, so that several oscillations of the limb may occur after the reflex is elicited. When muscles are contracted against resistance that is then removed, the antagonist muscle fails to check the movement and compensatory

muscular relaxation does not ensue promptly. This results in **rebound** movement of the limb.

B. Incoordination: In addition to hypotonia, cerebellar ataxia is associated with incoordination of voluntary movements. Simple movements are delayed in onset, and their rates of acceleration and deceleration are decreased. The rate, rhythm, amplitude, and force of movements fluctuate, producing a jerky appearance. Because these irregularities are most pronounced during initiation and termination of movement, their most obvious clinical manifestations include **terminal dysmetria,** or "overshoot," when the limb is directed at a target, and terminal **intention tremor** as the limb approaches the target. More complex movements tend to become decomposed into a succession of individual movements rather than a single smooth motor act **(asynergia).** Movements that involve rapid changes in direction or greater physiological complexity, such as walking, are most severely affected.

C. Associated Ocular Abnormalities: Because of the cerebellum's prominent role in the control of eye movements, ocular abnormalities are a frequent consequence of cerebellar disease. These include nystagmus and related ocular oscillations, gaze pareses, and defective saccadic and pursuit movements.

D. Anatomical Basis of Distribution of Clinical Signs: Various anatomical regions of the cerebellum (Figure 4–3) are functionally distinct, corresponding to the somatotopic organization of their motor, sensory, visual, and auditory connections (Figure 4–4).

1. Midline lesions–The middle zone of the cerebellum—the vermis and flocculonodular lobe and their associated subcortical (fastigial) nuclei—is involved in the control of axial functions, including eye movements, head and trunk posture, stance, and gait. Midline cerebellar disease therefore results in a clinical syndrome characterized by nystagmus and other disorders of ocular motility, oscillation of the head and trunk **(titubation),** instability of stance, and gait ataxia (Table 4–3). Selective involvement of the superior cerebellar vermis, as commonly occurs in alcoholic cerebellar degeneration, leads exclusively or

Table 4–2. Characteristics of vestibular, cerebellar, and sensory ataxia.

	Vestibular	Cerebellar	Sensory
Vertigo	Present.	May be present.	Absent.
Nystagmus	Present.	Often present.	Absent.
Dysarthria	Absent.	May be present.	Absent.
Limb ataxia	Absent.	Usually present (one limb, unilateral, legs only, or all limbs).	Present (typically legs only).
Stance	May be able to stand with feet together; typically worse with eyes closed.	Unable to stand with feet together and eyes either open or closed.	Often able to stand with feet together and eyes open but not with eyes closed (Romberg's sign).
Vibratory and position sense	Normal.	Normal.	Impaired.
Ankle reflexes	Normal.	Normal.	Depressed or absent.

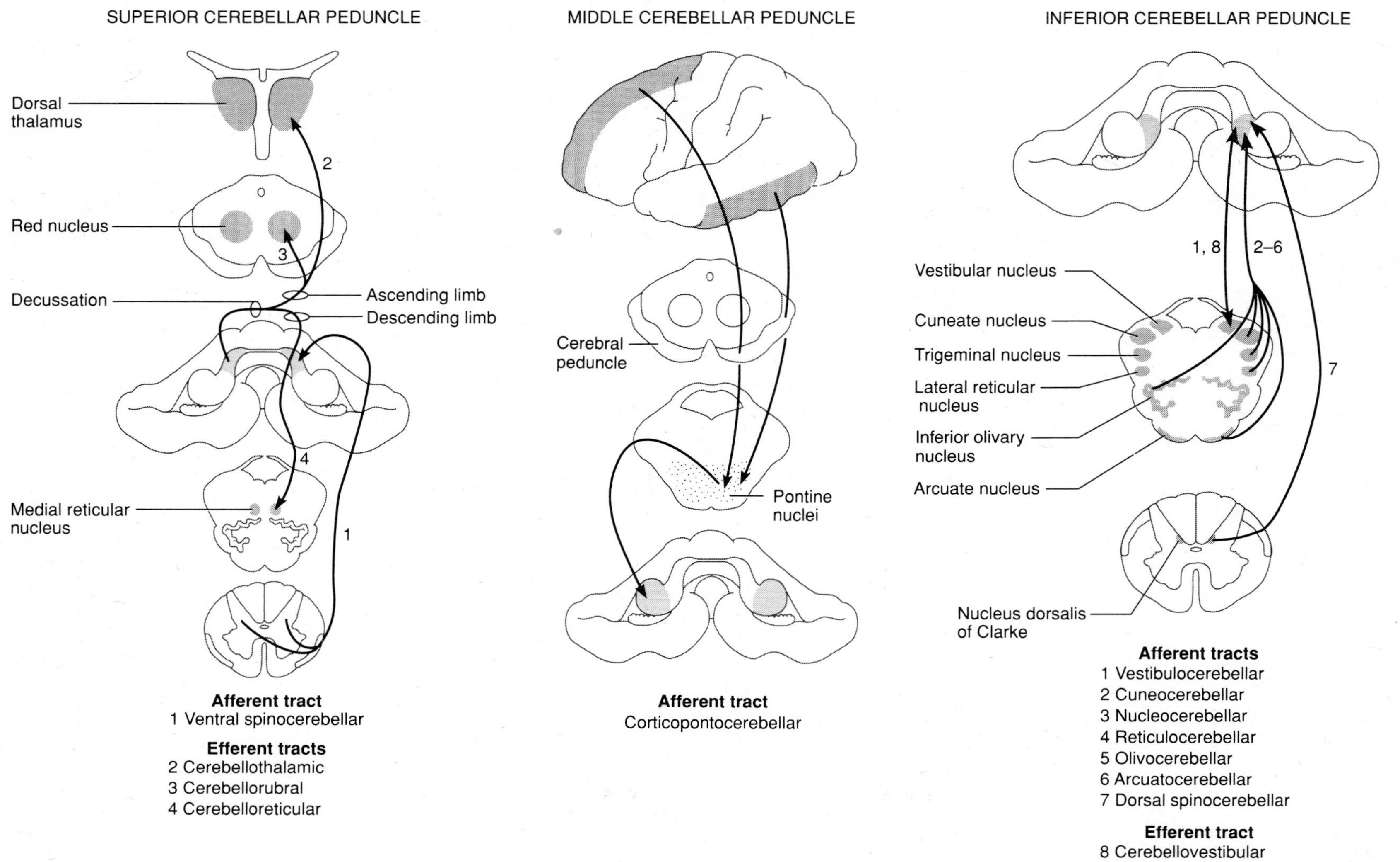

SUPERIOR CEREBELLAR PEDUNCLE

Dorsal thalamus

Red nucleus

Ascending limb
Descending limb

Decussation

Medial reticular nucleus

Afferent tract
1 Ventral spinocerebellar

Efferent tracts
2 Cerebellothalamic
3 Cerebellorubral
4 Cerebelloreticular

MIDDLE CEREBELLAR PEDUNCLE

Pontine nuclei

Cerebral peduncle

Afferent tract
Corticopontocerebellar

INFERIOR CEREBELLAR PEDUNCLE

Vestibular nucleus

Cuneate nucleus

Trigeminal nucleus

Lateral reticular nucleus

Inferior olivary nucleus

Arcuate nucleus

Nucleus dorsalis of Clarke

Afferent tracts
1 Vestibulocerebellar
2 Cuneocerebellar
3 Nucleocerebellar
4 Reticulocerebellar
5 Olivocerebellar
6 Arcuatocerebellar
7 Dorsal spinocerebellar

Efferent tract
8 Cerebellovestibular

8 The peduncles are

Figure 4–2. Cerebellar connections in the superior, middle, and inferior cerebellar peduncles. The peduncles are indicated by light shading and the areas to and from which they project by dark shading.

A

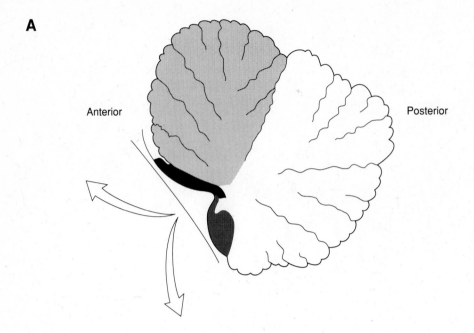

Anterior

Posterior

B

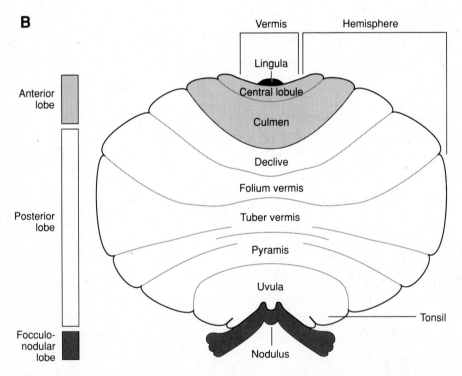

Vermis   Hemisphere

Lingula

Central lobule

Culmen

Declive

Folium vermis

Tuber vermis

Pyramis

Uvula

Tonsil

Nodulus

Anterior
lobe

Posterior
lobe

Focculo-
nodular
lobe

Figure 4–3. Anatomical divisions of the cerebellum in midsagittal view **(A)**; unfolded (arrows) and viewed from behind **(B)**.

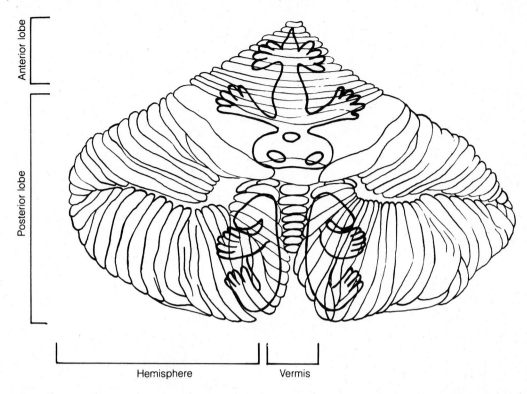

Figure 4–4. Functional organization of the cerebellum. The view is similar to that in Figure 4–3B, but is of a monkey rather than a human cerebellum. The three cerebellar homunculi represent areas to which proprioceptive and tactile stimuli project; the auditory and visual stimuli project to the head of the anterior (upper) homunculus and adjacent areas.

primarily to ataxia of gait, as would be predicted from the somatotopic map of the cerebellum (Figure 4–4).

2. Hemispheric lesions–The lateral zones of the cerebellum are represented by the cerebellar hemispheres, each of which helps to coordinate movements and maintain tone in the ipsilateral limbs. The hemispheres also have a role in regulating ipsilateral gaze. Disorders affecting one hemisphere

cause ipsilateral hemiataxia and hypotonia as well as nystagmus and transient ipsilateral gaze paresis (an inability to look voluntarily toward the affected side). Cerebellar dysarthria, traditionally considered a manifestation of midline cerebellar disease, may correlate more closely with paramedian lesions in the left cerebellar hemisphere.

3. Diffuse disease–Many cerebellar disorders —typically toxic, metabolic, and degenerative condi-

Table 4–3. Clinical patterns of cerebellar ataxia.

Pattern of Involvement	Signs	Causes
Midline	Nystagmus, head and trunk titubation, gait ataxia	Tumor, multiple sclerosis
Superior vermis	Gait ataxia	Wernicke's encephalopathy, alcoholic cerebellar degeneration, tumor, multiple sclerosis
Cerebellar hemisphere	Nystagmus, ipsilateral gaze paresis, dysarthria (especially left hemisphere lesion), ipsilateral hypotonia, ipsilateral limb ataxia, gait ataxia, falling to side of lesion	Infarction, hemorrhage, tumor, multiple sclerosis
Pancerebellar	Nystagmus, bilateral gaze paresis, dysarthria, bilateral hypotonia, bilateral limb ataxia, gait ataxia	Drug intoxications, hypothyroidism, idiopathic cerebellar degeneration, paraneoplastic cerebellar degeneration, Wilson's disease, infections and parainfectious encephalomyelitis, Creutzfeldt-Jakob disease, multiple sclerosis

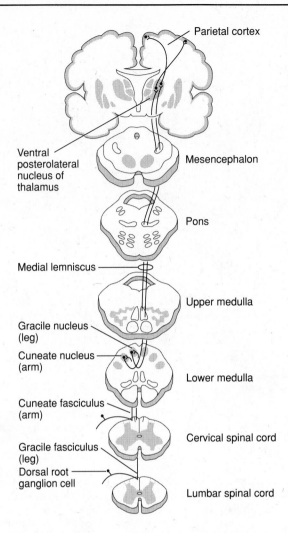

Parietal cortex

Ventral posterolateral nucleus of thalamus

Mesencephalon

Pons

Medial lemniscus

Upper medulla

Gracile nucleus (leg)

Cuneate nucleus (arm)

Lower medulla

Cuneate fasciculus (arm)

Cervical spinal cord

Gracile fasciculus (leg)

Dorsal root ganglion cell

Lumbar spinal cord

Figure 4–5. Pathway mediating proprioceptive sensation.

tions—affect the cerebellum diffusely. The clinical picture in such states combines the features of midline and bilateral hemisphere disease.

Sensory Ataxia

Sensory ataxia results from disorders that affect the proprioceptive pathways in peripheral sensory nerves, sensory roots, posterior columns of the spinal cord, or medial lemnisci. Thalamic and parietal lobe lesions are rare causes of contralateral sensory hemiataxia. Sensations of joint position and movement (**kinesthesis**) originate in pacinian corpuscles and unencapsulated nerve endings in joint capsules, ligaments, muscle, and periosteum. Such sensations are transmitted via heavily myelinated A fibers of primary afferent neurons, which enter the dorsal horn of the spinal cord and ascend uncrossed in the posterior columns (Figure 4–5). Proprioceptive information from the legs is conveyed in the medially placed fasciculus gracilis, that from the arms in the more laterally situated fasciculus cuneatus. These tracts synapse on second-order sensory neurons in the nucleus gracilis and nucleus cuneatus in the lower medulla. The second-order neurons decussate as internal arcuate fibers and ascend in the contralateral medial lemniscus. They terminate in the ventral posterior nucleus of the thalamus, from which third-order sensory neurons project to the parietal cortex.

Sensory ataxia from polyneuropathy or posterior column lesions typically affects the gait and legs in symmetric fashion; the arms are involved to a lesser extent or spared entirely. Examination reveals impaired sensations of joint position and movement in the affected limbs, and vibratory sense is also commonly disturbed. Vertigo, nystagmus, and dysarthria are characteristically absent.

HISTORY

Symptoms & Signs

A. Vertigo: True vertigo must be distinguished from a light-headed or presyncopal sensation. Vertigo is typically described as spinning, rotating, or moving, but when the description is vague, association with the illusion of movement must be asked about specifically. The circumstances under which symptoms occur may also be diagnostically helpful. Vertigo is often brought on by changes in head position. The occurrence of symptoms upon arising after prolonged recumbency is a common feature of orthostatic hypotension, and nonvertiginous dizziness related to pancerebral hypoperfusion may be immediately relieved by sitting or lying down. Such hypoperfusion states can lead to loss of consciousness, which is rarely associated with true vertigo. If the problem is identified as vertigo, associated symptoms may help to localize the site of involvement. Complaints of hearing loss or tinnitus strongly suggest a disorder of the peripheral vestibular apparatus (labyrinth or acoustic nerve). Dysarthria, dysphagia, diplopia, or focal weakness or sensory loss affecting the face or limbs indicates the likelihood of a central (brain stem) lesion.

B. Ataxia: Ataxia associated with vertigo suggests a vestibular disorder; whereas numbness or tingling in the legs is common in patients with sensory ataxia. Because proprioceptive deficits may, to some extent, be compensated for by other sensory cues, patients with sensory ataxia may report that their balance is improved by watching their feet when they walk or by using a cane or the arm of a companion for support. They thus find that they are much more unsteady in the dark and may experience particular difficulty in descending stairs.

Onset & Time Course

Establishing the time course of the disorder may suggest its cause. **Sudden** onset of disequilibrium occurs with infarcts and hemorrhages in the brain stem or cerebellum (eg, lateral medullary syndrome, cerebellar hemorrhage or infarction). **Episodic** disequilibrium of acute onset suggests transient ischemic attacks in the basilar artery distribution, benign positional vertigo, or Ménière's disease. Disequilibrium from transient ischemic attacks is usually accompanied by cranial nerve deficits, neurological signs in the limbs, or both. Ménière's disease is usually associated with hearing loss and tinnitus as well as vertigo.

Chronic, progressive disequilibrium evolving over weeks to months is most suggestive of a toxic or nutritional disorder (eg, vitamin B_{12} or vitamin E deficiency, nitrous oxide exposure). Evolution over months to years is characteristic of idiopathic spinocerebellar, olivopontocerebellar, or cerebellar parenchymal degeneration.

Prior Medical History

The medical history should be scrutinized for evidence of diseases that affect the sensory pathways (vitamin B_{12} deficiency, syphilis) or cerebellum (hypothyroidism, paraneoplastic syndromes, tumors), and drugs that produce disequilibrium by impairing vestibular or cerebellar function (ethanol, sedative drugs, phenytoin, aminoglycoside antibiotics, quinine, salicylates).

Family History

A hereditary degenerative disorder may be the cause of chronic, progressive cerebellar ataxia. Such disorders include idiopathic cerebellar and olivopontocerebellar degenerations, Friedreich's ataxia, ataxia-telangiectasia, and Wilson's disease.

GENERAL PHYSICAL EXAMINATION

Various features of the general physical examination may provide clues as to the underlying disorder. **Orthostatic hypotension** is associated with certain sensory disorders that produce ataxia—eg, tabes dorsalis, polyneuropathies—and with some cases of olivopontocerebellar degeneration. The **skin** may show oculocutaneous telangiectasia (ataxia-telangiectasia); it may be dry, with brittle hair (hypothyroidism) or have a lemon-yellow coloration (vitamin B_{12} deficiency). **Pigmented corneal (Kayser-Fleischer) rings** are seen in Wilson's disease (see Figure 8–10).

Skeletal abnormalities may be present. Kyphoscoliosis is typically present in Friedreich's ataxia; hypertrophic or hyperextensible joints are common in tabes dorsalis; and pes cavus is a feature of certain hereditary neuropathies. Abnormalities at the craniocervical junctions may be associated with Arnold-Chiari malformations or other congenital anomalies that involve the posterior fossa.

NEUROLOGICAL EXAMINATION

Mental Status Examination

An **acute confusional state** with ataxia characterizes ethanol, sedative, or hallucinogen intoxication and Wernicke's encephalopathy.

Dementia with cerebellar ataxia is seen in Wilson's disease, Creutzfeldt-Jakob disease, hypothyroidism, paraneoplastic syndromes, and some types of idiopathic cerebellar degeneration. Dementia with sensory ataxia suggests syphilitic taboparesis or vitamin B_{12} deficiency.

Korsakoff's amnestic syndrome and cerebellar ataxia are associated with chronic alcoholism.

Stance & Gait

Observation of stance and gait is helpful in distinguishing between cerebellar, vestibular, and sensory ataxias. In any ataxic patient, the stance and gait are wide-based and unsteady, often associated with reeling or lurching movements.

A. Stance: The ataxic patient asked to stand with the feet together may show great reluctance or an inability to do so. With persistent urging, the patient may gradually move the feet closer together but will leave some space between them. Patients with sensory ataxia and some with vestibular ataxia are able to stand with the feet together, compensating for the loss of one source of sensory input (proprioceptive or labyrinthine) with another (visual). Patients with cerebellar ataxia cannot. This compensation is demonstrated when the patient closes the eyes, eliminating visual cues. With sensory or vestibular disorders, unsteadiness increases and may result in falling (**Romberg's sign**). With a vestibular lesion, the tendency is to fall toward the side of the lesion. Patients with cerebellar ataxia are unstable on their feet whether the eyes are open or closed.

B. Gait:

1. The gait seen in **cerebellar ataxia** is wide-based, often with a staggering quality that might suggest drunkenness. Oscillation of the head or trunk (**titubation**) may be present. If a unilateral cerebellar hemisphere lesion is responsible, there is a tendency to deviate toward the side of the lesion when the patient attempts to walk in a straight line or circle or marches in place with eyes closed. Tandem (heel-to-toe) gait, which requires walking with an exaggeratedly narrow base, is always impaired.

2. In **sensory ataxia,** the gait is also wide-based and tandem gait is poor. In addition, walking is typically characterized by lifting the feet high off the ground and slapping them down heavily (**steppage gait**) because of impaired proprioception. Stability may be dramatically improved by letting the patient use a cane or lightly rest a hand on the examiner's arm for support. If the patient is made to walk in the dark or with eyes closed, gait is much more impaired.

3. Gait ataxia may also be a manifestation of **conversion disorder** or **malingering.** Determining this can be particularly difficult, since isolated gait ataxia without ataxia of individual limbs can also be produced by diseases that affect the superior cerebellar vermis. The most helpful observation in identifying factitious gait ataxia is that such patients often exhibit wildly reeling or lurching movements from which they are able to recover without falling. In fact, recovery of balance from such awkward positions requires excellent equilibratory function.

Oculomotor (III), Trochlear (IV), Abducens (VI), & Acoustic (VIII) Nerves

Abnormalities of ocular and vestibular nerve function are typically present with vestibular disease and often present with lesions of the cerebellum. (Examination of cranial nerves III, IV, and VI is discussed in more detail in Chapter 5.)

A. Ocular Alignment: The eyes are examined in the primary position of gaze (looking directly forward) to detect malalignment in the horizontal or vertical plane.

B. Nystagmus and Voluntary Eye Movements: The patient is asked to turn the eyes in each of the cardinal directions of gaze (left, up and left, down and left, right, up and right, down and right; see Figure 5–5) to determine whether gaze paresis (impaired ability to move the two eyes coordinately in any of the cardinal directions of gaze) or gaze-evoked nystagmus is present. Nystagmus—an abnormal involuntary oscillation of the eyes—is characterized in terms of the positions of gaze in which it occurs, its amplitude, and the direction of its fast phase. **Pendular nystagmus** has the same velocity in both directions of eye movement; **jerk nystagmus** is characterized by both fast (vestibular-induced) and slow (cortical) phases. The direction of jerk nystagmus is defined by the direction of the fast component. Fast voluntary eye movements (**saccades**) are elicited by having the patient rapidly shift gaze from one target to another placed in a different part of the visual field. Slow voluntary eye movements (**pursuits**) are assessed by having the patient track a slowly moving target such as the examiner's finger.

1. Peripheral vestibular disorders produce unidirectional horizontal jerk nystagmus that is maximal on gaze away from the involved side. Central vestibular disorders can cause unidirectional or bidirectional horizontal nystagmus, vertical nystagmus, or gaze paresis. Cerebellar lesions are associated with a wide range of ocular abnormalities, including gaze pareses, defective saccades or pursuits, nystagmus in any or all directions, and **ocular dysmetria** (overshoot of visual targets during saccadic eye movements).

2. Pendular nystagmus is usually the result of visual impairment that begins in infancy.

C. Hearing: Preliminary examination of the acoustic (VIII) nerve should include otoscopic inspection of the auditory canals and tympanic membranes, assessment of auditory acuity in each ear, and Weber and Rinne tests performed with a 256-Hz tuning fork.

1. In the **Weber test,** unilateral sensorineural hearing loss (from lesions of the cochlea or cochlear nerve) causes the patient to perceive the sound produced by a vibrating tuning fork placed at the vertex of the skull as coming from the normal ear. With a conductive (external or middle ear) disorder, sound is localized to the abnormal ear.

2. The **Rinne test** may also distinguish between sensorineural and conductive defects in the affected ear. Air conduction (tested by holding the vibrating tuning fork next to the external auditory canal) normally produces a louder sound than does bone conduction (tested by placing the base of the tuning fork over the mastoid bone). This pattern also occurs with

Table 4–4. Assessment of hearing loss.

	Weber Test	Rinne Test
Normal	Sound perceived as coming from midline	Air conduction > bone conduction
Sensorineural hearing loss	Sound perceived as coming from normal ear	Air conduction > bone conduction
Conductive hearing loss	Sound perceived as coming from affected ear	Bone conduction > air conduction on affected side

acoustic nerve lesions but is reversed in the case of conductive hearing loss (Table 4–4).

D. Positional Tests: When patients indicate that vertigo occurs with a change in position, the Nylen-Bárány maneuver (Figure 4–6) is used to try to reproduce the precipitating circumstance. The head, turned to the right, is rapidly lowered 30 degrees below horizontal while the gaze is maintained to the right. This process is repeated with the head and eyes turned first to the left and then straight ahead. The eyes are observed for nystagmus, and the patient is asked to note the onset, severity, and cessation of vertigo.

Positional nystagmus and **vertigo** are usually associated with peripheral vestibular lesions and are most often a feature of an idiopathic self-limited disorder termed **benign positional vertigo.** This is typically characterized by severe distress, a latency of several seconds between assumption of the position and the onset of vertigo and nystagmus, a tendency for the response to remit spontaneously (fatigue) as the position is maintained, and attenuation of the response (habituation) as the offending position is repeatedly assumed (Table 4–5). Positional vertigo can also occur with central vestibular disease.

E. Caloric Testing: Disorders of the vestibulo-ocular pathways can be detected by caloric testing. The patient is placed supine with the head elevated 30 degrees to bring the superficially situated lateral semicircular canal into the upright position. Each ear canal is irrigated in turn with cold (33°C) or warm (44°C) water for 40 seconds, with at least five minutes between tests. Warm water tends to produce less discomfort than cold. *Caution:* Caloric testing should be preceded by careful otoscopic examination; it is precluded if the tympanic membrane is perforated.

1. In the normal awake patient, cold-water caloric stimulation produces nystagmus with the slow phase toward and the fast phase away from the irrigated ear. Warm water irrigation produces the opposite response.

2. In patients with unilateral labyrinthine, vestibu-

Table 4–5. Characteristics of positional nystagmus.

Feature	Peripheral Lesion	Central Lesion
Vertigo	Severe	Mild
Latency	2–40 seconds	No
Fatigability	Yes	No
Habituation	Yes	No

lar nerve, or vestibular nuclear dysfunction, irrigation of the affected side fails to cause nystagmus or elicits nystagmus that is later in onset or briefer in duration than on the normal side.

Other Cranial Nerves

Papilledema associated with disequilibrium suggests an intracranial mass lesion, usually in the posterior fossa, that is causing increased intracranial pressure. Optic neuropathy may be present in multiple sclerosis, neurosyphilis, or vitamin B_{12} deficiency. A depressed corneal reflex or facial palsy ipsilateral to the lesion (and the ataxia) can accompany cerebellopontine angle tumor. Weakness of the tongue or palate, hoarseness, or dysphagia results from lower brain stem disease.

Motor System

Examination of motor function in the patient with a disorder of equilibrium should determine the pattern and severity of ataxia and disclose any associated pyramidal, extrapyramidal, or peripheral nerve involvement that might suggest a cause.

A. Ataxia and Disorders of Muscle Tone: Muscle tone is assessed as discussed in Chapter 6. Truncal stability is assessed with the patient in the sitting position, and the limbs are examined individually.

1. Movement of the patient's arm is observed as his or her finger tracks back and forth between his or her own nose or chin and the examiner's finger. With mild cerebellar ataxia, an intention tremor characteristically appears near the beginning and end of each such movement, and the patient may overshoot the target.

2. When the patient is asked to raise the arms rapidly to a given height—or when the arms, extended and outstretched in front of the patient, are displaced by a sudden force—there may be overshoot (rebound). Impaired ability to check the force of muscular contractions can also be demonstrated by having the patient forcefully flex the arm at the elbow against resistance—and then suddenly removing the resistance. If the limb is ataxic, continued contraction without resistance may cause the hand to strike the patient at the shoulder or in the face.

3. Ataxia of the legs is demonstrated by the supine patient's inability to run the heel of the foot smoothly up and down the opposite shin.

4. Ataxia of any limb is reflected by irregularity in

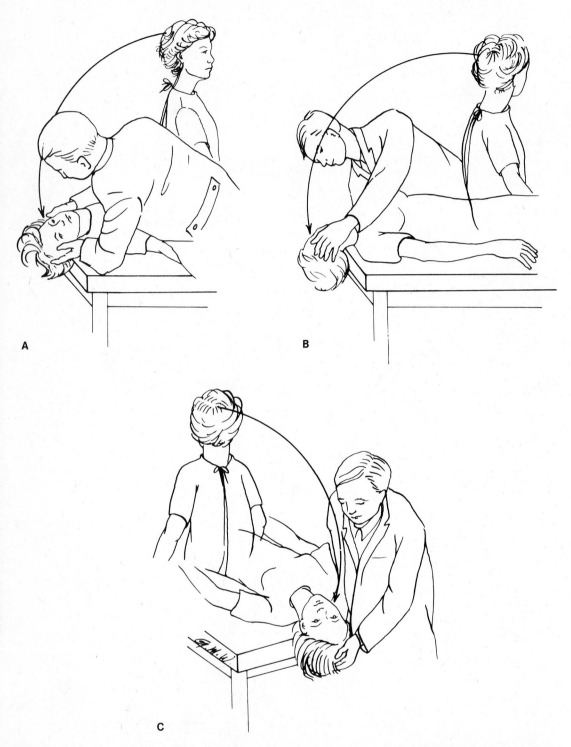

Figure 4–6. Test for positional vertigo and nystagmus. The patient is seated on a table with the head and eyes turned to the right **(A)**, and then quickly lowered to a supine position with the head over the table's edge, 30 degrees below horizontal. The patient's eyes are then observed for nystagmus, and the patient is asked to report any vertigo. The test is repeated with the patient's head and eyes turned to the left **(B)**, and again with the head and eyes straight ahead **(C)**.

the rate, rhythm, amplitude, and force of rapid successive tapping movements.

5. Hypotonia is characteristic of cerebellar disorders; with unilateral cerebellar hemispheric lesions, the ipsilateral limbs are hypotonic.

6. Extrapyramidal hypertonia (rigidity) occurs with cerebellar ataxia in Wilson's disease, acquired hepatocerebral degeneration, Creutzfeldt-Jakob disease, and certain types of olivopontocerebellar degeneration.

7. Ataxia with spasticity may be seen in multiple sclerosis, posterior fossa tumors or congenital anomalies, vertebrobasilar ischemia or infarction, olivopontocerebellar degeneration, Friedreich's and other hereditary ataxias, neurosyphilis, Creutzfeldt-Jakob disease, and vitamin B_{12} deficiency.

B. Weakness: The pattern of any weakness should be determined. **Distal neuropathic weakness** can be caused by disorders that produce sensory ataxia, such as polyneuropathies and Friedreich's ataxia. **Paraparesis** may be superimposed on ataxia in vitamin B_{12} deficiency, multiple sclerosis, foramen magnum lesions, or spinal cord tumors. **Ataxic quadriparesis, hemiataxia** with **contralateral hemiparesis,** or **ataxic hemiparesis** suggests a brain stem lesion.

C. Abnormal Involuntary Movements: Asterixis may occur in hepatic encephalopathy, acquired hepatocerebral degeneration, or other metabolic encephalopathies. **Myoclonus** occurs in the same conditions as asterixis and is a prominent manifestation of Creutzfeldt-Jakob disease. **Chorea** may be associated with cerebellar signs in Wilson's disease, acquired hepatocerebral degeneration, or ataxiatelangiectasia.

Sensory System

A. Joint Position Sense: In patients with sensory ataxia, joint position sense is always impaired in the legs and may be defective in the arms as well. Testing is accomplished by asking the patient to detect passive movement of the joints, beginning distally and moving proximally, to establish the upper level of deficit in each limb. Abnormalities of position sense can also be demonstrated by positioning one limb and having the patient, with eyes closed, place the opposite limb in the same position.

B. Vibratory Sense: Perception of vibratory sensation is frequently impaired in patients with sensory ataxia. The patient is asked to detect the vibration of a 128-Hz tuning fork placed over a bony prominence. Again, successively more proximal sites are tested to determine the upper level of the deficit in each limb or over the trunk. The patient's threshold for appreciating the vibration is compared with the examiner's own ability to detect it in the hand that holds the tuning fork.

Reflexes

Tendon reflexes are typically hypoactive, with a pendular quality, in cerebellar disorders; unilateral cerebellar lesions produce ipsilateral hyporeflexia. Hyporeflexia of the legs is a prominent manifestation of Friedreich's ataxia, tabes dorsalis, and polyneuropathies that cause sensory ataxia. Hyperactive reflexes and extensor plantar responses may accompany ataxia caused by multiple sclerosis, vitamin B_{12} deficiency, focal brain stem lesions, and certain olivopontocerebellar or spinocerebellar degenerations.

INVESTIGATIVE STUDIES

Blood Studies

Blood studies may disclose the hematological abnormalities associated with vitamin B_{12} deficiency, the decreased levels of thyroid hormones in hypothyroidism, the elevated hepatic enzymes and low ceruloplasmin and copper concentrations in Wilson's disease, or the immunoglobulin deficiency and elevated alpha-fetoprotein in ataxia-telangiectasia. It may also be possible to detect antibodies to Purkinje cell antigens in the blood of patients with paraneoplastic cerebellar degeneration.

Cerebrospinal Fluid Studies

The cerebrospinal fluid shows elevated protein with cerebellopontine angle tumors (eg, acoustic neuroma), brain stem or spinal cord tumors, hypothyroidism, and some polyneuropathies. Increased protein with pleocytosis is commonly found with infectious or parainfectious encephalitis, paraneoplastic cerebellar degeneration, and neurosyphilis. Although elevated pressure and bloody CSF characterize cerebellar hemorrhage, lumbar puncture is contraindicated if cerebellar hemorrhage is suspected. CSF VDRL is reactive in tabes dorsalis, and oligoclonal IgG bands may be present in multiple sclerosis or other inflammatory disorders.

Imaging

The **CT scan** is useful for demonstrating posterior fossa tumors or malformations, cerebellar infarction or hemorrhage, and cerebellar atrophy associated with degenerative disorders. **Magnetic resonance imaging** provides better visualization of posterior fossa lesions, including cerebellopontine angle tumors, and is superior to CT scanning for detecting the lesions of multiple sclerosis.

Evoked Potential Testing

Evoked potential testing, especially of optic pathways (visual evoked potentials), may be helpful in evaluating patients with suspected multiple sclerosis. Brain stem auditory evoked potentials may be abnormal in patients with cerebellopontine angle tumors even though CT scans show no abnormality.

Chest X-Ray & Echocardiography

The chest x-ray or echocardiogram may provide evidence of cardiomyopathy associated with Friedreich's ataxia. The chest x-ray may also show a lung tumor in paraneoplatic cerebellar degeneration.

Special Studies

In vestibular disorders, three additional special investigations may be of help.

A. Audiometry: This is useful when vestibular disorders are associated with auditory impairment; such testing can distinguish conductive, labyrinthine, acoustic nerve, and brain stem disease.

Tests of pure tone hearing are abnormal when sounds are transmitted through air with conductive hearing loss and when transmitted through either air or bone with labyrinthine or acoustic nerve disorders.

Speech discrimination is markedly impaired with acoustic nerve lesions, less so with disorders of the labyrinth. Speech discrimination is normal in conductive or brain stem involvement.

B. Electronystagmography (ENG): This test can be used to detect and characterize nystagmus, including that elicited by caloric stimulation.

C. Auditory Evoked Response: This test can localize vestibular disease to the peripheral vestibular pathways.

PERIPHERAL VESTIBULAR DISORDERS

A list of peripheral vestibular disorders and features helpful in the differential diagnosis is presented in Table 4–6.

BENIGN POSITIONAL VERTIGO

Positional vertigo is vertigo that occurs upon assuming a particular head position. It is usually associated with peripheral vestibular lesions but may also be due to central (brain stem or cerebellar) disease.

Benign positional vertigo is the most common cause of vertigo of peripheral origin, accounting for about 30% of cases. The most frequently identified cause is head trauma, but in most instances, no cause can be determined.

The syndrome is characterized by brief (seconds to minutes) episodes of severe vertigo that may be accompanied by nausea and vomiting. Symptoms may occur with any change in head position but are usu-

Table 4–6. Differential diagnosis of peripheral vestibular disorders.

	Hearing Loss		Other Cranial Nerve Palsies
	Conductive	Sensorineural	
Benign positional vertigo	–	–	–
Ménière's disease	–	+	–
Acute peripheral vestibulopathy	–	–	–
Otosclerosis	+	+	–
Head trauma	±	±	±
Cerebellopontine angle tumor	–	+	±
Toxic vestibulopathy			
Alcohol	–	–	–
Aminoglycosides	–	+	–
Salicylates	–	+	–
Quinine	–	+	–
Acoustic (VIII) neuropathy			
Basilar meningitis	–	+	±
Hypothyroidism	–	+	–
Diabetes	–	+	±
Paget's disease of the skull (osteitis deformans)	–	+	±

ally most severe in the lateral decubitus position with the affected ear down. Episodic vertigo typically continues for several weeks and then resolves spontaneously; in some cases it is recurrent. Hearing loss is not a feature.

Peripheral and central causes of positional vertigo can usually be distinguished on physical examination by means of the Nylen-Bárány maneuver (discussed earlier; see Figure 4–6). Positional nystagmus always accompanies vertigo in the benign disorder and is typically unidirectional, rotatory, and delayed in onset by several seconds after assumption of the precipitating head position. If the position is maintained, nystagmus and vertigo resolve within seconds to minutes. If the maneuver is repeated successively, the response is attenuated. In contrast, positional vertigo of central origin tends to be less severe, and positional nystagmus may be absent. There is no latency, fatigue, or habituation in central positional vertigo.

If treatment is required, the drugs listed in Table 4–7 can be used. It should be noted that antihistamines, anticholinergics, and benzodiazepines often produce sedation and that benzodiazepines and am-

Table 4–7. Drugs used in the treatment of vertigo.[1]

Drug	Dosage
Antihistamines	
Meclizine	25 mg PO q4–6h
Promethazine	25–50 mg PO, IM, or PR q4–6h
Dimenhydrinate	50 mg PO or IM q4–6h or 100 mg PR q8h
Anticholinergics	
Scopolamine	0.6 mg PO q4–6h or 0.5 mg transdermally q3d
Benzodiazepines	
Diazepam	5–10 mg PO or IM q4–6h
Sympathomimetics	
Amphetamine	5–10 mg PO q4–6h
Ephedrine	25 mg PO q4–6h

[1]Adapted from Baloh RW, Honrubia V: *Clinical Neurophysiology of the Vestibular System,* 2nd ed. Vol 32 of: Contemporary Neurology Series. Davis, 1990.

phetamines should be used for only brief periods because of their addictive potential.

MÉNIÈRE'S DISEASE

Ménière's disease is characterized by repeated episodes of vertigo lasting from minutes to days, accompanied by tinnitus and progressive sensorineural hearing loss. Onset is between the ages of 20 and 50 years in about three-fourths of cases, and men are affected more often than women. The cause is thought to be an increase in the volume of labyrinthine endolymph (endolymphatic hydrops), but the pathogenetic mechanism is unknown.

At the time of the first acute attack, patients may already have noted the insidious onset of tinnitus, hearing loss, and a sensation of fullness in the ear. Acute attacks are characterized by vertigo, nausea, and vomiting and recur at intervals ranging from weeks to years. Hearing deteriorates in a stepwise fashion, with bilateral involvement reported in 10–70% of patients. As hearing loss increases, vertigo tends to become less severe.

Physical examination during an acute episode shows spontaneous horizontal or rotatory nystagmus (or both) that may change direction. Although spontaneous nystagmus is characteristically absent between attacks, caloric testing usually reveals impaired vestibular function. The hearing deficit is not always sufficiently advanced to be detectable at the bedside. Audiometry shows low-frequency pure-tone hearing loss, however, that fluctuates in severity as well as impaired speech discrimination and increased sensitivity to loud sounds.

As has been noted, episodes of vertigo tend to resolve as hearing loss progresses. Therapies of value include the drugs listed in Table 4–7 and in persistent, disabling, drug-resistant cases, surgical proce-

dures such as endolymphatic shunting, labyrinthectomy, or vestibular nerve section.

ACUTE PERIPHERAL VESTIBULOPATHY

This term is used to describe a spontaneous attack of vertigo of inapparent cause that resolves spontaneously and is not accompanied by hearing loss or evidence of central nervous system dysfunction. It includes disorders diagnosed as acute labyrinthitis or vestibular neuronitis, which are based on unverifiable inferences about the site of disease and the pathogenetic mechanism. A recent antecedent febrile illness can sometimes be identified, however.

The disorder is characterized by vertigo, nausea, and vomiting of acute onset, typically lasting up to two weeks. Symptoms may recur, and some degree of vestibular dysfunction may be permanent.

During an attack, the patient—who appears ill—typically lies on one side with the affected ear upward and is reluctant to move his or her head. Nystagmus with the fast phase away from the affected ear is always present. The vestibular response to caloric testing is defective in one or both ears with about equal frequency. Auditory acuity is normal.

Acute peripheral vestibulopathy must be distinguished from central disorders that produce acute vertigo, such as stroke in the posterior cerebral circulation. Central disease is suggested by vertical nystagmus, altered consciousness, motor or sensory deficit, or dysarthria. Treatment is with the drugs listed in Table 4–7.

OTOSCLEROSIS

Otosclerosis is caused by bony changes in the tympanic cavity that result in immobility of the **stapes,** the ear ossicle that normally transmits sound-induced vibration of the tympanic membrane to the inner ear. Its most distinctive clinical feature is conductive hearing loss, but sensorineural hearing loss and vertigo are also common; tinnitus occurs less frequently. Auditory symptoms usually begin before 30 years of age, and familial occurrence is common.

Vestibular dysfunction in otosclerosis is most often characterized by recurrent episodic vertigo—with or without positional vertigo—and a sense of positional imbalance. More continuous symptoms may also occur, and the frequency and severity of attacks may increase with time.

Vestibular abnormalities that can be seen on examination include spontaneous or positional nystagmus of the peripheral type and attenuated caloric responses. Abnormalities shown by caloric testing are usually unilateral.

Hearing loss is always demonstrable by audiometry. Usually of mixed conductive-sensorineural character, the loss is bilateral in about two-thirds of patients.

In patients with episodic vertigo, progressive hearing loss, and tinnitus, otosclerosis must be distinguished from Ménière's disease. Otosclerosis (rather than Ménière's disease) is suggested by a positive family history, a tendency toward onset at an earlier age, the presence of conductive hearing loss, or bilateral symmetric auditory impairment. The CT scan may also be diagnostically useful.

Medical treatment with a combination of sodium fluoride, calcium gluconate, and vitamin D may be effective. If not, surgical stapedectomy should be considered.

HEAD TRAUMA

Head trauma is the most common identifiable cause of benign positional vertigo. Injury to the labyrinth is usually responsible for posttraumatic vertigo; however, fractures of the petrosal bone may lacerate the acoustic nerve, producing vertigo and hearing loss. Hemotympanum or CSF otorrhea suggests such a fracture.

CEREBELLOPONTINE ANGLE TUMOR

The cerebellopontine angle is a triangular region in the posterior fossa bordered by the cerebellum, the lateral pons, and the petrous ridge (Figure 4–7). By far the most common tumor in this area is the histologically benign **acoustic neuroma** (also termed **neurilemoma**, **neurinoma**, or **schwannoma**), which typically arises from the neurilemmal sheath of the vestibular portion of the acoustic nerve in the internal auditory canal. Less common tumors at this site include **meningiomas** and primary **cholesteatomas** (epidermoid cysts). Symptoms are produced by compression or displacement of the cranial nerves, brain stem, and cerebellum and by obstruction of CSF flow. Because of their anatomic relationship to the acoustic nerve (see Figure 4–7), the trigeminal (V) and facial (VII) nerves are often affected.

Acoustic neuromas occur most often as isolated lesions in patients 30–60 years old, but they may also be a manifestation of neurofibromatosis. **Neurofibromatosis 1 (von Recklinghausen's disease)** is a common autosomal dominant disorder related to a gene defect on chromosome 17 (17q11.2). In addition to unilateral acoustic neuromas, neurofibromatosis 1 is associated with cafe au lait spots on the skin, cutaneous neurofibromas, axillary or inguinal freckles, optic gliomas, iris hamartomas, and dysplastic bony lesions. **Neurofibromatosis 2** is a rare autosomal dominant disorder localized to chromosome 22 (22q11.1–13.1). Its hallmark is bilateral acoustic neuromas, which may be accompanied by other tumors of the central or peripheral nervous system, including neurofibromas, meningiomas, gliomas, and schwannomas.

Clinical Findings

A. Symptoms and Signs: Hearing loss of insidious onset is usually the initial symptom. Less often, patients present with headache, vertigo, gait ataxia, facial pain, tinnitus, a sensation of fullness in the ear, or facial weakness. Although vertigo ultimately develops in 20–30% of patients, a nonspecific feeling of unsteadiness is encountered more commonly. In contrast to Ménière's disease, there is a greater tendency for mild vestibular symptoms to persist between attacks. Symptoms may be stable or progress very slowly for months or years.

Unilateral hearing loss of the sensorineural type is the most common finding on physical examination. Other frequently noted abnormalities are ipsilateral facial palsy, depression or loss of the corneal reflex, and sensory loss over the face. Ataxia, spontaneous nystagmus, other lower cranial nerve palsies, and signs of increased intracranial pressure are less common. Unilateral vestibular dysfunction can usually be demonstrated with caloric testing.

Laboratory Findings: Audiometry shows a sensorineural pattern of deficit with high-frequency pure tone hearing loss, poor speech discrimination, and marked tone decay. CSF protein is elevated in about 70% of patients, usually in the range of 50–200 mg/dL. The most useful diagnostic radiologic study is MRI of the cerebellopontine angle. CT scanning is less sensitive. Acoustic neuromas sometimes can cause abnormalities of the brain stem auditory evoked potentials at a time when radiological studies show no abnormalities.

Differential Diagnosis

Acoustic neuroma must be distinguished from other cerebellopontine angle tumors, the most common being meningioma and cholesteatoma. Meningioma should be considered in patients whose initial symptoms indicate more than isolated acoustic nerve disease. Cholesteatoma is suggested by conductive hearing loss, early facial weakness, or facial twitching, with normal CSF protein. Metastatic carcinoma may also present as a lesion in the cerebellopontine angle.

Treatment

Treatment is complete surgical excision. In untreated cases, severe complications may result from brain stem compression or hydrocephalus.

TOXIC VESTIBULOPATHIES

Several drugs can produce vertigo by their effects on the peripheral vestibular system.

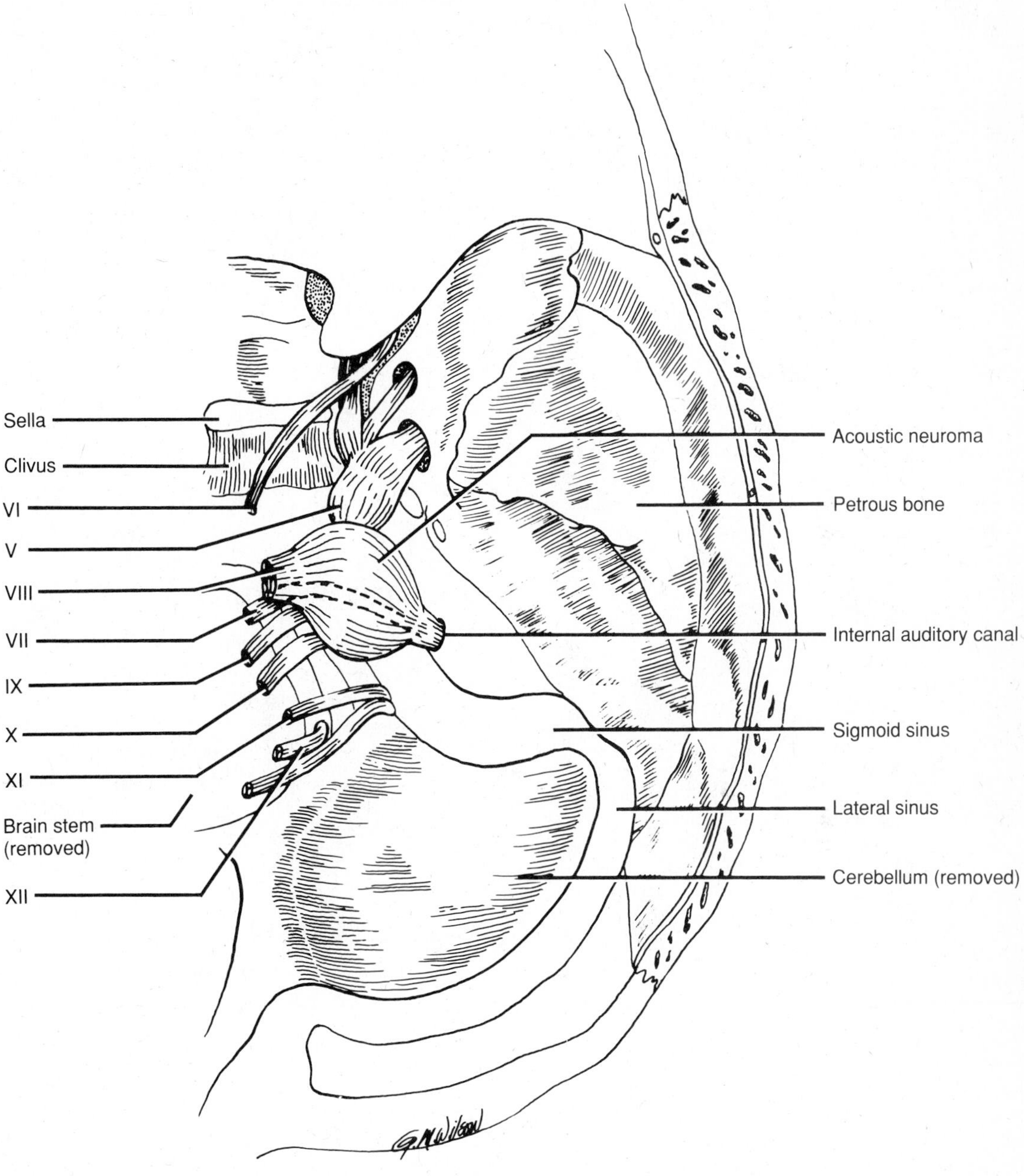

Figure 4–7. Cerebellopontine angle tumor, viewed from above, with the brain removed to show the cranial nerves and base of the skull. The tumor, a neuroma arising from the acoustic (VIII) nerve, can compress adjacent structures, including the trigeminal (V) and facial (VII) nerves, the brain stem and the cerebellum.

1. ALCOHOL

Alcohol causes an acute syndrome of positional vertigo because of its differential distribution between the cupula and endolymph of the inner ear. Alcohol initially diffuses into the cupula, reducing its density relative to the endolymph. This difference in density makes the peripheral vestibular apparatus un-

usually sensitive to gravity and thus to position. With time, alcohol also diffuses into the endolymph, and the densities of cupula and endolymph equalize, eliminating the gravitational sensitivity. As the blood alcohol level declines, alcohol leaves the cupula before it leaves the endolymph. This produces a second phase of gravitational sensitivity that persists until the alcohol diffuses out of the endolymph also.

Alcohol-induced positional vertigo typically occurs within two hours after ingesting ethanol in amounts sufficient to produce blood levels in excess of 40 mg/dL. It is characterized clinically by vertigo and nystagmus in the lateral recumbent position and is accentuated when the eyes are closed. The syndrome lasts up to about 12 hours and consists of two symptomatic phases separated by an asymptomatic interval of one to two hours. Other signs of alcohol intoxication, such as spontaneous nystagmus, dysarthria, and gait ataxia, are caused primarily by cerebellar dysfunction.

2. AMINOGLYCOSIDES

Aminoglycoside antibiotics are widely recognized ototoxins that can produce both vestibular and auditory symptoms. Streptomycin, gentamicin, and tobramycin are the agents most likely to cause vestibular toxicity, amikacin, kanamycin and tobramycin are associated with hearing loss. Aminoglycosides concentrate in the perilymph and endolymph and exert their ototoxic effects by destroying sensory hair cells. The risk of toxicity is related to drug dosage, plasma concentration, duration of therapy, conditions—such as renal failure—that impair drug clearance, preexisting vestibular or cochlear dysfunction, and concomitant administration of other ototoxic agents.

Symptoms of vertigo, nausea, vomiting, and gait ataxia may begin acutely; physical findings include spontaneous nystagmus and the presence of Romberg's sign. The acute phase typically lasts for one to two weeks and is followed by a period of gradual improvement. Prolonged or repeated aminoglycoside therapy may be associated with a chronic syndrome of progressive vestibular dysfunction.

3. SALICYLATES

Salicylates, when used chronically and in high doses, can cause vertigo, tinnitus, and sensorineural hearing loss—all usually reversible when the drug is discontinued. Symptoms result from cochlear and vestibular end-organ damage. Chronic salicylism is characterized by headache, tinnitus, hearing loss, vertigo, nausea, vomiting, thirst, hyperventilation, and sometimes a confusional state. Severe intoxication may be associated with fever, skin rash, hemorrhage, dehydration, seizures, psychosis, or coma. The characteristic laboratory findings are a high plasma salicylate level (about or above 0.35 mg/mL) and combined metabolic acidosis and respiratory alkalosis.

Measures for treating salicylate intoxication include gastric lavage, administration of activated charcoal, forced diuresis, peritoneal dialysis or hemodialysis, and hemoperfusion.

4. QUININE & QUINIDINE

Both quinine and quinidine can produce the syndrome of cinchonism, which resembles salicylate intoxication in many respects. The principal manifestations are tinnitus, impaired hearing, vertigo, visual deficits (including disorders of color vision), nausea, vomiting, abdominal pain, hot flushed skin, and sweating. Fever, encephalopathy, coma, and death can occur in severe cases. Symptoms result from either overdosage or idiosyncratic reactions (usually mild) to a single small dose of quinine.

5. *CIS*-PLATINUM

This antineoplastic drug causes ototoxicity in about 50% of patients. Tinnitus, hearing loss, and vestibular dysfunction are most likely to occur with cumulative doses of 3–4 mg/kg; they may be reversible if the drug is discontinued.

ACOUSTIC NEUROPATHY

Involvement of the acoustic nerve by systemic disease is an uncommon cause of vertigo. **Basilar meningitis** from bacterial, syphilitic, or tuberculous infection or sarcoidosis can lead to compression of the acoustic and other cranial nerves, but hearing loss is a more common consequence than vertigo. Metabolic disorders associated with acoustic neuropathy include **hypothyroidism, diabetes,** and **Paget's disease.**

CEREBELLAR & CENTRAL VESTIBULAR DISORDERS

Many disorders can produce acute or chronic cerebellar dysfunction (Table 4–8). Several of these conditions may also be associated with central vestibular disorders, particularly Wernicke's encephalopathy, vertebrobasilar ischemia or infarction, multiple sclerosis, and posterior fossa tumors.

Table 4–8. Differential diagnosis of cerebellar ataxia.

Acute
    Drug intoxications: ethanol, sedative-hypnotics, anticon-
        vulsants, hallucinogens
    Wernicke's encephalopathy[1]
    Vertebrobasilar ischemia or infarction[1]
    Cerebellar hemorrhage
    Inflammatory disorders

Chronic
    Multiple sclerosis[1,2]
    Alcoholic cerebellar degeneration
    Phenytoin-induced cerebellar degeneration
    Hypothyroidism
    Paraneoplastic cerebellar degeneration
    Idiopathic cerebellar and olivopontocerebellar
        degeneration
    Friedreich's ataxia[2]
    Ataxia-telangiectasia
    Wilson's disease
    Acquired hepatolenticular degeneration
    Creutzfeldt-Jakob disease
    Posterior fossa tumor[1]
    Posterior fossa malformations

[1]May also be associated with central vestibular dysfunction.
[2]May also produce sensory ataxia.

ACUTE DISORDERS

1. DRUG INTOXICATION

Pancerebellar dysfunction manifested by nystagmus, dysarthria, and limb and gait ataxia is a prominent feature of many drug intoxication syndromes. Agents that produce such syndromes include ethanol, sedative-hypnotics (eg, barbiturates, benzodiazepines, meprobamate, ethchlorvynol, methaqualone), anticonvulsants (such as phenytoin), and hallucinogens (especially phencyclidine). The severity of symptoms is dose-related; while therapeutic doses of sedatives or anticonvulsants commonly produce nystagmus, other cerebellar signs imply toxicity.

Drug-induced cerebellar ataxia is often associated with a confusional state, although cognitive function tends to be spared in phenytoin intoxication. The confusional state produced by ethanol and sedative drugs is characterized by somnolence, while hallucinogens are more often associated with agitated delirium. In most cases, only general supportive care is necessary. The distinctive features of intoxication with each of these groups of drugs are discussed in detail in Chapter 1.

2. WERNICKE'S ENCEPHALOPATHY

Wernicke's encephalopathy (see also Chapter 1) is an acute disorder comprising the clinical triad of ataxia, ophthalmoplegia, and confusion. It is caused by thiamine (vitamin B_1) deficiency and is most common in chronic alcoholics, although it may occur as a consequence of malnutrition from any cause. The major sites of pathological involvement are the medial thalamic nuclei, mammillary bodies, periaqueductal and periventricular brain stem nuclei (especially those of the oculomotor, abducens, and acoustic nerves), and superior cerebellar vermis. Cerebellar and vestibular involvement both contribute to the ataxia.

Ataxia affects gait primarily or exclusively; the legs themselves are ataxic in only about one-fifth of patients, and the arms in one-tenth. Dysarthria is rare. Other classic findings include an amnestic syndrome or global confusional state, horizontal or combined horizontal-vertical nystagmus, bilateral lateral rectus palsies, and absent ankle jerks. Caloric testing reveals bilateral or unilateral vestibular dysfunction. Conjugate gaze palsies, pupillary abnormalities, and hypothermia can also occur.

The diagnosis is established by the response to administration of thiamine, which is usually given initially in a dose of 100 mg intravenously. Ocular palsies tend to be the earliest deficits to improve and typically begin to do so within hours. Ataxia, nystagmus, and acute confusion start to resolve within a few days. Recovery from ocular palsies is invariably complete, but horizontal nystagmus may persist.

Ataxia is fully reversible in only about 40% of patients; where gait returns fully to normal, recovery typically takes several weeks to months.

3. VERTEBROBASILAR ISCHEMIA & INFARCTION

Transient ischemic attacks and strokes in the vertebrobasilar system are often associated with ataxia or vertigo.

Internal Auditory Artery Occlusion

Vertigo of central vestibular origin with unilateral hearing loss results from occlusion of the internal auditory artery (Figure 4–8), which supplies the acoustic nerve. This vessel may originate from the basilar or anterior inferior cerebellar artery. Vertigo is accompanied by nystagmus, with the fast phase directed away from the involved side. Hearing loss is unilateral and sensorineural.

Lateral Medullary Infarction

Lateral medullary infarction produces **Wallenberg's syndrome** (Figure 4–9) and is most often caused by proximal vertebral artery occlusion. Clinical manifestations vary, depending on the extent of infarction. They typically consist of vertigo, nausea, vomiting, dysphagia, hoarseness, and nystagmus in addition to ipsilateral Horner's syndrome, limb ataxia, impairment of all sensory modalities over the face, and loss of light touch and position sense in the limbs. There is also impairment of pinprick and temperature appreciation in the contralateral limbs. Ver-

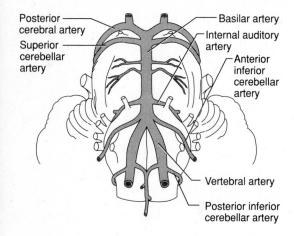

Posterior cerebral artery
Superior cerebellar artery
Basilar artery
Internal auditory artery
Anterior inferior cerebellar artery
Vertebral artery
Posterior inferior cerebellar artery

Figure 4–8. Principal arteries of the posterior fossa.

tigo results from involvement of the vestibular nuclei and hemiataxia from involvement of the inferior cerebellar peduncle.

Cerebellar Infarction

The cerebellum is supplied by three arteries: the superior cerebellar, anterior inferior cerebellar, and posterior inferior cerebellar. The territory supplied by each of these vessels is highly variable, both from one individual to another and between the two sides of the cerebellum in a given patient. The superior, middle, and inferior cerebellar peduncles are typically supplied by the superior, anterior inferior, and posterior inferior cerebellar arteries, respectively.

Cerebellar infarction results from occlusion of a cerebellar artery (Figure 4–10); the clinical syndromes produced can be distinguished only by the associated brain stem findings. In each case, cerebellar signs include ipsilateral limb ataxia and hypotonia. Other symptoms and signs such as headache, nausea, vomiting, vertigo, nystagmus, dysarthria, ocular or gaze palsies, facial weakness or sensory loss, and contralateral hemiparesis or hemisensory deficit may be present. Brain stem infarction or compression by cerebellar edema can result in coma and death.

The diagnosis of cerebellar infarction is made by CT scan or MRI, which allows differentiation between infarction and hemorrhage; it should be obtained promptly. When brain stem compression occurs, surgical decompression and resection of infarcted tissue can be lifesaving.

Paramedian Midbrain Infarction

Paramedian midbrain infarction caused by occlusion of the paramedian penetrating branches of the basilar artery affects the third nerve root fibers and red nucleus (Figure 4–11). The resulting clinical picture (**Benedikt's syndrome**) consists of ipsilateral medial rectus palsy with a fixed dilated pupil and contralateral

limb ataxia (typically affecting only the arm). Cerebellar signs result from involvement of the red nucleus, which receives a crossed projection from the cerebellum in the ascending limb of the superior cerebellar peduncle.

4. CEREBELLAR HEMORRHAGE

The vast majority of cerebellar hemorrhages are due to hypertensive vascular disease; less common causes include anticoagulation therapy, arteriovenous malformation, blood dyscrasia, tumor, and trauma. Hypertensive cerebellar hemorrhages are usually located in the deep white matter of the cerebellum and commonly extend into the fourth ventricle.

The classic clinical picture of hypertensive cerebellar hemorrhage consists of the sudden onset of headache, which may be accompanied by nausea, vomiting, and vertigo, followed by gait ataxia and impaired consciousness, usually evolving over a period of hours. At the time of presentation, patients can be fully alert, confused, or comatose. In alert patients, nausea and vomiting are often prominent. The blood pressure is typically elevated, and nuchal rigidity may be present. The pupils are often small and sluggishly reactive. Ipsilateral gaze palsy (with gaze preference away from the side of hemorrhage) and ipsilateral peripheral facial palsy are common. The gaze preference cannot be overcome by caloric stimulation. Nystagmus and ipsilateral depression of the corneal reflex may occur. The patient, if alert, exhibits ataxia of stance and gait; limb ataxia is less common. In the late stage of brain stem compression, the legs are spastic and extensor plantar responses are present.

The CSF is frequently bloody, but lumbar puncture should be avoided if cerebellar hemorrhage is suspected, because it may lead to a herniation syndrome. The diagnostic procedure of choice is a CT scan. Treatment consists of surgical evacuation of the hematoma, a procedure that can be lifesaving.

5. INFLAMMATORY DISORDERS

Acute inflammatory disorders of the cerebellum mediated by infection or immune mechanisms are important and often reversible causes of ataxia. Cerebellar ataxia caused by **viral infection** is one of the principal manifestations of St. Louis encephalitis. AIDS dementia complex and meningoencephalitis associated with varicella, mumps, poliomyelitis, infectious mononucleosis, and lymphocytic choriomeningitis can also produce cerebellar symptoms. **Bacterial infection** is a less common cause of cerebellar ataxia; 10–20% of brain abscesses are located in the cerebellum, however, and ataxia may be a feature of *Haemophilus influenzae* meningitis in children. A cerebellar syndrome has been described in legionnaires'

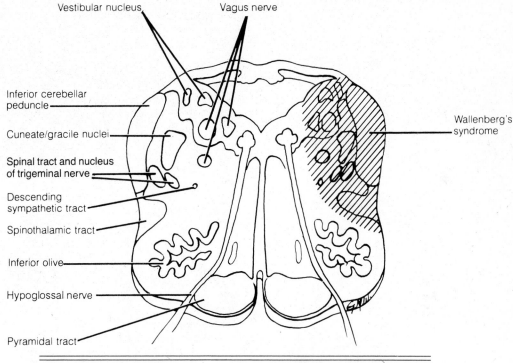

Figure 4–9. Lateral medullary infarction (Wallenberg's syndrome), showing the area of infarction (hatched), affected anatomical structures, and corresponding clinical features.

Structure Affected	Signs and Symptoms
Vestibular nucleus	Vertigo, nausea, vomiting, nystagmus
Cuneate or gracile nuclei	Ipsilateral loss of light touch over body
Inferior cerebellar peduncle and connections	Ipsilateral limb ataxia
Vagus (X) and glossopharyngeal (IX) nerves	Dysphagia, hoarseness
Spinal tract or nucleus of trigeminal (V) nerve	Ipsilateral loss of pain and temperature sensation over face
Descending sympathetic tract	Ipsilateral Horner's syndrome
Spinothalamic tract	Contralateral loss of pain and temperature sensation over body (and sometimes face)

disease, usually without clinical evidence of meningitis.

Several conditions that may occur following an acute febrile illness or vaccination produce cerebellar ataxia that is assumed to be of autoimmune origin.

Acute Cerebellar Ataxia of Childhood

Acute cerebellar ataxia of childhood is a syndrome characterized by severe gait ataxia that usually resolves completely within months. It generally follows an acute viral infection or inoculation. A full discussion of cerebellar ataxia in childhood is beyond the scope of this chapter.

Acute Disseminated Encephalomyelitis

This immune-mediated disorder may cause demyelination and inflammatory changes in the cerebellar white matter, producing ataxia that is often associated with impaired consciousness, seizures, focal neurological signs, or myelopathy.

Fisher Variant of Guillain-Barré Syndrome

Cerebellar ataxia, external ophthalmoplegia, and areflexia constitute this variant of Guillain-Barre syndrome. Symptoms develop over a few days. Ataxia primarily affects the gait and trunk, with lesser involvement of the individual limbs; dysarthria is uncommon. CSF protein may be elevated. Respiratory insufficiency occurs rarely, and the usual course is of gradual and often complete recovery over weeks to months. The ataxia is similar to that of cerebellar disease, but it is not yet known whether it arises centrally or peripherally.

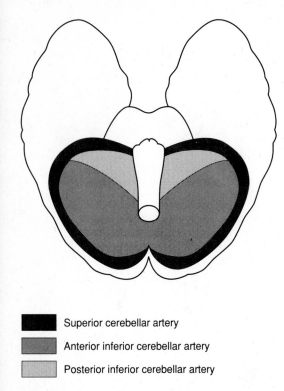

■	Superior cerebellar artery
▨	Anterior inferior cerebellar artery
▨	Posterior inferior cerebellar artery

Figure 4–10. Arterial supply of the cerebellum, viewed

CHRONIC DISORDERS

1. MULTIPLE SCLEROSIS

Multiple sclerosis can produce disorders of equilibrium of cerebellar, vestibular, or sensory origin. Cerebellar signs are associated with demyelinated areas (plaques) in the white matter of the cerebellum, cerebellar peduncles, or brain stem. As is the case with other manifestations of multiple sclerosis, these signs may remit and relapse.

Involvement of vestibular pathways in the brain stem produces vertigo, which may be acute in onset and sometimes positional. Vertigo, which is rarely the first symptom of multiple sclerosis, is not uncommon during the course of the disease.

Gait ataxia from cerebellar involvement is a presenting complaint in 10–15% of patients. Cerebellar signs are present in about one-third of patients on initial examination; they ultimately develop in twice that number.

Nystagmus is one of the most common physical findings; it can occur with or without other evidence of cerebellar dysfunction. Dysarthria also occurs frequently. When gait ataxia occurs, it is most often cerebellar rather than sensory in origin. Ataxia of the limbs is common; it is usually bilateral and tends to affect either both legs or all four limbs.

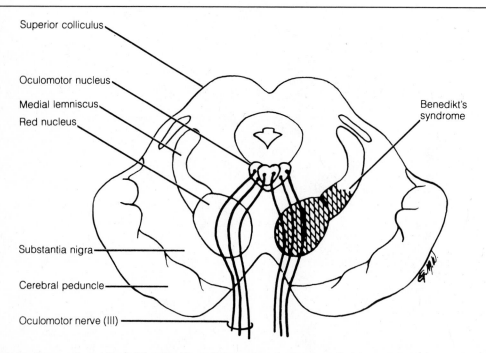

Figure 4–11. Paramedian midbrain infarction (Benedikt's syndrome). The area of infarction is indicated by cross-hatching.

Evidence that a cerebellar disorder is due to multiple sclerosis may be found in a history of remitting and relapsing neurological dysfunction that affects multiple sites in the central nervous system; from such associated abnormalities as optic neuritis, internuclear ophthalmoplegia, or pyramidal signs; or from laboratory investigations. CSF analysis may reveal oligoclonal bands, elevated IgG, increased protein, or a mild lymphocytic pleocytosis. Visual, auditory, or somatosensory evoked response recording can document subclinical sites of involvement. The CT scan or MRI may show areas of demyelination. It must be emphasized, however, that no laboratory finding is itself diagnostic of multiple sclerosis, and the history and neurological examination must be primarily relied upon in arriving at such a diagnosis.

No treatment has been shown to alter the eventual outcome. Short courses of corticosteroids may hasten recovery after an acute relapse. Approaches currently being evaluated include plasmapheresis; systemic or intrathecal administration of interferon; cytotoxic drugs such as cyclophosphamide and azathioprine; copolymer I; and total lymphoid irradiation. Multiple sclerosis is discussed in more detail in Chapter 6.

2. ALCOHOLIC CEREBELLAR DEGENERATION

A characteristic cerebellar syndrome may develop in chronic alcoholics, probably as a result of nutritional deficiency. Affected patients typically have a history of daily or binge drinking lasting ten or more years with associated dietary inadequacy. Most have experienced other medical complications of alcoholism: liver disease, delirium tremens, Wernicke's encephalopathy, or polyneuropathy. Alcoholic cerebellar degeneration is most common in men and usually has its onset between the ages of 40 and 60 years.

Degenerative changes in the cerebellum are largely restricted to the superior vermis (Figure 4–12); because this is also the site of cerebellar involvement in Wernicke's encephalopathy, both disorders may be part of the same clinical spectrum.

Alcoholic cerebellar degeneration is usually insidious in onset; it is gradually progressive, eventually reaching a stable level of deficit. Progression over weeks to months is more common than is deterioration over years; in occasional cases, ataxia appears abruptly or is mild and stable from the onset.

Gait ataxia is a universal feature and is almost always the problem that initially commands medical attention. The legs are also ataxic on heel-knee-shin testing in about 80% of patients. Commonly associated findings are distal sensory deficits in the feet and absent ankle reflexes—from polyneuropathy—and signs of malnutrition such as loss of subcutaneous tissue, generalized muscle atrophy, or glossitis. Less fre-

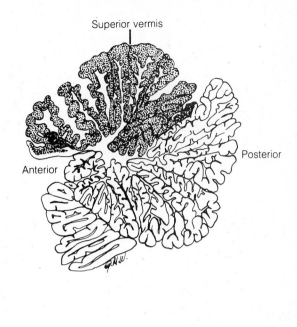

Figure 4–12. Distribution of disease in alcoholic cerebral degeneration. Midsagittal view of the cerebellum showing loss of Purkinje cells, confined largely to the superior vermis.

quent manifestations include ataxia of the arms, nystagmus, dysarthria, hypotonia, and truncal instability.

CT scan or MRI may show cerebellar atrophy (Figure 4–13), but this is a nonspecific finding that can be encountered in any degenerative disorder that affects the cerebellum.

Chronic cerebellar ataxia that begins in adulthood and primarily affects gait can also occur in hypothyroidism, paraneoplastic syndromes, idiopathic cerebellar degenerations, and anomalies at the craniocervical junction such as Arnold-Chiari malformation. The possibility of hypothyroidism or systemic cancer, which may be treatable, should be investigated with thyroid function tests, chest x-ray, and, in women, breast and pelvic examinations.

No specific treatment is available for alcoholic cerebellar degeneration. Nonetheless, all patients with this diagnosis should receive thiamine because of the apparent role of thiamine deficiency in the pathogenesis of Wernicke's encephalopathy, a closely related syndrome. Abstinence from alcohol, combined with adequate nutrition, leads to stabilization in most cases.

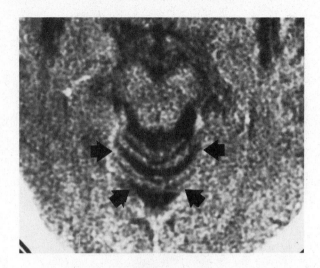

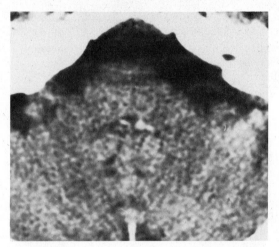

Figure 4–13. CT scan in alcoholic cerebellar degeneration, showing marked atrophy of the cerebellar vermis (**(A)**, arrows), with relative sparing of the cerebellar hemispheres **(B)**. (Courtesy of A Gean.)

3. PHENYTOIN-INDUCED CEREBELLAR DEGENERATION

Chronic therapy with phenytoin may produce cerebellar degeneration, probably the result of a toxic effect of the drug on cerebellar Purkinje cells. There is controversy, however, as to the relative importance of phenytoin and seizure-induced hypoxia in producing cerebellar damage in epileptic patients. Phenytoin-induced cerebellar degeneration affects the cerebellar hemispheres and inferior and posterior vermis most severely. The superior vermis, in contrast to alcoholic cerebellar degeneration, is relatively spared. Because of the more diffuse nature of cerebellar disease, phenytoin-induced cerebellar degeneration is associated with a pancerebellar syndrome consisting of nystagmus, dysarthria, and ataxia affecting the limbs, trunk, and gait. Polyneuropathy may be present.

The syndrome usually occurs following long-term treatment with phenytoin, often with drug levels in the toxic range. Unlike the symptoms of acute phenytoin intoxication, those caused by chronic ingestion are typically irreversible; they tend to stabilize when administration of the drug is discontinued, however.

4. HYPOTHYROIDISM

Among the neurological disorders associated with hypothyroidism is a subacute or chronically progressive cerebellar syndrome. This condition may complicate hypothyroidism (of various causes) and is most common in middle-aged or elderly women. Symptoms evolve over a period of months to years. Systemic symptoms of myxedema usually precede the appearance of the cerebellar disorder, but patients occasionally present first with ataxia.

Gait ataxia is the most prominent finding and is present in all patients; ataxia of the limbs, which is also common, may be asymmetric. Dysarthria and nystagmus occur less frequently. Patients may exhibit other neurological disorders related to hypothyroidism, including sensorineural hearing loss, carpal tunnel syndrome, neuropathy, or myopathy.

Laboratory studies show decreased blood levels of thyroid hormones, elevated TSH, and often increased CSF protein.

Replacement therapy with levothyroxine, 25–50 μg, increased gradually to 100–200 μg/d orally, usually produces definite but incomplete improvement.

5. PARANEOPLASTIC CEREBELLAR DEGENERATION

Cerebellar degeneration can also occur as a remote effect of systemic cancer. Carcinoma of the bronchus, breast, and ovary are the most commonly associated neoplasms, but other solid tumors or lymphoma can produce the same disorder.

Paraneoplastic degeneration affects the cerebellar vermis and hemispheres diffusely. While the pathogenetic mechanism has not been defined, elaboration of a neurotoxic substance, nutritional deficiency, autoimmune phenomena, and slow virus infection have all been proposed. The autoimmune theory has been bolstered in recent years by the finding that patients with this disorder produce antibodies to tumor cell antigens that cross-react with cerebellar Purkinje cells. Cerebellar symptoms may appear before or after the diagnosis of systemic cancer and typically develop over months. Although the disorder usually progresses steadily, it may stabilize; remission has been described with treatment of the underlying neoplasm.

Gait and limb ataxia are characteristically prominent, and dysarthria occurs in most cases. The limbs may be affected asymmetrically. Nystagmus is rare. Paraneoplastic involvement of other regions of the nervous system may produce associated dysphagia, dementia, memory disturbance, pyramidal signs, or neuropathy. Anti-Purkinje cell antibodies can sometimes be detected in the blood, and in some cases, the CSF shows a mild lymphocytic pleocytosis or elevated protein.

The diagnosis of paraneoplastic cerebellar degeneration is most difficult when the neurological symptoms precede the discovery of underlying cancer. The frequent occurrence of dysarthria and dysphagia helps to distinguish this condition from the cerebellar syndromes produced by chronic alcoholism or hypothyroidism. Ataxia of the arms also suggests that alcohol is an unlikely cause. Wernicke's encephalopathy should always be considered because of the susceptibility of patients with cancer to malnutrition.

6. IDIOPATHIC CEREBELLAR & OLIVOPONTOCEREBELLAR DEGENERATIONS

The idiopathic cerebellar and olivopontocerebellar degenerations comprise a heterogeneous group of disorders that, by virtue of their variable and overlapping clinical features and unknown pathogenesis, defy classification according to a universally accepted scheme. Two general subgroups are customarily identified on clinicopathological grounds.

Cerebellar cortical degenerations are characterized pathologically by prominent atrophy of the superior vermis, reminiscent of the distribution of involvement in alcoholic cerebellar degeneration, and by olivary atrophy in the brain stem, which may be due to secondary transsynaptic degeneration. **Olivopontocerebellar atrophies,** on the other hand, are associated with an early and striking loss of brain stem neurons in the pontine and olivary nuclei, atrophy of the cerebellar hemispheres, involvement of the deep cerebellar nuclei, and variable degeneration of the spinal cord (spinocerebellar tracts, corticospinal tracts, and posterior columns), basal ganglia, and thalamus (Figure 4–14). Cerebellar atrophy may be evident on CT or MRI scan, and the brain stem may also appear reduced in size.

Cerebellar and olivopontocerebellar degenerations exhibit different clinical features to some extent (Table 4–9), but they are often indistinguishable during life—unless a pathological diagnosis has previously been obtained in a family member. All such

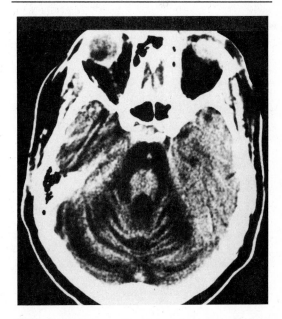

Figure 4–14. CT scan in olivopontocerebellar atrophy, showing an atrophic cerebellum and brain stem. (Courtesy of A Gean.)

Table 4–9. Classification of idiopathic cerebellar and olivopontocerebellar degenerations.[1]

Pathology	Syndrome	Age at Onset (mean)	Pyramidal Signs	Extrapyramidal Signs	Autonomic Insufficiency	Sensory Deficit
Cerebellar	Familial (autosomal dominant) cerebello-olivary atrophy (Holmes)	Infancy to age 70 (46)	−	−	−	−
	Late cortical cerebellar atrophy (Marie, Foix, and Alajouanine)[2]	40–75 (57)	±	−	−	−
Olivopontocerebellar	Hereditary (autosomal dominant; Menzel)[3]	14–73 (35)	+	+	±	±
	Sporadic (Dejerine and André-Thomas)[4]	17–66 (50)	+	+	±	−

[1]Modified and reproduced, with permission, from Maruyama S et al: CT scan study of spinocerebellar degeneration. Pages 67–82 in: *Spinocerebellar Degenerations.* Sobue I (editor). University Park Press, 1980.
[2]These may be cases of the Holmes syndrome with unrecognized heredity.
[3]Numerous variants of hereditary olivopontocerebellar atrophy have been described. These have been classified as type I (Menzel); type II (Fickler-Winkler), autosomal recessive; type III, autosomal dominant with retinal degeneration; type IV (Shut-Haymaker), autosomal dominant with sensory deficits and lower cranial nerve palsies; type V, autosomal dominant with parkinsonism, dementia, and ophthalmoplegia.
[4]These may be unrecognized hereditary cases.
+ = Present; − = Absent; ± = Can be present or absent.

disorders are characterized by slowly progressive cerebellar ataxia of gradual onset that affects gait early and severely and may eventually confine the patient to bed. Because involvement is more widespread in olivopontocerebellar atrophy, extrapyramidal and pyramidal dysfunction are commonly present, and dementia, autonomic insufficiency, or sensory impairment may occur.

Both cerebellar cortical degeneration and olivopontocerebellar atrophy can be either hereditary or sporadic; the mode of inheritance in the hereditary types is typically autosomal dominant.

7. FRIEDREICH'S ATAXIA

Among the idiopathic degenerative disorders that produce cerebellar ataxia, Friedreich's ataxia merits separate consideration because of its unique clinical and pathological features. The disorder is transmitted by autosomal recessive inheritance and appears to be due to a mutation on chromosome 9.

The pathological findings are localized, for the most part, to the spinal cord. These include degeneration of the spinocerebellar tracts, posterior columns, and dorsal roots as well as depletion of the neurons in Clarke's column that are the cells of origin of the dorsal spinocerebellar tracts. Large myelinated axons of peripheral nerves and cell bodies of primary sensory neurons in dorsal root ganglia are also involved.

Clinical Findings

Detailed clinical evaluation of relatively large numbers of patients has allowed certain diagnostic criteria to be established (Table 4–10). Clinical manifestations almost always appear after age four years and before the end of puberty.

The initial symptom is progressive gait ataxia, followed by ataxia of all limbs within two years. During

Table 4–10. Clinical features of Friedreich's ataxia.[1]

Obligatory features (present in 100% of cases and required for diagnosis)
Onset of symptoms by 20 years of age, almost always before the end of puberty
Gait ataxia
Progression of ataxia to involve all four limbs
Dysarthria
Impaired position or vibration sense in legs
Muscle weakness
Absent tendon reflexes in legs

Secondary features (present in ≥ 90% of cases but not required for diagnosis)
Extensor plantar responses
Pes cavus
Scoliosis
Cardiomyopathy (clinical or subclinical)

Accessory features (present in < 50% of cases)
Visual impairment (usually from optic atrophy)
Nystagmus
Paresthesia
Hearing loss
Essential tremor
Vertigo
Spasticity
Leg pains
Cognitive deficiency

[1]Criteria established by the Quebec Cooperative Study of Friedreich Ataxia, reported in Geoffroy G et al: Clinical description and roentgenologic evaluation of patients with Friedreich's ataxia. *Can J Neurol Sci* 1976;3:279.

the same early period, knee and ankle tendon reflexes are lost and cerebellar dysarthria appears; reflexes in the arms may be preserved. Joint position and vibration sense are impaired in the legs, typically adding a sensory component to the gait ataxia. Abnormalities of light touch, pain, and temperature sensation occur less frequently. Weakness of the legs—and less often the arms—is a later development and may be of the upper or lower motor neuron variety (or both).

Certain features are present in most but not all patients. Extensor plantar responses usually appear during the first five years of symptomatic disease. Pes cavus (high-arched feet with clawing of the toes caused by weakness and wasting of the intrinsic foot muscles) is a widely recognized sign, but it may also be an isolated finding in otherwise unaffected family members. It is also a classic feature of other neurological disorders, notably certain hereditary peripheral neuropathies (eg, Charcot-Marie-Tooth disease). Severe progressive kyphoscoliosis contributes to functional disability and may lead to chronic restrictive lung disease. While cardiomyopathy is sometimes detectable only by echocardiography or vectorcardiography, it may result in congestive heart failure and is a major cause of morbidity and death.

Other abnormalities that occur in only a few patients include visual impairment (usually from optic atrophy), nystagmus, paresthesias, postural tremor, hearing loss, vertigo, spasticity, leg pains, and clinically overt diabetes mellitus.

Differential Diagnosis

Friedreich's ataxia can usually be differentiated from cerebellar and olivopontocerebellar degenerations (see above) by its early onset and the presence of prominent sensory impairment, areflexia, skeletal abnormalities, and cardiomyopathy. A somewhat similar disorder may result from vitamin E deficiency. Cerebellar ataxia that begins in childhood can also be caused by ataxia-telangiectasia; the clinical features that distinguish Friedreich's ataxia from ataxia-telangiectasia are discussed below.

Prognosis

No treatment is available, but orthopedic procedures such as tenotomy may help to correct foot deformities. Advances in antimicrobial therapy have altered the ultimate course of the disorder, so that cardiomyopathy has become more frequent and infection less frequent as a cause of death. Neurological dysfunction typically results in the inability to walk unaided within five years after the onset of symptoms and in a bedridden state within 10 to 20 years. The average duration of symptomatic illness is about 25 years, with death occurring at a mean age of about 35 years.

8. ATAXIA-TELANGIECTASIA

Ataxia-telangiectasia is an inherited autosomal recessive disorder with its onset in infancy. It is characterized by progressive cerebellar ataxia, oculocutaneous telangiectasia, and immunological deficiency. All patients suffer from progressive pancerebellar degeneration—characterized by nystagmus, dysarthria, and gait, limb, and trunk ataxia—that begins in infancy. Choreoathetosis, loss of vibration and position sense in the legs, areflexia, and disorders of voluntary eye movement are almost universal findings. Mental deficiency is commonly observed in the second decade; oculocutaneous telangiectasia usually appears in the teen years. The bulbar conjunctivae are typically affected first, followed by sun-exposed areas of the skin, including the ears, nose, face, and antecubital and popliteal fossae. The vascular lesions, which rarely bleed, spare the central nervous system. Immunological impairment (decreased circulating IgA and IgE) usually becomes evident later in childhood and is manifested by recurrent sinopulmonary infections in more than 80% of patients.

Other common clinical findings are progeric changes of the skin and hair, hypogonadism, and insulin resistance. The characteristic laboratory abnormalities include those related to immunological deficiency and elevation of alpha-fetoprotein levels.

Because the vascular and immunological manifestations of ataxia-telangiectasia occur later than the neurological symptoms, the condition may be confused with Friedreich's ataxia, which also manifests in childhood (see above). Ataxia-telangiectasia can be distinguished by its earlier onset (before age four years), associated choreoathetosis, and the absence of such skeletal abnormalities as kyphoscoliosis.

9. WILSON'S DISEASE

Cerebellar symptoms may occur in Wilson's disease, a disorder of copper metabolism characterized by copper deposition in a variety of tissues. Wilson's disease is an inherited autosomal recessive disorder, with the defective gene on chromosome 13; it is discussed in Chapter 8.

10. CREUTZFELDT-JAKOB DISEASE

Creutzfeldt-Jakob disease is described in Chapter 2 as a transmissible disorder of the nervous system that causes dementia. Cerebellar signs present in about 60% of patients, and the patients present with ataxia in about 10% of cases. Cerebellar involvement is diffuse, but the vermis is often most severely affected. In contrast to most other cerebellar disorders, depletion of granule cells is frequently more striking than Purkinje cell loss.

Patients with cerebellar manifestations of Creutzfeldt-Jakob disease usually complain first of gait ataxia. Dementia is usually evident at this time, and cognitive dysfunction always develops eventually. Nystagmus, dysarthria, truncal ataxia, and limb ataxia are all present initially in about half the patients with the ataxic form of Creutzfeldt-Jakob disease. The course is characterized by progressive dementia, myoclonus, and extrapyramidal and pyramidal dysfunction. Death typically occurs within one year after onset.

11. POSTERIOR FOSSA TUMORS

Tumors of the posterior fossa cause cerebellar symptoms when they arise in the cerebellum or compress it from without. The most common cerebellar tumors of childhood are astrocytomas and medulloblastomas. Metastases from primary sites outside the nervous system predominate in adults (Table 4–11).

Patients with cerebellar tumors present with headache from the increased intracranial pressure or with ataxia. Nausea, vomiting, vertigo, cranial nerve palsies, and hydrocephalus are common. The nature of the clinical findings varies with the location of the tumor. Most metastases are located in the cerebellar hemispheres, causing asymmetric cerebellar signs. Medulloblastomas and ependymomas, on the other hand, tend to arise in the midline, with early involvement of the vermis and hydrocephalus.

As in the case of most brain tumors, the CT scan or—especially—MRI is extremely useful in diagnoses but biopsy may be required for histological characterization. Methods of treatment include surgical resection and irradiation. Corticosteroids are useful in controlling the associated edema.

Metastases from the lung and breast—and less commonly from other sites—are the most common tumors of the cerebellum, especially in adults. The site of the primary tumor may or may not be evident at the time the patient presents with central nervous system involvement. If the site is not evident, careful examination of the breasts and skin, chest x-ray, urinalysis, and tests for the presence of occult blood in the stool may lead to a diagnosis. The prognosis for patients with cerebellar metastases is usually worse than for patients with supratentorial lesions. Patients with carcinoma of the breast tend to survive longer than those with primary lung tumors.

Cerebellar astrocytomas usually occur between the ages of 2 and 20 years, but older patients can also be affected. These tumors are often histologically benign and cystic in appearance. Symptoms of increased intracranial pressure, including headache and vomiting, typically precede the onset of cerebellar dysfunction by several months. If complete surgical resection is possible, cerebellar astrocytoma is potentially curable.

Medulloblastoma is common in children but rare in adults. It is believed to originate from neuroectodermal rather than glial cells. In contrast to astrocytomas, medulloblastomas tend to be highly malignant. They often spread through the subarachnoid space and ventricles and may metastasize outside the nervous system. While most childhood medulloblastomas are located in the midline, adult-onset tumors usually arise laterally. Headache, vomiting, ataxia, and visual deterioration are common presenting symptoms. Hemiataxia is a frequent finding in adults because of the hemispheric location of most tumors. Gait ataxia, papilledema, nystagmus, facial palsy, and neck stiffness are also common. Without treatment, medulloblastoma causes death within a few months after presentation. Treatment with partial surgical resection, decompression, and craniospinal irradiation may prolong survival for years. Developing the tumors in adulthood and being female are favorable prognostic factors.

Acoustic neuromas have been discussed previously as a cause of vestibular nerve dysfunction. Growth of these or other less common tumors of the cerebellopontine angle may result in compression of the ipsilateral cerebellar hemisphere, causing hemiataxia in addition to the earlier symptoms of vertigo and hearing loss. These tumors are histologically benign and often fully resectable. Unilateral acoustic neuromas can occur in **neurofibromatosis 1** (von Recklinghausen's disease); whereas bilateral acoustic neuromas are characteristic of **neurofibromatosis 2.** These disorders are discussed in more detail in the section on cerebellopontine angle tumors (above).

Hemangioblastoma is a rare benign tumor that usually affects adults. It can be an isolated abnormality or a feature of von Hippel-Lindau disease. In the latter case, associated features include retinal hemangioblastoma; cysts of the kidney, pancreas, or

Table 4–11. Tumors of the cerebellum.[1]

Type	Percentage of All Cerebellar Tumors	Percentage of Cerebellar Tumors in Adults (≥ 20 years)
Metastasis	36	56
Astrocytoma	28	10
Medulloblastoma	16	9
Schwannoma	4	7
Hemangioblastoma	4	5
Meningioma	4	5
Ependymoma	2	1
Other	6	7

[1]Data from Gilman S, Bloedel JR, Lechtenberg R: Page 334 in: *Disorders of the Cerebellum.* Vol 21 of: *Contemporary Neurology Series.* Davis, 1981.

other viscera; and polycythemia. Patients typically present with headache, and common examination findings include papilledema, nystagmus, and ataxia. Treatment is by surgical resection.

Meningiomas of the posterior fossa constitute 9% of all meningiomas. They are benign tumors, derived from arachnoidal cap cells, that involve the cerebellum indirectly by compression. The locations of posterior fossa meningiomas (in decreasing order of frequency) include the posterior surface of the petrous bone, the tentorium cerebelli, the clivus, the cerebellar convexities, and the foramen magnum. Meningiomas grow slowly and usually present with headache, although tumors of the cerebellopontine angle or clivus may come to attention when they give rise to cranial nerve or brain stem symptoms. Where possible, complete surgical resection is curative.

Ependymomas most commonly arise from the walls or choroid plexus of the fourth ventricle. Like medulloblastomas, they are malignant tumors that seed through the ventricular system and usually occur in children. Because of their location they produce early hydrocephalus; cerebellar signs caused by compression are late or minor manifestations. Surgical resection, craniospinal irradiation, and shunting procedures to relieve hydrocephalus may prolong survival, but widespread dissemination of the tumors and postoperative recurrences are common.

12. POSTERIOR FOSSA MALFORMATIONS

Developmental anomalies affecting the cerebellum and brain stem may present with vestibular or cerebellar symptoms in adulthood. This occurs most commonly with type I (adult) **Arnold-Chiari malformation,** which consists of downward displacement of the cerebellar tonsils through the foramen magnum.

Table 4–12. Causes of sensory ataxia.

Polyneuropathy[1]
  Cisplatin (*cis*-platinum)
  Dejerine-Sottas disease (HMSN[2] type III)
  Diabetes
  Diphtheria
  Hypothyroidism
  Isoniazid
  Paraneoplastic sensory neuronopathy
  Pyridoxine
  Refsum's disease
Myelopathy[3]
  Acute transverse myelitis
  AIDS (vacuolar myelopathy)
  Multiple sclerosis
  Tumor or cord compression
  Vascular malformations
Polyneuropathy or myelopathy
  Friedreich's ataxia
  Neurosyphilis (tabes dorsalis)
  Nitrous oxide
  Vitamin B_{12} deficiency
  Vitmain E deficiency

[1]Involving large, myelinated sensory fibers.
[2]Hereditary motor and sensory neuropathy.
[3]Involving posterior columns.

The clinical manifestations of this malformation are related to cerebellar involvement, obstructive hydrocephalus, brain stem compression, and syringomyelia. Type II Arnold-Chiari malformation is associated with meningomyelocele (protrusion of the spinal cord, nerve roots, and meninges through a fusion defect in the vertebral column) and has its onset in childhood.

Cerebellar ataxia in the type I malformation usually affects the gait and is bilateral; in some cases it is asymmetrical. Hydrocephalus leads to headache and vomiting. Compression of the brain stem by herniated cerebellar tissue may be associated with vertigo,

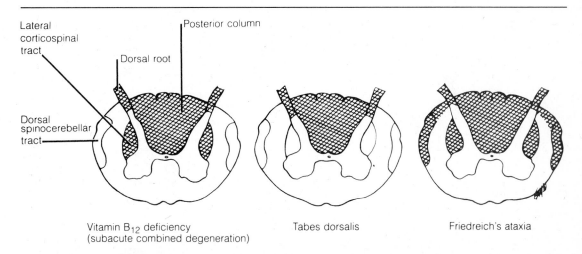

Lateral corticospinal tract

Posterior column

Dorsal root

Dorsal spinocerebellar tract

Vitamin B_{12} deficiency (subacute combined degeneration)

Tabes dorsalis

Friedreich's ataxia

Figure 4–15. Principal sites of spinal cord disease in disorders producing sensory ataxias.

nystagmus, and lower cranial nerve palsies. Syringo-myelia typically produces a capelike distribution of defective pain and temperature sensation.

Arnold-Chiari malformation can be diagnosed by CT or MRI studies that demonstrate cerebellar tonsil-lar herniation. High cervical laminectomy with decompression of the posterior fossa may be of therapeutic benefit.

SENSORY ATAXIAS

Sensory ataxia results from impaired propriocep-tive sensation at the level of peripheral nerves or roots, posterior columns of the spinal cord, or sensory pathways in the brain. Clinical findings include defective joint position and vibration sense in the legs and sometimes the arms, unstable stance with Romberg's sign, and a gait of slapping or steppage quality. Sensory ataxia can be produced by polyneuropathies that prominently affect large, myelinated sensory fibers (Table 4–12) and by myelopathies, including those resulting from Friedreich's ataxia, neurosyphilis (tabes dorsalis), or vitamin B_{12} deficiency (Figure 4–15). Polyneuropathies, tabes dorsalis and vitamin B_{12} deficiency are discussed in detail in Chapter 7.

REFERENCES

Baloh RW, Honrubia V: Clinical Neurophysiology of the Vestibular System, 2nd ed. Vol 32 of: *Contemporary Neurology Series.* Davis, 1990.

Brandt T, Daroff RB: The multisensory physiological and pathological vertigo syndromes. *Ann Neurol* 1980;7: 195–203.

Charness ME, Simon RP, Greenberg DA: Ethanol and the nervous system. *N Engl J Med* 1989;321:442–454.

Daroff RB: Vertigo. *Am Fam Pract* 1977;16:143–150.

Drachman DA, Hart CW: An approach to the dizzy patient. *Neurology* 1972;22:323–334.

Furneaux HM et al: Selective expression of Purkinje-cell antigens in tumor tissue from patients with paraneoplastic cerebellar degeneration. *N Engl J Med* 1990;322: 1844–1851.

Geoffroy G et al: Clinical description and roentgenological evaluation of patients with Friedreich's ataxia. *Can J Neurol Sci* 1976;3:279–286.

Gilman S, Bloedel JR, Lechtenberg R: Disorders of the Cerebellum. Vol 21 of: *Contemporary Neurology Series.* Davis, 1981.

Harner SG, Laws ER Jr: Clinical findings in patients with acoustic neurinoma. *Mayo Clin Proc* 1983;58:721–728.

Hart RG, Gardner DP, Howieson J: Acoustic tumors: Atypical features and recent diagnostic tests. *Neurology* 1983;33:211–221.

Haye R, Quist-Hanssen S: The natural course of Ménière's disease. *Acta Otolaryngol* 1976;82:289–293.

Healy GB: Hearing loss and vertigo secondary to head injury. *N Engl J Med* 1982;306:1029–1031.

Luxon LM: Diseases of the eighth cranial nerve. In: *Peripheral Neuropathy* 2nd ed. Dyck PJ, et al (editors). Saunders, 1984.

Martuza RL, Eldridge R: Neurofibromatosis 2 (bilateral acoustic neurofibromatosis). *N Engl J Med* 1988;318: 684–688.

Matthews WB (editor): *McAlpine's Multiple Sclerosis, 2nd ed.* Churchill Livingstone, 1991.

McFarlin DE, Strober W, Waldmann TA: Ataxia-telangiectasia. *Medicine* 1972;51:281–314.

Ott KH et al: Cerebellar hemorrhage: Diagnosis and treatment. *Arch Neurol* 1974;31:160–167.

Scotti G et al: Cerebellar softening. *Ann Neurol* 1980;8: 133–140.

Thomas JE, Cody DT: Neurological perspectives of otosclerosis. *Mayo Clin Proc* 1981;56:17–21.

Disturbances of Vision

5

APPROACH TO DIAGNOSIS

Disorders that affect the ocular muscles, cranial nerves, or visual or ocular motor pathways in the brain produce a wide variety of neuro-ophthalmologic disturbances. Because the anatomic and functional features of the visual and ocular motor pathways have been well characterized, neuro-ophthalmologic signs are often of great value in the anatomic localization of neurological disease. Familiarity with the organization of these systems allows the formulation of an anatomic diagnosis, which in turn suggests possible etiologies.

FUNCTIONAL ANATOMY OF THE VISUAL SYSTEM

Reception of Visual Information

Visual information enters the nervous system when light, refracted and focused by the **lens,** creates a visual image on the **retina** at the posterior pole of the eye (Figure 5–1). The action of the lens causes this image to be reversed in the horizontal and vertical planes. Thus, the superior portion of the visual image falls on the inferior retina and vice versa, and the temporal (lateral) and nasal (medial) fields are likewise reversed (Figure 5–2). The center of the visual field is focused at the **fovea,** where the retina's perceptual sensitivity is greatest. Within the retina, photoreceptor cells **(rods** and **cones)** transduce of incident light into neuronal impulses, which are transmitted by retinal neurons to the **optic (II) nerve.** At this and all other levels of the visual system, the topographic relations of the visual field are preserved.

Peripheral Visual Pathways

Each optic nerve contains fibers from one eye, but as shown in Figure 5–2, the nasal (medial) fibers, conveying information from the temporal (lateral)

visual fields, cross in the **optic chiasm**. As a result, each **optic tract** contains fibers not from one eye but from one half of the visual field. Because of this arrangement, **prechiasmal lesions** affect vision in the ipsilateral eye and **retrochiasmal lesions** produce defects in the contralateral half of the visual field of *both* eyes.

Central Visual Pathways

The optic tracts terminate in the **lateral geniculate nuclei,** where their neurons synapse on neurons that project through the **optic radiations** to the primary visual or **calcarine cortex** (area 17), located near the posterior poles of the occipital lobes, and visual association areas (areas 18 and 19). Here, too, the visual image is represented in such a way that its topographic organization is preserved (Figure 5–3). The central region of the visual field **(macula)** projects to the most posterior portion of the visual cortex, while the inferior and superior parts of the field are represented above and below the calcarine fissure, respectively.

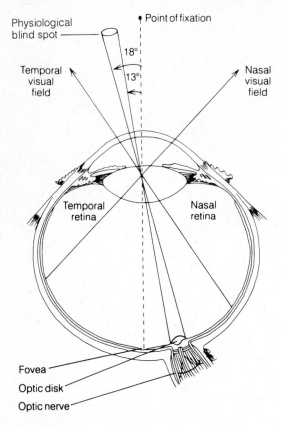

Figure 5–1. Representation of the visual field at the level of the retina. The point of fixation is focused on the fovea, the physiological blind spot on the optic disk, the temporal half of the visual field on the nasal side of the retina, and the nasal half of the visual field on the temporal side of the retina.

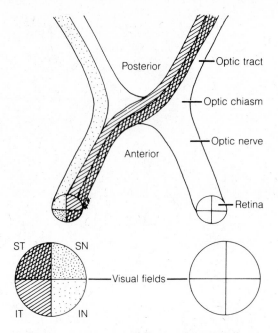

Figure 5–2. Representation of the visual field at the level of the optic nerve, chiasm, and tract. Quadrants of the visual field are designated ST (superior temporal), IT (inferior temporal), SN (superior nasal), and IN (inferior nasal).

Vascular Supply

The vascular supply of the visual system is derived from the ophthalmic, middle cerebral, and posterior cerebral arteries (Figure 5–4); thus, ischemia or infarction in the territory of any of these vessels can produce visual field defects.

A. Retina: The retina is supplied by the central retinal artery, a branch of the ophthalmic artery. Because the central retinal artery subsequently divides into superior and inferior retinal branches, vascular disease of the retina tends to produce altitudinal (ie, superior or inferior) visual field deficits.

B. Optic Nerve: The optic nerve receives arterial blood primarily from the ophthalmic artery and its branches.

C. Optic Radiations: As the optic radiations course backward toward the visual cortex, they are supplied by branches of the middle cerebral artery. Ischemia or infarction in the distribution of the middle cerebral artery may thus cause loss of vision in the contralateral visual field.

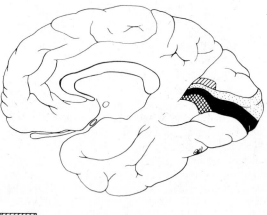

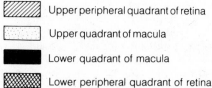
Upper peripheral quadrant of retina

Upper quadrant of macula

Lower quadrant of macula

Lower peripheral quadrant of retina

Figure 5–3. Representation of the visual field at the level of the primary visual cortex, midsagittal view, shows the medial surface of the right occipital lobe, which receives visual input from the left side of the visual field of both eyes.

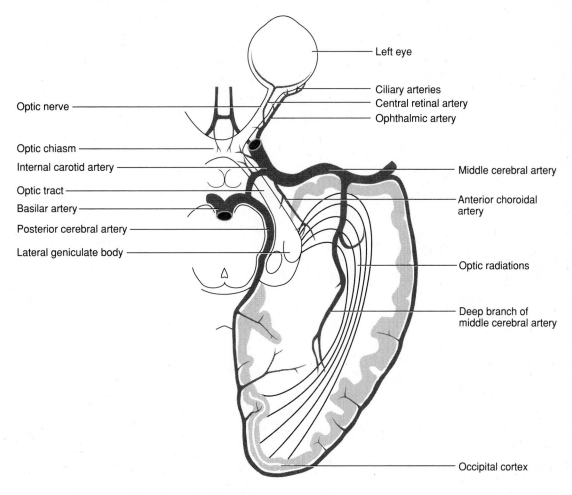

Figure 5–4. Arterial supply of the visual system, viewed from below.

D. Primary Visual Cortex: The principal source of arterial blood for the primary visual cortex is the posterior cerebral arteries. Occlusion of one posterior cerebral artery produces blindness in the contralateral visual field, although the dual (middle and posterior cerebral) arterial supply to the macular region of the visual cortex (see Figure 5–4) may spare central (macular) vision. Because the posterior cerebral arteries arise together from the basilar artery, occlusion at the tip of the basilar artery can cause bilateral occipital infarction and complete cortical blindness—although, in some cases, macular vision is spared.

FUNCTIONAL ANATOMY OF THE OCULAR MOTOR SYSTEM

Extraocular Muscles

Movement of the eyes is accomplished by the action of six muscles attached to each globe. These muscles act to move the eye into each of six cardinal positions of gaze (Figure 5–5). Equal and opposed actions of these six muscles in the resting state place the eye in mid or primary position, ie, looking directly forward. When the function of one extraocular muscle is disrupted, the eye is unable to move in the direction of action of the affected muscle (**ophthalmoplegia**) and may deviate in the opposite direction because of the unopposed action of other extraocular muscles. When the eyes are thus misaligned, visual images of perceived objects fall on a different region of each retina, creating the illusion of double vision, or **diplopia.**

Cranial Nerves

The extraocular muscles are innervated by the oculomotor (III), trochlear (IV), and abducens (VI) nerves. Because of this differential innervation of the ocular muscles, the pattern of their involvement in pathological conditions can help to distinguish a dis-

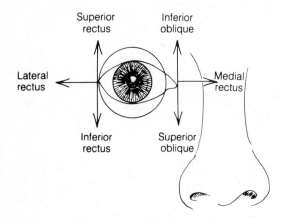

Figure 5–5. Extraocular muscles subserving the six cardinal positions of gaze. The eye is adducted by the medial rectus and abducted by the lateral rectus. The adducted eye is elevated by the inferior oblique and depressed by the superior oblique; the abducted eye is elevated by the superior rectus and depressed by the inferior rectus.

order of the ocular muscles per se from a disorder that is affecting a cranial nerve. Cranial nerves that control eye movement traverse long distances to pass from the brain stem to the eye; they are thereby rendered vulnerable to injury by a variety of pathological processes.

A. Nerve III: The oculomotor nerve supplies the medial rectus, superior and inferior rectus, and inferior oblique muscles and carries fibers to the levator palpebrae (which raises the eyelid). It also supplies the parasympathetic fibers responsible for pupillary constriction. With a complete nerve III lesion, the eye is partially abducted and there is an inability to adduct, elevate, and depress the eye; the eyelid droops **(ptosis),** and the pupil is nonreactive.

B. Nerve IV: The trochlear nerve innervates the superior oblique muscle. Lesions of this nerve result in defective depression of the adducted eye.

C. Nerve VI: Lesions of the abducens nerve cause lateral rectus palsy, with impaired abduction of the affected eye.

Cranial Nerve Nuclei

The nuclei of the oculomotor and trochlear nerves are located in the dorsal midbrain, ventral to the cerebral aqueduct (of Sylvius), while the abducens nerve nucleus occupies a similarly dorsal and periventricular position in the pons.

Lesions involving these nuclei give rise to clinical abnormalities similar to those produced by involvement of their respective cranial nerves; in some cases, nuclear and nerve lesions can be distinguished.

A. Nerve III Nucleus: Familiarity with the organization of the oculomotor nerve nucleus sometimes makes it possible to distinguish nuclear from nerve lesions: While each oculomotor nerve supplies muscles of the ipsilateral eye only, fibers to the superior rectus originate in the contralateral oculomotor nerve nucleus, and the levator palpebrae receives bilateral nuclear innervation. Thus, ophthalmoplegia affecting only one eye with ipsilateral ptosis or superior rectus palsy suggests oculomotor nerve disease, whereas ophthalmoplegia accompanied by bilateral ptosis or a contralateral superior rectus palsy is probably due to a nuclear lesion.

B. Nerve IV Nucleus: It is not possible to distinguish clinically between lesions of the trochlear nerve and those of its nucleus.

C. Nerve VI Nucleus: In disorders affecting the abducens nerve nucleus rather than the nerve itself, lateral rectus paresis is often associated with facial weakness, paresis of ipsilateral conjugate gaze, or a depressed level of consciousness. This is because of the proximity of the abducens nerve nucleus to the facial (VII) nerve fasciculus, lateral gaze center, and ascending reticular activating system, respectively.

Supranuclear Control of Eye Movements

Supranuclear control of eye movements enables the two eyes to act in concert to produce **version (conjugate gaze)** or **vergence (convergence and divergence)** movements.

A. Brain Stem Gaze Centers: Centers that control horizontal and vertical gaze are located in the pons and in the pretectal region of the midbrain, respectively, and receive descending inputs from the cerebral cortex that allow voluntary control of gaze (Figure 5–6). Each **lateral gaze center,** located in the paramedian pontine reticular formation (PPRF) adjacent to the abducens nerve nucleus, mediates ipsilateral conjugate horizontal gaze via its connections to the ipsilateral abducens and contralateral oculomotor nerve nucleus. A lesion in the pons affecting the PPRF therefore produces a **gaze preference** away from the side of the lesion—and toward the side of an associated hemiparesis, if present.

B. Cortical Input: The PPRF receives cortical input from the contralateral frontal lobe, which regulates rapid eye movements **(saccades),** and from the ipsilateral parieto-occipital lobe, which regulates slow eye movements **(pursuits).** Therefore, a destructive lesion affecting the frontal cortex interferes with the mechanism for contralateral horizontal gaze and may result in a gaze preference toward the side of the lesion (and away from the side of associated hemiparesis). By contrast, an irritative (seizure) focus in the frontal lobe may cause a gaze preference away from the side of the focus.

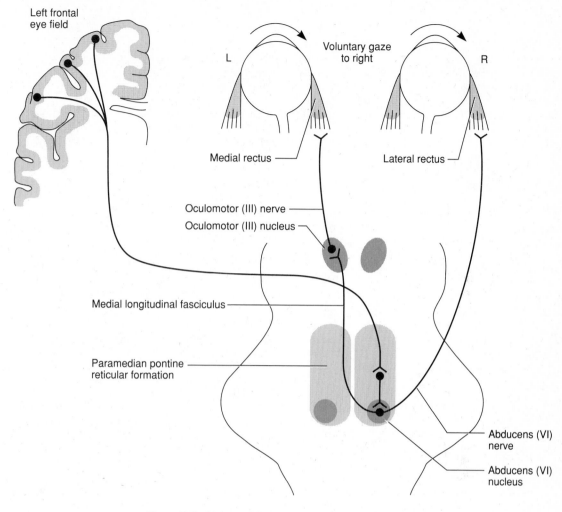

Figure 5–6. Neuronal pathways involved in horizontal gaze.

HISTORY

Nature of Complaint

The first step in evaluating a neuro-ophthalmologic disorder is to obtain a clear description of the complaint. Patients often complain only of vague symptoms, such as blurred vision, which provide little diagnostic information. An attempt must be made to determine exactly what the patient means to convey—decreased visual acuity in one or both eyes, loss of vision in part of the visual field, diplopia, an unstable visual image, pain in or about the eye, or some other problem.

Temporal Pattern of Symptoms

Once the nature of the complaint has been established, inquiries regarding its temporal pattern can provide clues to the underlying pathological process.

A. Sudden Onset: Vascular disorders that affect the eye or its connections in the brain tend to produce symptoms of sudden onset.

B. Slow Onset: With inflammatory or neoplastic disease, symptoms usually evolve over a longer period of time.

C. Transient, Recurrent Symptoms: Symptoms that are transient and recurrent suggest a select group of pathological processes, including ischemia, demyelinating disease, and myasthenia gravis.

Associated Neurological Abnormalities

The nature of any associated neurological abnormalities, such as impaired facial sensation, weakness, ataxia, or aphasia, can be valuable in localizing the anatomic site of involvement.

Medical History

The history should be scrutinized for conditions that predispose the patient to neuro-ophthalmologic problems.

Multiple sclerosis often involves the optic nerve or brain stem, leading to a variety of neuro-ophthalmologic disorders. A history of disturbances that also involve other parts of the central nervous system should suggest this diagnosis.

Atherosclerosis, hypertension, and diabetes can be complicated by vascular disorders of the eye, cranial nerves, or visual or ocular motor pathways in the brain.

Endocrine disorders (eg, hyperthyroidism) can cause ocular myopathy.

Connective tissue disease and systemic cancer can affect the visual and ocular motor systems at a variety of sites.

Patients with nutritional deficiencies may present with neuro-ophthalmologic symptoms, as in the amblyopia (decreased visual acuity) associated with malnutrition and the ophthalmoplegia of Wernicke's encephalopathy.

Numerous drugs (eg, ethambutol, isoniazid, digitalis, clioquinol) are known to be toxic to the visual system, and others (sedative drugs, anticonvulsants) commonly produce ocular motor disorders.

NEURO-OPHTHALMOLOGIC EXAMINATION

Visual Acuity

A. Assessment: To assess visual acuity from a neurological standpoint, vision is tested under conditions that eliminate refractive errors. Therefore, patients who wear glasses should be examined while wearing them (a pinhole can be substituted if the corrective lenses usually worn are not available at the time of testing). Visual acuity must be assessed for each eye separately. Distant vision is tested using a Snellen eye chart, with the patient 6 meters (20 feet) away. Near vision is tested with the Rosenbaum pocket eye chart held about 36 cm (14 inches) from the patient. In each case, the smallest line of print that can be read is noted.

B. Recording: Visual acuity is expressed as a fraction (eg, 20/20, 20/40, 20/200). The numerator is the distance (in feet) from the test figures at which the examination is performed, and the denominator is the distance (in feet) at which figures of a given size can be correctly identified by persons with normal vision. For example, if a patient standing 20 feet away from the eye chart is unable to identify figures that can normally be seen from that distance but can identify the larger figures that would be visible 40 feet away with normal acuity, the visual acuity is recorded as 20/40. If the patient can read most of a given line but makes some errors, acuity may be recorded as 20/40 − 1, for example, indicating that all but one letter on the 20/40 line were correctly identified. When visual acuity is markedly reduced, it can still be quantified, though less precisely, in terms of the distance at which the patient can count fingers (CF), discern hand movement (HM), or perceive light. If an eye is totally blind, the examination will reveal no light perception (NLP).

C. Red-Green Color Vision: Red-green color vision is often disproportionately impaired in optic nerve lesions and can be tested with colored objects such as pens or hatpins or with color vision plates.

Visual Fields

Evaluating the visual fields can be a lengthy and tedious procedure if conducted in an undirected fashion. Familiarity with the common types of visual field defects is important if testing is to be reasonably rapid and yield useful information. The most common visual field abnormalities are illustrated in Figure 5–7.

A. Extent of Visual Fields: The normal monocular visual field subtends an angle of about 160 degrees in the horizontal plane and about 135 degrees in the vertical plane (Figure 5–8). With binocular vision, the horizontal range of vision exceeds 180 degrees.

B. Physiological Blind Spot: Within the normal field of each eye is a 5-degree blind spot, corresponding to the region of space projected onto the optic disk, which lacks receptor cells.

C. Measurement Techniques: Numerous techniques exist for measuring the visual field—which, like visual acuity, must be examined separately for each eye.

1. The simplest method for visual field testing is the **confrontation** technique (Figure 5–9). The examiner stands at about arm's length from the patient, with the eyes of both patient and examiner aligned in the horizontal plane. The eye not being tested is covered by the patient's hand or an eye patch. The examiner closes the eye opposite the patient's covered eye, and the patient is instructed to fix on the examiner's open eye. Now the monocular fields of patient and examiner are superimposed, which allows comparison of the patient's field with the examiner's presumably normal field. The examiner uses the index fingers of both hands to locate the boundaries of the patient's field, moving them slowly inward from the periphery in all directions until the patient detects them. The boundaries are then defined more carefully by determining the farthest peripheral sites at which the patient can detect slight movements of the fingertips or the white head of a pin. The patient's blind spot can be located in the region of the examiner's own blind spot, and the sizes of these spots can be compared using a pin with a white head as the target. The procedure is then repeated for the other eye.

2. Subtle field defects may be detected by asking the patient to compare the brightness of colored objects presented at different sites in the field or by measuring the fields using a pin with a red head as the target.

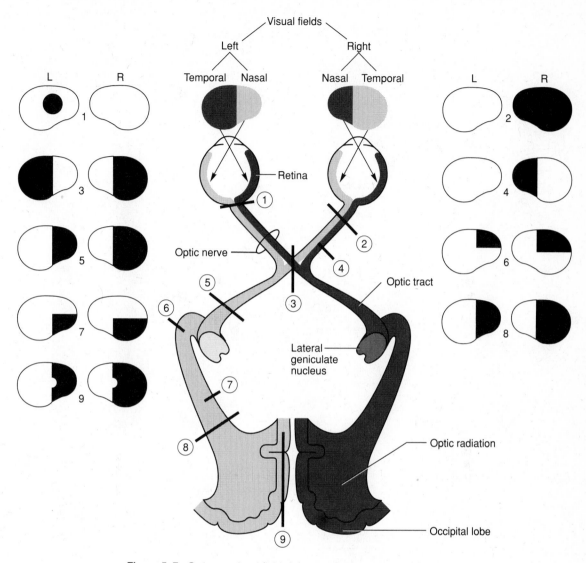

Figure 5–7. Common visual field defects and their anatomical bases.

1. **Central scotoma** caused by inflammation of the optic disk (optic neuritis) or optic nerve (retrobulbar neuritis).
2. **Total blindness of the right eye** from a complete lesion of the right optic nerve.
3. **Bitemporal hemianopia** caused by pressure exerted on the optic chiasm by a pituitary tumor.
4. **Right nasal hemianopia** caused by a perichiasmal lesion (eg, calcified internal carotid artery).
5. **Right homonymous hemianopia** from a lesion of the left optic tract.
6. **Right homonymous superior quadrantanopia** caused by partial involvement of the optic radiation by a lesion in the left temporal lobe (Meyer's loop).
7. **Right homonymous inferior quadrantanopia** caused by partial involvement of the optic radiation by a lesion in the left parietal lobe.
8. **Right homonymous hemianopia** from a complete lesion of the left optic radiation. (A similar defect may also result from lesion 9.)
9. **Right homonymous hemianopia (with macular sparing)** resulting from posterior cerebral artery occlusion.

3. In young children, the fields may be assessed by standing behind the child and bringing an attention-getting object, such as a toy, forward around the child's head in various directions until it is first noticed.

4. A gross indication of visual field abnormalities may be obtained in obtunded patients by determining whether they blink in response to a visual threat—typically the examiner's finger—brought toward the patient's eye in various regions of the field.

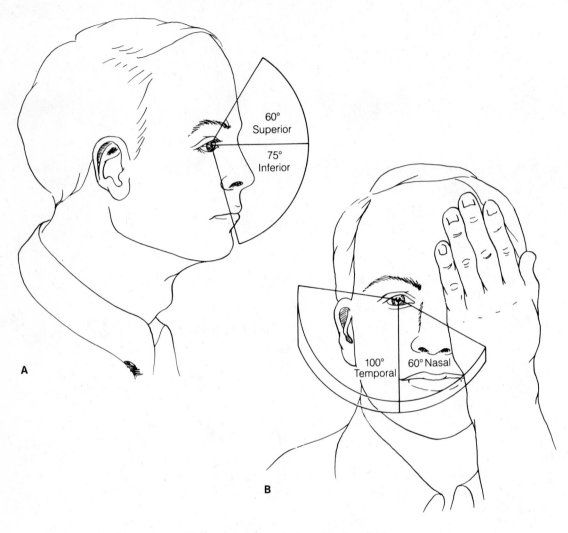

Figure 5–8. Normal limits of the visual field.

5. While many visual field deficits are detectable by these screening procedures, more precise mapping of the fields requires the use of one of many perimetry techniques. In **tangent screen testing,** the patient typically sits 1 meter from the screen with one eye covered, and the examiner places pins of various sizes and colors on the surface of the screen. The field is plotted for each eye, indicating the sizes of the test objects and the distance of the patient from the screen.

Ophthalmoscopy

A. Preparation of the Patient: Ophthalmoscopic examination of the optic fundus is particularly important in evaluating neuro-ophthalmologic disorders that affect the retina or optic disk and in the evaluation of patients with a suspected increase in intracranial pressure. The examination should be con-

ducted in a dark room so that the pupils are dilated; in some patients, the use of mydriatic (sympathomimetic or anticholinergic) eye drops is necessary. In the latter case, visual acuity and pupillary reflexes should always be assessed before instilling the drops. Mydriatic agents should be avoided in patients with glaucoma and in situations—such as impending or ongoing transtentorial herniation—in which the state of pupillary reactivity is an important guide to management.

B. Examination of the Fundus: Familiarity with the normal appearance of the optic fundus (Figure 5–10) is necessary if abnormalities are to be appreciated.

1. Optic disk–

a. Normal appearance–The optic disk is usually easily recognizable as a yellowish, slightly oval structure situated nasally at the posterior pole of the eye. The temporal side of the disk is often paler than

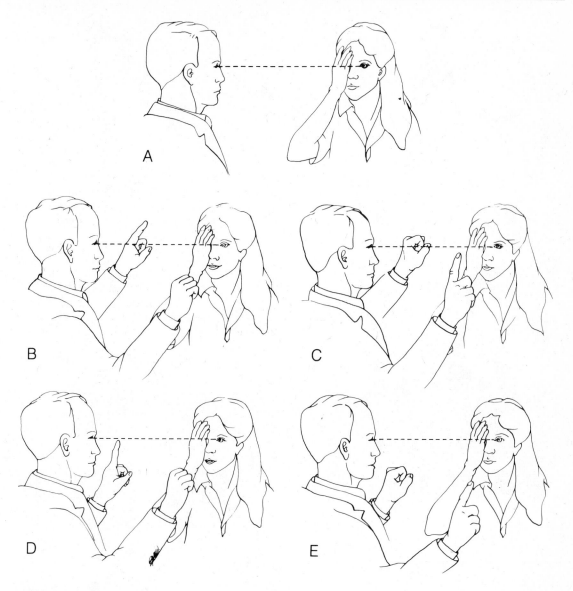

Figure 5–9. Confrontation testing of the visual field. **A**: The left eye of the patient and the right eye of the examiner are aligned. **B**: Testing the superior nasal quadrant. **C**: Testing the superior temporal quadrant. **D**: Testing the inferior nasal quadrant. **E**: Testing the inferior temporal quadrant. The procedure is then repeated for the patient's other eye.

the nasal side. The disk margins should be sharply demarcated, though the nasal edge is commonly somewhat less distinct than the temporal edge. The disk is normally in the same plane as the surrounding retina.

b. Optic disk swelling–Among the many ophthalmoscopic findings that provide useful diagnostic information, the abnormality that most often requires prompt interpretation and attention is optic nerve swelling **(papilledema).** While this condition implies increased intracranial pressure, it must be differentiated from swelling that is due to other causes, such as local inflammation (papillitis) and ischemic optic neuropathy. In making this distinction, it is most helpful to bear in mind that papilledema is almost always bilateral; it does not typically impair vision, except for enlargement of the blind spot; and it is not associated with eye pain. Papilledema can also be simulated by disk abnormalities such as drusen (colloid or hyaline bodies).

Increased intracranial pressure is thought to cause papilledema by transmitting the increased pressure through the intravaginal space surrounding the optic nerve. Because this compartment communicates with the subarachnoid space, disorders associ-

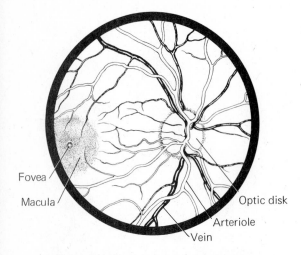

Fovea

Macula

Optic disk

Arteriole

Vein

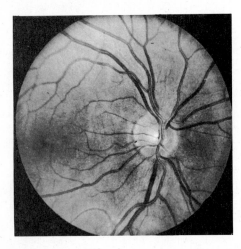

Figure 5–10. The normal fundus. The diagram shows landmarks corresponding to the photograph. (Photo by Diane Beeston; reproduced with permission, from Vaughan D, Asbury T, Riordan-Eva P: *General Ophthalmology,* 13th ed. Appleton & Lange, 1992.)

ated with increased intracranial pressure that also obstruct the subarachnoid space, such as meningitis, are less likely to cause papilledema. The ophthalmoscopic changes in papilledema typically develop over days or weeks but may become apparent within hours following a sudden increase in intracranial pressure— as, for example, following intracranial hemorrhage. In early papilledema (Figure 5–11), the retinal veins appear engorged and spontaneous venous pulsations are absent. The disk may be hyperemic, and linear hemorrhages may be seen at its borders. The disk margins become blurred, with the temporal edge last to be affected. In fully developed papilledema, the optic disk is elevated above the plane of the retina.

c. Optic disk pallor–Optic disk pallor with impaired visual acuity, visual fields, or pupillary reac-

tivity is associated with a wide variety of disorders that affect the optic nerve, including inflammatory conditions, nutritional deficiencies, and heredodegenerative diseases. Note that a pale optic disk with normal visual function can occur as a congenital variant.

2. Arteries and veins–To determine the caliber of the retinal arteries and veins, they are observed at the point where they arise from the disk and pass over its edges onto the retina. Observations include whether they are easily visible throughout their course, whether they appear engorged, and whether spontaneous venous pulsations are present. The remainder of the visible retina is inspected, noting the presence of hemorrhages, exudates, or other abnormalities.

3. Macula–The macula, a somewhat paler area than the rest of the retina, is located about two disk diameters temporal to the temporal margin of the optic disk. It can be visualized quickly by having the patient look at the light from the ophthalmoscope. Ophthalmoscopic examination of the macula can reveal abnormalities related to visual loss from age-related macular degeneration, from macular holes, or from hereditary cerebromacular degenerations.

Pupils

A. Size: Assessing the size and reactivity of the pupils provides an evaluation of nervous system pathways from the optic nerve to the midbrain (Figure 5–12). The normal pupil is round, regular, and centered within the iris; its size varies with age and with the intensity of ambient light. In a brightly illuminated examining room, normal pupils are about 3 mm in diameter in adults. They are often smaller in the elderly and commonly 5 mm or more in diameter in children. Pupillary size may be asymmetric in as much as 20% of the population (physiological **anisocoria**), but the difference in size is not more than 1 mm. Symmetrically rapid constriction in response to a bright light indicates that the size difference is not due to oculomotor nerve compression.

B. Reaction to Light: Direct (ipsilateral) and **consensual (contralateral)** pupillary constriction in response to a bright light shined in one eye demonstrates the integrity of the pathways shown in Figure 5–12. Normally, the direct response to light is slightly brisker and more pronounced than the consensual response.

C. Reaction to Accommodation: When the eyes converge to focus on a nearer object, the pupils normally constrict. The reaction to accommodation is tested by having the patient focus alternately on a distant object and a finger held just in front of his or her nose.

D. Pupillary Abnormalities:

1. Nonreactive pupils–Unilateral disorders of pupillary constriction are seen with local disease of the iris (trauma, iritis, glaucoma), oculomotor nerve

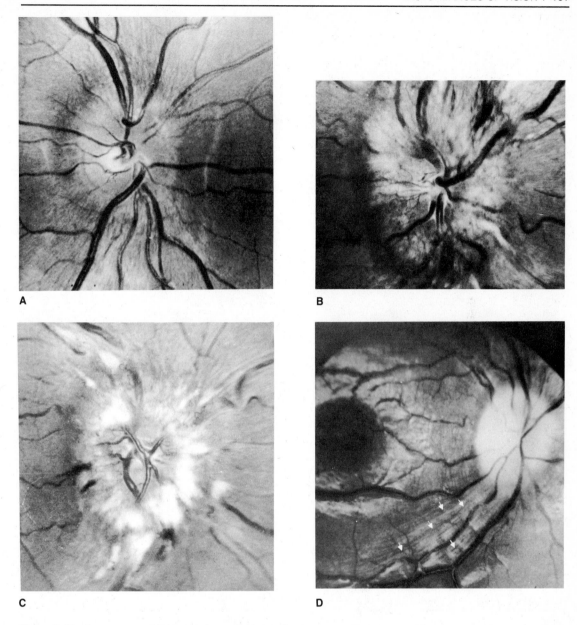

Figure 5–11. Appearance of the fundus in papilledema. **A:** In early papilledema, the superior and inferior margins of the optic disk are blurred by the thickened layer of nerve fibers entering the disk. **B:** Swollen nerve fibers (white patches) and hemorrhages can be seen. **C:** In fully developed papilledema, the optic disk is swollen, elevated, and congested, and the retinal veins are markedly dilated. **D:** In chronic atrophic papilledema, the optic disk is pale and slightly elevated and its margins are blurred. The white areas surrounding the macula are reflected light from the vitreoretinal interface. The inferior temporal nerve fiber bundles are partially atrophic (arrows). (Photos courtesy of WF Hoyt.)

compression (tumor, aneurysm), and optic nerve disorders (optic neuritis, multiple sclerosis).

2. Light-near dissociation–Impaired pupillary reactivity to light with preserved constriction during accommodation (light-near dissociation) is usually bilateral and may result from neurosyphilis, diabetes, optic nerve disorders, and tumors compressing the midbrain tectum.

3. Argyll Robertson pupils–These pupils are small, poorly reactive in shape, often irregular in shape, and unequal in size; they show light-near dissociation (see Table 5–1). Neurosyphilis is the usual cause.

4. Tonic pupil–The tonic (**Adie's**) pupil (Table 5–1) is larger than the contralateral unaffected pupil and reacts sluggishly to changes in illumination.

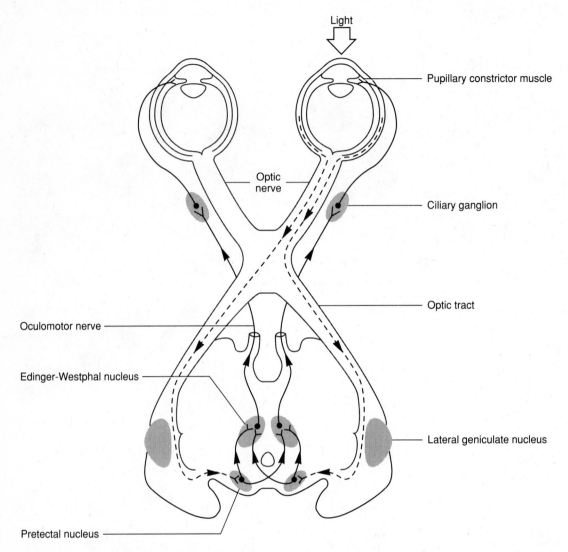

Light

Pupillary constrictor muscle

Optic nerve

Ciliary ganglion

Optic tract

Oculomotor nerve

Edinger-Westphal nucleus

Lateral geniculate nucleus

Pretectal nucleus

Figure 5–12. Anatomical basis of the pupillary light reflex. The afferent visual pathways from the retina to the prectectal nuclei of the midbrain are represented by dashed lines; the efferent pupilloconstrictor pathways from the midbrain to the retinas by solid lines. Note that illumination of one eye results in bilateral pupillary constriction.

Since the tonic pupil does eventually react, anisocoria becomes less marked with time. This abnormality is most commonly a manifestation of a benign, often familial disorder that frequently affects young women **(Holmes-Adie syndrome)** and may be associated with depressed deep tendon reflexes (especially in the legs), segmental anhidrosis (localized lack of sweating), orthostatic hypotension, or cardiovascular autonomic instability. The pupillary abnormality may be caused by degeneration of the ciliary ganglion, followed by aberrant reinnervation of the pupilloconstrictor muscles.

5. Horner's syndrome–Horner's syndrome (Tables 5–1 and 5–2) results from a lesion of the cen-

tral or peripheral sympathetic nervous system and consists of a small (miotic) pupil associated with ptosis and sometimes loss of sweating **(anhidrosis).**

a. Oculosympathetic pathways–The sympathetic pathway controlling pupillary dilation (Figure 5–13) consists of an uncrossed three-neuron arc: **hypothalamic neurons,** the axons of which descend through the brain stem to the intermediolateral column of the spinal cord at the T1 level; **preganglionic sympathetic neurons** projecting from the spinal cord to the superior cervical ganglion; and **postganglionic sympathetic neurons** that originate in the superior cervical ganglion, ascend in the neck along the internal carotid artery, and enter the orbit with the first

Table 5–1. Common pupillary abnormalities.

	Appearance	Response	Differential Diagnosis
Tonic (Adie's) pupil	Unilateral (rarely bilateral) dilated pupil	Reacts sluggishly and only to persistent bright light or 0.125% pilocarpine eye drops; accommodation less affected.	Holmes-Adie syndrome, ocular trauma, autonomic neuropathy
Horner's syndrome	Unilateral small pupil and slight ptosis	Normal response to light and accommodation.	Lateral medullary infarcts, cervical cord lesions, pulmonary apical or mediastinal tumors, neck - trauma or masses, carotid artery thrombosis, intrapartum brachial plexus injury, cluster headache
Argyll Robertson pupil	Unequal irregular pupils less than 3 mm in diameter (usually bilateral)	Poorly reactive to light; more responsive to accommodation.	Neurosyphilis; mimicked by diabetes, pineal region tumors

(ophthalmic) division of the trigeminal (V) nerve. Horner's syndrome is caused by interruption of these pathways at any site.

b. Clinical features–The lesions—and the pupillary abnormality produced—are usually unilateral. The pupillary diameter on the involved side is typically reduced by 0.5–1 mm compared with the normal side. This inequality is most marked in dim illumination and in other situations in which the pupils are normally dilated, such as during a painful stimulus or startle. The pupillary abnormality is accompanied by mild to moderate ptosis (see below) of the upper lid, often associated with elevation of the lower lid. When Horner's syndrome has been present since infancy, the ipsilateral iris is lighter and blue in color (**heterochromia iridis).**

Deficits in the pattern of sweating, which are most

Table 5–2. Causes of Horner's syndrome in 100 hospitalized patients.[1]

	Percentage
Central (first) neuron	63
Brain stem infarction	36
Cerebral hemorrhage/infarction	12
Multiple sclerosis	3
Intracranial tumor	2
Trauma (including surgery)	2
Syrinx	2
Transverse myelopathy	2
Other or unknown	4
Preganglionic (second) neuron	21
Thoracic and neck tumor	14
Trauma	
Nonsurgical	4
Surgical	3
Other or unknown	0
Postganglionic (third) neuron	13
Intracranial tumor (cavernous sinus)	7
Trauma (including surgical)	2
Vascular headache	2
Other or unknown	2
Unknown localization	3

[1]Data from Keane JR: *Arch Neurol* 1979;36:13–16.

prominent in acute-onset Horner's syndrome, can help localize the lesion. If sweating is decreased on an entire half of the body and face, the lesion is in the central nervous system. Cervical lesions produce anhidrosis of the face, neck, and arm only. Sweating is unimpaired if the lesion is above the bifurcation of the carotid artery. The differential diagnosis of Horner's syndrome is presented in Table 5–2.

6. Relative afferent pupillary defect–In this condition, one pupil constricts less markedly in response to direct illumination than to illumination of the contralateral pupil. The abnormality is detected by rapidly moving a bright flashlight back and forth between the eyes while continuously observing the suspect pupil (**Gunn's pupillary test).** Relative afferent pupillary defect is commonly associated with disorders of the ipsilateral optic nerve, which interrupt the afferent limb and affect the pupillary light reflex (see Figure 5–12). Such disorders also commonly impair vision (especially color vision) in the involved eye.

Optokinetic Response

Optokinetic nystagmus consists of eye movements elicited by sequential fixation on a series of targets passing in front of a patient's eyes, such as telephone poles seen from a moving train. For clinical testing, a revolving drum with vertical stripes or a vertically striped strip of cloth moved across the visual field is used to generate these movements. Testing produces a slow following phase in the direction of the target's movement, followed by a rapid return jerk in the opposite direction. The slow (pursuit) phase tests ipsilateral parieto-occipital pathways; the rapid (saccadic) movement tests pathways originating in the contralateral frontal lobe. The presence of an optokinetic response reflects the ability to perceive movement or contour and is sometimes useful for documenting visual perception in newborns or in psychogenic blindness. Visual acuity required to produce the optokinetic response is minimal, however (20/400, or finger counting at 3–5 feet). Unilateral

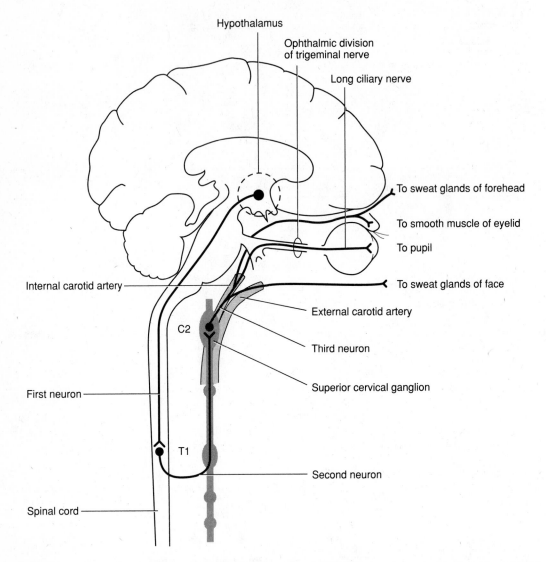

Figure 5–13. Oculosympathetic pathway involved in Horner's syndrome. This three-neuron pathway projects from the hypothalamus to the intermediolateral column of the spinal cord, then to the superior cervical (sympathetic) ganglion, and finally to the pupil, smooth muscle of the eyelid, and sweat glands of the forehead and face.

impairment of the optokinetic response may be found when targets are moved toward the side of a parietal lobe lesion.

Eyelids

The eyelids **(palpebrae)** should be examined with the patient's eyes open. The distance between the upper and lower lids (interpalpebral fissure) is usually about 10 mm and equal in both eyes, though physiological asymmetries do occur. The position of the inferior margin of the upper lid relative to the superior border of the iris should be noted in order to detect drooping **(ptosis)** or abnormal elevation of the eyelid **(lid retraction).** The upper lid normally covers 1–2 mm of the iris.

Unilateral ptosis is seen with paralysis of the levator palpebrae muscle itself, lesions of the oculomotor nerve or its superior branch, and Horner's syndrome. In the last condition, ptosis is customarily associated with miosis and may be momentarily overcome by effortful eye opening.

Bilateral ptosis suggests disease affecting the oculomotor nerve nucleus; a disorder of the neuromuscular junction, such as myasthenia gravis; or a disorder of muscle, such as myotonic, ocular, or oculopharyngeal dystrophy.

Lid retraction (abnormal elevation of the upper lid) is seen in hyperthyroidism; in **Parinaud's syndrome,** it is caused by tumors in the pineal region.

Exophthalmos

Abnormal protrusion of the eye from the orbit (**exophthalmos** or **proptosis**) is best detected by standing behind the seated patient and looking down at his or her eyes. The causes include hyperthyroidism, orbital tumor or pseudotumor, and carotid artery-cavernous sinus fistula. A bruit may be audible on auscultation over the proptotic eye in patients with carotid artery-cavernous sinus fistula or other vascular anomalies.

Eye Movements

A. Ocular Excursion and Gaze: Ocular palsies and gaze palsies are detected by having the patient gaze in each of the six cardinal positions (see Figure 5–5). If voluntary eye movement is impaired or the patient is unable to cooperate with the examination (eg, is comatose), reflex eye movements can be induced by one of two maneuvers. The **doll's head (oculocephalic) maneuver** is performed by rotating the head horizontally, to elicit horizontal eye movements, and vertically, to elicit vertical movements. The eyes should move in the direction opposite to that of head rotation. This may be an inadequate stimulus for inducing eye movements, however, and the reflex is usually suppressed in conscious patients. **Caloric (oculovestibular) stimulation** is a more potent stimulus and is performed by irrigating the tympanic membrane with cold or warm water. Otoscopic examination should always be undertaken before this maneuver is attempted: it is contraindicated if the tympanic membrane is perforated. In conscious patients, unilateral cold water irrigation produces nystagmus with the fast phase directed away from the irrigated side. Because this procedure may produce discomfort and nausea or vomiting, only small volumes (eg, 1 mL) of water should be used in conscious patients. In comatose patients with intact brain stem function, unilateral cold water irrigation results in tonic deviation of the eyes toward the irrigated side. Bilateral irrigation with cold water causes tonic downward deviation, whereas bilateral stimulation with hot water induces tonic upward deviation. An absent or impaired response to caloric stimulation with large volumes (eg, 50 mL) of cold water is indicative of peripheral vestibular disease, a structural lesion in the posterior fossa (cerebellum or brain stem), or intoxication with sedative drugs. If limitations in movement are observed, the muscles involved are noted and the nature of the abnormality is determined according to the following scheme.

1. Ocular palsy–This weakness of one or more eye muscles results from nuclear or infranuclear (nerve, neuromuscular junction, or muscle) lesions. An ocular palsy cannot be overcome by caloric stim-

ulation of reflex eye movement. Nerve lesions produce distinctive patterns of ocular muscle involvement.

a. Oculomotor (III) nerve palsy–A complete lesion of the oculomotor nerve produces closure of the affected eye because of impaired levator function. Passively elevating the paralyzed lid (Figure 5–14) shows the involved eye to be laterally deviated because of the unopposed action of the lateral rectus muscle, which is not innervated by the oculomotor nerve. Diplopia is present in all directions of gaze except for lateral gaze toward the side of involvement. The pupil's function may be normal (pupillary sparing) or impaired.

b. Trochlear (IV) nerve palsy–With trochlear nerve lesions, which paralyze the superior oblique muscle, the involved eye is elevated during primary (forward) gaze; the extent of elevation increases during adduction and decreases during abduction. Elevation is greatest when the head is tilted toward the side of the involved eye and abolished by tilt in the opposite direction (Bielschowsky's head-tilt test; Figure 5–15). Diplopia is most pronounced when the patient looks downward with the affected eye adducted (as in looking at the end of one's nose). Spontaneous head tilting, intended to decrease or correct the diplopia, is present in about half the patients with unilateral palsies and in an even greater number with bilateral palsies.

c. Abducens (VI) nerve palsy–An abducens nerve lesion causes paralysis of the lateral rectus muscle, resulting in adduction of the involved eye at rest and failure of attempted abduction (Figure 5–16). Diplopia occurs on lateral gaze to the side of the affected eye.

2. Gaze palsy–Gaze palsy is the diminished ability of a pair of yoked muscles (muscles that operate in concert to move the two eyes in a given direction) to move the eyes in voluntary gaze; it is caused by supranuclear lesions in the brain stem or cerebral hemisphere. Gaze palsy, unlike ocular palsies, affects both eyes and can usually be overcome by caloric stimulation. Its pathophysiology and causes are dis-

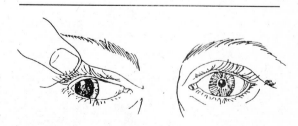

Figure 5–14. Clinical findings with oculomotor (III) nerve lesion. With the ptotic lid passively elevated, the affected (right) eye is abducted. On attempted downgaze, the unaffected superior oblique muscle, which is innervated by the trochlear (IV) nerve, causes the eye to turn inward.

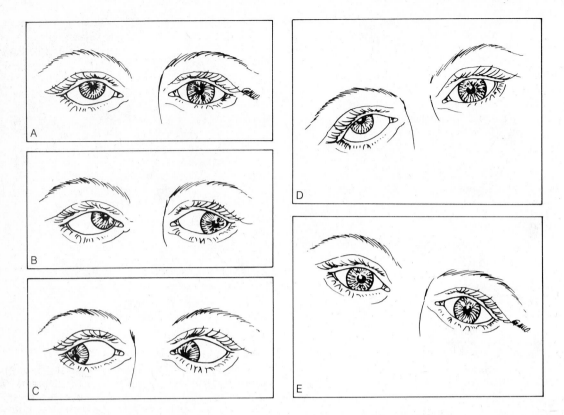

Figure 5–15. Clinical findings with trochlear (IV) nerve lesion. The affected (right) eye is elevated on forward gaze *(A)*. The extent of elevation is increased with adduction *(B)* and decreased with abduction *(C)*. Elevation is maximal with head tilting to the affected side *(D)* and disappears with head tilting in the opposite direction *(E)*.

cussed more fully in the section on gaze palsy. Mild impairment of upgaze is not uncommon in asymptomatic elderly subjects.

3. Internuclear ophthalmoplegia–This disorder results from a lesion of the medial longitudinal fasciculus, an ascending pathway in the brain stem that projects from the abducens to the contralateral oculomotor nerve nucleus. As a consequence, the actions of the abducens and oculomotor nerves during voluntary gaze or caloric-induced movement are uncoupled. Excursion of the abducting eye is full, but adduction of the contralateral eye is impaired (Figure 5–17). Internuclear ophthalmoplegia cannot be overcome by caloric stimulation; it can be distinguished from oculomotor nerve palsy by noting preservation of adduction with convergence. Its causes are discussed later (see *Internuclear Ophthalmoplegia*).

4. One-and-a-half syndrome–A pontine lesion affecting both the medial longitudinal fasciculus and the ipsilateral paramedian pontine reticular formation (lateral gaze center) produces a syndrome that combines internuclear ophthalmoplegia with an inability to gaze toward the side of the lesion (Figure 5–18). The ipsilateral eye is immobile in the horizontal plane and movement of the contralateral eye is restricted to abduction, which may be associated with nystagmus. The causes include pontine infarct, multiple sclerosis, and pontine hemorrhage.

B. Diplopia Testing: When the patient complains of diplopia, maneuvers to test eye movement should be used to determine its anatomical basis. The patient is asked to fix his or her vision on an object, such as a flashlight, in each of the six cardinal positions of gaze. With normal conjugate gaze, light from the flashlight falls at the same spot on both corneas; a lack of such congruency confirms that gaze is disconjugate. When the patient notes diplopia in a given direction of gaze, each eye should be covered in turn and the patient asked to report which of the two images disappears. The image displaced farther in the direction of gaze is always referable to the weak eye. A variation of this procedure is the **red glass test,** in which one eye is covered with translucent red glass, plastic, or cellophane; this allows the eye responsible for each image to be identified.

C. Nystagmus: Nystagmus is rhythmic oscillation of the eyes. **Pendular nystagmus,** which usually has its onset in infancy, occurs with equal velocity in

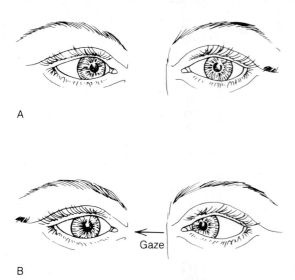

A

B

Figure 5–16. Clinical findings with abducens (VI) nerve lesion. The affected (right) eye is adducted at rest **(A)** and cannot be abducted **(B)**.

both directions. **Jerk nystagmus** is characterized by a slow phase of movement followed by a fast phase in the opposite direction; the direction of jerk nystagmus is specified by stating the direction of the fast phase (eg, leftward-beating nystagmus). Jerk nystagmus usually increases in amplitude with gaze in the direction of the fast phase.

Nystagmus, a normal component of both the optokinetic response and the response to caloric stimulation of reflex eye movements, can also occur at the extremes of voluntary gaze in normal subjects. In other settings, however, it is commonly due to anticonvulsant or sedative drugs or is a sign of disease in the peripheral vestibular apparatus, central vestibular pathways, or cerebellum.

To detect nystagmus, the eyes are observed in the primary position and in each of the cardinal positions of gaze (see Figure 5–5). Nystagmus is described in terms of the position of gaze in which it occurs, its direction and amplitude, precipitating factors such as changes in head position, and associated symptoms, such as vertigo.

Many forms of nystagmus and related ocular oscillations have been described, but two syndromes of acquired **pathological jerk nystagmus** are by far the most common.

1. Gaze-evoked nystagmus–As its name implies, gaze-evoked nystagmus occurs when the patient attempts to gaze in one or more directions away from the primary position. The fast phase is in the direction of gaze. Nystagmus evoked by gaze in a single direction is a common sign of early or mild residual ocular palsy. Multidirectional gaze-evoked nystagmus is most often an adverse effect of anticonvulsant or sedative drugs, but it can also result from cerebellar or central vestibular dysfunction.

2. Vestibular nystagmus–Vestibular nystagmus increases with gaze toward the fast phase and is usually accompanied by vertigo. When caused by a lesion of the **peripheral vestibular apparatus,** vestibular nystagmus is characteristically unidirectional, horizontal, or horizontal and rotatory and associated with severe vertigo. In contrast, **central vestibular nystagmus** may be bidirectional and purely horizontal, vertical, or rotatory, and the accompanying vertigo is typically mild. **Positional nystagmus**— elicited by changes in head position—can occur with either peripheral or central vestibular lesions. The most helpful distinguishing features are the presence of hearing loss or tinnitus with peripheral lesions and of corticospinal tract or additional cranial nerve abnormalities with central lesions.

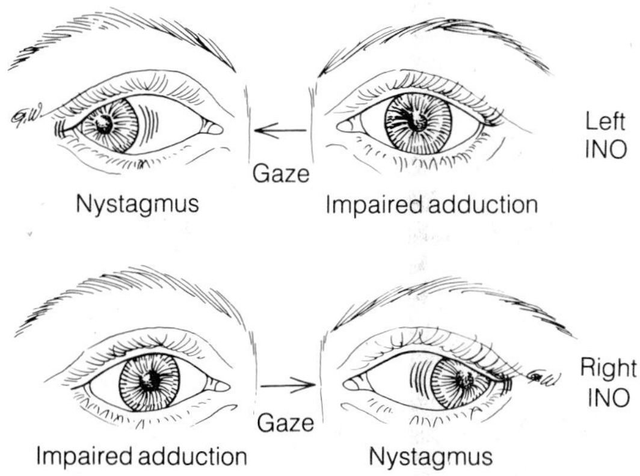

DISORDERS OF THE VISUAL SYSTEM

MONOCULAR DISORDERS

Common syndromes of monocular visual loss include two reversible and two irreversible disorders. **Transient monocular blindness** caused by optic nerve ischemia is sudden in onset and resolves rapidly. Subacute, painful, unilateral visual loss with partial resolution is associated with **optic neuritis.** Irreversible visual loss of sudden onset occurs in idiopathic **ischemic optic neuropathy** and in **giant cell (temporal) arteritis.**

Figure 5–17. Eye movements in internuclear ophthalmoplegia (INO) resulting from a lesion of the medial longitudinal fasciculus.

Left INO

Nystagmus | Gaze | Impaired adduction

Right INO

Impaired adduction | Gaze | Nystagmus

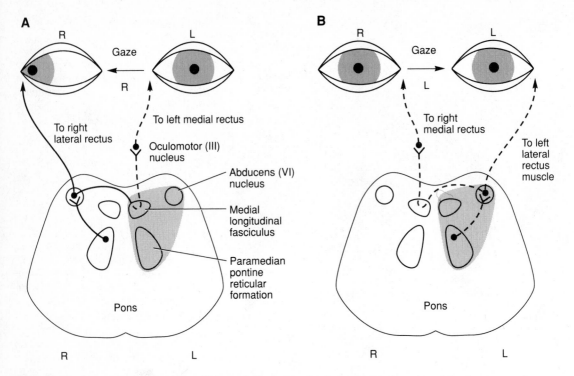

Figure 5–18. One-and-a-half syndrome. This results from a pontine lesion (shaded area) involving the paramedian pontine recticular formation (lateral gaze center) and medial longitudinal fasciculus, and sometimes also the abducens (VI) nucleus, and affecting the neuronal pathways indicated by dotted lines. In **(A)**, attempted gaze away from the lesion activates the uninvolved right lateral gaze center and abducens (VI) nucleus; the right lateral rectus muscle contracts and the right eye abducts normally. Involvement of the medial longitudinal fasciculus interrupts the pathway to the left oculomotor (III) nucleus, and the left eye fails to adduct. On attempted gaze toward the lesion **(B)**, the left lateral gaze center cannot be activated, and the eyes do not move. There is a complete (bilateral) gaze palsy in one direction (toward the lesion) and one-half (unilateral) gaze palsy in the other direction (away from the lesion), accounting for the name of the syndrome.

1. TRANSIENT MONOCULAR BLINDNESS

This condition, sometimes called **amaurosis fugax,** is characterized by unilateral transient diminution or loss of vision that develops over seconds, remains maximal for 1–5 minutes, and resolves over 10–20 minutes. Although the cause of these episodes often remains uncertain, the presence of what appears to be embolic material in retinal arteries during episodes suggests that emboli are the cause. The major site of origin of such emboli appears to be atherosclerotic lesions at the carotid bifurcation. Mitral valve prolapse and other cardiac sources of emboli can produce a similar syndrome. The risk for subsequent hemispheric infarction is increased (14% within seven years) in patients with a history of transient monocular blindness but is only about one-half that in patients with hemispheric transient ischemic attacks (TIAs).

Diagnostic evaluation and treatment of patients with transient monocular blindness resembles that recommended for patients with hemispheric TIAs (see Chapter 10). Recent studies have shown that in patients with transient monocular blindness or TIAs and high-grade (>70%) stenosis of the carotid artery at angiography, the combination of aspirin plus surgical removal of thrombus (endarterectomy) is superior to aspirin alone.

2. OPTIC NEURITIS

Inflammation of the optic nerve produces the syndrome of optic neuritis, which can be idiopathic; caused by demyelination or parameningeal, meningeal, or intraocular inflammation; or associated with viral infections or post-viral-infection syndromes. Unilateral impairment of visual acuity occurs over hours to days, becoming maximal within one week. The visual loss is associated with headache, globe tenderness, or eye pain; the last is typically exacerbated by eye movement.

On visual field testing, there is usually a central scotoma (blind spot). Examination of the fundus is often normal, since the inflammatory process is posterior to the optic disk (retrobulbar neuritis), but unilateral disk swelling may be seen. The pupils are equal in size but show a diminished reaction to illumination of the affected eye (relative afferent pupillary defect; discussed above). Visual acuity usually improves over two to three weeks, sometimes returning to normal, although actual recovery may take longer—and may never be complete. Systemic steroids have been used to hasten recovery but do not alter the final outcome. The frequency with which optic neuritis is the first sign of more widespread central nervous system demyelination (multiple sclerosis) remains uncertain and varies with the length of follow-up studies. Most prospective and retrospective series, however, report progression to definite multiple sclerosis in 15–20% of cases.

Rare causes of optic neuropathy include toxins (eg, methanol), neurosyphilis, and vitamin B_{12} deficiency.

3. ISCHEMIC OPTIC NEUROPATHY

Idiopathic infarction of the anterior portion of the optic nerve is termed ischemic optic neuropathy. Such visual loss is sudden in onset, painless, always monocular, and without premonitory ocular symptoms. Visual loss is maximal at onset and frequently subtotal, producing a field defect that is typically **altitudinal** (superior or inferior) in configuration. Examination reveals ipsilateral disk swelling. In the absence of this finding, the diagnosis is tenuous, and other causes, such as a rapidly expanding intracranial mass or neoplastic meningitis, should be sought. Although ischemic optic neuropathy is often assumed to be atherosclerotic in origin, there is no consistent association with other risk factors for cerebrovascular disease, such as hypertension, diabetes, or atherosclerotic carotid artery disease.

Attempts at treatment have been uniformly unsuccessful. As disk swelling resolves, ophthalmoscopic evaluation shows optic atrophy.

4. GIANT CELL (TEMPORAL) ARTERITIS

Arteritic infarction of the anterior portion of the optic nerve is the most devastating complication of giant cell, or temporal, arteritis. This disorder is usually accompanied by systemic symptoms such as fever, malaise, and headache and often by **polymyalgia rheumatica.** Transient retinal ischemia may precede optic nerve infarction. The visual loss is sudden, most often total, and may be simultaneously bilateral. On examination, the optic disk may appear swollen or normal. Immediate treatment with corticosteroids (prednisone, 60–80 mg/d orally) is urgently required to protect what vision remains.

Because giant cell arteritis is treatable, it is most important to distinguish it from ischemic optic neuropathy as the cause of monocular visual loss. Patients with giant cell arteritis tend to be slightly older (aged 70–80 years), and they may have premonitory symptoms. In addition, simultaneous bilateral involvement is essentially limited to giant cell arteritis.

Ischemic optic neuropathy is unilateral at presentation, but contralateral involvement follows in months to years in 30–50% of cases. The most helpful differential feature is the erythrocyte sedimentation rate, which is greater than 50 mm/h (Westergren) in most patients with giant cell arteritis.

BINOCULAR DISORDERS

1. PAPILLEDEMA

Papilledema is the passive bilateral disk swelling that is associated with increased intracranial pressure. Less common causes include congenital cyanotic heart disease and disorders associated with increased cerebrospinal fluid protein content, including spinal cord tumor and idiopathic inflammatory polyneuropathy (Guillain-Barré syndrome).

The speed with which papilledema develops is dictated by the underlying cause. When intracranial pressure increases suddenly, as in subarachnoid or intracerebral hemorrhage, disk swelling may be seen within hours, but it most often evolves over days. Papilledema may require two to three months to resolve following restoration of normal intracranial pressure. Associated nonspecific symptoms of raised intracranial pressure include headache, nausea, vomiting, and diplopia from abducens nerve palsy. Funduscopic examination (see Figure 5–11) reveals (in order of onset) blurring of the nerve fiber layer, absence of venous pulsations (signifying intracranial pressure greater than approximately 200 mm Hg), hemorrhages in the nerve fiber layer, elevation of the disk surface with blurring of the margins, and disk hyperemia.

Papilledema requires urgent evaluation to search for an intracranial mass and to exclude papillitis from syphilis, carcinoma, or sarcoidosis, which may produce a similar ophthalmoscopic appearance. In the history and examination, attention should be directed at symptoms and signs of intracranial masses, such as hemiparesis, hemianopia or seizures, and signs of meningeal irritation.

If an intracranial mass lesion is ruled out by the history, examination, and CT scanning or MRI; if inflammatory meningeal processes are excluded by spinal fluid examination; and if CSF pressure is elevated, a diagnosis of **pseudotumor cerebri** is established by exclusion. The idiopathic form, which is the most common, occurs most often in obese women during the childbearing years. Although this disorder is usually self-limited, prolonged elevation of intracranial pressure can lead to permanent visual loss (see discussion in Chapter 3).

2. CHIASMAL LESIONS

The major lesions that produce visual impairment at the level of the optic chiasm are tumors, especially those of pituitary origin. Other causes include trauma, demyelinating disease, and expanding berry aneurysms. The classic pattern of visual deficit caused by lesions of the optic chiasm is **bitemporal hemianopia** (see Figure 5–7). Chiasmal visual loss is gradual in onset, and the resulting impairment in depth perception or in the lateral visual fields may remain asymptomatic for some time. Associated involvement of the oculomotor, trochlear, trigeminal, or abducens nerve suggests tumor expansion into the cavernous sinus. Nonophthalmologic manifestations of pituitary tumors include headache, acromegaly, amenorrhea, galactorrhea, and Cushing's syndrome.

Headache, endocrine abnormalities, and occasionally blurred or double vision may occur in patients with an enlarged sella turcica (shown on radiographic examination), but in whom neither tumor nor increased intracranial pressure is found. This **empty sella syndrome** is most common in women and occurs mainly between the fourth and seventh decades of life. Treatment is symptomatic.

3. RETROCHIASMAL LESIONS

Optic Tract & Lateral Geniculate Body

Lesions of the optic tract and lateral geniculate body are usually due to infarction. The resulting visual field abnormality is typically a **noncongruous homonymous hemianopia,** ie, the field defect is not the same in the two eyes. Associated hemisensory loss may occur with thalamic lesions.

Optic Radiations

Lesions of the optic radiations produce field deficits that are congruous and homonymous (bilaterally symmetric). Visual acuity is normal in the unaffected portion of the field. With lesions in the **temporal lobe,** where tumors are the most common cause, the field deficit is denser superiorly than inferiorly, resulting in a **superior quadrantanopia** (pie in the sky deficit; see Figure 5–7).

Lesions affecting the optic radiations in the **parietal lobe** may be due to tumor or vascular disease and are usually associated with contralateral weakness and sensory loss. A gaze preference is common, with the eyes conjugately deviated to the side of the parietal lesion. The visual field abnormality is either complete **homonymous hemianopia** or **inferior quadrantanopia** (see Figure 5–7). The optokinetic response to a visual stimulus moved toward the side of the lesion is impaired, which is not the case with pure temporal or occipital lobe lesions.

Occipital Cortex

Lesions in the occipital cortex usually produce **homonymous hemianopias** affecting the contralateral visual field. The patient may be unaware of the visual deficit. Since the region of the occipital cortex in which the macula is represented is often supplied by branches of both the posterior and middle cerebral arteries (see Figure 5–4), visual field abnormalities caused by vascular lesions in the occipital lobe may show **sparing of macular vision** (see Figure 5–7). It has also been suggested that in some cases, macular sparing may result from bilateral cortical representation of the macular region of the visual field.

The most common cause of visual impairment in the occipital lobe is infarction in the posterior cerebral artery territory (90% of cases). Occipital lobe arteriovenous malformations (AVMs), vertebral angiography, and watershed infarction following cardiac arrest are less common causes. Additional symptoms and signs of basilar artery ischemia may occur. Tumors and occipital lobe AVMs are often associated with unformed visual hallucinations that are typically unilateral, stationary or moving, and often brief or flickering; they can be colored or not colored.

Bilateral occipital lobe involvement produces cortical blindness. Pupillary reactions are normal, and bilateral macular sparing may preserve central (tunnel) vision. With more extensive lesions, denial of blindness may occur (**Anton's syndrome).**

DISORDERS OF OCULAR MOTILITY

GAZE PALSY

Lesions in the cortex or brain stem above the level of the ocular motor nuclei may impair conjugate (yoked) movement of the eyes, producing gaze disorders.

Hemispheric Lesions

Acutely, hemispheric lesions produce tonic deviation of both eyes toward the side of the lesion and away from the side of the hemiparesis (Figure 5–19A). This gaze deviation lasts for up to several days in alert patients—somewhat longer in comatose patients. Seizure discharges involving the frontal gaze centers can also produce gaze deviation by driving the eyes away from the discharging focus. When the ipsilateral motor cortex is also involved, producing focal motor seizures, the patient gazes toward the side of the motor activity (Figure 5–19B).

Midbrain Lesions

Lesions of the dorsal midbrain affect the center responsible for upward gaze and may therefore produce upgaze paralysis. In addition, all or some of the features of **Parinaud's syndrome** may occur. These include normal vertical eye movements with the doll's head maneuver or Bell's phenomenon (elevation of the eye with eyelid closure), nystagmus (especially on downward gaze and typically associated with retraction of the eyes), paralysis of accommodation, midposition pupils, and light-near dissociation.

Pontine Lesions

Brain stem lesions at the level of the pontine gaze centers produce disorders of conjugate horizontal gaze. Gaze palsies from pontine involvement (unlike those from hemispheric lesions) cause eye deviation toward—rather than away from—the side of the hemiparesis (see Figure 5–19C). This occurs because, at this level of the brain stem, the corticobulbar pathways that regulate gaze have decussated, but the descending motor pathways have not. Brain stem gaze pareses are characteristically far more resistant to attempts to move the eyes (via the doll's eye ma-

neuver or caloric stimulation) than are supratentorial gaze pareses and are commonly associated with abducens nerve dysfunction because of the involvement of the abducens nerve nucleus.

INTERNUCLEAR OPHTHALMOPLEGIA

Internuclear ophthalmoplegia results from lesions of the **medial longitudinal fasciculus** between the midpons and the oculomotor nerve nucleus that disconnect the abducens nerve nucleus from the contralateral oculomotor nucleus (see Figure 5–6). The site of the internuclear ophthalmoplegia is named according to the side on which oculomotor nerve function is impaired. There is a characteristic abnormality consisting of disconjugate gaze with impaired adduction and nystagmus of the abducting eye (Figure 5–17). Such a finding strongly supports a diagnosis of intrinsic brain stem disease. The most common cause, especially in young adults or in patients with bilateral involvement, is multiple sclerosis. In older patients

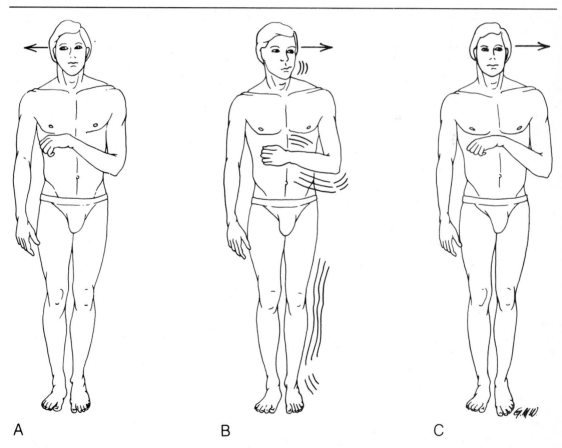

A   B   C

Figure 5–19. Disorders of gaze associated with hemispheric and brain stem lesions. **A:** Destructive lesion in the frontal lobe of the right cerebral hemisphere. **B:** Seizure arising from the frontal lobe of the right cerebral hemisphere. **C:** Destructive lesion in the right pons. Arrows indicate the direction of gaze preference (away from the hemiparetic side in **A** and toward the convulsing or hemiparetic side in **B** and **C**).

and those with unilateral involvement, vascular disease is likely. These two diagnoses encompass 80% or more of all cases in reported series. Rarer causes include brain stem encephalitis, intrinsic brain stem tumors, syringobulbia, sedative drug intoxication, and Wernicke's encephalopathy. Because the oculomotor abnormalities of myasthenia gravis can closely mimic a lesion of the medial longitudinal fasciculus, myasthenia must be ruled out in patients with isolated internuclear ophthalmoplegia.

OCULOMOTOR (III) NERVE LESIONS

Lesions of the oculomotor nerve can occur at any of several levels. The most common causes are listed in Table 5–3; oculomotor disorders resulting from diabetes are discussed separately below.

Brain Stem

Within the brain stem, associated neurological signs permit localization of the lesion; associated contralateral hemiplegia (Weber's syndrome) and contralateral ataxia (Benedikt's syndrome) are the most common vascular syndromes.

Subarachnoid Space

As the oculomotor nerve exits the brain stem in the interpeduncular space, it is susceptible to injury from trauma and from aneurysms of the posterior communicating artery. The latter often cause acute oculomotor palsy from aneurysmal expansion with a characteristic impairment of the pupillary light reflex.

Cavernous Sinus

In the cavernous sinus (Figure 5–20), the oculomotor nerve is usually involved along with the trochlear and abducens nerves and the first and sometimes the second division of the trigeminal nerve. Horner's syndrome may occur. Oculomotor nerve lesions in the cavernous sinus tend to produce partial deficits that may or may not spare the pupil.

Orbit

Unlike cavernous sinus lesions, orbital lesions that affect the oculomotor nerve are often associated with optic nerve involvement and exophthalmos; however, disorders of the orbit and cavernous sinus may be clinically indistinguishable except by CT scanning or MRI.

TROCHLEAR (IV) NERVE LESIONS

Head trauma, often minor, is the most common cause of an isolated trochlear nerve palsy (Table 5–3). While trochlear palsies in middle-aged and elderly patients are also frequently attributed to vascular disease or diabetes, they often occur without obvi-

Table 5–3. Causes of oculomotor (III) trochlear (IV) and abducens (VI) nerve lesions.[1]

Cause	Nerve III (%)	Nerve IV (%)	Nerve VI (%)
Unknown	23	29	26
Vasculopathy[2]	20	21	17
Aneurysm	19	1	3
Trauma	14	32	14
Neoplasm[3]	12	7	20
Syphilis	2	...	1
Multiple sclerosis	...	...	6
Other	10[4]	10[5]	13[6]

[1]Data are from several series, as compiled in Burde RM, Savino PJ, Trobe JD: *Clinical Decisions in Neuro-ophthalmology.* Mosby, 1984.
[2]Includes diabetes, hypertension, and atherosclerosis.
[3]Includes pituitary and parapituitary tumors, cavernous sinus meningioma, and primary and metastatic tumors of the brain stem.
[4]Includes sinusitis, Hodgkin's disease, herpes zoster, giant cell arteritis, meningitis, encephalitis, collagen vascular diseases, Paget's disease, and postoperative neurosurgical complications.
[5]Includes herpes zoster, collagen vascular disease, hypoxia, hydrocephalus, postoperative complications, and encephalitis.
[6]Includes raised intracranial pressure from any cause, Wernicke's encephalopathy, cervical manipulation, meningitis, sarcoidosis, post-lumbar-puncture complications, postoperative complications, migraine, and sinusitis.

ous cause. For patients with isolated trochlear nerve palsies without a history of trauma, in whom diabetes, myasthenia, thyroid disease, and orbital mass lesions have been excluded, observation is the appropriate clinical approach.

ABDUCENS (VI) NERVE LESIONS

Patients with abducens nerve lesions complain of horizontal diplopia due to weakness of the lateral rectus muscle (see Figure 5–16). Lateral rectus palsies can occur as a result of disorders of either the muscle itself or the abducens nerve, and each of these possibilities should be investigated in turn. The causes of abducens nerve lesions are summarized in Table 5–3. In elderly patients, abducens nerve involvement is most often idiopathic or caused by vascular disease or diabetes, but the erythrocyte sedimentation rate should be determined to exclude a rare presentation of giant cell arteritis. Radiographic investigation of the base of the skull is indicated to exclude nasopharyngeal carcinoma or other tumors. In painless abducens palsy—when the above studies are normal, other systemic and neurological symptoms are absent, and intracranial pressure is not elevated—patients can be followed conservatively. A trial of prednisone (60 mg/d orally for five days) may pro-

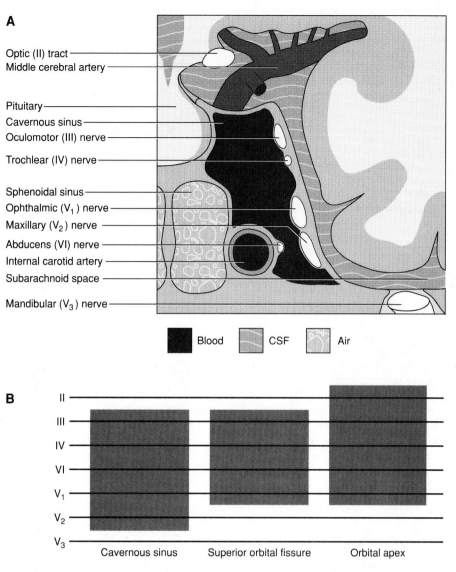

Figure 5–20. Position of cranial nerves in the cavernous sinus and adjacent structures. **A:** Coronal view through the cavernous sinus, with the midline at left and the temporal lobe at right. **B:** Location of cranial nerves as they course anteriorly (left to right) in relation to the cavernous sinus, superior orbital fissure and orbital apex. Note that a lesion in the cavernous sinus spares the optic (II) and mandibular (V₃) nerves, a lesion in the superior orbital fissure additionally spares the maxillary (V₂) nerve, and a lesion in the orbital apex spares both V₂ and V₃, but may involve II.

duce dramatic relief in painful abducens nerve palsy, giving support to a tentative diagnosis of idiopathic inflammation of the superior orbital fissure (**superior orbital fissure syndrome**) or cavernous sinus (**Tolosa-Hunt syndrome**). Persistent pain despite treatment with steroids should prompt investigation of the cavernous sinus by CT scanning or MRI, followed, in some cases, by angiography.

DIABETIC OPHTHALMOPLEGIAS

An isolated oculomotor, trochlear, or abducens nerve lesion may occur in patients with diabetes mellitus, and noninvasive imaging procedures (CT scanning or MRI) reveal no abnormality. Such oculomotor nerve lesions are characterized by **pupillary sparing** with or without pain. Pain, when present, may be severe enough to suggest aneurysmal expansion as a likely diagnosis. The lack of pupillary involvement is commonly attributed to infarction of the central portion of the nerve with sparing of the more peripherally situated fibers that mediate pupillary constriction. Pupil-sparing oculomotor palsies can also be seen occasionally, however, with compressive, infiltrative, or inflammatory lesions of the oculomotor nerve or with infarcts, hemorhages or tumors that affect the oculomotor nucleus or fascicle within the midbrain.

In known diabetics, painful ophthalmoplegia with exophthalmos and metabolic acidosis requires urgent attention to determine the possibility of fungal infection in the paranasal sinus, orbit, or cavernous sinus by **mucormycosis** (see Chapter 1). The diagnosis is usually made by biopsy of the nasal mucosa. Failure to make a prompt diagnosis and to institute treatment at once with amphotericin B and surgical debridement of necrotic tissue may lead to a fatal outcome.

PAINFUL OPHTHALMOPLEGIAS

Dysfunction of one or more of the ocular motor nerves with accompanying pain may be produced by lesions located anywhere from the posterior fossa to the orbit (Table 5–4). The evaluation should consist of careful documentation of the clinical course, inspection and palpation of the globe for proptosis (localizing the process to the orbit or anterior cavernous sinus), auscultation over the globe to detect a bruit (which would strongly support a diagnosis of carotid artery-cavernous sinus fistula or another vascular anomaly), and evaluation for diabetes. Useful laboratory studies include an orbital CT scan or MRI, carotid arteriography, and orbital venography.

Therapy for these disorders is dictated by the specific diagnosis. Idiopathic inflammation of the orbit (orbital pseudotumor) or cavernous sinus (Tolosa-Hunt syndrome) responds dramatically to corticosteroids (prednisone, 60–100 mg/d orally). However, the pain and ocular signs of some neoplasms may also improve transiently during corticosteroid therapy so that a specific etiological diagnosis depends on biopsy.

MYASTHENIA GRAVIS

Myasthenia eventually involves the ocular muscles in approximately 90% of patients; more than 60% present with ocular involvement. The syndrome is painless; pupillary responses are always normal, and there are no sensory abnormalities. The diagnosis is confirmed by a positive response to intravenous edrophonium (Tensilon). Details of this disorder are discussed in Chapter 6.

Table 5–4. Causes of painful ophthalmoplegia.

Orbit
Orbital pseudotumor
Sinusitis
Tumor (primary or metastatic)
Infections (bacterial or fungal)
Cavernous sinus
Tolosa-Hunt syndrome (idiopathic granulomatous inflammation)
Tumor (primary or metastatic)
Carotid artery-cavernous sinus fistula or thrombosis
Aneurysm
Sella and posterior fossa
Pituitary tumor or apoplexy
Aneurysm
Metastatic tumor
Other
Diabetes
Migraine
Giant cell arteritis

OCULAR MYOPATHIES

Ocular myopathies are painless syndromes that spare pupillary function and are usually bilateral. The most common is the myopathy of **hyperthyroidism,** a common cause of double vision beginning in midlife or later. Note that many patients are otherwise clinically euthyroid at the time of diagnosis. Double vision on attempted elevation of the globe is the most common symptom, but in mild cases there is lid retraction during staring or lid lag during rapid up-and-down movements of the eye. Exophthalmos is a characteristic finding, especially in advanced cases. The diagnosis can be confirmed by the forced duction test, which detects mechanical resistance to forced movement of the anesthetized globe in the orbit. This restrictive ocular myopathy is usually self-limited. The patient should be referred for testing of thyroid function and treated for hyperthyroidism as appropriate.

The **progressive external ophthalmoplegias** are a group of syndromes characterized by slowly progressive, symmetric impairment of ocular movement that cannot be overcome by caloric stimulation. Pupillary function is spared, and there is no pain; ptosis may be prominent. This clinical picture can be produced by **ocular** or **oculopharyngeal muscular dystrophy.** Progressive external ophthalmoplegia associated with myotonic contraction on percussion of muscle groups (classically, the thenar group in the palm) suggests the diagnosis of **myotonic dystrophy.** In **Kearns-Sayre-Daroff syndrome,** which has been associated with deletions in muscle mitochondrial DNA, progressive external ophthalmoplegia is accompanied by pigmentary degeneration of the retina, cardiac conduction defects, cerebellar ataxia, and elevated CSF protein. The muscle biopsy shows ragged red fibers that reflect the presence of abnormal mitochondria. Disorders that simulate progressive external ophthalmoplegia include progressive supranuclear palsy and Parkinson's disease, but in these conditions the impairment of (usually vertical) eye movements can be overcome by oculocephalic or caloric stimulation.

REFERENCES

Ash PR, Keltner JL: Neuro-ophthalmic signs in pontine lesions. *Medicine* 1979;58:304–320.

Brazis PW: Localization of lesions of the oculomotor nerve: Recent concepts. *Mayo Clin Proc* 1991;66:1029–1035.

Fisher CM: Some neuro-ophthalmological observations. *J Neurol Neurosurg Psychiatry* 1967;30:383–392.

Giles CL, Henderson JW: Horner's syndrome: An analysis of 216 cases. *Am J Ophthalmol* 1958;46:289–296.

Glaser JS: *Neuro-ophthalmology*, 2nd ed. Lippincott, 1990.

Grove AS Jr: Evaluation of exophthalmos. *N Engl J Med* 1975;292:1005–1013.

Hunt, WE, Brightman RP: The Tolosa-Hunt syndrome: A problem in differential diagnosis. *Acta Neurochirurgica* 1988;Suppl 42:248–252.

Hurwitz BJ et al: Comparison of amaurosis fugax and transient cerebral ischemia: A prospective clinical and arteriographic study. *Ann Neurol* 1985;18:698–704.

Keane JR: Acute bilateral ophthalmoplegia: 60 Cases. *Neurology* 1986;36:279–281.

Keane JR: Bilateral sixth nerve palsy: Analysis of 125 cases. *Arch Neurol* 1976;33:681–683.

Keane JR: Oculosympathetic paresis: Analysis of 100 hospitalized patients. *Arch Neurol* 1979;36:13–16.

Keane JR: The prectectal syndrome: 206 patients. *Neurology* 1990;40:684–690.

Lessell S: Optic neuropathies. *N Engl J Med* 1978;299:533–536.

Miller NR: *Walsh and Hoyt's Clinical Neuro-ophthalmology*, 4th ed. William & Wilkins, 1984.

Moraes CT et al: Mitochondrial DNA deletions in progressive external ophthalmoplegia and Kearns-Sayre syndrome. *N Engl J Med* 1989;320:1293–1299.

Nadeau SE, Trobe JD: Pupil sparing in oculomotor palsy: A brief review. *Ann Neurol* 1983;13:143–148.

Rush JA, Younge BR: Paralysis of cranial nerves III, IV, and VI: Cause and prognosis in 1000 cases. *Arch Ophthalmol* 1981;99:76–79.

Smigiel MR Jr, MacCarty CS: Exophthalmos: The more commonly encountered neurosurgical lesions. *Mayo Clin Proc* 1975;50:345–355.

Wall M, Wray SH: The one-and-a-half syndrome—A unilateral disorder of the pontine tegmentum: a study of 20 cases and review of the literature. *Neurology* 1983;33:971–980.

Younge BR, Sutula F: Analysis of trochlear nerve palsies: Diagnosis, etiology, and treatment. *Mayo Clin Proc* 1977;52:11–18.

Motor Deficits

APPROACH TO DIAGNOSIS

Motor function can be impaired by a lesion that involves the nervous system either centrally or peripherally. Several parts of the central nervous system are involved in the regulation of motor activity; these include the pyramidal and extrapyramidal pathways, the cerebellum, and the lower motor neurons of the brain stem and spinal cord.

The **pyramidal system** consists of fibers that descend from the cerebral cortex through the internal capsule, traverse the medullary pyramid, and then mostly decussate, to descend in the lateral corticospinal tract on the side opposite that of their origin, where they synapse on lower motor neurons in the spinal cord. All other descending influences on lower motor neurons belong to the **extrapyramidal system** and originate primarily in the basal ganglia and cerebellum. Disorders of the basal ganglia (see Chapter 8) and cerebellum (see Chapter 4) are considered separately.

The motor fibers that make up the cranial and peripheral nerves have their origin in the **lower motor neurons** (Figure 6–1). A disturbance of function at any point in the peripheral nervous system (anterior horn cell, nerve root, limb plexus, peripheral nerve, or neuromuscular junction) can disturb motor func-

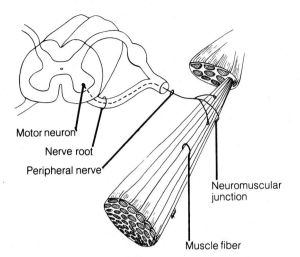

Figure 6–1. Anatomical components of the motor unit.

tion, as can disease that primarily affects the muscles themselves.

HISTORY & EXAMINATION

Patients with motor deficits generally complain of weakness, heaviness, stiffness, clumsiness, impaired muscular control, or difficulty in executing movements. The term *weakness* is sometimes used in a nonspecific way to denote loss of energy, drive, or enthusiasm, and care must be taken to clarify what the patient means. The word is properly used to mean loss of muscle power, and it is in this sense that it is employed here.

History of Present Illness

Several aspects of the present complaint must be documented.

A. Mode of Onset: An abrupt onset suggests a vascular disturbance, such as a stroke, or certain toxic or metabolic disturbances, whereas subacute onset of days to weeks is commonly associated with a neoplastic, infective, or inflammatory process (Table 6–1). Weakness that evolves slowly over several months or years often has a hereditary, degenerative, endocrinological, or neoplastic basis.

B. Course: A progressive increase in the motor deficit from its onset suggests continuing activity of the underlying process. Episodic progression suggests a vascular or inflammatory origin; a steadily progressive course is more suggestive of neoplastic disorder or such degenerative conditions as motor neuron disease. Rapid fluctuation of symptoms over short periods (eg, activity leads to fatigue and an exacerbation of weakness; rest is followed by recovery of strength) is characteristic of myasthenia gravis.

C. Associated Symptoms: The distribution of weakness and the presence of associated symptoms may indicate the approximate site of the lesion. For example, weakness in the right arm and leg may result from a lesion of the contralateral motor cortex or the corticospinal pathway at any point above the fifth cervical segment of the spinal cord. Associated right facial weakness indicates that the lesion must be above the level of the facial (VII) nerve nucleus in the brain stem, and an accompanying aphasia (see Chapter 1) or visual field defect (see Chapter 5) localizes it to the cerebral hemisphere.

The character of the associated symptoms may suggest the nature of the lesion at any given site in the nervous system. Thus, progressive leg weakness caused by myelopathy is often preceded or accompanied by pain in the back or legs when the myelopathy is due to a compressive lesion—but not when it has a metabolic or hereditary basis.

D. Severity of Symptoms: An attempt must be made to evaluate the functional severity of any motor deficit by determining whether there has been any restriction of daily activities, difficulty in performing previously easy tasks, or reduction in exercise tolerance. The nature of the functional disturbance depends on the muscles involved.

Weakness of proximal muscles in the legs leads to difficulty in climbing or descending stairs or in getting up from a squatting position, while weakness in the arms leads to difficulty with such tasks as combing the hair. Distal weakness in the arms may lead to clumsiness, difficulty with such fine motor tasks as doing up buttons or tying shoelaces, and eventually the inability to pick up or grasp objects with the hands, so that even eating becomes difficult or impossible.

Table 6–1. Causes of weakness of acute or subacute onset.

Supraspinal lesions
  Stroke
  Other structural lesions
Spinal cord lesions
  Infective: poliomyelitis, coxsackievirus infection
  Inflammatory: transverse myelitis, multiple sclerosis
  Compressive: tumor, disk protrusion, abscess
  Vascular: infarction, hematomyelia
Peripheral neuropathy
  Guillain-Barré syndrome
  Diphtheria
  Shellfish poisoning
  Porphyria
  Arsenic poisoning
  Organophosphate toxicity
Disorders of neuromuscular transmission
  Myasthenia gravis
  Botulism
  Aminoglycoside toxicity
Muscle disorders
  Necrotizing myopathies
  Acute hypo- or hyperkalemia
  Periodic paralyses

Involvement of the muscles supplied by the cranial nerves may lead to diplopia (oculomotor [III], trochlear [IV], and abducens [VI] cranial nerves; see Chapter 5); difficulty in chewing (trigeminal [V] nerve) or sucking, blowing, or using the facial muscles (facial [VII] nerve); and difficulty in swallowing, with nasal regurgitation and dysarthria (glossopharyngeal [IX], vagus [X], and hypoglossal [XII] nerves).

Weakness of the respiratory muscles leads to tachypnea, the use of accessory muscles of respiration, and anxiety at a stage when arterial blood gases are usually still normal. A vital capacity of less than 1 L in an adult generally calls for ventilatory support, especially if weakness is increasing.

Medical History

The importance of the history depends upon the patient's present complaint and the nature of any previous illnesses. For example, in a patient with known carcinoma of the lung, limb weakness may be due to metastasis or to a remote (nonmetastatic) complication of cancer. Leg weakness in a diabetic may reflect peripheral nerve, plexus, or multiple root involvement, and hand weakness in a myxedematous patient may be associated with carpal tunnel syndrome.

The history should include careful note of all drugs taken by the patient. Drugs can cause peripheral neuropathy, impair neuromuscular transmission, or lead to myopathy (Table 6–2).

Developmental History

When symptoms develop during infancy, childhood, or early adult life, it is particularly important to obtain a full developmental history, including details of the delivery, birth weight, the patient's condition

Table 6–2. Motor disorders associated with drugs.

Drugs that cause motor (or predominantly motor) peripheral neuropathy[1]
Dapsone
Imipramine
Certain sulfonamides

Drugs that can impair neuromuscular transmission

ACTH	Penicillamine
Aminoglycoside antibiotics	Phenothiazines
β-blockers	Phenytoin
Chloroquine	Polymyxin
Colistin	Procainamide
Corticosteroids	Quinidine, quinine
Lithium	Tetracycline
Magnesium-containing cathartics	

Drugs associated with myopathy

β-blockers	Emetine
Chloroquine	Epsilon aminocaproic acid
Clofibrate	Penicillamine
Corticosteroids	Zidovudine
Drugs causing hypokalemia	

[1]A number of drugs cause mixed sensory and motor neuropathies, as shown in Table 7–2.

in the neonatal period, and the dates at which motor milestones were attained. Congenital or perinatal cerebral disease accounts for most causes of infantile diplegia (weakness of all four limbs, with the legs more severely affected than the arms).

Family History

Hereditary factors may be important, and the patient's family background must therefore be explored. Some types of myopathy and peripheral neuropathy have a genetic basis, as do some spinocerebellar degenerations, hereditary spastic paraparesis, and certain other neurological disorders.

Examination of the Motor System

In examining the motor system, a systematic approach will help to avoid overlooking important abnormalities. A sequential routine for the examination should be developed.

A. Muscle Appearance: Wasting, or muscle **atrophy,** suggests that weakness is due to a lesion of the lower motor neurons or of the muscle itself. The distribution of wasting may help to localize the underlying disorder. Upper motor neuron disorders are not usually accompanied by muscle wasting, though muscle atrophy may occasionally occur with prolonged disuse. **Pseudohypertrophy** of muscles occurs in certain forms of myopathy, but the apparently enlarged muscles are weak and flabby.

The presence of **fasciculations**—visible irregular flickerings over the surface of the affected muscle caused by spontaneous contractions of individual motor units—suggests that weakness is due to a lower motor neuron lesion. Fasciculations are most apt to be seen in anterior horn cell disorders. While such activity does not occur with upper motor neuron disorders, **flexor or extensor spasms** of the limbs are sometimes seen in these latter conditions as a result of impaired supraspinal control of reflex activity.

B. Muscle Tone: For clinical purposes, tone can be defined as the resistance of muscle to passive movement of a joint. Tone depends on the degree of muscle contraction and on the mechanical properties of muscle and connective tissue. The degree of muscle contraction depends, in turn, on the activity of anterior horn cells, which is governed by spinal and supraspinal mechanisms. Tone is assessed by observing the position of the extremities at rest, by palpating the muscle belly, and particularly by determining the resistance to passive stretch and movement. Postural abnormalities may result from the increased activity of certain muscle groups caused by disturbances of reflex function, as exemplified by the typical hemiplegic posture—flexion of the upper limb and extension of the ipsilateral lower limb—of many patients who have had a stroke. To assess resistance to passive movement, the patient is asked to relax while each limb is examined in turn by passively taking the major joints through their full range of movement at different speeds and estimating whether the force required is more or less than normal.

1. Hypertonia–Two types of increased tone can be distinguished.

a. Spasticity consists of an increase in tone that affects different muscle groups to different extents. In the arms, tone is increased to a greater extent in the flexor muscles than in the extensors; in the legs, tone is increased to a greater extent in the extensor muscles than in the flexors. Moreover, the resistance of affected muscle is not the same throughout the range of movement but tends to be most marked when passive movement is initiated and then diminishes as the movement continues (the **clasp-knife phenomenon**). The increase in tone is velocity–dependent, so that passive movement at a high velocity—but not at lower velocities—may be met with increased resistance. Spasticity is caused by an upper motor neuron lesion, such as a stroke that involves the supplementary motor cortex or corticospinal tract. Spasticity may not become apparent for several days following the onset of an acute lesion, however.

b. Rigidity consists of increased resistance to passive movement that is independent of the direction of the movement—ie, it affects agonist and antagonist muscle groups equally. The term **lead-pipe rigidity** is sometimes used for descriptive purposes, while **cogwheel rigidity** is used when there are superimposed ratchetlike interruptions in the passive movement, which probably relate to underlying tremor. In general, rigidity indicates extrapyramidal dysfunction and is due to a lesion of the basal ganglia (eg, Parkinson's disease).

2. Hypotonia (flaccidity)–This is characterized by excessive floppiness—a reduced resistance to passive movement—so that the distal portion of the limb is easily waved to and fro when the extremity is passively shaken. In hypotonic limbs it is often possible to hyperextend the joints, and the muscle belly may look flattened and feel less firm than usual. While hypotonia usually relates to pathological involvement of the lower motor neuron supply to the affected muscles, it can also occur with primary muscle disorders, disruption of the sensory (afferent) limb of the reflex arc, cerebellar disease, and certain extrapyramidal disorders such as Huntington's disease as well as in the acute stage of a pyramidal lesion.

3. Paratonia–Some patients give the impression of being unable to relax and will move the limb being examined as the physician moves it, despite instructions to the contrary. In more advanced cases, there seems to be rigidity when the examiner moves the limb rapidly but normal tone when the limb is moved slowly. This phenomenon—paratonia—is particularly apt to occur in patients with frontal lobe or diffuse cerebral disease.

C. Muscle Power: When muscle power is to be tested, the patient is asked to resist pressure exerted by the examiner. Selected individual muscles are tested in turn, and strength on the two sides is compared so that minor degrees of weakness can be recognized. Weakness can result from a disturbance in function of the upper or the lower motor neurons; the distribution of weakness is of paramount importance in distinguishing between these two possibilities. Upper motor neuron lesions (eg, stroke) lead to weakness that characteristically involves the extensors and abductors more than the flexors and adductors of the arms—and the flexors more than the extensors of the legs. Lower motor neuron lesions produce weakness of the muscles supplied by the affected neurons; the particular distribution of the weakness may point to lower motor neuron involvement at the spinal cord, nerve root, plexus, or peripheral nerve level.

On the basis of the history and other findings, muscles that are particularly likely to be affected are selected for initial evaluation, and other muscles are subsequently examined to determine the distribution of the weakness more fully and to shorten the list of diagnostic possibilities. For instance, if an upper motor neuron (pyramidal) lesion is suspected, the extensors and abductors of the upper extremity and the flexors of the lower extremity are tested in the most detail, since these muscles will be the most affected.

Weakness may also result from a primary muscle disorder (myopathy) or from a disorder of neuromuscular transmission. In patients with a motor deficit in all limbs that is not due to an upper motor neuron lesion, proximal distribution of weakness suggests a myopathic disorder, whereas predominantly distal involvement suggests a lower motor neuron disturbance. Marked variability in the severity and distribution of weakness over short periods of time suggests myasthenia gravis, a disorder of neuromuscular transmission. Apparent weakness that is not organic in nature also shows a characteristic variability; it is often more severe on formal testing than is consistent with the patient's daily activities. Moreover, palpation of antagonist muscles commonly reveals that they contract each time the patient is asked to activate the agonist.

For practical and comparative purposes, power is best graded in the manner shown in Table 6–3.

Table 6–3. Grading of muscle power according to the system suggested by the Medical Research Council.[1]

Grade	Muscle Power
5	Normal power
4	Active movement against resistance and gravity
3	Active movement against gravity but not resistance
2	Active movement possible only with gravity eliminated
1	Flicker or trace of contraction
0	No contraction

[1]Reproduced, with permission, from *Aids to the Investigation of Peripheral Nerve Injuries.* HMSO, 1943.

Monoplegia denotes paralysis or severe weakness of the muscles in one limb, and **monoparesis** denotes less severe weakness in one limb, although the two words are often used interchangeably. **Hemiplegia** or **hemiparesis** is weakness in both limbs (and sometimes the face) on one side of the body; **paraplegia** or **paraparesis** is weakness of both legs; and **quadriplegia** or **quadriparesis** (also **tetraplegia, tetraparesis**) is weakness of all four limbs.

D. Coordination: The coordination of motor activity can be impaired by weakness, sensory disturbances, or cerebellar disease and requires careful evaluation.

Voluntary activity is observed with regard to its accuracy, velocity, range, and regularity, and the manner in which individual actions are integrated to produce a smooth complex movement. In the finger-nose test, the patient moves the index finger to touch the tip of his or her nose and then the tip of the examiner's index finger; the examiner can move his or her own finger about during the test to change the location of the target and should position it so that the patient's arm must extend fully to reach it. In the heel-knee-shin test, the recumbent patient lifts one leg off the bed, flexes it at the knee, places the heel on the other knee, and runs the heel up and down the shin as smoothly and rapidly as possible.

The patient should also be asked to tap repetitively with one hand on the back of the other; to tap alternately with the palm and back of one hand on the back of the other hand or on the knee; to screw an imaginary light bulb into the ceiling with each arm in turn; and to rub the fingers of one hand in a circular polishing movement on the back of the other hand. Other tests of rapid alternating movement include tapping on the ball of the thumb with the tip of the index finger or tapping the floor as rapidly as possible with the sole while keeping the heel of the foot in place. During all these tests, the examiner looks for irregularities of rate, amplitude, and rhythm and for precision of movements. With pyramidal lesions, fine voluntary movements are performed slowly. With cerebellar lesions, the rate, rhythm, and amplitude of such movements are irregular.

If weakness or impaired sensation is responsible for impaired coordination, the underlying deficits are generally clearly evident on neurological examination. In patients with cerebellar disease, the main complaint and physical finding are often of incoordination, and examination may reveal little else. Further discussion of the ataxia of cerebellar disease and the various terms used to describe aspects of it will be found in Chapter 4.

E. Tendon Reflexes: Changes in the tendon reflexes may accompany disturbances in motor (or sensory) function and provide a guide to the cause of the motor deficit. The tendon is tapped with a reflex hammer to produce a sudden brisk stretch of the muscle and its contained spindles. The clinically important stretch reflexes and the nerves, roots, and spinal segments subserving them are indicated in Table 6–4. When the reflexes are tested, the limbs on each side should be placed in identical positions and the reflexes elicited in the same manner.

1. Areflexia–Apparent loss of the tendon reflexes in a patient may merely reflect a lack of clinical expertise on the part of the examiner. Performance of Jendrassik's maneuver (an attempt by the patient to pull apart the fingers of the two hands when they are hooked together) or some similar action (such as making a fist with the hand that is not being tested) may elicit the reflex response when it is otherwise unobtainable. A reflex may be lost or depressed by any lesion that interrupts the structural or functional continuity of its reflex arc, as in a root lesion or peripheral neuropathy. In addition, reflexes are often depressed during the acute stage of an upper motor neuron lesion, in patients who are deeply comatose, and in patients with cerebellar disease.

2. Hyperreflexia–Increased reflexes occur with upper motor neuron lesions, but they may also occur with symmetrical distribution in certain healthy subjects and in patients under emotional tension. The presence of reflex asymmetry is therefore of particular clinical significance. **Clonus** consists of a series of rhythmic reflex contractions of a muscle that is suddenly subjected to sustained stretch, with each beat caused by renewed stretch of the muscle during relaxation from its previous contracted state. Sustained clonus—more than three or four beats in response to sudden sustained stretch—is always pathological and is associated with an abnormally brisk reflex. In hyperreflexic states, there may be spread of the region from which a particular reflex response can be elicited. For example, elicitation of the biceps reflex may be accompanied by reflex finger flexion, or eliciting the finger flexion reflex may cause flexion of the thumb (Hoffmann's sign).

3. Reflex asymmetry–Although the intensity of reflex responses varies considerably among subjects, reflexes should be symmetrical in any individual. Several general points can be made regarding reflex asymmetries.

Table 6–4. Muscle stretch reflexes.

Reflex	Segmental Innervation	Nerve
Jaw jerk	Pons	Mandibular branch, trigeminal
Biceps jerk	C5, C6	Musculocutaneous
Brachioradialis jerk	C5, C6	Radial
Triceps jerk	C7, C8	Radial
Finger jerk	C8, T1	Median
Knee jerk	L3, L4	Femoral
Ankle jerk	S1, S2	Tibial

a. Lateralized asymmetries of response—ie, reflexes that are brisker on one side of the body than on the other—usually indicate an upper motor neuron disturbance.

b. Focal reflex deficits often relate to root, plexus, or peripheral nerve lesions. For example, unilateral depression of the ankle jerk commonly reflects an S1 radiculopathy resulting from a lumbosacral disk lesion.

c. Loss of distal tendon reflexes (especially ankle jerks), with preservation of more proximal ones, is common in polyneuropathies.

F. Superficial Reflexes:

1. The polysynaptic superficial abdominal reflexes, which depend on the integrity of the T8–12 spinal cord segments, are elicited by gently stroking each quadrant of the abdominal wall with a blunt object such as a wooden stick. A normal response consists of contraction of the muscle in the quadrant stimulated, with a brief movement of the umbilicus toward the stimulus. Asymmetric loss of the response may be of diagnostic significance.

a. The response may be depressed or lost on one side in patients with an upper motor neuron disturbance from a lesion of the contralateral motor cortex or its descending pathways.

b. Segmental loss of the response may relate to local disease of the abdominal wall or its innervation, as in a radiculopathy.

c. The cutaneous abdominal reflexes are frequently absent bilaterally in the elderly, in the obese, in multiparous women, and in patients who have had abdominal surgery.

2. The **cremasteric reflex,** mediated through the L1 and L2 reflex arcs, consists of retraction of the ipsilateral testis when the inner aspect of the thigh is lightly stroked; it is lost in patients with a lesion involving these nerve roots. It is also lost in patients with contralateral upper motor neuron disturbances.

3. Stimulation of the lateral border of the foot in a normal adult leads to plantar flexion of the toes and dorsiflexion of the ankle. The **Babinski response** consists of dorsiflexion of the big toe and fanning of the other toes in response to stroking the lateral border of the foot, which is part of the S1 dermatome; flexion at the hip and knee may also occur. Such an extensor plantar response indicates an upper motor neuron lesion involving the contralateral motor cortex or the corticospinal tract. It can also be found in anesthetized or comatose subjects, in patients who have had a seizure, and in normal infants. An extensor plantar response can also be elicited, though less reliably, by such maneuvers as pricking the dorsal surface of the big toe with a pin (Bing's sign), firmly stroking down the anterior border of the tibia from knee to ankle (Oppenheim's maneuver), squeezing the calf muscle (Gordon's maneuver) or Achilles tendon (Schafer's maneuver), flicking the little toe (Gonda's maneuver), or stroking the back of the foot just below

the lateral malleolus (Chaddock's maneuver). In interpreting responses, attention must be focused only on the direction in which the big toe first moves.

G. Gait: In evaluating gait, the examiner first observes the patient walking at a comfortable pace. Attention is directed at the stance and posture; the facility with which the patient starts and stops walking and turns to either side; the length of the stride; the rhythm of walking; the presence of normally associated movements, such as swinging of the arms; and any involuntary movements. Subtle gait disorders become apparent only when the patient is asked to run, walk on the balls of the feet or the heels, hop on either foot, or walk heel-to-toe along a straight line. Gait disorders occur in many neurological disturbances and in other contexts that are beyond the scope of this chapter. A motor or sensory disturbance may lead to an abnormal gait whose nature depends upon the site of pathological involvement. Accordingly, the causes and clinical types of gait disturbance are best considered together.

1. Apraxic gait–Apraxic gait occurs in some patients with disturbances, usually bilateral, of frontal lobe function, such as may occur in hydrocephalus or progressive dementing disorders. There is no weakness or incoordination of the limbs, but the patient is unable to walk properly—the feet seem glued to the ground. If walking is possible at all, the gait is unsteady, uncertain, and short-stepped.

2. Corticospinal lesions–A corticospinal lesion, irrespective of its cause, can lead to a gait disturbance that varies in character depending on whether there is unilateral or bilateral involvement. In patients with hemiparesis, the selective weakness and spasticity lead to a gait in which the affected leg must be **circumducted** to be advanced. The patient tilts at the waist toward the normal side and swings the affected leg outward as well as forward, thus compensating for any tendency to drag or catch the foot on the ground because of weakness in the hip and knee flexors or the ankle dorsiflexors. The arm on the affected side is usually held flexed and adducted. In mild cases, there may be no more than a tendency to drag the affected leg, so that the sole of that shoe tends to be excessively worn.

With severe bilateral spasticity, the legs are brought stiffly forward and adducted, often with compensatory movements of the trunk. Such a gait is commonly described as **scissorslike.** This gait is seen in its most extreme form in children with spastic diplegia from perinatally acquired static encephalopathy. In patients with mild spastic paraparesis, the gait is shuffling, slow, stiff, and awkward, with the feet tending to drag.

3. Extrapyramidal disorders–Extrapyramidal disorders can produce characteristic gait disturbances.

a. In advanced parkinsonism, the patient is often stooped and has difficulty in beginning to walk. Indeed, the patient may need to lean farther and farther forward while walking in place in order to advance; once in motion, there may be unsteadiness in turning and difficulty in stopping. The gait itself is characterized by small strides, often taken at an increasing rate until the patient is almost running **(festination),** and by loss of the arm swinging that normally accompanies locomotion. In mild parkinsonism, a mildly slowed or unsteady gait, flexed posture, or reduced arm swinging may be the only abnormality found.

b. Abnormal posturing of the limbs or trunk is a feature of dystonia; it can interfere with locomotion or lead to a distorted and bizarre gait.

c. Chorea can cause an irregular, unpredictable, and unsteady gait, as the patient dips or lurches from side to side. Choreiform movements of the face and extremities are usually well in evidence.

4. Cerebellar disorders–In cerebellar disorders (see Chapter 4), the gait may be disturbed in several ways.

a. Truncal ataxia results from involvement of midline cerebellar structures, especially the vermis. The gait is irregular, clumsy, unsteady, uncertain, and broad-based, with the patient walking with the feet wide apart for additional support. Turning and heel-to-toe walking are especially difficult. There are often few accompanying signs of a cerebellar disturbance in the limbs. Causes include midline cerebellar tumors and the cerebellar degeneration that can occur with alcoholism or hypothyroidism, as a nonmetastatic complication of cancer, and with certain hereditary disorders.

b. In extreme cases, with gross involvement of midline cerebellar structures (especially the vermis), the patient cannot stand without falling.

c. A lesion of one cerebellar hemisphere leads to an unsteady gait in which the patient consistently falls or lurches toward the affected side.

5. Impaired sensation–Impaired sensation, especially disturbed proprioception, also leads to an unsteady gait, which is aggravated by walking in the dark or with the eyes closed, since visual input cannot then compensate for the sensory loss. Because of their defective position sense, many patients lift their feet higher than necessary when walking, producing a **steppage** gait. Causes include tabes dorsalis, sensory neuropathies, vitamin B_{12} deficiency, and certain hereditary disorders (discussed in Chapter 7).

6. Anterior horn cell, peripheral motor nerve, or voluntary muscle disorders–These disorders lead to gait disturbances if the muscles involved in locomotion are affected. Weakness of the anterior tibial muscles leads to **foot drop;** to avoid catching or scuffing the foot on the ground, the patient must lift the affected leg higher than the other, in a characteristic steppage gait. Weakness of the calf muscles leads to an inability to walk on the balls of the feet. Weakness of the trunk and girdle muscles, such as occurs in muscular dystrophy, other myopathic disor-

ders, and Kugelberg-Welander syndrome, leads to a **waddling gait** because the pelvis tends to slump toward the non-weight-bearing side.

CLINICAL LOCALIZATION OF THE LESION

The findings on examination should indicate whether the weakness or other motor deficit is due to an upper or lower motor neuron disturbance, a disorder of neuromuscular transmission, or a primary muscle disorder. In the case of an upper or lower motor neuron disturbance, the clinical findings may also help to localize the lesion more precisely to a single level of the nervous system. Such localization helps to reduce the number of diagnostic possibilities.

Upper Motor Neuron Lesions
A. Signs:
–Weakness or paralysis.
– Spasticity.
– Increased tendon reflexes.
– An extensor plantar (Babinski) response.
– Loss of superficial abdominal reflexes.
– Little, if any, muscle atrophy.

Such signs occur with involvement of the upper motor neuron at any point, but further clinical findings depend upon the actual site of the lesion. Note that it may not be possible to localize a lesion by its motor signs alone.

B. Localization of Underlying Lesion:
1. A parasagittal intracranial lesion produces an upper motor neuron deficit that characteristically affects both legs and may later involve the arms.

2. A discrete lesion of the cerebral cortex or its projections may produce a focal motor deficit involving, for example, the contralateral hand. Weakness may be restricted to the contralateral leg in patients with anterior cerebral artery occlusion or to the contralateral face and arm if the middle cerebral artery is involved. A more extensive cortical or subcortical lesion will produce weakness or paralysis of the contralateral face, arm, and leg and may be accompanied by aphasia, a visual field defect, or a sensory disturbance of cortical type.

3. A lesion at the level of the internal capsule, where the descending fibers from the cerebral cortex are closely packed, commonly results in a severe hemiparesis that involves the contralateral limbs and face.

4. A brain stem lesion commonly—but not invariably—leads to bilateral motor deficits, often with accompanying sensory and cranial nerve disturbances, and disequilibrium. A more limited lesion involving the brain stem characteristically leads to a cranial nerve disturbance on the ipsilateral side and a contralateral hemiparesis; the cranial nerves affected depend on the level at which the brain stem is involved.

5. A unilateral spinal cord lesion above the fifth cervical segment (C5) causes an ipsilateral hemiparesis that spares the face and cranial nerves. Lesions between C5 and the first thoracic segment (T1) affect the ipsilateral arm to a variable extent as well as the ipsilateral leg; a lesion below T1 will affect only the ipsilateral leg. Because, in practice, both sides of the cord are commonly involved, quadriparesis or paraparesis usually results. If there is an extensive but unilateral cord lesion, the motor deficit is accompanied by ipsilateral impairment of vibration and position sense and by contralateral loss of pain and temperature appreciation (**Brown-Séquard syndrome**). With compressive and other focal lesions that involve the anterior horn cells in addition to the fiber tracts traversing the cord, the muscles innervated by the affected cord segment weaken and atrophy. Therefore, a focal lower motor neuron deficit exists at the level of the lesion and an upper motor neuron deficit exists below it—in addition to any associated sensory disturbance.

Lower Motor Neuron Lesions
A. Signs:
–Weakness or paralysis.
–Wasting of involved muscles.
–Hypotonia (flaccidity).
–Loss of tendon reflexes when neurons subserving them are affected.
–Normal abdominal and plantar reflexes—unless the neurons subserving them are directly involved, in which case reflex responses are lost.
–Fasciculations over affected muscles.

B. Localization of the Underlying Lesion: In
distinguishing weakness from a root, plexus, or peripheral nerve lesion, the distribution of the motor deficit is of particular importance. Only those muscles supplied wholly or partly by the involved struc-

ture are weak (Tables 6–5 and 6–6). The distribution of any accompanying sensory deficit similarly reflects the location of the underlying lesion (see Figure 7–1). It may be impossible to distinguish a radicular (root) lesion from discrete focal involvement of the spinal cord. In the latter situation, however, there is more often a bilateral motor deficit at the level of the lesion, a corticospinal or sensory deficit below it, or a disturbance of bladder, bowel, or sexual function. Certain disorders selectively affect the anterior horn cells of the spinal cord diffusely (see *Anterior Horn Cell Diseases*); the extensive lower motor neuron deficit without sensory changes helps to indicate the site and nature of the pathological involvement.

Cerebellar Dysfunction
A. Signs:
–Hypotonia.
–Depressed or pendular tendon reflexes.
–Ataxia.
–Gait disorder.
–Disturbances of eye movement.
–Dysarthria.

Ataxia is a complex movement disorder caused, at least in part, by impaired coordination. It occurs in the limbs on the same side as a lesion affecting the cerebellar hemisphere. With midline lesions, incoordination may not be evident in the limbs at all, but there is marked truncal ataxia that becomes evident on walking. The term **dysmetria** is used when movements are not adjusted accurately for range, so that—for example—a moving finger overshoots a target at which it is aimed. **Dysdiadochokinesia** denotes rapid alternating movements that are clumsy and irregular in terms of rhythm and amplitude. **Asynergia** or **dys-**

Table 6–5. Innervation of selected muscles of upper limbs.

Muscle	Main Root	Peripheral Nerve	Main Action
Supraspinatus	C5	Suprascapular	Abduction of arm
Infraspinatus	C5	Suprascapular	External rotation of arm at shoulder
Deltoid	C5	Circumflex	Abduction of arm
Biceps	C5, C6	Musculocutaneous	Elbow flexion
Brachioradialis	C5, C6	Radial	Elbow flexion
Extensor carpi radialis longus	C6, C7	Radial	Wrist extension
Flexor carpi radialis	C6, C7	Median	Wrist flexion
Extensor carpi ulnaris	C7	Radial	Wrist extension
Extensor digitorum	C7	Radial	Finger extension
Triceps	C8	Radial	Extension of forearm
Flexor carpi ulnaris	C8	Ulnar	Wrist flexion
Abductor pollicis brevis	T1	Median	Abduction of thumb
Opponens pollicis	T1	Median	Opposition of thumb
First dorsal interosseous	T1	Ulnar	Abduction of index finger
Abductor digiti minimi	T1	Ulnar	Abduction of little finger

Table 6–6. Innervation of selected muscles of lower limbs.

Muscle	Main Root	Peripheral Nerve	Main Action
Iliopsoas	L2, L3	Femoral	Hip flexion
Quadriceps femoris	L3, L4	Femoral	Knee extension
Adductors	L2, L3, L4	Obturator	Adduction of thigh
Gluteus maximus	L4, L5, S1	Inferior gluteal	Hip extension
Gluteus medius and minimus, tensor fasciae latae	L4, L5, S1	Superior gluteal	Hip abduction
Hamstrings	L5, S1	Sciatic	Knee flexion
Tibialis anterior	L4, L5	Peroneal	Dorsiflexion of ankle
Extensor digitorum longus	L5, S1	Peroneal	Dorsiflexion of toes
Extensor digitorum brevis	S1	Peroneal	Dorsiflexion of toes
Peronei	L5, S1	Peroneal	Eversion of foot
Tibialis posterior	L4	Tibial	Inversion of foot
Gastrocnemius	S1, S2	Tibial	Plantar flexion of ankle
Soleus	S1, S2	Tibial	Plantar flexion of ankle

ynergia denotes the breakdown of complex actions into the individual movements composing them; when asked to touch the tip of the nose with a finger, for example, the patient may first flex the elbow and then bring the hand up to the nose instead of combining the maneuvers into one action. **Intention tremor** occurs during activity and is often most marked as the target is neared. The **rebound phenomenon** is the overshooting of the limb when resistance to a movement or posture is suddenly withdrawn.

The gait becomes unsteady in patients with disturbances of either the cerebellar hemispheres or midline structures, as discussed in Chapter 4.

Jerk nystagmus, which is commonly seen in patients with a unilateral lesion of the cerebellar hemisphere, is slowest and of greatest amplitude when the eyes are turned to the side of the lesion. Nystagmus is not present in patients with lesions of the anterior cerebellar vermis.

Speech becomes dysarthric and takes on an irregular and explosive quality in patients with lesions that involve the cerebellar hemispheres. Speech is usually unremarkable when only the midline structures are involved.

B. Localization of the Underlying Lesion: The relationship of symptoms and signs to lesions of different parts of the cerebellum is considered in Chapter 4.

Neuromuscular-Transmission Disorders
A. Signs:
–Normal or reduced muscle tone.
–Normal or depressed tendon and superficial reflexes.
–No sensory changes.
–Weakness, often patchy in distribution, not conforming to the distribution of any single anatomical structure; frequently involves the cranial

muscles and may fluctuate in severity over short periods, particularly in relation to activity.

B. Localization of the Underlying Lesion: Pathological involvement of either the pre- or postsynaptic portion of the neuromuscular junction may impair neuromuscular transmission. Disorders affecting neuromuscular transmission are discussed below.

Myopathic Disorders
A. Signs:
–Weakness, usually most marked proximally rather than distally.
–No muscle wasting or depression of tendon reflexes until at least an advanced stage of the disorder.
–Normal abdominal and plantar reflexes.
–No sensory loss or sphincter disturbances.

B. Differentiation: In distinguishing the various myopathic disorders, it is important to determine whether the weakness is congenital or acquired, whether there is a family history of a similar disorder, and whether there is any clinical evidence that a systemic disease may be responsible. The distribution of affected muscles is often especially important in distinguishing the various hereditary myopathies (see *Myopathic Disorders,* below, and Table 6–11).

INVESTIGATIVE STUDIES

Investigative studies of patients with weakness from focal cerebral deficits are considered in Chapter 12. The investigations discussed here may be helpful in evaluating patients with weakness from other causes (Table 6–7).

Imaging
A. Plain X-Rays of the Spine: Congenital ab-

Table 6–7. Investigation of patients with weakness.

Test	Spinal Cord	Anterior Horn Cell Disorders	Peripheral Nerve or Plexus	Neuromuscular Junction	Myopathy
Serum enzymes	Normal.	Normal.	Normal.	Normal.	Normal or increased.
Electromyography	Reduced number of motor units under voluntary control. With lesions causing axonal degeneration, may be abnormal spontaneous activity (eg, fasciculations, fibrillations) if sufficient time has elapsed after onset; with reinnervation, motor units may be large, long, and polyphasic.			Often normal, but individual motor units may show abnormal variability in size.	Small, short, abundant polyphasic motor unit potentials. Abnormal spontaneous activity may be conspicuous in myositis.
Nerve conduction velocity	Normal.	Normal.	Slowed, especially in demyelinative neuropathies. May be normal in axonal neuropathies.	Normal.	Normal.
Muscle response to repetitive motor nerve stimulation	Normal.	Normal, except in active stage of disease.	Normal.	Abnormal decrement or increment depending on stimulus frequency and disease.	Normal.
Muscle biopsy	May be normal in acute stage but subsequently suggestive of denervation.			Normal.	Changes suggestive of myopathy.
Myelography or spinal MRI	May be helpful.	Helpful in excluding other disorders.	Not helpful.	Not helpful.	Not helpful.

normalities and degenerative, inflammatory, neoplastic, or traumatic changes may be revealed by plain x-rays of the spine, which should therefore be undertaken in the evaluation of patients with suspected cord or root lesions.

B. Myelography: Radiological study of the spinal subarachnoid space with injection of a contrast medium is an important means of visualizing intramedullary tumors and extramedullary lesions that compress the spinal cord or nerve roots. It can also permit detection of congenital or acquired structural abnormalities, especially in the region of the foramen magnum. For most purposes, however, spinal MRI is superior to myelography (see Chapter 12).

C. CT Scan or MRI: A CT scan of the spine, especially when performed after instilling water-soluble contrast material into the subarachnoid space, may also reveal disease involving the spinal cord or nerve roots. MRI is superior to CT scanning in this regard (see Chapter 12).

Electrodiagnostic Studies

The function of the normal motor unit, which consists of a lower motor neuron and all of the muscle fibers it innervates, may be disturbed at any of several sites in patients with weakness. A lesion may, for example, affect the anterior horn cell or its axon, interfere with neuromuscular transmission, or involve the muscle fibers directly so that they cannot respond normally to neural activation. In each circumstance, characteristic changes in the electrical activity can be recorded from affected muscle by a needle electrode

inserted into it and connected to an oscilloscope (electromyography). Depending on the site of pathology, nerve conduction studies or the muscle responses to repetitive nerve stimulation may also be abnormal. See Chapter 12 for further details.

Serum Enzymes

Damage to muscle fibers may lead to the release of certain enzymes (creatine phosphokinase [CPK], aldolase, lactic acid dehydrogenase, and the transaminases) that can then be detected in increased amounts in serum. CPK shows the greatest increase and is the most useful for following the course of muscle disease. It is also present in high concentrations in the heart and brain, however, and damage to these structures can lead to increased serum CPK levels. Fractionation of serum CPK into isoenzyme forms is useful for determining the tissue of origin. In patients with weakness, elevated serum CPK levels are generally indicative of a primary myopathy, especially one that is evolving rapidly. A mildly elevated serum CPK may also occur in motor neuron disease, however, and more marked elevations can follow trauma, surgery, intramuscular injections, or vigorous activity.

Muscle Biopsy

Histopathological examination of a specimen of weak muscle can be important in determining whether the underlying weakness is neurogenic or myopathic in origin. With neurogenic disorders, muscle biopsy specimens show atrophied fibers occurring in groups, with adjacent groups of larger, uninvolved fibers. In myopathies, atrophy occurs in a random pattern; nuclei of muscle cells may be centrally situated, in contrast to their normal peripheral location; and fibrosis or fatty infiltration may be seen. In addition, examination of a muscle biopsy specimen may permit recognition of certain inflammatory muscle diseases (eg, polymyositis) for which specific treatment is available—helping to differentiate them from muscle disorders that have no specific treatment.

SPINAL CORD DISORDERS

Cord lesions can lead to motor, sensory, or sphincter disturbances or to some combination of these deficits. Depending upon whether it is unilateral or bilateral, a lesion above C5 may cause either an ipsilateral hemiparesis or quadriparesis. With lesions located lower in the cervical cord, involvement of the upper limbs is partial, and a lesion below T1 affects only the lower limbs on one or both sides. Disturbances of sensation are considered in detail in Chapter 7, but it should be noted here that unilateral involvement of the posterior columns of the cord leads to ipsilateral loss of position and vibration sense. In addition, any disturbance in function of the spinothalamic tracts in the anterolateral columns impairs contralateral pain and temperature appreciation below the level of the lesion.

TRAUMATIC MYELOPATHY

While cord damage may result from whiplash (recoil) injury, severe injury to the cord usually relates to fracture-dislocation in the cervical, lower thoracic, or upper lumbar region.

Clinical Findings
A. Total Cord Transection: Total transection results in immediate permanent paralysis and loss of sensation below the level of the lesion. Although reflex activity is lost for a variable period after the injury, a persistent increase in reflex function follows.

1. In the acute stage, there is flaccid paralysis with loss of tendon and other reflexes, accompanied by sensory loss and by urinary and fecal retention. This is the stage of **spinal shock.**

2. Over the following weeks, as reflex function returns, the clinical picture of a spastic paraplegia or quadriplegia emerges, with brisk tendon reflexes and extensor plantar responses; however a flaccid, atrophic (lower motor neuron) paralysis may affect muscles innervated by spinal cord segments at the level of the lesion, where anterior horn cells are dam-

aged. The bladder and bowel now regain some reflex function, so that urine and feces are expelled at intervals.

3. Flexor or extensor spasms of the legs may become increasingly troublesome and are ultimately elicited by even the slightest cutaneous stimulus, especially in the presence of bedsores or a urinary tract infection. Eventually, the patient assumes a posture with the legs in flexion or extension, the former being especially likely with cervical or complete cord lesions.

B. Less Severe Injury: With lesser degrees of injury, the neurological deficit is less severe and less complete, but patients may be left with a mild paraparesis or quadriparesis or a distal sensory disturbance. Sphincter function may also be impaired—urinary urgency and urgency incontinence are especially common. Hyperextension injuries of the neck can lead to focal cord ischemia that causes bibrachial paresis (weakness of both arms) with sparing of the legs and variable sensory signs.

Treatment
A. Immobilization: Initial treatment consists of immobilization until the nature and extent of the injury are determined. If there is cord compression, urgent decompressive surgery will be necessary. An unstable spine may require surgical fixation, and vertebral dislocation may necessitate spinal traction.

B. Corticosteroids: Corticosteroids (eg, methylprednisolone, 30 mg/kg intravenous bolus, followed by intravenous infusion at 5.4 mg/kg/h for 24 hours) can improve motor and sensory function at six months when treatment is begun within eight hours of traumatic spinal cord injury. The mechanism of the action is unknown, but it may involve the inhibition of lipid peroxidation and the improvement of blood flow to the injured spinal cord.

C. Painful Spasms: Painful flexor or extensor spasms can be treated with drugs that enhance spinal inhibitory mechanisms (baclofen, diazepam) or uncouple muscle excitation from contraction (dantrolene). Baclofen should be given 5 mg orally twice daily to 20 mg four times daily; diazepam, 2 mg orally twice daily to 20 mg three times daily; and dantrolene, 25 mg/d orally to 100 mg four times daily. Patients who fail to benefit from oral medications may respond to intrathecal infusion of baclofen.

All these drugs may increase functional disability by reducing tone. Dantrolene may also increase weakness and should be avoided in patients with severely compromised respiratory function.

D. Skin Care: Particular attention must be given to skin care, avoiding continued pressure on any single area.

E. Bladder and Bowel Disorders: Depending on the severity of the injury, catheterization may be necessary initially. Subsequently, the urgency and frequency of the spastic bladder may respond to a parasympatholytic drug such as propantheline bromide, 15–30 mg three or four times daily. Suppositories and enemas will help maintain regular bowel movements and may prevent or control fecal incontinence.

DEMYELINATING MYELOPATHIES

1. MULTIPLE SCLEROSIS

Multiple sclerosis is one of the most common neurological disorders, and its highest incidence is in young adults. Initial symptoms generally commence before the age of 55 years, with a peak incidence between ages 20 and 40; women are affected somewhat more commonly than men. It is defined clinically by the involvement of different parts of the central nervous system at different times—provided that other disorders causing multifocal central dysfunction have been excluded. The cause is unknown, but an immune mechanism directed against myelin antigens is suspected. The disorder is characterized pathologically by the development of focal—often perivenular—scattered areas of demyelination followed by a reactive gliosis. These lesions occur in the white matter of the brain and cord and in the optic (II) nerve.

Epidemiological studies show that the prevalence of the disease rises with increasing distance from the equator, and no population with a high risk for the disease exists between latitudes 40°N and 40°S. Incidence may occasionally be familial, and there is a strong association between it and specific HLA antigens (HLA-DR2). Present evidence supports an immunological basis for the disease.

Clinical Findings

A. Initial or Presenting Symptoms: Patients can present with any of a variety of symptoms (Table 6–8). Common initial complaints are focal weakness, numbness, tingling, or unsteadiness in a limb; sudden loss or blurring of vision in one eye (optic neuritis); diplopia; disequilibrium; or a bladder-function disturbance (urinary urgency or hesitancy). Such symptoms are often transient, disappearing after a few days or weeks, even though some residual deficit may be found on careful neurological examination. Other patients present with an acute or gradually progressive spastic paraparesis and sensory deficit; this should raise concern about the possibility of an underlying structural lesion unless there is evidence on clinical examination of more widespread disease.

B. Subsequent Course: There may be an interval of months or years after the initial episode before further neurological symptoms appear. New symptoms may then develop, or the original ones may recur and progress. Relapses may be triggered by infection and, in women, are more likely in the three months or so following childbirth. A rise in body temperature can cause transient deterioration in patients with a fixed and stable deficit. With time—and after a number of relapses and usually incomplete remissions—the patient may become increasingly disabled by weakness, stiffness, sensory disturbances, unsteadiness of the limbs, impaired vision, and urinary incontinence.

Examination in advanced cases commonly reveals optic atrophy, nystagmus, dysarthria, and upper motor neuron, sensory, or cerebellar deficits in some or all of the limbs (Table 6–8). Note that the diagnosis cannot be based on any single symptom or sign but only on a total clinical picture that indicates involvement of different parts of the central nervous system at different times.

Investigative Studies

These may help to support the clinical diagnosis and exclude other disorders but do not themselves justify a definitive diagnosis of multiple sclerosis.

The CSF is commonly abnormal, with mild lymphocytosis or a slightly increased protein concentration, especially if examined soon after an acute relapse. CSF protein electrophoresis shows the presence of discrete bands in the IgG region (**oligoclonal bands**) in many patients. The antigens responsible for these antibodies are not known.

If clinical evidence of a lesion exists at only one site in the central nervous system, a diagnosis of multiple sclerosis cannot properly be made unless it can

Table 6–8. Symptoms and signs of multiple sclerosis.[1]

	Percentage of Patients
Symptoms (at presentation)	
Paresthesia	37
Gait disorder	35
Lower extremity weakness or incoordination	17
Visual loss	15
Upper extremity weakness or incoordination	10
Diplopia	10
Signs	
Absent abdominal reflexes	81
Hyperreflexia	76
Lower extremity ataxia	57
Extensor plantar responses	54
Impaired rapid alternating movements	49
Impaired vibratory sense	47
Optic neuropathy	38
Nystagmus	35
Impaired joint position sense	33
Intention tremor	32
Spasticity	31
Impaired pain or temperature sense	22
Dysarthria	19
Paraparesis	17
Internuclear ophthalmoplegia	11

[1]Adapted from Swanson JW: Multiple Sclerosis: Update in diagnosis and review of prognostic factors. *Mayo Clin Proc* 1989;64:577–586.

be shown that other regions have been affected subclinically, as detected by the electrocerebral responses evoked by one or more of the following: monocular visual stimulation with a checkerboard pattern (**visual evoked potentials**); monaural stimulation with repetitive clicks (**brain stem auditory evoked potentials**); and electrical stimulation of a peripheral nerve (**somatosensory evoked potentials**).

Magnetic resonance imaging or CT scan may also detect subclinical lesions; MRI is considerably more sensitive in this regard.

In patients presenting with the spinal form of the disorder and no evidence of disseminated disease, myelography may be necessary to exclude the possibility of a single congenital or acquired surgically treatable lesion. The region of the foramen magnum must be visualized to exclude the possibility of a lesion such as Arnold-Chiari malformation, in which part of the cerebellum and the lower brain stem are displaced into the cervical canal, producing mixed pyramidal and cerebellar deficits in the limbs.

Treatment

There is no proved means of preventing the progression of this disorder. General health care is important. Excessive fatigue must be avoided, and patients should rest during periods of acute relapse.

Corticosteroids may hasten recovery from acute relapses, but the extent of the recovery itself is unchanged, and long-term steroid management does not prevent relapses. There is no standard schedule of treatment with corticosteroids. ACTH in high doses (eg, repository corticotropin gel, 80 units intramuscularly) can be given daily for one week and tapered over the following two or three weeks. Some clinicians have advocated the use of methylprednisolone, 15–20 mg/kg/d intravenously for three days, followed by tapering over two weeks. Alternatively, prednisone, 60 or 80 mg/d orally, or dexamethasone, 16 mg/d, can be given for one week, and tapered over the following two or three weeks.

Cytotoxic drugs such as cyclophosphamide (in a total dose of 80–100 mg/kg intravenously over 10–14 days) or azathioprine (1–2.5 mg/kg/d), sometimes given in combination with corticosteroids, have been reported to slow progression of the disease in the short term in some studies. Plasmapheresis may enhance the benefits of immunosuppression, at least temporarily, but its role in management is unclear. The role of interferon therapy in multiple sclerosis is currently under investigation, as is that of cyclosporine. In preliminary studies, Cop 1, a polymer that mimics the structure of myelin basic protein, reduced the frequency of exacerbation in patients with multiple sclerosis. Treatment for spasticity (discussed above) may be needed in advanced cases.

Prognosis

At least partial recovery from an acute episode can be anticipated, but it is impossible to predict when the next relapse will occur. Features that tend to imply a more favorable prognosis include female sex, onset before age 40, and presentation with visual or somatosensory, rather than pyramidal or cerebellar, dysfunction. Although some degree of disability is likely to result eventually, about half of all patients are without significant disability ten years after the onset of symptoms.

2. ACUTE DISSEMINATED ENCEPHALOMYELITIS

This occurs as a single episode of neurological symptoms and signs that develop over a few days in association with a viral infection, especially measles or chickenpox. The neurological deficit resolves, at least in part, over the succeeding few weeks. Pathologically, perivascular areas of demyelination are scattered throughout the brain and spinal cord, with an associated inflammatory reaction. A similar disorder may also occur independently, with no apparent infection; it may then represent the initial manifestation of multiple sclerosis.

The initial symptoms often consist of headache, fever, and confusion; seizures may also occur, and examination reveals signs of meningeal irritation. Flaccid weakness and sensory disturbance of the legs, extensor plantar responses, and urinary retention are common manifestations of cord involvement. Other neurological signs may indicate involvement of the optic nerves, cerebral hemispheres, brain stem, or cerebellum.

Examination of the CSF may show an increased mononuclear cell count, with normal protein and glucose concentrations.

Corticosteroids are often prescribed, but there is little evidence of benefit. A mortality rate of 5–30% is reported, and survivors often have severe residual deficits.

OTHER INFECTIVE OR INFLAMMATORY MYELOPATHIES

Epidural Abscess

Epidural abscess may occur as a sequel to skin infection, septicemia, vertebral osteomyelitis, back trauma or surgery, or lumbar puncture. The most common causative organisms are *Staphylococcus aureus,* streptococci, gram-negative bacilli, and anaerobes. Fever, backache and tenderness, pain in the distribution of a spinal nerve root, headache, and malaise are early symptoms, followed by rapidly progressive paraparesis, sensory disturbances in the legs, and urinary and fecal retention.

Spinal epidural abscess is a neurological emergency that requires prompt diagnosis and treatment. Investigations reveal peripheral leukocytosis, an increased erythrocyte sedimentation rate, mild CSF pleocytosis with increased protein but normal glucose concentration, a positive Queckenstedt test, and a block at myelography. The role of CT scanning and MRI, compared to myelography, awaits full delineation.

Treatment involves surgery and antibiotics. In the absence of cord compression, treatment with antibiotics alone has been successful. Semisynthetic penicillins (eg, nafcillin or oxacillin) are administered to cover staphylococcal or streptococcal infection, and other agents are added or substituted based on the results of Gram's stain of excised material. The results of culture of the necrotic material that makes up the abscess may subsequently alter the antibiotic regimen. The antibiotic dosages are those used to treat bacterial meningitis, as given in Chapter 1.

Syphilis

Syphilis can produce meningovasculitis of the cord, resulting in spinal cord infarction. Vascular myelopathies are discussed later in this chapter.

Tuberculosis

Tuberculosis may lead to vertebral disease **(Pott's disease)** with secondary compression of the cord, to meningitis with secondary arteritis and cord infarction, or to cord compression by a tuberculoma. Such complications assume great importance in certain parts of the world, especially Asia and Africa, and among such groups as the homeless and intravenous drug users. Tuberculous meningitis is considered in more detail in Chapter 1.

AIDS

A disorder of the spinal cord, **vacuolar myelopathy,** is found at autopsy in about 20% of patients with AIDS. This disorder is characterized by vacuolation of white matter in the spinal cord, which is most pronounced in the lateral and posterior columns of the thoracic cord. Direct involvement of the spinal cord by human immunodeficiency virus-1 (HIV-1), the etiological agent in AIDS, is thought to be the cause.

Most patients with vacuolar myelopathy have coexisting AIDS dementia complex (see Chapter 2). Symptoms progress over weeks to months and include leg weakness, ataxia, incontinence, and paresthesias. Examination shows paraparesis, lower extremity monoparesis, or quadriparesis; spasticity; increased or decreased tendon reflexes; Babinski signs; and diminished vibration and position sense. MRI of the spinal cord is typically normal. It is unknown whether treatment with zidovudine or other antiviral drugs is helpful. Vacuolar myelopathy in AIDS resembles myelopathy caused by vitamin B_{12} deficiency, but it tends to produce earlier incontinence and less conspicuous sensory abnormalities. Myelopathy in patients with AIDS may also be caused by lymphoma, cryptococcal infection, or herpesviruses.

Other Viral Infections

A retrovirus, human T-lymphotropic virus type I (HTLV-I) appears to be the cause of **tropical spastic paraparesis,** a disorder found in the Caribbean, off the Pacific coast of Colombia, and in the Seychelles. Clinical features include spastic paraparesis, impaired vibration and joint position sense, and bowel and bladder dysfunction.

Herpesviruses can also produce myelopathy, which commonly affects spinal nerve roots as well as the cord **(radiculomyelopathy),** especially in immunocompromised patients, such as those with AIDS. Cytomegalovirus causes a myelopathy characterized by demyelination of the posterior columns of the spinal cord and by cytomegalic cells that contain Cowdry's type A inclusion bodies. The value of treatment with antiviral drugs such as ganciclovir and foscarnet is still uncertain. Herpes zoster and herpes simplex types 1 and 2 can also cause myelopathy, which may respond to treatment with acyclovir (see Chapter 1).

Tetanus

Tetanus is a disorder of neurotransmission associated with infection by *Clostridium tetani*. The organism typically becomes established in a wound where it elaborates a toxin that is transported retrogradely along motor nerves into the spinal cord or, with wounds to the face or head, the brain stem. The toxin is also disseminated through the bloodstream to skeletal muscle, where it gains access to additional motor nerves. In the spinal cord and brain stem, tetanus toxin interferes with the release of inhibitory neurotransmitters, including glycine and GABA, resulting in motor nerve hyperactivity. Autonomic nerves are also disinhibited.

After an incubation period of up to three weeks, tetanus usually presents with **trismus** (lockjaw), difficulty in swallowing, or spasm of the facial muscles that resembles a contorted smile **(risus sardonicus).** Painful muscle spasms and rigidity progress to involve both axial and limb musculature and may give rise to hyperextended posturing **(opisthotonos).** Laryngospasm and autonomic instability are potential life-threatening complications.

Although the diagnosis is usually made on clinical grounds, the presence of continuous motor unit activity or absence of the normal silent period in the masseter muscle following elicitation of the jaw-jerk reflex are helpful electromyographic findings. The serum CPK may be elevated, and myoglobinuria may occur. The organisms can be cultured from a wound in only a minority of cases.

Tetanus is preventable through immunization with tetanus toxoid. Tetanus toxoid is usually administered routinely to infants and children in the United Staes, in combination with pertussis vaccine and diphtheria toxoids. In children under age seven years, three doses of tetanus toxoid are administered at intervals of at least one month, followed by a booster dose one year later. For older children and adults, the third dose is delayed for at least six months after the second, and no fourth dose is required. Immunization lasts for five to ten years.

Debridement of wounds is an important preventive measure. Patients with open wounds should receive an additional dose of tetanus toxoid if they have not received a booster dose within ten years—or if the last booster dose was more than five years ago and the risk of infection with *C tetani* is moderate or high. A moderate likelihood of infection is associated with wounds that penetrate muscle, those sustained on wood or pavement, human bites, and nonabdominal bullet wounds. High-risk wounds include those acquired in barnyards, near sewers or other sources of waste material, and abdominal bullet wounds. Patients with moderate or high-risk wounds should also be given tetanus immune globulin.

The treatment of tetanus includes hospitalization in an intensive care unit to monitor respiratory and circulatory function, tetanus immune globulin to neutralize the toxin, and penicillin for the infection itself. Diazepam, 10–20 mg intravenously or intramuscularly every four to six hours, and chlorpromazine, 25–50 mg intravenously or intramuscularly every eight hours, are useful for treating painful spasms and rigidity. Neuromuscular blockade with curare or pancuronium may be required when these measures fail; if so, mechanical ventilation must be used.

Fatality rates of 10–60% are reported. Lower fatality rates are most likely to be achieved by early diagnosis, prompt institution of appropriate treatment before the onset of spasms, and the use of intrathecal—in addition to intramuscular—tetanus immune globulin. Among patients who recover, about 95% do so without long-term sequelae.

Chronic Adhesive Arachnoiditis

This inflammatory disorder is usually idiopathic but can follow subarachnoid hemorrhage; meningitis; intrathecal administration of penicillin, radiological contrast materials, and certain forms of spinal anesthetic; trauma; and surgery.

The usual initial complaint is of constant radicular pain, but in other cases there is lower motor neuron weakness because of the involvement of anterior nerve roots. Eventually, a spastic ataxic paraparesis develops, with sphincter involvement. Lumbar puncture reveals a partial or complete block on **Queckenstedt's test** (compression of the jugular vein fails to elevate CSF pressure); CSF protein is elevated, and the cell count may be increased. Myelography shows a characteristic fragmentation of the contrast material into pockets.

Treating this aseptic inflammatory leptomeningeal process with steroids or with non-steroidal anti-inflammatory analgesics may be helpful. Surgery may be indicated in cases with localized cord involvement.

VASCULAR MYELOPATHIES

Infarction of the Spinal Cord

This rare event generally occurs only in the territory of the anterior spinal artery (Figure 6–2). This artery, which supplies the anterior two-thirds of the cord, is itself supplied by only a limited number of feeding vessels, while the paired posterior spinal arteries are supplied by numerous feeders at many different levels. Thus, anterior spinal artery syndrome usually results from interrupted flow in one of its feeders. Causes include trauma, dissecting aortic aneurysm, aortography, polyarteritis nodosa, and hypotensive crisis. Since the anterior spinal artery is particularly well supplied in the cervical region, infarcts almost always occur more caudally.

The typical clinical presentation is with the acute onset of a flaccid, areflexic paraparesis that, as spinal shock wears off after a few days or weeks, evolves into a spastic paraparesis with brisk tendon reflexes and extensor plantar responses. In addition, there is dissociated sensory impairment—pain and temperature appreciation are lost, but there is sparing of vibration and position sense because the posterior columns are supplied by the posterior spinal arteries.

Treatment is symptomatic.

Hematomyelia

Hemorrhage into the spinal cord is rare; it is caused by trauma, a vascular anomaly, a bleeding disorder, or anticoagulant therapy. A severe cord syndrome develops acutely and is usually associated with blood in the CSF. The prognosis depends on the extent of the hemorrhage and the rapidity with which it occurs.

Epidural or Subdural Hemorrhage

Spinal epidural or subdural hemorrhage can occur in relation to trauma or tumor and as a complication of anticoagulation, aspirin therapy, thrombocytopenia, coagulopathy, or lumbar puncture. The likelihood of hemorrhage following lumbar puncture—usually epidural in location—is increased when a disorder of coagulation is present. Therefore, the platelet count, prothrombin time, and partial thromboplastin time should be determined before lumbar puncture is performed, and if anticoagulant therapy is to be instituted, it should be delayed for at least one hour following the procedure. Spinal epidural hemorrhage usually presents with back pain that may radiate in the distribution of one or more spinal nerve roots; it is occasionally painless. Paraparesis or quadriparesis, sensory disturbances in the lower limbs, and bowel and bladder dysfunction may de-

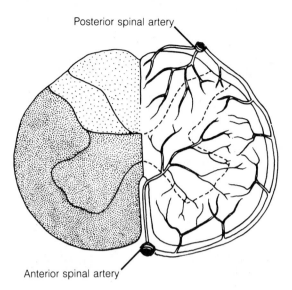

Posterior spinal artery

Anterior spinal artery

Figure 6–2. Blood supply to the spinal cord (shown in transverse section). Territories supplied by the anterior spinal artery (dark stippling) and the posterior spinal artery (light stippling) are shown on the left. The pattern of supply by intramedullary arteries is shown on the right. From the pial vessels (around the circumference of the cord), radially oriented branches supply much of the white matter and the posterior horns of gray matter. The remaining gray matter and the innermost portion of the white matter are supplied by the central artery (located in the anterior median fissure), which arises from the anterior spinal artery.

velop rapidly, necessitating urgent CT scan, MRI, or myelography, and surgical evacuation of the hematoma.

Arteriovenous Malformation

This may present with subarachnoid hemorrhage or with myelopathy. Most of these lesions involve the lower part of the cord. Symptoms include motor and sensory disturbances in the legs and disorders of sphincter function. Pain in the legs or back is often conspicuous. On examination, there may be an upper, a lower, or a mixed motor deficit in the legs, while sensory deficits are usually extensive but occasionally radicular; the signs indicate an extensive lesion in the longitudinal axis of the cord. In patients with cervical lesions, symptoms and signs may also be present in the arms. A bruit is sometimes audible over the spine, and there may be a cutaneous angioma. The diagnosis is suggested by the myelographic finding of serpiginous filling defects caused by enlarged vessels and is confirmed by selective spinal arteriography. Spinal MRI is sometimes normal despite the presence of an arteriovenous malformation and therefore cannot be relied upon to exclude this diagnosis.

Most lesions are extramedullary and posterior to the cord; they can be treated by ligation of feeding vessels and excision of the anomalous arteriovenous nidus of the malformation, which is usually dural in location. Left untreated, the patient is likely to become increasingly disabled until chair- or bed-bound.

DEFICIENCY DISORDERS

Subacute combined degeneration of the cord as a result of vitamin B_{12} deficiency is characterized by an upper motor neuron deficit in the limbs that is usually preceded by sensory symptoms and signs caused by posterior column involvement (see Chapter 7). In addition to the myelopathy, there may be optic atrophy, mental changes, or peripheral neuropathy.

CERVICAL SPONDYLOSIS

Cervical spondylosis is characterized by any or all of the following: pain and stiffness in the neck; pain in the arms, with or without a segmental motor or sensory deficit in the arms; and an upper motor neuron deficit in the legs. It results from chronic cervical disk degeneration, with herniation of disk material, secondary calcification, and associated osteophytic outgrowths. It can lead to involvement of one or more nerve roots on either or both sides and to myelopathy related to compression, vascular insufficiency, or recurrent minor trauma to the cord.

Clinical Findings

Patients often present with neck pain and limitation of head movement or with occipital headache. In some cases, radicular pain and other sensory disturbances occur in the arms, and there may be weakness of the arms or legs. Examination commonly reveals restricted lateral flexion and rotation of the neck. There may be a segmental pattern of weakness or dermatomal sensory loss in one or both arms, along with depression of those tendon reflexes mediated by the affected root(s). Cervical spondylosis tends to affect particularly the C5 and C6 nerve roots, so there is commonly weakness of muscles (eg, deltoid, supra- and infraspinatus, biceps, brachioradialis) supplied from these segments, pain or sensory loss about the shoulder and outer border of the arm and forearm, and depressed biceps and brachioradialis reflexes. If there is an associated myelopathy, upper motor neuron weakness develops in one or both legs, with concomitant changes in tone and reflexes. There may also be posterior column or spinothalamic sensory deficits.

Investigative Studies

Plain x-rays show osteophyte formation, narrowing of disk spaces, and encroachment on the intervertebral foramina. Myelography, CT scanning, or MRI may be necessary to confirm the diagnosis and exclude other structural causes of myelopathy. The CSF obtained at the time of myelography is usually normal, but the protein concentration may be increased, especially if there is a block in the subarachnoid space.

Differential Diagnosis

Spondylotic myelopathy may resemble myelopathy caused by such disorders as multiple sclerosis, motor neuron disease, subacute combined degeneration, cord tumor, syringomyelia, or hereditary spastic paraplegia. Moreover, degenerative changes in the spine are common in the middle-aged and elderly and may coincide with one of these other disorders.

Treatment

Treatment with a cervical collar to restrict neck movements may relieve any pain. Operative treatment may be necessary to prevent further progression if there is a significant neurological deficit; it may also be required if the root pain is severe, persistent, and unresponsive to conservative measures.

CONGENITAL ANOMALIES

A combination of corticospinal and cerebellar signs may be found in the limbs of patients with congenital skeletal abnormalities such as **platybasia** (flattening of the base of the skull) or **basilar invagination** (an upward bulging of the margins of the foramen magnum). **Syringomyelia** (cavitation of the cord), which can be congenital or acquired, may lead to a lower motor neuron deficit, a dissociated sensory loss in the arms, and upper motor neuron signs in the legs. Because the sensory findings are so characteristic, this disorder, which is frequently associated with Arnold-Chiari malformation, is discussed in detail in Chapter 7.

TUMORS & CORD COMPRESSION

Common causes of cord compression are disk protrusion, trauma, and tumors; in certain parts of the world, tuberculous disease of the spine is also a frequent cause. Rare but important causes include epidural abscess and hematoma. The present section will be restricted to a consideration of tumors, and other causes will be considered elsewhere.

Classification

Tumors can be divided into two groups: **intramedullary** (10%) and **extramedullary** (90%). **Ependymomas** are the most common type of intramedullary tumor, and the various types of **gliomas** make up the remainder. Extramedullary tumors can be either extradural or intradural in location. Among the primary extramedullary tumors, **neurofibromas**

and **meningiomas** are relatively common and are benign; they can be intra- or extradural. Carcinomatous metastases (especially from bronchus, breast, or prostate), lymphomatous or leukemic deposits, and myeloma are usually extradural.

Clinical Findings

Irrespective of its nature, a tumor can lead to cord dysfunction and a neurological deficit by direct compression, ischemia secondary to arterial or venous obstruction, or, in the case of intramedullary lesions, by invasive infiltration.

A. Symptoms: Symptoms may develop insidiously and progress gradually or—as is often the case with spinal cord compression from metastatic carcinoma—exhibit a rapid course.

Pain is a conspicuous feature—and usually the initial abnormality—in many patients with extradural lesions; it can be radicular, localized to the back, or experienced diffusely in an extremity and is characteristically aggravated by coughing or straining (Table 6–9).

Motor symptoms (heaviness, weakness, stiffness, or focal wasting of one or more limbs) may develop, or there may be paresthesias or numbness, especially in the legs. When sphincter disturbances occur, they usually are particularly disabling.

B. Signs: Examination sometimes reveals localized spinal tenderness. Involvement of anterior roots leads to an appropriate lower motor neuron deficit, and involvement of posterior roots leads to dermatomal sensory changes at the level of the lesion. Involvement of pathways traversing the cord may cause an upper motor neuron deficit below the level of the lesion and a sensory deficit with an upper level on the trunk. The distribution of signs varies with the level of the lesion and may take the form of Brown-Séquard or central cord syndrome (see Figure 7–7).

Investigative Studies

The CSF is often xanthochromic, with a greatly increased protein concentration, a normal or elevated white blood cell count, and normal or depressed glucose concentration; Queckenstedt's test at lumbar puncture may reveal a partial or complete block. A plain x-ray of the spine may or may not be abnormal, and myelography, CT scanning, or MRI is necessary to delineate the lesion and localize it accurately.

Table 6–9. Clinical features of spinal cord compression by extradural metastasis.[1]

Sign or Symptom	Initial Feature (%)	Present at Diagnosis (%)
Pain	96	96
Weakness	2	76
Sensory disturbance	0	51
Sphincter dysfunction	0	57

[1]Adapted from Byrne TN, Waxman SG: *Spinal Cord Compression.* Vol 33 of: *Contemporary Neurology Series.* Davis, 1990.

Treatment

Treatment depends upon the nature of the lesion. Extradural metastases must be treated urgently. Depending upon the nature of the primary neoplasm, they are best managed by analgesics, corticosteroids, radiotherapy, and hormonal treatment; decompressive laminectomy is often unnecessary. Intradural (but extramedullary) lesions are best removed if possible. Intramedullary tumors are treated by decompression and surgical excision when feasible and by radiotherapy.

Prognosis

The prognosis depends upon the cause and severity of the cord compression before it is relieved. Cord compression by extradural metastasis is usually manifested first by pain alone and may progress rapidly to cause permanent impairment of motor, sensory, and sphincter function. Therefore, the diagnosis must be suspected early in any patient with cancer and spinal or radicular pain, who must be investigated immediately. Reliance on motor, sensory, or sphincter disturbances to make the diagnosis will unnecessarily delay treatment and worsen the outcome.

ANTERIOR HORN CELL DISEASES

Disorders that predominantly affect the anterior horn cells are characterized clinically by wasting and weakness of the affected muscles without accompanying sensory changes. Electromyography shows changes that are characteristic of chronic partial denervation, with abnormal spontaneous activity in resting muscle and a reduction in the number of motor units under voluntary control; signs of reinnervation may also be present. Motor conduction velocity is usually normal but may be slightly reduced, and sensory conduction studies are normal. Muscle biopsy shows the histological changes of denervation. Serum CPK may be slightly elevated, but it never reaches the extremely high values seen in some muscular dystrophies.

IDIOPATHIC ANTERIOR HORN CELL DISORDERS

The clinical features and outlook depend in part on the patient's age at onset.

1. MOTOR NEURON DISEASE IN CHILDREN

Infantile Spinal Muscular Atrophy (Werdnig-Hoffmann Disease)

This autosomal recessive disorder usually manifests itself within the first 3 months of life. The infant is floppy and may have difficulty with sucking, swallowing, or ventilation. In established cases, examination reveals impaired swallowing or sucking, atrophy and fasciculation of the tongue, and muscle wasting in the limbs that is sometimes obscured by subcutaneous fat. The tendon reflexes are normal or depressed, and the plantar responses may be absent. There is no sensory deficit. The disorder is rapidly progressive, generally leading to death from respiratory complications by about age 3 years.

The cause is unknown, and there is no effective treatment.

Intermediate Spinal Muscular Atrophy (Chronic Werdnig-Hoffmann Disease)

This also has an autosomal recessive mode of inheritance but usually begins in the latter half of the first year of life. Its main clinical features are wasting and weakness of the extremities; bulbar weakness occurs less commonly. The disorder progresses slowly, ultimately leading to severe disability with kyphoscoliosis and contractures, but its course is more benign than the infantile variety described above, and many patients survive into adulthood.

Treatment is essentially supportive and directed particularly at the prevention of scoliosis and other deformities.

Juvenile Spinal Muscular Atrophy (Kugelberg-Welander Disease)

Generally this disorder develops in childhood or early adolescence, on either a hereditary or sporadic basis. The usual mode of inheritance is autosomal recessive, but cases with autosomal dominant or X-linked recessive inheritance also occur. It particularly tends to affect the proximal limb muscles, while there is generally little involvement of the bulbar musculature. It follows a gradually progressive course, leading to disability in early adult life. The proximal weakness may lead to a mistaken diagnosis of muscular dystrophy, but serum CPK determination, electromyography, and muscle biopsy will differentiate the disorders.

There is no effective treatment.

2. MOTOR NEURON DISEASE IN ADULTS

Motor neuron disease in adults generally begins between the ages of 30 and 60 years and is characterized by degeneration of anterior horn cells in the spinal cord, motor nuclei of the lower cranial nerves in the brain stem, and corticospinal and corticobulbar pathways. The disorder usually occurs sporadically but may also be familial. A gene associated with autosomal-dominant familial motor neuron disease has been localized to the long arm of chromosome 21 (21q22.1–22.2). Five varieties of the disorder can be distinguished by their predominant distribution (limb or bulbar musculature) and the nature of their clinical deficits (upper or lower motor neuron).

Classification

A. Progressive Bulbar Palsy: Bulbar involvement predominates and is due to lesions affecting the motor nuclei of cranial nerves (ie, lower motor neurons) in the brain stem.

B. Pseudobulbar Palsy: This term is used when bulbar involvement predominates and is due primarily to upper motor neuron disease, ie, to bilateral involvement of corticobulbar pathways. A pseudobulbar palsy can occur in any disorder that causes bilateral corticobulbar disease, however, and the use of the term must not be taken to imply that the underlying cause is *necessarily* motor neuron disease.

C. Progressive Spinal Muscular Atrophy: There is primarily a lower motor neuron deficit in the limbs, caused by anterior horn cell degeneration in the spinal cord.

D. Primary Lateral Sclerosis: In this rare disorder, a purely upper motor neuron (corticospinal) deficit is found in the limbs.

E. Amyotrophic Lateral Sclerosis: A mixed upper and lower motor neuron deficit is found in the limbs. There may also be bulbar involvement of the upper or lower motor neuron type.

Clinical Findings

In about 20% of the patients, the initial symptoms are related to weakness of bulbar muscles. Bulbar involvement is generally characterized by difficulty in swallowing, chewing, coughing, breathing, and speaking (dysarthria). In progressive bulbar palsy, examination may reveal drooping of the palate, a depressed gag reflex, a pool of saliva in the pharynx, a weak cough, and a wasted and fasciculating tongue. The tongue is contracted and spastic in pseudobulbar palsy and cannot be moved rapidly from side to side.

Weakness of the upper extremity muscles is the presenting complaint in about 40% of patients; lower extremity muscles are first affected in a similar proportion of patients. Limb involvement is characterized by easy fatigability, weakness, stiffness, twitching, wasting, and muscle cramps, and there may be vague sensory complaints and weight loss. Examination reveals no sensory deficit, but only upper or lower motor neuron signs, as indicated above.

There is generally no involvement of extraocular muscles or sphincters. The CSF is normal.

Treatment

There is no specific treatment for the idiopathic disorder. Symptomatic measures may include anticholinergic drugs (eg, trihexyphenidyl, amitriptyline, atropine) if drooling of saliva is troublesome. Braces or a walker may improve mobility, and physical therapy may prevent contractures.

A semiliquid diet or feeding via nasogastric tube may be required for severe dysphagia. Gastrostomy or cricopharyngomyotomy is sometimes necessary in extreme cases, and tracheostomy may be necessary if respiratory muscles are severely affected.

Prognosis

Motor neuron disease is progressive and usually has a fatal outcome within three to five years, most commonly from pulmonary infections. In general, patients with bulbar involvement have a poorer prognosis than those in whom dysfunction is limited to the extremities.

OTHER NONINFECTIVE DISORDERS OF ANTERIOR HORN CELLS

Juvenile spinal muscular atrophy can occur in patients with hexosaminidase deficiency. Rectal biopsy may be abnormal, and reduced hexosaminidase A is found in serum and leukocytes.

Patients with monoclonal gammopathy may present with pure motor syndromes. Plasmapheresis and immunosuppressive drug treatment (with dexamethasone and cyclophosphamide) may be beneficial in such cases.

Anterior horn cell disease may occur as a rare complication of lymphoma. Both men and women are affected, and the symptoms typically have their onset after the diagnosis of lymphoma has been established. The principal manifestation is weakness, which primarily affects the legs, may be patchy in its distribution, and spares bulbar and respiratory muscles. The reflexes are depressed, and sensory abnormalities are minor or absent. Neurological deficits usually progress over months, followed by spontaneous improvement and, in some cases, resolution.

INFECTIVE DISORDERS OF ANTERIOR HORN CELLS

Poliomyelitis—still common in certain parts of the world—has become rare in developed countries since the introduction of immunization programs. It is caused by an RNA virus of the picornavirus group. The usual route of infection is fecal-oral, and the incubation period varies between 5 and 35 days.

Neurological involvement follows a prodromal phase of fever, myalgia, malaise, and upper respiratory or gastrointestinal symptoms in a small number of cases. This involvement may consist merely of aseptic meningitis but in some instances leads to weakness or paralysis. Weakness develops over the course of one or a few days, sometimes in association with recrudescence of fever, and is accompanied by myalgia and signs of meningeal irritation. The weakness is asymmetrical in distribution and can be focal or unilateral; the bulbar and respiratory muscles may be affected either alone or in association with limb muscles. Tone is reduced in the affected muscles, and tendon reflexes may be lost. There is no sensory deficit.

CSF pressure is often mildly increased, and spinal fluid analysis characteristically shows an increased numbers of cells, a slightly elevated protein concentration, and a normal glucose level. Diagnosis may be confirmed by virus isolation from the stool or nasopharyngeal secretions—and less commonly from the CSF. A rise in viral antibody titer in convalescent serum, compared with serum obtained during the acute phase of the illness, is also diagnostically helpful. A clinically similar disorder is produced by coxsackievirus infection.

There is no specific treatment, and management is purely supportive, with attention directed particularly to the maintenance of respiratory function. With time, there is often useful recovery of strength even in severely weakened muscles.

NERVE ROOT LESIONS

ACUTE INTERVERTEBRAL DISK PROLAPSE

Lumbar Disk Prolapse

Acute prolapse of a lumbar disk (Figure 6–3) generally leads to pain in the back and in a radicular distribution (L5 or S1) in the leg, where it is often accompanied by numbness and paresthesias. A motor deficit may also be found; this depends on the root affected. An L5 radiculopathy causes weakness of dorsiflexion of the foot and toes, while S1 root involvement produces weakness of eversion and plantar flexion of the foot and a depressed ankle jerk. Movement of the spine is restricted, and there is local back tenderness. Straight-leg raising in the supine position is restricted, often to about 20 or 30 degrees of hip flexion, from a normal value of about 80 or 90 degrees, because of reflex spasm of the hamstring muscles (**Lasegue's sign**). A centrally prolapsed disk can lead to bilateral symptoms and signs and to sphincter involvement.

The symptoms and signs of a prolapsed lumbar intervertebral disk can be either sudden or insidious in onset and may follow trauma. Pelvic and rectal examination and plain x-rays of the spine help to exclude lesions such as tumors.

Bed rest on a firm mattress for two to four weeks (or longer) often permits symptoms to settle, but persisting pain, an increasing neurological deficit, or any evidence of sphincter dysfunction should lead to myelography, CT, or MRI followed by surgical treatment. Drug treatment for pain includes aspirin or acetaminophen with 30 mg of codeine, two doses three or four times daily, or other nonsteroidal analgesics such as ibuprofen or naproxen. Muscle spasm may respond to cyclobenzaprine, 10 mg orally three times daily or as needed and tolerated, or diazepam, 5–10 mg orally three times daily or as tolerated.

Cervical Disk Prolapse

Acute protrusion of a cervical disk can occur at any age, often with no preceding trauma, and leads to pain in the neck and radicular pain in the arm. The pain is exacerbated by head movement. With lateral herniation of the disk, a motor, sensory, or reflex deficit may be found in a radicular (usually C6 or C7) distribution on the affected side; with more centrally directed herniations, the spinal cord may also be involved, leading to a spastic paraparesis and sensory disturbance in the legs, sometimes accompanied by impaired sphincter function. The diagnosis is confirmed by myelography, CT scanning, or MRI.

Surgical treatment may be needed.

CERVICAL SPONDYLOSIS

This disorder has been described on p 161.

TRAUMATIC AVULSION OF NERVE ROOTS

Erb-Duchenne Paralysis

Traumatic avulsion of the C5 and C6 roots can occur at birth as a result of traction on the head during delivery of the shoulder. It can also be the result of injuries causing excessive separation of the head and shoulder. It leads to loss of shoulder abduction and elbow flexion. In consequence, the affected arm is held internally rotated at the shoulder, with a pronated forearm and extended elbow. The biceps and brachioradialis jerks are lost, but sensory impairment is usually inconspicuous, since it is confined to a small area overlying the deltoid muscle.

Klumpke's Paralysis

Involvement of the C8 and T1 roots causes paralysis and wasting of the small muscles of the hand and of the long finger flexors and extensors. Horner's syndrome is sometimes an associated finding. This kind of lower plexus paralysis often follows a fall that

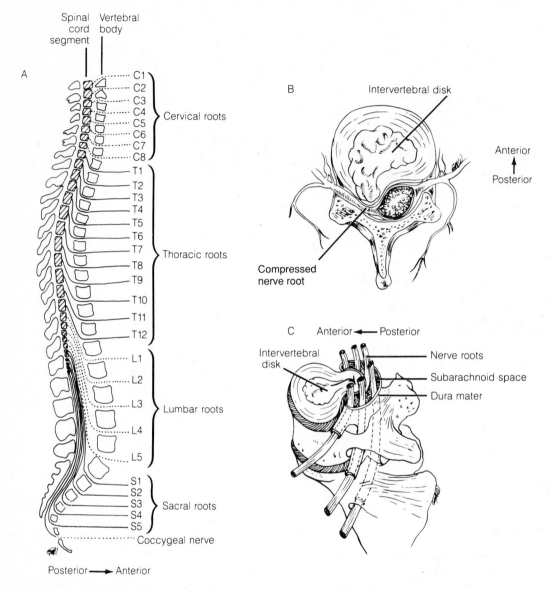

Figure 6–3. **A:** Lateral view of the vertebral column, showing the levels at which the various nerve roots exit. **B:** Lateral disk prolapse, causing compression of a nerve root. **C:** Central disk prolapse, causing bilateral root compression.

has been arrested by grasping a fixed object with one hand or may result from traction on the abducted arm.

NEURALGIC AMYOTROPHY
(Idiopathic Brachial Plexopathy)

This disorder typically begins with severe pain about the shoulder followed within a few days by weakness, reflex changes, and sensory disturbances in the arm, often involving the C5 and C6 segments especially. Symptoms and signs are usually unilateral but may be bilateral, and wasting of the affected muscles is often profound. The disorder relates to disturbed function of cervical roots or part of the brachial plexus, but its precise cause is unknown. It sometimes occurs shortly after minor injury, injections, inoculations, or minor systemic infections, but whether these are of etiological relevance is unclear. Familial cases occur occasionally.

Treatment is symptomatic. Recovery over the ensuing weeks and months is the rule—but it is sometimes incomplete.

CERVICAL RIB SYNDROME

The C8 and T1 roots or the lower trunk of the brachial plexus may be compressed by a cervical rib or band arising from the seventh cervical vertebra. This leads to weakness and wasting of intrinsic hand muscles, especially those in the thenar eminence, accompanied by pain and numbness in the appropriate dermatomal distribution (often like that of an ulnar nerve lesion but extending up the medial border of the forearm). The subclavian artery may also be compressed; this forms the basis of **Adson's test** for diagnosing the disorder. The radial pulse decreases in amplitude when the seated patient turns the head to the affected side and inhales deeply. A positive Adson's test, however, can also be seen in normal subjects; a supraclavicular bruit during the maneuver supports the diagnosis of subclavian artery compromise.

X-rays may show the cervical rib or a long transverse process of the seventh cervical vertebra, but normal findings do not exclude the possibility of a cervical band. Electromyography shows evidence of chronic partial denervation in the hand—in a territory beyond that of any individual peripheral nerve. Nerve conduction studies show no evidence of peripheral nerve disease, but there is a small or absent ulnar sensory nerve action potential on stimulation of the little finger.

Treatment is by surgical excision of the rib or band.

DISORDERS OF PERIPHERAL NERVES

The term **peripheral neuropathy** designates a disturbance in function of one or more peripheral nerves. Several types of peripheral neuropathy are distinguishable by the extent of involvement.

Depending upon the underlying cause, there may be selective involvement of motor, sensory, or autonomic fibers or more diffuse involvement of all fibers in the peripheral nerve.

The clinical deficit is usually a mixed one, and sensory symptoms and signs are often the initial—and most conspicuous—feature of peripheral nerve involvement. Further discussion of these disorders and their treatment is therefore deferred to Chapter 7, except in those instances in which presentation is typically with acute motor deficits. For convenience, however, the root and peripheral nerve supply of the major limb muscles is set forth in Tables 6–5 and 6–6. Reference to the tables should facilitate evaluation of patients presenting with focal weakness of lower motor neuron type.

POLYNEUROPATHY

In polyneuropathy, because there is symmetrical and simultaneous involvement of various nerves, the deficits resulting from individual nerves cannot be recognized clinically. Polyneuropathies are discussed in Chapter 7, but brief mention is made here of those neuropathies in which patients present with acute weakness.

Acute Inflammatory Polyradiculoneuropathy (Guillain-Barré Syndrome)

This disorder commonly presents with weakness that is often symmetrical and most commonly begins in the legs. The speed and extent of progression vary, but in severe cases there is marked weakness of all limbs in addition to bilateral facial weakness. There may also be subjective sensory complaints, although objective sensory disturbances are usually far less conspicuous than motor deficits. Autonomic involvement is common and may lead to a fatal outcome, as may aspiration pneumonia or impaired respiration from weakness. Further details about this disorder are given in Chapter 7.

Diphtheritic Polyneuritis

Infection with *Corynebacterium diphtheriae* can occur either in the upper respiratory tract or by infection of a skin wound, and neuropathy results from a neurotoxin that is released by the organism. Palatal weakness may develop two to three weeks after infection of the throat, and cutaneous diphtheria may be followed by focal weakness of neighboring muscles after a similar interval. Impaired pupillary responses to accommodation may occur about four or five weeks after infection and a generalized sensorimotor polyneuropathy after one to three months. The weakness may be asymmetric and is often more marked proximally than distally. Respiratory paralysis occurs in severe cases. Recovery usually occurs over the following two to three months but may take longer in severe cases.

In patients with polyneuropathy, CSF protein content is usually increased, and there may be a mild pleocytosis. Electrophysiological studies show a slowing of nerve conduction velocity, but this is often not manifest until the patient has begun to improve clinically. Treatment consists of early administration of equine diphtheria antitoxin without awaiting the results of bacterial culture, provided the patient is not hypersensitive to horse serum. A two-week course of penicillin or erythromycin will usually eradicate the infection but does not alter the incidence of serious complications. In patients with marked weakness, supportive measures, including ventilatory support, are necessary.

Paralytic Shellfish Poisoning

Mussels and clams found on the East and West Coasts of the United States may be dangerous to eat, especially in the summer months. They feed on poisonous varieties of plankton and come to contain saxitoxin, which blocks sodium channels—and therefore action potentials—in motor and sensory nerves and in muscle. A rapidly progressive acute peripheral neuropathy, with sensory symptoms and a rapidly ascending paralysis, begins within 30 minutes after eating affected shellfish and may lead to respiratory paralysis and death. There is no available antitoxin, but with proper supportive care (including mechanical ventilation if necessary) the patient recovers completely. A cathartic or enema may help remove unabsorbed toxin.

Porphyria

Acute polyneuropathy may occur with the hereditary hepatic porphyrias. Attacks can be precipitated by drugs (eg, barbiturates, estrogens, sulfonamides, griseofulvin, phenytoin, succinimides) that can induce the enzyme δ-aminolevulinic acid synthetase, or by infection, a period of fasting, or, occasionally, menses or pregnancy. Colicky abdominal pain frequently precedes neurological involvement, and there may also be acute confusion or delirium and convulsions. Weakness is the major neurological manifestation and is due to a predominantly motor polyneuropathy that causes a symmetrical disturbance that is sometimes more marked proximally than distally. It may begin in the upper limbs and progress to involve the lower limbs or trunk. Progression occurs at a variable rate and can lead to complete flaccid quadriparesis with respiratory paralysis over a few days. Sensory loss occurs also but is less conspicuous and extensive. The tendon reflexes may be depressed or absent. The disorder may be accompanied by fever, persistent tachycardia, hypertension, hyponatremia, and peripheral leukocytosis. The CSF may show a slight increase in protein concentration and a slight pleocytosis. The diagnosis is confirmed by demonstrating increased levels of porphobilinogen and δ-aminolevulinic acid in the urine or deficiency of uroporphyrinogen I synthetase in red blood cells (**acute intermittent porphyria**) or of coproporphyrinogen oxidase in lymphocytes (**hereditary coproporphyria**).

Treatment is with intravenous dextrose to suppress the heme biosynthetic pathway and propranolol to control tachycardia and hypertension. Hematin, 4 mg/kg by intravenous infusion over 15 minutes once or twice daily, is also effective in improving the clinical state. The best index of progress is the heart rate. The abdominal and mental symptoms (but not the neuropathy) may be helped by chlorpromazine or another phenothiazine. Respiratory failure may necessitate tracheostomy and mechanical ventilation. Preventing acute attacks by avoiding known precipitants is important.

Acute Arsenic or Thallium Poisoning

Acute arsenic or thallium poisoning can produce a rapidly evolving sensorimotor polyneuropathy, often with an accompanying or preceding gastrointestinal disturbance. Arsenic may also cause a skin rash, with increased skin pigmentation and marked exfoliation, together with the presence of Mees lines (transverse white lines) on the nails in long-standing cases. Thallium can produce a scaly rash and hair loss. Sensory symptoms are often the earliest manifestation of polyneuropathy; this is followed by symmetrical motor impairment, which is usually more marked distally than proximally and occurs in the legs rather than the arms. The CSF protein may be increased, with little or no change in cell content, and the electrophysiological findings sometimes resemble those of Guillain-Barré syndrome, especially in the acute phase of the disorder. The diagnosis of arsenic toxicity is best established by measuring the arsenic content of hair protected from external contamination (eg, hair from the pubic region). Urine also contains arsenic in the acute phase. The diagnosis of thallium poisoning is made by finding thallium in body tissues or fluids, especially in urine. The degree of neurological recovery depends upon the severity of the intoxication.

Chelating agents are of uncertain value.

Organophosphate Polyneuropathy

Organophosphate compounds are widely used as insecticides and are also the active principles in the nerve gas of chemical warfare. They have a variety of acute toxic effects, particularly manifestations of cholinergic crisis caused by inhibition of acetylcholinesterase. Some organophosphates, however, also induce a delayed polyneuropathy that generally begins about one to three weeks after acute exposure. Cramping muscle pain in the legs is usually the initial symptom of neuropathy, sometimes followed by distal numbness and paresthesias. Progressive leg weakness then occurs, along with depression of the tendon reflexes. Similar deficits may develop in the upper limbs after several days. Sensory disturbances also develop in some instances, initially in the legs and then in the arms, but these disturbances are often mild or inconspicuous. Examination shows a distal symmetric, predominantly motor polyneuropathy, with wasting and flaccid weakness of distal leg muscles. In some patients, this may be severe enough to cause quadriplegia, whereas in others the weakness is much milder. Mild pyramidal signs may also be present. Objective evidence of sensory loss is usually slight. The acute effects of organophosphate poisoning may be prevented by the use of protective masks and clothing or by pretreatment with pyridostigmine, a short-acting acetylcholinesterase inhibitor. Treatment after exposure includes decontamination of the skin with bleach or soap and water and administration of atropine, 2–6 mg every five minutes, and pralidoxime, 1 g every hour for up to three hours, both given intramuscularly or intravenously. Recovery of peripheral nerve function may occur with time, but central deficits are usually permanent and may govern the extent of ultimate functional recovery. There is no treatment for the neuropathy other than supportive care.

MONONEUROPATHY MULTIPLEX

This term signifies that there is involvement of various nerves but in an asymmetric manner and at different times, so that the individual nerves involved can usually be identified until the disorder reaches an advanced stage. Comment here will be restricted to the disorder produced by lead, because of the selective motor involvement characteristic of lead poisoning.

Lead Toxicity

Lead toxicity is common among persons involved in the manufacture or repair of storage batteries or other lead-containing products, the smelting of lead or lead-containing ores, and the shipbreaking industry. It may also occur in persons using lead-containing paints or those who ingest contaminated alcohol. Inorganic lead can produce dysfunction of both the central and peripheral nervous systems. In children, who can develop toxicity by ingesting lead-containing paints that flake off old buildings or furniture, acute encephalopathy is the major neurological feature. The peripheral neuropathy is predominantly motor, and in adults it is more severe in the arms than in the legs. It typically affects the radial nerves, although other nerves may also be affected, leading to an asymmetric progressive motor disturbance. Sensory loss is usually inconspicuous or absent. There may be loss or depression of tendon reflexes. Systemic manifestations of lead toxicity include anemia, constipation, colicky abdominal pain, gum discoloration, and nephropathy. The extent to which exposed workers develop minor degrees of peripheral nerve damage as a result of lead toxicity is not clear. Similarly, there is no agreement about the lowest concentration of blood lead that is associated with damage to the peripheral nerves.

The optimal approach to treatment is not known, but intravenous or intramuscular edetate calcium disodium (EDTA) and oral penicillamine have been used, as has dimercaprol (BAL).

MONONEUROPATHY SIMPLEX

In mononeuropathy simplex there is involvement of a single peripheral nerve. Most of the common mononeuropathies entail both motor and sensory involvement (as discussed in Chapter 7). Accordingly, only Bell's palsy, which leads primarily to a motor deficit, is discussed here.

Bell's Palsy

Facial weakness of the lower motor neuron type caused by idiopathic facial nerve involvement outside the central nervous system, without evidence of aural or more widespread neurological disease, has been designated Bell's palsy. The cause is unclear, but the disorder occurs more commonly in pregnant women and diabetics. Facial weakness is often preceded or accompanied by pain about the ear. Weakness generally comes on abruptly but may progress over several hours or even a day or so. Depending upon the site of the lesion, there may be associated impairment of taste, lacrimation, or hyperacusis. There may be paralysis of all muscles supplied by the affected nerve (**complete palsy**) or variable weakness in different muscles (**incomplete palsy.**) Clinical examination reveals no abnormalities beyond the territory of the facial nerve. Most patients recover completely without treatment, but this may take several days in some instances and several months in others. A poor prognosis for complete recovery is suggested by severe pain at onset and complete palsy when the patient is first seen. Even if recovery is incomplete, permanent disfigurement or some other complication affects only about 10% of patients. Treatment with corticosteroids (prednisone, 60 mg/d orally for three days, tapering over the next seven days), beginning within five days after the onset of palsy, is said to increase the proportion of patients who recover completely. It should therefore be prescribed in patients who have a poor prognosis. However, it should be noted that the evidence that corticosteroids are indeed beneficial is incomplete, and they may have unpleasant side effects. Other conditions that can produce facial palsy include tumors, herpes zoster infection of the geniculate ganglion (Ramsay Hunt syndrome), Lyme disease, AIDS, and sarcoidosis.

DISORDERS OF NEUROMUSCULAR TRANSMISSION

MYASTHENIA GRAVIS

Myasthenia gravis can occur at any age and is sometimes associated with thymic tumor, thyrotoxicosis, rheumatoid arthritis, or disseminated lupus erythematosus. More common in females than males, it is characterized by fluctuating weakness and easy fatigability of voluntary muscles; muscle activity cannot be maintained, and initially powerful movements weaken readily. There is a predilection for the external ocular muscles and certain other cranial muscles, including the masticatory, facial, pharyngeal, and laryngeal muscles. Respiratory and limb muscles may also be affected. Weakness is due to a variable block of neuromuscular transmission related to an immune-mediated decrease in the number of functioning acetylcholine receptors (Figure 6–4).

A similar disorder in patients receiving penicillamine for rheumatoid arthritis frequently remits when the drug is discontinued.

Clinical Findings

Although the onset of the disease is usually insidious, the disorder is sometimes unmasked by a concurrent infection, which leads to an exacerbation of symptoms. Exacerbations may also occur in pregnancy or before menses. Symptoms may be worsened by quinine, quinidine, procainamide, propranolol, phenytoin, lithium, tetracycline, and aminoglycoside antibiotics, which should therefore be avoided in such patients. Myasthenia follows a slowly progressive course. Patients present with ptosis, diplopia, difficulty in chewing or swallowing, nasal speech, respiratory difficulties, or weakness of the limbs (Table

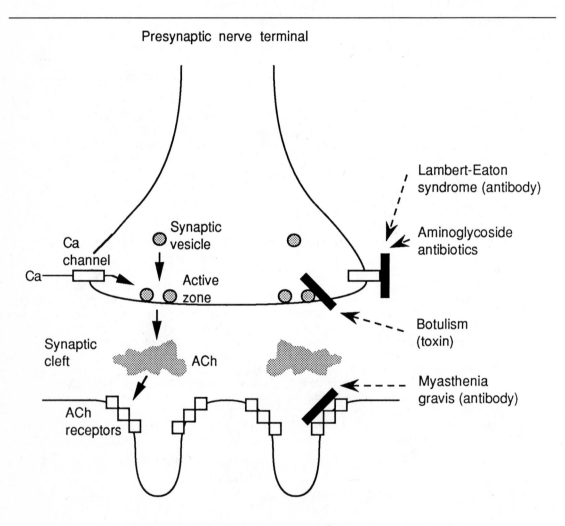

Figure 6–4. Sites of involvement in disorders of neuromuscular transmission. At left, normal transmission involves depolarization-induced influx of calcium (Ca) through voltage-gated channels. This stimulates release of acetylcholine (ACh) from synaptic vesicles at the active zone and into the synaptic cleft. ACh binds to ACh receptors and depolarizes the postsynaptic muscle membrane. At right, disorders of neuromuscular transmission result from blockage of Ca channels (Lambert-Eaton syndrome or aminoglycoside antibiotics), impairment of Ca-mediated ACh release (botulinum toxin), or antibody-induced internalization and degradation of ACh receptors (myasthenia gravis).

Table 6–10. Presenting symptoms in myasthenia gravis.[1]

Symptom	Percentage of Patients
Diplopia	41
Ptosis	25
Dysarthria	16
Lower extremity weakness	13
Generalized weakness	11
Dysphagia	10
Upper extremity weakness	7
Masticatory weakness	7

[1]Adapted from Herrmann C Jr: Myasthenia gravis—Current concepts. *West J Med* 1985;142:797–809.

6–10). These symptoms often fluctuate in intensity during the day, and this diurnal variation is superimposed on longer-term spontaneous relapses and remissions that may last for weeks.

Clinical examination confirms the weakness and fatigability of affected muscles. The weakness does not conform to the distribution of any single nerve, root, or level of the central nervous system. In more than 90% of cases the extraocular muscles are involved, leading to often asymmetric ocular palsies and ptosis. Pupillary responses are not affected. The characteristic feature of the disorder is that sustained activity of affected muscles leads to temporarily increased weakness. Thus, sustained upgaze for two minutes can lead to increased ptosis, with power in the affected muscles improving after a brief rest. In advanced cases, there may be some mild atrophy of affected muscles. Sensation is normal, and there are usually no reflex changes.

Diagnosis

The diagnosis of myasthenia gravis can generally be confirmed by the benefit that follows administration of anticholinesterase drugs; the power of affected muscles is influenced at a dose that has no effect on normal muscles and slight, if any, effect on muscles weakened by other causes.

The most commonly used pharmacological test is the **edrophonium (Tensilon) test.** Edrophonium is given intravenously in a dose of 10 mg (1 mL), of which 2 mg is given initially and the remaining 8 mg about 30 seconds later if the test dose is well tolerated. In myasthenic patients, there is an obvious improvement in the strength of weak muscles that lasts for about five minutes.

Alternatively, 1.5 mg of **neostigmine** can be given intramuscularly, with a response that lasts for about two hours; atropine sulfate (0.6 mg) should be available to counteract the muscarinic cholinergic side effects of increased salivation, diarrhea, and nausea. Atropine does not affect nicotinic cholinergic function at the neuromuscular junction. The longer-acting neostigmine reduces the incidence of false-negative evaluations.

Investigative Studies

X-rays and CT scans of the chest may reveal a coexisting thymoma. Impaired neuromuscular transmission can be detected electrophysiologically by a decremental response of muscle to repetitive supramaximal stimulation (at 2 or 3 Hz) of its motor nerve, but normal findings do not exclude the diagnosis. Single-fiber electromyography shows increased variability in the interval between two muscle fiber action potentials from the same motor unit in clinically weak muscles. Measuring serum acetylcholine receptor antibody levels may be helpful, since increased values are found in 80–90% of patients with myasthenia gravis.

Treatment

The following approaches to treatment are recommended.

A. Anticholinesterase Drugs: Treatment with these drugs provides symptomatic benefit without influencing the course of the underlying disease. Neostigmine, pyridostigmine, or both, can be used, with the dose being determined on an individual basis. The oral dose of neostigmine is usually between 7.5 and 30 mg (average, 15 mg) taken four to eight times daily; pyridostigmine is often taken in a dose of 30–180 mg (average, 60 mg) four times daily. Overmedication can lead to increased weakness, which, unlike myasthenic weakness, is unaffected or enhanced by intravenous edrophonium. Such a **cholinergic crisis** may be accompanied by pallor, sweating, nausea, vomiting, salivation, colicky abdominal pain, and miosis.

B. Thymectomy: Thymectomy should be performed in patients under 60 years of age with weakness that is not restricted to the extraocular muscles. Although thymectomy usually leads to symptomatic benefit or remission, the mechanism by which it confers benefit is unclear, and its beneficial effect may not be evident immediately.

C. Corticosteroids: Corticosteroids are indicated for patients who have responded poorly to anticholinesterase drugs and have already undergone thymectomy. Treatment is initiated with the patient in the hospital, since weakness may initially be exacerbated. An initial high dose of prednisone (60–100 mg/d orally) can gradually be tapered to a relatively low maintenance level (5–15 mg/d) as improvement occurs. Alternate-day treatment is helpful in reducing the incidence of side effects, which are described (as clinical findings) in the section on hyperadrenalism in Chapter 1.

D. Azathioprine: This drug can be used in patients with severe or progressive disease despite thymectomy and treatment with anticholinesterases and corticosteroids. It can also be given in place of high doses of corticosteroids to patients who show no sustained benefit with low doses. The usual dose is 2–3 mg/kg/d, increased from a lower initial dose.

E. Plasmapheresis: Plasmapheresis may be used to achieve temporary improvement in certain situations, such as prior to surgery that is likely to produce postoperative respiratory compromise.

Prognosis

Most patients can be managed successfully with drug treatment. The disease may have a fatal outcome because of respiratory complications such as aspiration pneumonia.

MYASTHENIC SYNDROME (Lambert-Eaton Syndrome)

This disorder has a well-recognized association with an underlying neoplasm and may occasionally be associated with such autoimmune diseases as pernicious anemia. In the paraneoplastic disorder, antibodies directed against tumor antigens cross-react with voltage-gated calcium channels involved in acetylcholine release, leading to a disturbance of neuromuscular transmission (see Figure 6–4).

Clinically there is weakness, especially of the proximal muscles of the limbs. Unlike myasthenia gravis, however, the extraocular muscles are characteristically spared, and power steadily increases if a contraction is maintained. Autonomic disturbances, such as dry mouth, constipation and impotence, may also occur.

The diagnosis is confirmed electrophysiologically by the response to repetitive nerve stimulation. There is a remarkable increase in the size of the muscle response to stimulation of its motor nerve at high rates—even in muscles that are not clinically weak.

Immunosuppressive drug therapy (corticosteroids and azathioprine as described above for myasthenia gravis) and plasmapheresis may lead to improvement. Guanidine hydrochloride, 25–50 mg/kg/d in three or four divided doses, is sometimes helpful in seriously disabled patients, but adverse effects of the drug include bone marrow suppression and renal failure. The response to treatment with anticholinesterase drugs such as pyridostigmine or neostigmine, alone or in combination with guanidine, is variable. 3,4-Diaminopyridine (investigational), at doses up to 25 mg orally four times daily, may improve weakness and autonomic dysfunction; paresthesia is a common side effect, and seizures may occur.

BOTULISM

The toxin of *Clostridium botulinum* can cause neuromuscular paralysis. It acts by preventing the release of acetylcholine at neuromuscular junctions and autonomic synapses (see Figure 6–4). Botulism occurs most commonly following ingestion of home-canned food that is contaminated with the toxin; it occurs rarely from infected wounds. The shorter the latent period between ingestion of the toxin and the onset of symptoms, the greater the dose of toxin and the risk for further involvement of the nervous system.

Clinical Findings

Fulminating weakness begins 12–72 hours after ingestion of the toxin and characteristically is manifested by diplopia, ptosis, facial weakness, dysphagia, nasal speech, and then difficulty with respiration; weakness usually appears last in the limbs. In addition to the motor deficit, blurring of vision is characteristic, and there may be dryness of the mouth, paralytic ileus, and postural hypotension. There is no sensory deficit, and the tendon reflexes are usually unchanged unless the involved muscles are quite weak. Symptoms can progress for several days after their onset.

Investigative Studies

Once the diagnosis is suspected, the local health authority should be notified and samples of the patient's serum and the contaminated food (if available) sent to be assayed for toxin. The most common types of toxin encountered clinically are A, B, and E. Electrophysiological studies may help confirm the diagnosis, since the evoked muscle response tends to increase in size progressively with repetitive stimulation of motor nerves at fast rates.

Treatment

Patients should be hospitalized, since respiratory insufficiency can develop rapidly and necessitates ventilatory assistance. Treatment with trivalent antitoxin (ABE) is commenced once it is established that the patient is not allergic to horse serum, but the effect on the course of the disease is unclear.

Guanidine hydrochloride (25–50 mg/kg/d in divided doses), a drug that facilitates release of acetylcholine from nerve endings, is sometimes helpful in improving muscle strength; anticholinesterase drugs are generally of no value. Nursing and supportive care are important.

AMINOGLYCOSIDE ANTIBIOTICS

Large doses of antibiotics such as kanamycin and gentamicin can produce a clinical syndrome rather like botulism, because the release of acetylcholine from nerve endings is prevented. This effect may be related to calcium channel blockade (Figure 6–4). Symptoms resolve rapidly as the responsible drug is eliminated from the body. Note that these antibiotics are particularly dangerous in patients with preexisting disturbances of neuromuscular transmission and are therefore best avoided in patients with myasthenia gravis.

MYOPATHIC DISORDERS

MUSCULAR DYSTROPHIES

The muscular dystrophies are a group of inherited myopathic disorders characterized by progressive muscle weakness and wasting. They are subdivided by their mode of inheritance, age at onset, distribution of involved muscles, rate of progression, and long-term outlook (Table 6–11).

There is no specific treatment for the muscular dystrophies. It is important to encourage patients to lead as normal a life as possible. Deformities and contractures can often be prevented or ameliorated by physical therapy and orthopedic procedures. Prolonged bed rest must be avoided, as inactivity often leads to worsening of disability.

A. Duchenne's Dystrophy: The most common form of muscular dystrophy, it is an X-linked disorder that affects predominantly males. Symptoms begin by age five years, and patients are typically severely disabled by adolescence, with death occurring in the third decade. Toe walking, waddling gait, and an inability to run are early symptoms. Weakness is most pronounced in the proximal lower extremities but also affects the proximal upper extremities. In attempting to rise to stand from a supine position, patients characteristically must use their arms to climb up their bodies **(Gowers' sign). Pseudohypertrophy** of the calves caused by fatty infiltration of muscle is common. The heart is involved late in the course, and mental retardation is a frequent accompaniment. Serum CPK levels are exceptionally high.

No definitive treatment is available, but some studies suggest that prednisone, 1.5 mg/kg/d orally, may improve muscle strength in the short term (up to six months). Side effects include weight gain, cushingoid appearance, and hirsutism; the long-term effects of prednisone in this disorder are uncertain.

A genetic defect that may be responsible for Duchenne's dystrophy has been identified. The gene in question is located on the short arm of the X chromosome and codes for the protein **dystrophin,** which is absent or profoundly reduced in muscle from patients with the disorder. The absence of dystrophin from synaptic regions of cerebral cortical neurons might contribute to mental retardation in patients with Duchenne's dystrophy.

B. Becker's Dystrophy: This is also X-linked and associated with a pattern of weakness similar to that observed in Duchenne's dystrophy. Its average onset (11 years) and age at death (42 years) are later, however. Cardiac and cognitive impairment do not occur, and CPK levels are less strikingly elevated than in Duchenne's dystrophy. In contrast to Duchenne's dystrophy, dystrophin levels in muscle are normal in Becker's dystrophy, but the protein is qualitatively altered.

C. Limb-Girdle Dystrophy: Previously a catch-all designation that probably subsumed a variety of disorders, including undiagnosed cases of other dystrophies, it is (in classic form) inherited in autosomal recessive fashion and begins between late childhood and early adulthood. In contrast to Duchenne's and Becker's dystrophies, the shoulder and pelvic girdle muscles are affected to a more nearly equal extent. Pseudohypertrophy is not seen, and CPK levels are less elevated.

D. Facioscapulohumeral Dystrophy: An autosomal dominant disorder that usually has its onset in adolescence, this is compatible with a normal life span. Its clinical severity is highly variable. Weakness is typically confined to the face, neck, and shoulder girdle, but foot drop can occur. Winged scapula is common. The heart is not involved, and serum CPK levels are normal or only slightly elevated.

E. Distal myopathy: This autosomal dominant dystrophy typically presents after age 40, although onset may be earlier and symptoms more severe in homozygotes. Small muscles of the hands and feet, wrist extensors, and the dorsiflexors of the foot are affected. The course is slowly progressive.

F. Ocular Dystrophy: This is typically an autosomal dominant disorder, although recessive and sporadic cases also occur. Some cases are associated with deletions in mitochondrial DNA. Onset is usually before age 30 years. Ptosis is the earliest manifestation, but progressive external ophthalmoplegia subsequently develops; facial weakness is also common, and subclinical involvement of limb muscles may occur. The course is slowly progressive. The extent to which ocular dystrophy is distinct from oculopharyngeal dystrophy (see below) is unclear in many cases.

G. Oculopharyngeal Dystrophy: An autosomal dominant disorder, this is found with increased frequency in certain geographic areas, including Quebec and the American southwest. It most often begins in the third to fifth decade. Findings include ptosis, total external ophthalmoplegia, dysphagia, facial weakness, and often proximal limb weakness. CPK is mildly elevated. Dysphagia is particularly incapacitating and may require nasogastric feeding or gastrostomy.

CONGENITAL MYOPATHIES

The congenital myopathies are a heterogeneous group of rare and relatively nonprogressive disorders that usually begin in infancy or childhood, but may not become clinically apparent until adulthood. Most are characterized by predominantly proximal muscle weakness, hypotonia, hyporeflexia, and normal CPK;

Table 6–11. The muscular dystrophies.

Disorder	Inheritance	Onset (Years)	Distribution	Prognosis	CPK	Notes
Duchenne's	X-linked recessive	1–5	Pelvic, then shoulder girdle; later, limb and respiratory muscles.	Rapid progression. Die within about 15 years after onset.	Marked increase.	May be pseudohypertrophy of muscles at some stage. Cardiac involvement, skeletal deformities, and muscle contractures occur. Intellectual retardation is common.
Becker's	X-linked recessive	5–25	Pelvic, then shoulder girdle.	Slow progression. May have normal life span.	Increase.	Usually no cardiac involvement, skeletal deformities, or contractures.
Limb-girdle (Erb)	Autosomal recessive or dominant, or sporadic	10–30	Pelvic or shoulder girdle initially, with later spread to other muscles.	Variable severity and rate of progression. May be severe disability in middle life.	Mild increase.	Variable clinical expression. May be hypertrophy of calves. Normal intellectual function. Cardiac involvement is rare.
Facioscapulohumeral	Autosomal dominant	Any age	Face and shoulder girdle initially; later, pelvic girdle and legs.	Slow progression. Minor disability. Usually normal life span.	Often normal.	Aborted or mild cases are common. Muscle hypertrophy, contractures, and deformities are rare.
Distal	Autosomal dominant	40–60	Onset distally in extremities; proximal involvement later.	Slow progression.	Often normal.	
Ocular	Autosomal dominant (may be recessive)	Any age (usually 5–30)	External ocular muscles. Mild weakness of face, neck, and arms may occur.	Not known.	Often normal.	
Oculopharyngeal	Autosomal dominant	Any age	As in the ocular form, but with dysphagia.	Not known.	Often normal.	
Myotonic dystrophy	Autosomal dominant	Any age (usually 20–40)	Facial and sternomastoid muscles and distal muscles in the extremities.	Variable severity and progression.	Normal or mild increase.	Associated features include myotonia, cataracts, gonadal atrophy, endocrinopathies, cardiac abnormalities, intellectual changes. Asymptomatic carriers of the gene may sometimes be detected by clinical examination, slit lamp examination for lenticular abnormalities, or electromyography.

many are inherited. They are classified according to ultrastructural histopathological features and are diagnosed by muscle biopsy. They include **nemaline** myopathy, characterized by rod-shaped bodies in muscle fibers, which are also seen in some patients with AIDS-related myopathy (see below); **central core** disease, which may be associated with malignant hyperthermia as a complication of general anesthesia; **myotubular** or **centronuclear** myopathy; and **mitochondrial** myopathies, such as Kearns-Sayre-Daroff syndrome, a cause of progressive external ophthalmoplegia (see Chapter 5). No treatment is available for any of these disorders.

MYOTONIC DISORDERS

In **myotonia**, an abnormality of the muscle fiber membrane (**sarcolemma**) leads to marked delay before the affected muscles can relax after a contraction; this leads to apparent muscle stiffness. In at least some cases, the disorder appears to be related to a decrease in chloride ion conductance across the sarcolemma. On examination, it is frequently possible to demonstrate myotonia by difficulty in relaxing the hand after sustained grip or by persistent contraction after percussion of the belly of a muscle. Electromyography of affected muscles may reveal characteristic high-frequency discharges of potentials that wax and wane in amplitude and frequency, producing over the EMG loudspeaker a sound like that of a dive bomber.

Myotonic Dystrophy

Myotonic dystrophy is a dominantly inherited disorder that usually is manifest in the third or fourth decade, although it may appear in early childhood. The gene defect has been localized to the centromeric region of chromosome 19 (19cen-q13.2). Myotonia accompanies weakness and wasting of the facial, sternomastoid, and distal limb muscles (Figure 6–5). There may also be cataracts, frontal baldness, testicular atrophy, diabetes mellitus, cardiac abnormalities, and intellectual changes.

Myotonia can be treated with quinine sulfate, 300–400 mg three times daily; procainamide, 0.5–1 g four times daily; or phenytoin, 100 mg three times daily. In myotonic dystrophy, phenytoin is perhaps the drug of choice, since the other drugs may have undesirable effects on cardiac conduction. There is no treatment for the weakness that occurs, and pharmacological maneuvers do not influence the natural history.

Myotonia Congenita

Myotonia congenita is usually inherited as a dominant trait. Generalized myotonia without weakness is usually present from birth, but symptoms may not develop until early childhood. Muscle stiffness is enhanced by cold and inactivity and relieved by exer-

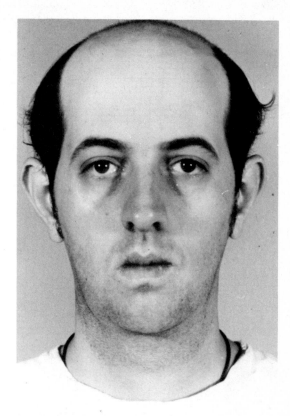

Figure 6–5. Photograph of a 37-year-old man with myotonic dystrophy, showing frontal baldness, bilateral ptosis, and wasting of the temporalis, facial, and sternocleidomastoid muscles. (Courtesy of R Griggs.)

cise. Muscle hypertrophy, sometimes pronounced, is also a feature. A recessive form with later onset is associated with slight weakness and atrophy of distal muscles.

Treatment with quinine sulfate, procainamide, tocainide, or phenytoin may help the myotonia.

INFLAMMATORY MYOPATHIES

Trichinosis, Toxoplasmosis, & Sarcoidosis

These disorders may lead to an inflammatory disorder of muscle, but this is uncommon.

Polymyositis & Dermatomyositis

Polymyositis and dermatomyositis are characterized by destruction of muscle fibers and inflammatory infiltration of muscles. Polymyositis can occur at any age; it progresses at a variable rate and leads to weakness and wasting, especially of the proximal limb and girdle muscles (Table 6–12). It is often associated with muscle pain, tenderness, dysphagia, and respiratory difficulties. Raynaud's phenomenon, arthralgia, malaise, weight loss, and a low-grade fever

Table 6–12. Symptoms and signs of polymyositis.[1]

	Percentage of Patients
Initial symptom	
Lower extremity weakness	42
Skin rash	25
Myalgia or arthralgia	15
Upper extremity weakness	8
Dysphagia	2
Other	2
Neurological signs	
Proximal upper extremity weakness	99
Proximal lower extremity weakness	80
Neck flexor weakness	65
Dysphagia	62
Muscle pain or tenderness	48
Distal limb weakness	35
Muscle atrophy	35
Contractures	35
Facial weakness	5
Extraocular muscle weakness	2
Nonneurological signs	
Heliotrope rash	40
Arthropathy	35
Raynaud's phenomenon	30
Other rash	20

[1]Adapted from Barwick DD, Walton JN: Polymyositis. *Am J Med* 1963;35:646.

round out the clinical picture. Dermatomyositis is the term used if an erythematous rash is present over the eyelids, about the eyes **(heliotrope rash),** or on the extensor surfaces of the joints.

Polymyositis has been reported in association with various autoimmune disorders, including scleroderma, lupus erythematosus, rheumatoid arthritis, and Sjögren's syndrome. In addition, there is a definite correlation between adult-onset dermatomyositis and cancer. The serum CPK is generally elevated in patients with polymyositis or dermatomyositis, sometimes to very high levels. At electromyography, an abundance of short, low-amplitude, polyphasic motor unit potentials is found, as in any myopathic process; but abnormal spontaneous activity is often conspicuous as well. Muscle biopsy usually shows muscle fiber necrosis and infiltration with inflammatory cells.

Treatment is with anti-inflammatory drugs. Prednisone is commonly used in an initial dose of 60 or 80 mg/d, along with potassium supplements and frequent antacids if necessary. As improvement occurs and serum CPK values decline, the dose is gradually tapered to maintenance levels that usually range between 10 and 20 mg/d. Patients may need to continue this regimen for two to three years, however; too rapid a reduction in dose may lead to relapse.

Cytotoxic drugs such as azathioprine have also been used, either alone or in combination with corticosteroids. Methotrexate may be useful in corticosteroid-resistant patients. Physical therapy may help to prevent contractures and, as the patient responds to anti-inflammatory drugs, active exercise may hasten recovery.

AIDS

Several forms of myopathy can occur in patients with otherwise asymptomatic HIV-1 infection or with AIDS (Table 6–13). These disorders can be distinguished by muscle biopsy. The most common is **polymyositis,** which may be caused by autoimmune mechanisms triggered by HIV-1 infection. It resembles polymyositis in patients without HIV-1 infection (see above), and may respond to treatment with corticosteroids. Patients with AIDS may also develop a myopathy associated with **type II muscle fiber atrophy.** Malnutrition, cachexia, immobility, or remote effects of AIDS-related tumors may have a pathogenetic role. Proximal muscle weakness is the major finding, and serum CPK is normal. **Rod-body myopathy** is a noninflammatory disorder characterized by rod-shaped bodies in type I muscle fibers. Clinical features include proximal muscle weakness and moderate elevation of CPK. Treatment with corticosteroids may be helpful. A **mitochondrial myopathy** (in which muscle biopsy specimens show the ragged red fibers indicative of damaged mitochondria) can occur in patients receiving zidovudine for treatment of AIDS and may coexist with polymyositis. The disorder is characterized clinically by proximal muscle weakness, myalgia, and moderate to marked elevation of serum CPK; it is thought to result from a toxic effect of zidovudine on muscle. Mild symptoms may be controlled with non-steroidal anti-inflammatory drugs or corticosteroids, and more severe involvement may respond to discontinuing zidovudine. If there is no response, a muscle biopsy should be performed to look for other causes of myopathy.

Polymyalgia Rheumatica

Polymyalgia rheumatica, which is more common in women than in men, generally occurs in patients over the age of 50 years and is best regarded as a variant of giant cell arteritis. It is characterized by muscle pain and stiffness, particularly about the neck and girdle muscles. Headache, anorexia, weight loss, and low-grade fever may be conjoined, and the erythrocyte sedimentation rate is increased. Serum enzymes, electromyography, and muscle biopsy are normal.

There is usually a dramatic response to treatment with corticosteroids in low dosage (eg, prednisone, 10–15 mg/d orally). Treatment is monitored by clinical parameters and sedimentation rate and may need

Table 6–13. AIDS-related myopathies.

Polymyositis
Type II muscle fiber atrophy
Rod-body myopathy
Zidovudine-induced mitochondrial myopathy

to be continued for one year or more if serious complications are to be avoided, as indicated in Chapter 3 in the discussion on giant cell arteritis.

Eosinophilia-Myalgia Syndrome

Eosinophilia-myalgia syndrome produces muscle pain and weakness associated with inflammation of skin and other soft tissues, but little direct involvement of muscle. Because the prominent symptoms are sensory, this disorder is discussed in Chapter 7.

METABOLIC MYOPATHIES

Proximal myopathic weakness may result from **chronic hypokalemia,** and once the metabolic disturbance has been corrected, power usually returns to normal within a few weeks. **Acute hypo- or hyperkalemia** may also lead to muscle weakness that is rapidly reversed by correcting the metabolic disturbance.

The **periodic paralysis syndromes,** which may be familial (dominant inheritance), are characterized by episodes of flaccid weakness or paralysis that may be associated with abnormalities of the plasma potassium level. Strength is normal between attacks. In the **hypokalemic** form, sometimes associated with **thyrotoxicosis,** attacks tend to occur on awakening, after exercise, or after a heavy meal—and may last for several days. Oral potassium supplements often prevent attacks, while ongoing attacks may be aborted by potassium chloride given orally or even intravenously. If hyperthyroidism is associated, its treatment may prevent recurrences. Attacks associated with **hyperkalemia** also tend to come on after exercise but are usually much briefer, lasting less than one hour. Severe attacks may be terminated by intravenous calcium gluconate, intravenous diuretics (furosemide, 20–40 mg), or glucose, while daily acetazolamide or chlorothiazide may help prevent further episodes. **Normokalemic** periodic paralysis is sometimes unresponsive to treatment; in severe attacks, it may be impossible to move the limbs, but respiration and swallowing are rarely affected.

Proximal muscle weakness may also occur in **osteomalacia,** often with associated bone pain and tenderness, mild hypocalcemia, and elevated serum alkaline phosphatase. Strength improves following treatment with vitamin D.

ENDOCRINE MYOPATHIES

Myopathy may occur in association with hyper- or hypothyroidism, hyper- or hypoparathyroidism, hyper- or hypoadrenalism, hypopituitarism, and acromegaly. Treatment is that of the underlying endocrine disorder.

ALCOHOLIC MYOPATHIES

Acute Necrotizing Myopathy

Heavy binge drinking may result in an acute necrotizing myopathy that develops over one or two days. Presenting symptoms include muscle pain, weakness, and sometimes dysphagia. On examination, the affected muscles are swollen, tender, and weak. Weakness is proximal in distribution and may be asymmetric or focal. Serum CPK is moderately to severely elevated, and myoglobinuria may occur. Since hypokalemia and hypophosphatemia can produce a similar syndrome in alcoholic patients, serum potassium and phosphorus concentrations should be determined. With abstinence from alcohol and a nutritionally adequate diet, recovery can be expected over a period of weeks to months.

Chronic Myopathy

Chronic myopathy characterized by proximal weakness of the lower limbs may develop insidiously over weeks to months in alcoholic patients. Muscle pain is not a prominent feature. Cessation of drinking and an improved diet are associated with clinical improvement over several months in most cases.

DRUG-INDUCED MYOPATHIES

Myopathy can occur in association with administration of corticosteroids, chloroquine, clofibrate, emetine, aminocaproic acid, certain β-blockers, bretylium tosylate, colchicine, zidovudine, or drugs that cause potassium depletion.

MYOGLOBINURIA

This can result from muscle injury or ischemia (irrespective of its cause) and leads to a urine that is dark red. The following causes are important:

–Excessive unaccustomed exercise, leading to muscle necrosis (rhabdomyolysis) and thus to myoglobinuria, sometimes on a familial basis.
–Crush injuries.
–Muscle infarction.
–Prolonged tonic-clonic convulsions.
–Polymyositis.
–Chronic potassium depletion.
–An acute alcoholic binge.
–Certain viral infections associated with muscle weakness and pain.
–Hyperthermia.

Serum CPK levels are elevated, often greatly. Myoglobin can be detected in the urine by the dipstick test for heme pigment; a positive test indicates the presence of myoglobin in the urine unless red blood cells are present. In severe cases, myoglobinuria may lead to renal failure, and peritoneal dialysis or hemodialysis may then be necessary. Otherwise, treatment consists of increasing the urine volume by hydration. The serum potassium level must be monitored, since it may rise rapidly.

MOTOR-UNIT HYPERACTIVITY STATES

Disorders affecting the central or peripheral nervous system at a variety of sites can produce abnormal, increased activity in the motor unit (Table 6–14).

CENTRAL DISORDERS

Stiff-Man Syndrome

This is a rare, usually sporadic, and slowly progressive disorder manifested by tightness, stiffness, and rigidity of axial and proximal limb muscles with superimposed painful spasms. Examination may show tight muscles, a slow or cautious gait, and hyperreflexia. Many patients also have diabetes. Stiff-man syndrome can be distinguished from tetanus by its more gradual onset and by the absence of trismus (lockjaw). In some cases, the blood contains autoantibodies against glutamic acid decarboxylase, which is involved in synthesis of the neurotransmitter γ-aminobutyric acid (GABA), and is concentrated in pancreatic β-cells and in GABAergic neurons of the central nervous system. A defect in central GABA-ergic transmission has been proposed as the cause of the disorder, and treatment is with drugs that enhance GABAergic transmission, such as diazepam, 5–75 mg orally four times daily. Physical therapy is also beneficial.

Tetanus

Tetanus, a disorder of central inhibitory neurotransmission caused by a toxin produced by *Clostridium tetani,* is discussed earlier in this chapter.

PERIPHERAL NERVE DISORDERS

Cramps

These involuntary and typically painful contractions of a muscle or portion of a muscle are thought to arise distally in the motor neuron. Palpable knotlike hardening of the muscle may occur. Cramps are characteristically relieved by passive stretching of the affected muscle. They usually represent a benign condition, and are common at night or during or after exercise. However, cramps may also be a manifestation of motor neuron disease or polyneuropathy, metabolic disturbances (pregnancy, uremia, hypothyroidism, adrenal insufficiency), or fluid or electrolyte disorders (dehydration, hemodialysis). If a reversible underlying cause cannot be found, daytime cramps may respond to treatment with phenytoin, 300–400 mg/d orally, or carbamazepine, 200–400 mg orally three times a day. Nocturnal cramps may respond to a single oral bedtime dose of quinine sulfate (325 mg), phenytoin (100–300 mg), carbamazepine (200–400 mg), or diazepam (5–10 mg).

Neuromyotonia

Neuromyotonia **(Isaacs' syndrome)** is a rare, sporadic disorder that produces continuous muscle stiffness, rippling muscle movements **(myokymia),** and delayed relaxation following muscle contraction. Symptoms may be controlled with phenytoin, 300–400 mg/d orally, or carbamazepine, 200–400 mg orally three times a day.

Table 6–14. Motor-unit hyperactivity states.

Site of Pathology	Syndrome	Clinical Features	Treatment
Central nervous system	Stiff-man syndrome	Rigidity, spasms	Diazepam
	Tetanus	Rigidity, spasms	Diazepam
Peripheral nerve	Cramps	Painful contraction of single muscle relieved by passive stretch	Quinine Phenytoin Carbamazepine
	Neuromyotonia	Stiffness, myokymia, delayed relaxation	Phenytoin Carbamazepine
	Tetany	Chvostek's sign Trousseau's sign Carpopedal spasm	Calcium Magnesium Correction of alkalosis
Muscle	Myotonia	Delayed relaxation, percussion myotonia	Phenytoin Carbamazepine Procainamide
	Malignant hyperthermia	Rigidity, fever	Dantrolene

Tetany

Tetany—not to be confused with tetanus (see above)—is a hyperexcitable state of peripheral nerves usually associated with hypocalcemia, hypomagnesemia, or alkalosis. Signs of tetany (Chvostek's sign, Trousseau's sign, carpopedal spasm) are described in the section on hypocalcemia in Chapter 1. Treatment is by correction of the underlying electrolyte disorder.

MUSCLE DISORDERS

Myotonia

Disorders that produce myotonia are discussed on p 175.

Malignant Hyperthermia

This disorder, which is often inherited in autosomal dominant fashion, is thought to result from abnormal excitation-contraction coupling in skeletal muscle. Symptoms are usually precipitated by admin- istration of neuromuscular blocking agents (eg, suc- cinylcholine) or inhalational anesthetics. Clinical features include rigidity, hyperthermia, metabolic acidosis, and myoglobinuria. Mortality rates as high as 70% have been reported. Treatment includes prompt cessation of anesthesia; administration of the excitation-contraction uncoupler dantrolene, 1–2 mg/kg intravenously every five to ten minutes as needed, to a maximum dose of 10 mg/kg; reduction of body temperature; and correction of acidosis with intravenous bicarbonate. Patients who require surgery and are known or suspected to have malignant hyperthermia should be pretreated with dantrolene (four 1-mg/kg oral doses) on the day prior to surgery. Preoperative administration of atropine (which can also cause hyperthermia) should be avoided, and the anesthetics used should be restricted to those known to be safe in this condition (nitrous oxide, opiates, barbiturates, droperidol).

REFERENCES

General

Aminoff MJ: *Electromyography in Clinical Practice,* 2nd ed. Churchill Livingstone, 1987.

Layzer RB: *Neuromuscular Manifestations of Systemic Disease.* Vol 25 of: *Contemporary Neurology Series.* Davis, 1984.

Sudarsky L: Geriatrics: Gait disorders in the elderly. *N Engl J Med* 1990;322:1441–1446.

Spinal Cord Disorders

Aminoff MJ: *Spinal Angiomas.* Blackwell, 1976.

Baker AS et al: Spinal epidural abscess. *N Engl J Med* 1975;293:463–468.

Bracken MB et al: A randomized, controlled trial of methylprednisolone or naloxone in the treatment of acute spinal-cord injury. *N Engl J Med* 1990;322:1405–1411.

Byrne TN, Waxman SG: *Spinal Cord Compression.* Vol 33 of: *Contemporary Neurology Series.* Davis, 1990.

Erickson RP, Lie MR, Wineinger MA: Rehabilitation in multiple sclerosis. *Mayo Clin Proc* 1989;64:818–828.

McFarlin DE, McFarland HF: Multiple sclerosis. (2 parts.) *N Engl J Med* 1982;307:1183–1188, 1246–1251.

Petito CK et al: Vacuolar myelopathy pathologically resembling subacute combined degeneration in patients with the acquired immunodeficiency syndrome. *N Engl J Med* 1985;312:874–879.

Rodichok LD et al: Early diagnosis of spinal epidural metastases. *Am J Med* 1981;70:1181–1188.

Rodriguez M.: Multiple sclerosis: Basic concepts and hypothesis. *Mayo Clin Proc* 1989;64:570–576.

Sandson TA, Friedman JH: Spinal cord infarction: Report of 8 cases and review of the literature. *Medicine* 1989;68:282–292.

Swanson JW: Multiple sclerosis: Update in diagnosis and review of prognostic factors. *Mayo Clin Proc* 1989;64:577–586.

Wynn DR et al: Update on the epidemiology of multiple sclerosis. *Mayo Clin Proc* 1989;64:808–817.

Anterior Horn Cell Disease

Siddique T et al: Linkage of a gene causing familial amyotrophic lateral sclerosis to chromosome 21 and evidence of genetic-locus heterogeneity. *N Engl J Med* 1991;324:1381–1384.

Tandan R, Bradley WG: Amyotrophic lateral sclerosis. (2 parts.) *Ann Neurol* 1985;18: 271–280, 419–431.

Williams DB, Windebank AJ: Motor neuron disease (amyotrophic lateral sclerosis). *Mayo Clin Proc* 1991; 66:54–82.

Nerve Root Lesions

Tsairis P, Dyck PJ, Mulder DW: Natural history of brachial plexus neuropathy: Report on 99 patients. *Arch Neurol* 1972;27:109–117.

Disorders of Peripheral Nerves

Schaumburg HH, Berger AK, Thomas PK: *Disorders of Peripheral Nerves,* 2nd ed. Vol 36 of: *Contemporary Neurology Series.* Davis, 1992.

Disorders of Neuromuscular Transmission

Engel AG: Myasthenia gravis and myasthenic syndromes. *Ann Neurol* 1984;16:519–534.

Finley JC, Pascuzzi RM: Rational therapy of myasthenia gravis. *Semin Neurol* 1990;10:70–82.

Howard JF Jr: Adverse drug effects on neuromuscular transmission. *Semin Neurol* 1990;10:89–102.

Hughes JM et al: Clinical features of types A and B food-borne botulism. *Ann Intern Med* 1981;95:442–445.

McEvoy KM et al: 3,4-Diaminopyridine in the treatment

of Lambert-Eaton myasthenic syndrome. *N Engl J Med* 1989;321:1567–1571.

Vincent A, Lang B, Newsom-Davis J.: Autoimmunity to the voltage-gated calcium channel underlies the Lambert-Eaton syndrome, a paraneoplastic disorder. *Trends in Neurosci* 1989;12:496–502.

Myopathic Disorders

Bunch TW: Polymyositis: A case history approach to the differential diagnosis and treatment. *Mayo Clin Proc* 1990;65:1480–1497.

Charness ME, Simon RP, Greenberg DA: Ethanol and the nervous system. *N Engl J Med* 1989;321:442–454.

Chuang TY et al: Polymyalgia rheumatica: A 10-year epidemiologic and clinical study. *Ann Intern Med* 1982; 97:672–680.

Dalakas MC: Polymyositis, dermatomyositis, and inclusion-body myositis. *N Engl J Med* 1991;325:1487–1498.

Dalakas MC et al: Mitochondrial myopathy caused by long-term zidovudine therapy. *N Engl J Med* 1990; 322:1098–1105.

Gutmann DH, Fischbeck KH: Molecular biology of Duchenne and Becker's muscular dystrophy: Clinical applications. *Ann Neurol* 1989;26:189–194.

Mastaglia FL, Ojeda VJ: Inflammatory myopathies. (2 parts.) *Ann Neurol* 1985;17:215–227, 317–323.

Mendell JR et al: Randomized, double-blind six-month trial of prednisone in Duchenne's muscular dystrophy. *N Engl J Med* 1989;320:1592–1597.

Simpson DM, Bender AN: Human immunodeficiency virus-associated myopathy: Analysis of 11 patients. *Ann Neurol* 1988;24:79–84.

Urbano-Marquez A et al: The effects of alcoholism on skeletal and cardiac muscle. *N Engl J Med* 1989; 320:409–415.

Motor-Unit Hyperactivity States

Lorish TR, Thorsteinsson G, Howard FM Jr: Stiff-man syndrome updated. *Mayo Clin Proc* 1989;64:629–636.

Solimena M et al: Autoantibodies to GABA–ergic neurons and pancreatic beta cells in stiff-man syndrome. *N Engl J Med* 1990;322:1555–1560.

Disorders of Somatic Sensation

APPROACH TO DIAGNOSIS

An appreciation of the functional anatomy of the sensory components of the nervous system is essential for properly interpreting the history and clinical signs of patients with disorders of **somatic sensation.** As used here, the term includes sensations of touch or pressure, vibration, joint position, pain, temperature, and more complex functions that rely on these primary sensory modalities (eg, two-point discrimination, stereognosis, graphesthesia); it excludes special senses such as smell, vision, taste, and hearing.

FUNCTIONAL ANATOMY OF THE SOMATIC SENSORY PATHWAYS

The sensory pathway between the skin and deeper structures and the cerebral cortex involves three neurons, with two synapses occurring centrally. The cell body of the first sensory neuron of the spinal nerve is in the dorsal root ganglion (Figure 7–1). Each cell located there sends a peripheral process that terminates in a free nerve ending or encapsulated sensory receptor and a central process that enters the spinal cord. Sensory receptors are relatively specialized for particular sensations and, in addition to free nerve endings (pain), include Meissner's corpuscles, Merkel's corpuscles, and hair cells (touch); Krause's end-bulbs (cold); and Ruffini's corpuscles (heat). The location of the first central synapse depends upon the type of sensation but is either in the posterior gray column of the spinal cord or in the upward extension of this column in the lower brain stem. The second synapse is located in the anterior part of the anterolateral nucleus of the thalamus, from which there is sensory radiation to the cerebral cortex. In the spinal cord, fibers mediating touch, pressure, and postural sensation ascend in the posterior white columns to the medulla, where they synapse in the gracile and cuneate

nuclei (Figure 7–1). From these nuclei, fibers cross the midline and ascend in the medial lemniscus to the thalamus. Other fibers that mediate touch and those subserving pain and temperature appreciation synapse on neurons in the posterior horns of the spinal

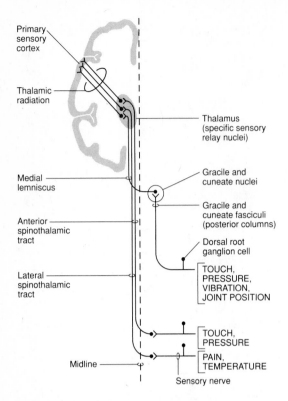

Figure 7–1. Sensory pathways conveying touch, pressure, vibration, joint position, pain, and temperature sensation.

cord, particularly in the substantia gelatinosa. The fibers from these neurons then cross the midline and ascend in the anterolateral part of the cord; fibers mediating touch pass upward in the anterior spinothalamic tract, whereas pain and temperature fibers generally travel in the lateral spinothalamic tract (Figure 7–1). Fibers from this anterolateral system pass to the thalamic relay nuclei and to nonspecific thalamic projection nuclei and the mesencephalic reticular formation. Fibers from the lemniscal and anterolateral systems are joined in the brain stem by fibers subserving sensation from the head. Cephalic pain and temperature sensation are dependent upon the spinal nucleus of the trigeminal (V) nerve; touch, pressure, and postural sensation are conveyed mostly by the main sensory and mesencephalic nuclei of this nerve.

HISTORY

Sensory disturbances may consist of loss of sensation, the occurrence of abnormal sensations, or pain.

The term **paresthesia** is used to denote abnormal spontaneous sensations, such as burning, tingling, or pins and needles. The term **dysesthesia** denotes any unpleasant sensation produced by a stimulus that is usually painless. The term **numbness** is often used by patients to describe a sense of heaviness, weakness, or deadness in the affected part of the body—and sometimes to signify any sensory impairment; its meaning must be clarified whenever the word is used.

In obtaining a history of sensory complaints, it is important to determine the location of the symptoms; the mode of onset and progression of the symptoms; whether the symptoms are constant or episodic in nature; whether any factors specifically produce, enhance, or relieve symptoms; and whether there are any accompanying symptoms.

The **location** of symptoms may provide a clue to their origin. For example, sensory disturbances involving all the limbs suggest peripheral neuropathy, a cervical cord or brain stem lesion, or a metabolic disturbance such as hyperventilation syndrome. Involvement of one entire limb—or of one side of the body—suggests a central (brain or spinal cord) lesion. A hemispheric or brain stem lesion may lead to lateralized sensory symptoms, but the face is also commonly affected. In addition, there may be other symptoms and signs, such as aphasia, apraxia, and visual field defects with hemispheric disease, or dysarthria, weakness, vertigo, diplopia, disequilibrium, and ataxia with brain stem disorders. Involvement of part of a limb or a discrete region of the trunk raises the possibility of a nerve or root lesion, depending upon the precise distribution. With a root lesion, symptoms may show some relationship to neck or back movements, and pain is often conspicuous.

The **course** of sensory complaints provides a guide to their cause. Intermittent or repetitive transient symptoms may represent sensory seizures, ischemic phenomena, or metabolic disturbances such as those accompanying hyperventilation. Intermittent localized symptoms that occur at a consistent time may suggest the diagnosis or an exogenous precipitating factor. For example, the pain and paresthesias of carpal tunnel syndrome (of median nerve compression), characteristically occur at night and awaken the patient from sleep.

SENSORY EXAMINATION

In the investigation of sensory complaints, various modalities are tested in turn, and the distribution of any abnormality is plotted with particular reference to the normal root and peripheral nerve territories. Complete loss of touch appreciation is **anesthesia,** partial loss is **hypesthesia,** and increased sensitivity is **hyperesthesia.** The corresponding terms for pain appreciation are **analgesia, hypalgesia,** and **hyperalgesia** or **hyperpathia.**

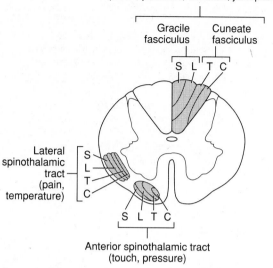

Posterior column
(touch, pressure, vibration, joint position)

Gracile fasciculus | Cuneate fasciculus

Lateral spinothalamic tract (pain, temperature)

Anterior spinothalamic tract
(touch, pressure)

Figure 7–2. Location and lamination of sensory pathways in the spinal cord. C (cervical), T (thoracic), L (lumbar), and S (sacral) indicate the level of origin of fibers within each tract.

1. PRIMARY SENSORY MODALITIES

Light Touch

The appreciation of light touch is evaluated with a wisp of cotton wool, which is brought down carefully on a small region of skin. The patient lies quietly, with the eyes closed, and makes a signal each time the stimulus is felt. The appreciation of light touch depends on fibers that traverse the posterior column of the spinal cord in the gracile (leg) and cuneate (arm) fasciculi ipsilaterally (Figures 7–1 and 7–2), passing to the medial lemniscus of the brain stem (Figure 7–3), and on fibers in the contralateral anterior spinothalamic tract.

Pinprick & Temperature

Pinprick appreciation is tested by asking the patient to indicate whether the point of a pin (not a hypodermic needle, which is likely to puncture the skin and draw blood) feels sharp or blunt. Appreciation of pressure or touch by the pinpoint must not be confused with the appreciation of sharpness. Temperature appreciation is evaluated by application to the skin of containers of hot or cold water. Pinprick and temperature appreciation depend upon the integrity of the lateral spinothalamic tracts (Figures 7–1 and 7–2). The afferent fibers cross in front of the central canal after ascending for two or three segments from their level of entry into the cord.

Deep Pressure

Deep pressure sensibility is evaluated by pressure on the tendons, such as the Achilles tendon at the ankle.

Vibration

Vibration appreciation is evaluated with a tuning fork (128 Hz) that is set in motion and then placed over a bony prominence; the patient is asked to indicate whether vibration, rather than simple pressure, is felt. Many elderly patients have impaired appreciation of vibration below the knees.

Joint Position

Joint position sense is tested by asking the patient to indicate the direction of small passive movements of the terminal interphalangeal joints of the fingers and toes. Patients with severe impairment of joint position sense may exhibit slow, continuous movement of the fingers (**pseudoathetoid movement**) when attempting to hold the hands outstretched with the eyes closed. For clinical purposes, both joint position sense and the ability to appreciate vibration are considered to depend on fibers carried in the posterior columns of the cord, although there is evidence that this is not true for vibration.

2. COMPLEX SENSORY FUNCTIONS

Romberg's Test

The patient is asked to assume a steady stance with feet together, arms outstretched, and eyes closed and is observed for any tendency to sway or fall. The test is positive (abnormal) if unsteadiness is markedly increased by eye closure—as occurs, for example, in tabes dorsalis. A positive test is indicative of grossly impaired joint position sense in the legs.

A. MIDBRAIN

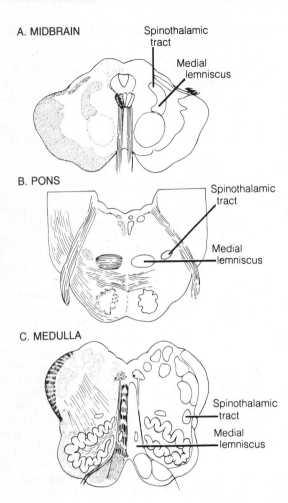

B. PONS

C. MEDULLA

Figure 7–3. Sensory pathways in the brain stem. In the medulla, spinothalamic fibers conveying pain and temperature sensation are widely separated from medial lemniscal fibers mediating touch and pressure; these pathways converge as they ascend in the pons and midbrain.

Two-Point Discrimination

The ability to distinguish simultaneous touch at two neighboring points depends upon the integrity of the central and peripheral nervous system, the degree of separation of the two points, and the part of the body that is stimulated. The patient is required to indicate whether he or she is touched by one or two compass points, while the distance between the points is varied in order to determine the shortest distance at which they are recognized as different points. The threshold for two-point discrimination approximates 4 mm at the fingertips and may be several centimeters on the back. When peripheral sensory function is intact, impaired two-point discrimination suggests a disorder affecting the sensory cortex.

Graphesthesia, Stereognosis, & Barognosis

Agraphesthesia, the inability to identify a number traced on the skin of the palm of the hand despite normal cutaneous sensation, implies a lesion involving the contralateral parietal lobe. The same is true of inability to distinguish between various shapes or textures by touch (**astereognosis**) or impaired ability to distinguish between different weights (**abarognosis**).

Bilateral Sensory Discrimination

In some patients with apparently normal sensation, simultaneous stimulation of the two sides of the body reveals an apparent neglect of (or inattention to) sensation from one side, usually because of some underlying contralateral cerebral lesion.

SENSORY CHANGES & THEIR SIGNIFICANCE

It is important to determine the nature and distribution of any sensory change. Failure to find clinical evidence of sensory loss in patients with sensory symptoms must *never* be taken to imply that the symptoms have a psychogenic basis. Sensory symptoms often develop well before the onset of sensory signs.

Peripheral Nerve Lesions

A. Mononeuropathy: In patients with a lesion of a single peripheral nerve, sensory loss is usually less than would have been predicted on anatomical grounds because of overlap from adjacent nerves. Moreover, depending upon the type of lesion, the fibers in a sensory nerve may be affected differently. Compressive lesions, for example, tend to affect preferentially the large fibers that subserve touch.

B. Polyneuropathy: In patients with polyneuropathies, sensory loss is generally symmetrical and is greater distally than proximally—as suggested by the term **glove-and-stocking sensory loss.** This term is misleading, however, because sensory loss generally commences in the legs and is greater there than in the arms—in fact, there may be little or no sensory disturbance in the upper limbs, depending upon the stage of the disorder at the time the patient is examined. Certain metabolic disorders (such as **Tangier disease,** a recessive trait characterized by the near absence of high-density lipoproteins) preferentially involve small nerve fibers that subserve pain and temperature appreciation. Sensory loss may be accompanied by a motor deficit and reflex changes.

Root Involvement

Nerve root involvement produces impairment of cutaneous sensation in a segmental pattern (Figures 7–4A and 7–4B), but because of overlap there is generally no loss of sensation unless two or more adjacent roots are affected. Pain is often a conspicuous feature in patients with compressive root lesions. Depending on the level affected, there may be loss of tendon reflexes (C5–6, biceps and brachioradialis; C7–8, triceps; L3–4, knee; S1, ankle), and if the anterior roots are also involved there may be weakness and muscle atrophy.

Cord Lesion

In patients with a cord lesion, there may be a transverse sensory level. Physiological areas of increased sensitivity do occur, however, at the costal margin, over the breasts, and in the groin, and these must not be taken as abnormal. Therefore, the level of a sensory deficit affecting the trunk is best determined by careful sensory testing over the back rather than the chest and abdomen.

A. Central Cord Lesion: With a central cord lesion—such as occurs in syringomyelia, following trauma, and with certain cord tumors—there is characteristically a loss of pain and temperature appreciation with sparing of other modalities. This loss is due to the interruption of fibers conveying pain and temperature that cross from one side of the cord to the spinothalamic tract on the other. Such a loss is usually bilateral, may be asymmetrical, and involves only the fibers of the involved segments. It may be accompanied by lower motor neuron weakness in the muscles supplied by the affected segments and sometimes by a pyramidal and posterior column deficit below the lesion (Figure 7–5).

B. Anterolateral Cord Lesion: Lesions involving the anterolateral portion of the spinal cord (lateral spinothalamic tract) can cause contralateral impairment of pain and temperature appreciation in segments below the level of the lesion. The spinothalamic tract is laminated, with fibers from the sacral segments the outermost; this has important clinical implications. Intrinsic cord (intramedullary) lesions often spare the sacral fibers, while extramedullary lesions, which compress the cord, tend to involve these fibers as well as those arising from more rostral levels.

C. Anterior Cord Lesion: With destructive lesions involving predominantly the anterior portion of the spinal cord, pain and temperature appreciation are impaired below the level of the lesion from lateral spinothalamic tract involvement. In addition, weakness or paralysis of muscles supplied by the involved segments of the cord results from damage to motor neurons in the anterior horn. With more extensive disease, involvement of the corticospinal tracts in the lateral funiculi may cause a pyramidal deficit below the lesion. There is relative preservation of posterior column function (Figure 7–6). Ischemic myelopathies caused by occlusion of the anterior spinal artery take the form of anterior cord lesions.

D. Posterior Column Lesion: A patient with a posterior column lesion may complain of a tight or bandlike sensation in the regions corresponding to

the level of spinal involvement and sometimes also of paresthesias (like electric shocks) radiating down the extremities on neck flexion (**Lhermitte's sign**). There is loss of vibration and joint position sense below the level of the lesion, with preservation of other sensory modalities. The deficit may resemble that resulting from involvement of large fibers in the posterior roots.

E. Cord Hemisection: Hemisection of the cord leads to **Brown-Séquard's syndrome.** Below the lesion, there is an ipsilateral pyramidal deficit and disturbed appreciation of vibration and joint position sense, with contralateral loss of pain and temperature appreciation that begins two or three segments below the lesion (Figure 7–7).

Brain Stem Lesion

Sensory disturbances may be accompanied by a motor deficit, cerebellar signs, and cranial nerve palsies when the lesion is in the brain stem.

In patients with lesions involving the spinothalamic tract in the dorsolateral medulla and pons, pain and temperature appreciation are lost in the limbs and trunk on the opposite side of the body. When such a lesion is located in the medulla, it also typically involves the spinal trigeminal nucleus, impairing pain and temperature sensation on the same side of the face as the lesion. The result is a crossed sensory deficit that affects the ipsilateral face and contralateral limbs. In contrast, spinothalamic lesions above the spinal trigeminal nucleus affect the face, limbs, and trunk contralateral to the lesion. With lesions affecting the medial lemniscus, there is loss of touch and proprioception on the opposite side of the body. In the upper brain stem, the spinothalamic tract and medial lemniscus run together so that a single lesion may cause loss of all superficial and deep sensation over the contralateral side of the body (Figure 7–3).

Thalamic Lesions

Thalamic lesions may lead to loss or impairment of all forms of sensation on the contralateral side of the body. Spontaneous pain, sometimes with a particularly unpleasant quality, may occur on the affected side. Patients may describe it as burning, tearing, knifelike, or stabbing, but often have difficulty characterizing it. Any form of cutaneous stimulation can lead to painful or unpleasant sensations. Such a thalamic syndrome (**Dejerine-Roussy syndrome**) can also occasionally result from lesions of the white matter of the parietal lobe or from cord lesions.

Lesions of the Sensory Cortex

Disease limited to the sensory cortex impairs discriminative sensory function on the opposite side of the body. Thus, patients may be unable to localize stimuli on the affected side or to recognize the position of different parts of the body. They may not be

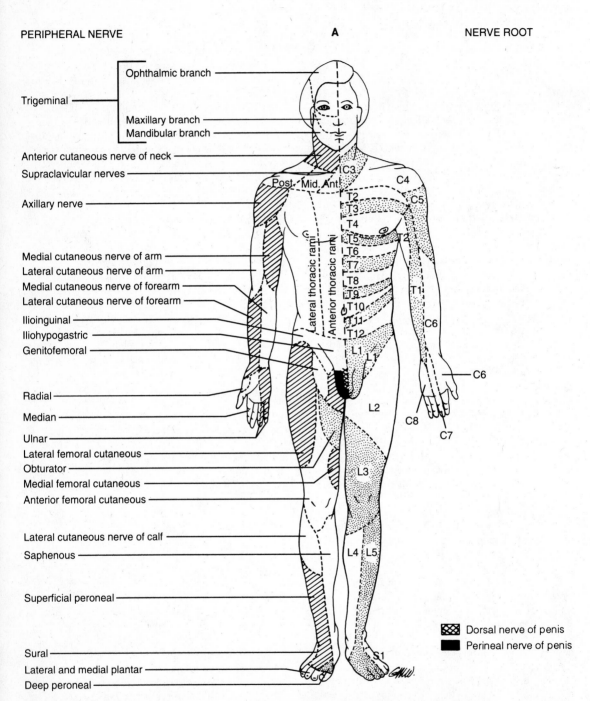

PERIPHERAL NERVE **A** NERVE ROOT

Trigeminal
- Ophthalmic branch
- Maxillary branch
- Mandibular branch

Anterior cutaneous nerve of neck
Supraclavicular nerves

Axillary nerve

Medial cutaneous nerve of arm
Lateral cutaneous nerve of arm
Medial cutaneous nerve of forearm
Lateral cutaneous nerve of forearm
Ilioinguinal
Iliohypogastric
Genitofemoral

Radial

Median

Ulnar
Lateral femoral cutaneous
Obturator
Medial femoral cutaneous
Anterior femoral cutaneous

Lateral cutaneous nerve of calf

Saphenous

Superficial peroneal

Sural
Lateral and medial plantar
Deep peroneal

Post. Mid. Ant

C3
C4
C5
T2
T3
T4
T5
T6
T7
T8
T9
T10
T11
T12
L1
L1
L2
L3
L4 L5

T2
T1
C6
C6
C8
C7
S1

Lateral thoracic rami
Anterior thoracic rami

▨ Dorsal nerve of penis
■ Perineal nerve of penis

Figure 7–4 A. Cutaneous innervation (anterior view). The segmental or radicular (nerve root) distribution is shown on the left side of the body, and the peripheral nerve distribution on the right side of the body. (continued)

NERVE ROOT **B** PERIPHERAL NERVE

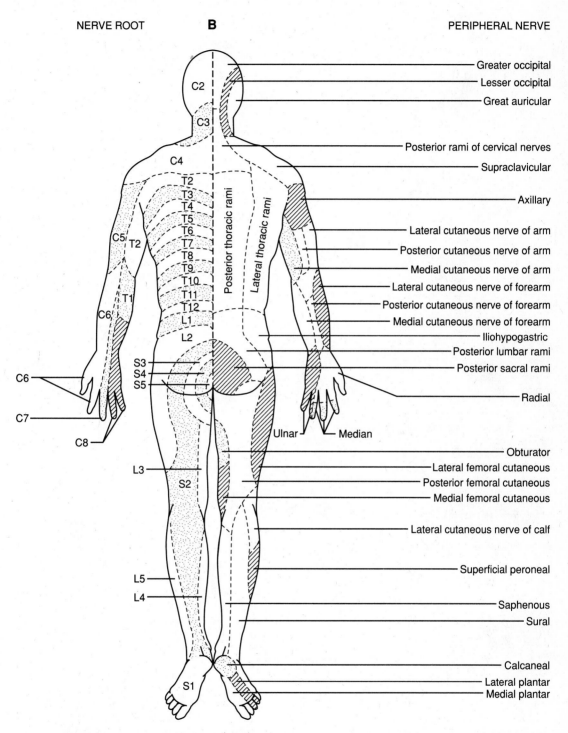

Greater occipital
Lesser occipital
Great auricular
Posterior rami of cervical nerves
Supraclavicular
Axillary
Lateral cutaneous nerve of arm
Posterior cutaneous nerve of arm
Medial cutaneous nerve of arm
Lateral cutaneous nerve of forearm
Posterior cutaneous nerve of forearm
Medial cutaneous nerve of forearm
Iliohypogastric
Posterior lumbar rami
Posterior sacral rami
Radial
Obturator
Lateral femoral cutaneous
Posterior femoral cutaneous
Medial femoral cutaneous
Lateral cutaneous nerve of calf
Superficial peroneal
Saphenous
Sural
Calcaneal
Lateral plantar
Medial plantar

Ulnar Median

C2, C3, C4, C5, T2, C6, T1, C6, C7, C8, L3, L5, L4

T2, T3, T4, T5, T6, T7, T8, T9, T10, T11, T12, L1, L2, S3, S4, S5, S2, S1

Posterior thoracic rami
Lateral thoracic rami

Figure 7–4B. Cutaneous innervation (posterior view). The segmental or radicular (nerve root) distribution is shown on the left side of the body, and the peripheral nerve distribution on the right side of the body.)

A

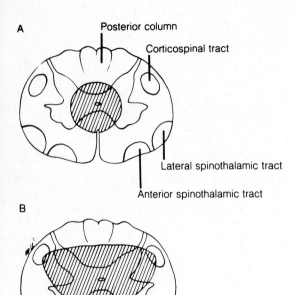

Posterior column

Corticospinal tract

Lateral spinothalamic tract

Anterior spinothalamic tract

B

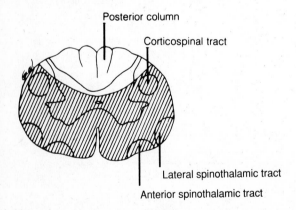

Posterior column

Corticospinal tract

Lateral spinothalamic tract

Anterior spinothalamic tract

Figure 7–5. Central cord lesions (hatched area) of moderate *(A)* or marked *(B)* extent. Less extensive lesions impair pain and temperature appreciation by interrupting incoming sensory fibers as they cross to the contralateral spinothalamic tract; involvement of anterior horn cells causes lower motor neuron weakness. These deficits are restricted to dermatomes and muscles innervated by the involved spinal cord segments. More extensive lesions also produce disturbances of touch, pressure, vibration, and joint position sense because of involvement of the posterior columns and cause pyramidal signs because of corticospinal tract involvement. These deficits occur below the level of the lesion.

Posterior column

Corticospinal tract

Lateral spinothalamic tract

Anterior spinothalamic tract

Figure 7–6. Anterior cord lesion (hatched area) associated with occlusion of the anterior spinal artery. Clinical features are similar to those seen with severe central cord lesions (Figure 7–5B), except that posterior column sensory functions are spared and the defect in pain and temperature sensation extends to sacral levels.

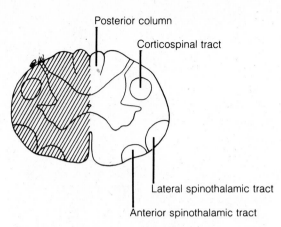

Posterior column

Corticospinal tract

Lateral spinothalamic tract

Anterior spinothalamic tract

Figure 7–7. Cord lesion (hatched area) in Brown-Séquard syndrome. Hemisection of the cord causes ipsilateral pyramidal dysfunction and impairment of posterior column sensory function below the level of the lesion, and contralateral impairment of pain and temperature sensation with an upper limit slightly below the level of the lesion.

able to recognize objects by touch or to estimate their size, weight, consistency, or texture. Cortical sensory disturbances are usually more conspicuous in the hands than in the trunk or proximal portions of the limbs.

DISTINCTION OF ORGANIC & PSYCHOGENIC SENSORY DISTURBANCES

Psychogenic disturbances of sensation may be associated with such psychiatric disturbances as conversion disorder. They may take any form but most often are restricted to loss of cutaneous sensation. There may be several characteristic features.

Nonorganic sensory loss does not conform in its distribution to any specific neuroanatomical pattern. It may surround a bony landmark or involve an area defined by surface landmarks rather than innervation. Indeed, it is not uncommon for there to be an apparent loss of sensation in one or more extremities, with the margin occurring circumferentially in the axilla or groin; organic sensory loss with such a margin is unusual. Organic peripheral sensory loss over the trunk or face does not usually extend to the midline but stops 3–5 cm before it, because of overlap in the innervation on the two sides; with nonorganic disturbances, apparent sensory loss commonly stops precisely at the midline.

There is often a sudden transition between areas of nonorganic sensory loss and areas with normal sensation. By contrast, with organic disturbances, there is usually an area of altered sensation between insensitive areas and adjacent areas with normal sensibility.

In nonorganic disturbances, there may be a dissociated loss that is difficult to interpret on an anatomical basis. For example, there may be a total loss of pinprick appreciation but preserved temperature sensation. Moreover, despite the apparent loss of posterior column function, the patient may be able to walk normally or maintain the arms outstretched without difficulty or pseudoathetoid movements.

In nonorganic sensory disturbances, appreciation of vibration may be impaired on one side but not the other side of a bony midline structure, such as the skull or sternum. The vibrations are in fact conducted to both sides by the bone, so that even if there is a hemisensory disturbance, the vibrations are appreciated on either side in patients with organic sensory disorders.

Finally, it should be noted that sensory disturbances are often suggested to the patient by the examiner's own expectations. Such findings can be particularly misleading because they may be neuroanatomically correct. One helpful approach is to have the patient outline on the body the extent of any perceived sensory disturbance before formal sensory testing is undertaken.

PERIPHERAL NERVE LESIONS

Sensory symptoms are usually a conspicuous feature in patients with peripheral nerve lesions (Table 7–1). Sensory impairment may be in a distal glove-and-stocking pattern in patients with polyneuropathies or may follow the pattern of individual peripheral nerves in patients with mononeuropathies.

Classification

A. Mononeuropathy Simplex: This term signifies involvement of a single peripheral nerve.

B. Mononeuropathy Multiplex: In this disorder, several individual nerves are affected, usually at random and noncontiguously. Clinical examination reveals a clinical deficit attributable to involvement of one or more isolated peripheral nerves, except when mononeuropathy multiplex is extensive and the resulting deficits become confluent.

C. Polyneuropathy: This term denotes a disorder in which the function of numerous peripheral nerves is affected at the same time. This leads to a predominantly distal and symmetrical deficit with loss of tendon reflexes. Polyneuropathies are sometimes subclassified according to the primary site at which the nerve is affected. In **distal axonopathies,** the axon is the principal pathological target; most

Table 7–1. Causes of peripheral neuropathy.

Idiopathic inflammatory neuropathies
Acute idiopathic polyneuropathy (Guillain-Barré syndrome)
Chronic inflammatory demyelinating polyneuropathy
Metabolic and nutritional neuropathies
Diabetes
Other endocrinopathies
Hypothyroidism
Acromegaly
Uremia
Liver disease
Vitamin B_{12} deficiency
Infective and granulomatous neuropathies
AIDS
Leprosy
Diphtherihia
Sarcoidosis
Vasculitic neuropathies
Polyarteritis nodosa
Rheumatoid arthritis
Systemic lupus erythematosus
Neoplastic and paraproteinemic neuropathies
Compression and infiltration by tumor
Paraneoplastic syndromes
Paraproteinemias
Amyloidosis
Drug-induced and toxic neuropathies
Alcohol
Other drugs
Dapsone
Hydralazine
Isoniazid
Phenytoin
Pyridoxine
Vincristine
Toxins
Organic compounds
Hexacarbons
Organophosphates
Heavy metals
Arsenic
Lead
Thallium
Gold
Platinum
Tryptophan (contaminant)
Hereditary neuropathies
Idiopathic
Hereditary motor and sensory neuropathies
Hereditary sensory neuropathies
Friedreich's ataxia
Familial amyloidosis
Metabolic
Porphyria
Metachromatic leukodystrophy
Krabbe's disease
Abetalipoproteinemia
Tangier's disease
Refsum's disease
Fabry's disease
Entrapment neuropathies

polyneuropathies fall into this category. **Myelinopathies** are conditions that involve the myelin sheath surrounding the axon. These disorders include acute idiopathic polyneuropathy (Guillain-Barré syndrome), chronic inflammatory demyelinating neuropathy, diphtheria, certain paraneoplastic and paraproteinemic states, and some hereditary metabolic conditions (metachromatic leukodystrophy, type III hereditary motor and sensory neuropathy, Krabbe's disease). Finally, certain disorders—termed **neuronopathies**—principally affect nerve cell bodies in the anterior horn of the spinal cord or dorsal root ganglion. Examples are type II hereditary motor and sensory neuropathy, pyridoxine-induced neuropathy, and some paraneoplastic syndromes.

Clinical Findings

A. Sensory Disturbances: Involvement of sensory fibers can lead to numbness and impaired sensation. It can also lead to abnormal spontaneous sensations, such as pain and paresthesias, and to perverted sensations such as hyperpathia.

1. Pain is a conspicuous feature of certain neuropathies, especially if small fibers within the nerves are affected. The precise mechanism of its genesis is unclear. Polyneuropathies associated with prominent pain include those related to diabetes, alcoholism, porphyria, Fabry's disease, amyloidosis, rheumatoid arthritis, and AIDS, as well as dominantly inherited sensory neuropathy and paraneoplastic sensory neuronopathy. Pain is also a feature of many entrapment neuropathies and of idiopathic brachial plexopathy.

2. Dissociated sensory loss is impairment of some sensory modalities, such as pain and temperature, with preservation of others, such as light touch, vibration, and joint position sense. Although the presence of a dissociated sensory loss often indicates a spinal cord lesion, it also occurs in peripheral neuropathies when there is selective involvement of peripheral nerve fibers of a certain size, such as occurs in amyloid neuropathy, leprous neuritis, or hereditary sensory neuropathy. In such cases, preferential involvement of small fibers is commonly associated with disproportionate impairment of pain and temperature appreciation, spontaneous pain, and autonomic dysfunction. Large-fiber disease, on the other hand, results in defective touch, vibration, and joint position sense, early loss of tendon reflexes, and prominent motor symptoms.

B. Motor Deficits: The motor deficit that occurs with a peripheral nerve lesion consists of weakness of muscles innervated by the nerve, accompanied in severe cases by wasting and fasciculation. There may be difficulty in the performance of fine tasks; this is compounded by any accompanying sensory loss. The clinical findings reflect a lower motor neuron deficit, and it is the distribution of these signs and the presence of accompanying sensory and reflex changes that suggest they may be due to peripheral nerve involvement.

C. Tendon Reflexes: These are impaired or lost if reflex arcs are interrupted on either the afferent or efferent side (C5–6, biceps and brachioradialis; C7–8, triceps; L3–4, knee; S1, ankle). The ankle jerks are usually the first to be lost in patients with polyneuropathies.

D. Autonomic Disturbances: Autonomic disturbances may be particularly conspicuous in some

peripheral neuropathies—especially Guillain-Barré syndrome and neuropathies related to diabetes, renal failure, porphyria, or amyloidosis. Symptoms include postural hypotension, coldness of the extremities, impaired thermoregulatory sweating, disturbances of bladder and bowel function, and impotence.

E. Enlarged Nerves: Palpably enlarged peripheral nerves raise the possibility of leprosy, amyloidosis, hereditary motor and sensory neuropathies, Refsum's disease, acromegaly, or chronic inflammatory demyelinating polyneuropathy.

Evaluation of Patients

A. Time Course: Polyneuropathy that develops acutely over a few days usually relates to an inflammatory process, as in the Guillain-Barré syndrome. It may also relate to an underlying neoplasm, to infections such as diphtheria, to metabolic disorders such as acute intermittent porphyria, or to exposure to such toxic substances as thallium or triorthocresyl phosphate. A chronic course with a gradual evolution over several years is typical of many hereditary or metabolic polyneuropathies but also characterizes chronic inflammatory demyelinating polyneuropathy.

Mononeuropathy of acute onset is likely to be traumatic or ischemic in origin, while one evolving gradually is more likely to relate to entrapment (ie, compression by neighboring anatomical structures) or to recurrent minor trauma.

B. Age at Onset: Polyneuropathies that develop during childhood or early adult life often have a hereditary basis, but they may also relate to an underlying inflammatory disorder. Those developing in later life are more likely to be due to a metabolic, toxic, or inflammatory disorder or to an underlying neoplasm.

Mononeuropathy presenting in the neonatal period is likely to be developmental in origin or related to birth injury; one developing in later life may relate to entrapment or injury that is often occupationally determined.

C. Occupational History: Various industrial substances can lead to peripheral neuropathy, including carbon disulfide, *n*-hexane, ethylene oxide, methyl bromide, acrylamide, triorthocresyl phosphate and certain other organophosphates, DDT, arsenic, lead, and thallium. A mononeuropathy is sometimes the first clinical manifestation of an occupationally related polyneuropathy, but it may also develop in response to entrapment or recurrent minor occupational trauma. For example, carpal tunnel syndrome is more common in persons who do heavy manual labor, and a lesion of the deep palmar branch of the ulnar nerve may relate to repeated pressure on the palm of the hand by, for example, punching down heavily on a stapler or using heavy equipment such as a pneumatic road drill.

D. Medical History:

1. Peripheral neuropathy may relate to **metabolic disorders** such as diabetes mellitus, uremia, liver disease, myxedema, acromegaly, metachromatic leukodystrophy, or Fabry's disease. That caused by diabetes is especially important and may take the form of an entrapment mononeuropathy, acute ischemic mononeuritis, distal sensorimotor polyneuropathy, subacute proximal motor polyradiculopathy (diabetic amyotrophy), thoracoabdominal radiculopathy, or autonomic neuropathy.

2. A peripheral neuropathy may also relate to an underlying malignant **neoplasm.** The peripheral nerves, spinal nerves, and limb plexuses may be compressed or infiltrated by extension of primary tumors or metastatic lymph nodes. Neoplastic disease can also lead to a nonmetastatic (paraneoplastic) sensory or sensorimotor polyneuropathy or to Lambert-Eaton syndrome, a disorder of neuromuscular transmission discussed in Chapter 6.

3. Certain **connective tissue disorders,** especially polyarteritis nodosa, rheumatoid arthritis, Churg-Strauss syndrome, and Wegener's granulomatosis, may be associated with mononeuropathy multiplex or, less commonly, polyneuropathy or cranial neuropathy. Polyneuropathy is more common in systemic lupus erythematosus. Patients with rheumatoid arthritis are particularly likely to develop focal entrapment or compressive mononeuropathies in the vicinity of the affected joints.

4. **AIDS** is commonly associated with a distal, symmetrical, primarily sensory polyneuropathy. Peripheral nerve involvement in AIDS less frequently takes the form of an acute or chronic inflammatory demyelinating polyneuropathy, polyradiculopathy, mononeuropathy multiplex, or autonomic neuropathy. Neuropathies are also seen in patients with AIDS-related complex, asymptomatic human immunodeficiency virus-1 (HIV-1) infection, and HIV-1 seroconversion.

E. Drug and Alcohol History: Some of the drugs that cause peripheral neuropathy are shown in Table 7–2; there may be selective involvement of motor or sensory fibers with some drugs.

F. Family Background: Certain polyneuropathies have a hereditary basis. These are discussed later in this chapter in the section on hereditary neuropathies.

Differential Diagnosis

Peripheral neuropathies can lead to a motor or sensory deficit or both. The preservation of sensation and tendon reflexes distinguishes the motor deficit that results from pure pyramidal lesions or is associated with spinal muscular atrophies, myopathies, or disorders of neuromuscular transmission from that caused by peripheral nerve involvement. Other distinguishing features are discussed in Chapter 6.

Myelopathies are characterized by a pyramidal deficit below the level of the lesion as well as by distal sensory loss.

In tabes dorsalis, there is often a history of syphi-

Table 7–2. Drugs inducing peripheral neuropathy.[1]

Sensory neuropathy
  Chloramphenicol
  Cisplatin
  Pyridoxine
Predominantly sensory neuropathy
  Ethambutol
  Hydralazine
  Misonidazole
  Metronidazole
Motor neuropathy
  Dapsone
  Imipramine
  Certain sulfonamides
Mixed sensory and motor neuropathy
  Amiodarone
  Chloroquine
  Disulfiram
  Gold
  Indomethacin
  Isoniazid
  Nitrofurantoin
  Penicillamine
  Perhexilene
  Phenytoin
  Tryptophan (contaminant)
  Vincristine

[1]Selected drugs.

litic infection, and examination reveals other stigmas of syphilis. In addition, tactile sensation is preserved.

Radiculopathies are distinguished from peripheral neuropathies by the distribution of motor or sensory deficits (Figures 7–4A and 7–4B). The presence of neck or back pain that radiates to the extremities in a radicular distribution also suggests a root lesion.

Investigative Studies

Laboratory studies in patients with peripheral neuropathy are directed at confirming the diagnosis and revealing any underlying cause. Electromyography may reveal evidence of denervation in the affected muscles and can be used to determine whether any motor units remain under voluntary control. Nerve conduction studies permit conduction velocity to be measured in motor and sensory fibers. On the basis of electrodiagnostic or histopathological studies, peripheral neuropathies can be divided into demyelinating or axonal neuropathies. In the former, electromyography typically reveals little or no evidence of denervation but there is marked slowing of maximal conduction velocity in affected nerves. In the axonal neuropathies, electromyography shows that denervation has occurred, especially distally in the extremities, but maximal nerve conduction velocity is normal or slowed only slightly.

In patients with electrophysiologically confirmed peripheral neuropathy, laboratory studies should include a complete blood count; erythrocyte sedimentation rate; serum urea nitrogen and creatinine, fasting blood glucose, and serum vitamin B_{12}; serum protein, protein electrophoresis, and immunoelectrophoresis;

liver and thyroid function blood tests; serological tests for syphilis (FTA or MHA-TP), rheumatoid factor, and antinuclear antibody; and chest x-ray. If toxic causes are suspected, a 24-hour urine collection followed by analysis for heavy metals may be necessary, and hair and fingernail clippings can be analyzed for arsenic. Examination of a fresh specimen of urine for porphobilinogen and δ-aminolevulinic acid is necessary if porphyria is suspected.

Treatment

Treatment of the underlying cause may limit the progression of or even reverse the neuropathy. Nursing care is important in patients with severe motor or sensory deficits to prevent decubitus ulcers, joint contractures, and additional compressive peripheral nerve damage. Respiratory function must also be monitored carefully—particularly in acute idiopathic polyneuropathy (Guillain-Barré syndrome), chronic inflammatory demyelinating polyneuropathy, and diphtheritic neuropathy—and preparations must be made to assist ventilation if the vital capacity falls below about 1 L. In patients with severe dysesthesia, a cradle (inverted metal bar frame) can be used to keep the bedclothes from touching sensitive areas of the skin. Treatment with phenytoin, 300 mg/d; carbamazepine, up to 1200 mg/d; or amitriptyline, 25–100 mg at bedtime, is sometimes helpful in relieving the lancinating pain of certain neuropathies when the response to simple analgesics has not been adequate.

Extremities with sensory loss must be protected from repeated minor trauma, such as thermal injury, that can destroy tissues. The temperature of hot surfaces should be checked with a part of the body in which sensation is preserved, and the setting of water heaters must be reduced to prevent scalding. The skin and nails must be cared for meticulously.

Dysautonomic symptoms may be troublesome, especially in diabetic or alcoholic polyneuropathy. Waist-high elastic hosiery, dietary salt supplementation, and treatment with fludrocortisone, 0.1—1 mg/d orally, may help relieve postural hypotension, but the patient must be monitored carefully to prevent recumbent hypertension. Instructing the patient to sleep in a semierect rather than a recumbent position is helpful because dysautonomic patients are often unable to conserve salt and water when recumbent at night.

POLYNEUROPATHIES

IDIOPATHIC INFLAMMATORY NEUROPATHIES

Acute Idiopathic Polyneuropathy (Guillain-Barré Syndrome)

Guillain-Barré syndrome is an acute or subacute polyneuropathy that can follow minor infective illnesses, inoculations, or surgical procedures—or may occur without obvious precipitants. Its precise cause is unclear, but it appears to have an immunological basis.

A. Clinical Features: The features useful for diagnosing Guillain-Barré syndrome are summarized in Table 7–3. Patients generally present with weakness that is symmetrical, usually begins in the legs, is often more marked proximally than distally, and is sometimes so severe that it is life-threatening, especially if the muscles of respiration or swallowing are involved. Sensory complaints, while usually less marked than motor symptoms, are also frequent. The deep tendon reflexes are usually absent. There may be marked autonomic dysfunction, with tachycardia, cardiac irregularities, labile blood pressure, disturbed sweating, impaired pulmonary function, sphincter disturbances, paralytic ileus, and other abnormalities.

B. Investigative Studies: The cerebrospinal fluid often shows a characteristic abnormality, with increased protein concentration but a normal cell count; abnormalities may not be found in the first

Table 7–3. Diagnostic criteria for Guillain-Barré syndrome.[1]

Required for diagnosis
    Progressive weakness of more than one limb
    Distal areflexia with proximal areflexia or hyporeflexia
Supportive of diagnosis
    Progression for up to four weeks
    Relatively symmetrical deficits
    Mild sensory involvement
    Cranial nerve (especially VII) involvement
    Recovery beginning within four weeks after progression stops
    Autonomic dysfunction
    No fever at onset
    Increased CSF protein after one week
    CSF white blood cell count ≤10/μl
    Nerve conduction slowing or block by several weeks
Against diagnosis
    Markedly asymmetrical weakness
    Bowel or bladder dysfunction (at onset or persistent)
    CSF white blood cell count >50 or PMN count >0/μL
    Well-demarcated sensory level
Excluding diagnosis
    Isolated sensory involvement
    Another polyneuropathy that explains clinical picture

[1]Adapted from Asbury AK, Cornblath DR: Assessment of current diagnostic criteria for Guillain-Barré syndrome. *Ann Neurol* 1990;27(Suppl):S21–S24.

week, however. Electrophysiological studies may reveal marked slowing of motor and sensory conduction velocity, but with a time course that does not necessarily parallel any clinical developments.

C. Treatment: Plasmapheresis appears to reduce the time required for recovery and may decrease the likelihood of residual neurological deficits. Where plasmapheresis is unavailable, plasma exchange can be substituted.

In the past, corticosteroids were often prescribed for patients with a progressive downhill course, but recent studies have shown that these agents may affect the outcome adversely and even increase the time necessary for recovery. Therapy is otherwise symptomatic, the aim being to prevent such complications as respiratory failure or vascular collapse. For this reason, patients who are severely affected are best managed in intensive care units, where facilities are available for monitoring and assisted respiration if necessary (eg, if the vital capacity falls below about 1 L, the patient is short of breath, or the blood oxygen saturation declines).

D. Prognosis: Symptoms and signs cease to progress by about four weeks into the illness. The disorder is self-limiting, and improvement occurs over the weeks or months following onset. About 70–75% of patients recover completely, 25% are left with mild neurological deficits, and 5% die, usually as a result of respiratory failure. Advanced age, the need for ventilatory support, or more rapid onset of symptoms may predict a poorer prognosis.

Chronic Inflammatory Demyelinating Polyneuropathy

Chronic inflammatory demyelinating polyneuropathy is clinically similar to Guillain-Barré syndrome except that it follows a chronic progressive course—or a course characterized by relapses—and no improvement is apparent within the six months after onset. Its cause is not known. Its clinical features are summarized in Table 7–4. Examination of the CSF reveals findings resembling those in Guillain-Barré syndrome. The electrophysiological findings indicate a demyelinative neuropathy with superimposed axonal degeneration. The disorder is often responsive to treatment with corticosteroids (prednisone, 60–100 mg/d for two to four weeks, then gradually tapered to 5–20 mg every other day) and sometimes to plasmapheresis.

METABOLIC & NUTRITIONAL NEUROPATHIES

Diabetes Mellitus

Peripheral nerve involvement in diabetes is common and may be characterized by polyneuropathy, which is of mixed (sensory, motor, and autonomic) character in about 70% of cases and predominantly

sensory in about 30%; mononeuropathy multiplex; or mononeuropathy simplex (Table 7–5). Such clinical manifestations can occur in isolation or in any combination. The incidence of peripheral nerve involvement may be influenced by the adequacy of diabetes control, which should, in any event, be optimal.

A. Clinical Features: The most common manifestation is a distal sensory or mixed **polyneuropathy,** which is sometimes diagnosed, before it becomes symptomatic, from the presence of depressed tendon reflexes and impaired appreciation of vibration in the legs. Symptoms are generally more common in the legs than in the arms and consist of numbness, pain, or paresthesias. In severe cases, there is distal sensory loss in all limbs and some accompanying motor disturbance. Diabetic dysautonomia leads to many symptoms, including postural hypotension, disturbances of cardiac rhythm, impaired thermoregulatory sweating, and disturbances of bladder, bowel, gastric, and sexual function. Diabetic **mononeuropathy multiplex (diabetic amyotrophy)** is usually associated with pain, weakness, and atrophy of pelvic girdle and thigh muscles; absent quadriceps reflexes; and little sensory loss. Diabetic amyotrophy may also relate to **plexopathy** or **polyradiculopathy.** Diabetic **mononeuropathy simplex** is typically abrupt in onset and often painful. CSF protein is typically increased in diabetic polyneuropathy and mononeuropathy multiplex.

B. Treatment and Prognosis: No specific treatment exists for the peripheral nerve complications of diabetes except when the patient has an entrapment

Table 7–4. Clinical features of chronic inflammatory demyelinating polyneuropathy.[1]

	Percentage of Patients
Hyporeflexia or areflexia	94
Weakness	
Distal upper extremity	85
Distal lower extremity	85
Proximal upper extremity	74
Proximal lower extremity	68
Respiratory muscles	11
Neck	4
Face	2
Sensory deficit on examination	
Distal lower extremity	83
Distal upper extremity	68
Paresthesia	
Upper extremity	79
Lower extremity	72
Face	6
Pain	
Lower extremity	17
Upper extremity	15
Dysarthria	9
Dysphagia	9
Impotence	4
Incontinence	2

[1]Adapted from Dyck PJ et al: Chronic inflammatory polyradiculopathy. *Mayo Clin Proc* 1975;**50:**621–637.

Table 7–5. Neuropathies associated with diabetes.

Type	Distribution
Polyneuropathy	
Mixed sensory, motor and autonomic	Symmetrical, distal, lower > upper limbs
Primarily sensory	
Mononeuropathy multiplex	
(Diabetic amyotrophy)	Asymmetrical, proximal (pelvic girdle and thighs)
Mononeuropathy simplex	
Peripheral	Ulnar, median, radial, lateral femoral cutaneous, sciatic, peroneal, other nerves
Cranial	Oculomotor (III) > abducens (VI) > trochlear (IV) nerve

neuropathy and may benefit from a decompressive procedure. Phenytoin (200–400 mg/d orally) or carbamazepine (100–600 mg orally twice daily) may help to relieve shooting or stabbing neuropathic pain, while amitriptyline (75–150 mg orally at bedtime) or a combination of amitriptyline and fluphenazine may be useful for treating deep, constant, aching pain.

Postural hypotension may respond to treatment with salt supplementation; sleeping in an upright position; wearing waist-high elastic hosiery; fludrocortisone, 0.1–1 mg/d; and indomethacin, 25–50 mg three times daily. Treatment is otherwise symptomatic. Diabetic amyotrophy and mononeuropathy simplex usually improve or resolve spontaneously.

Other Endocrinopathies

Hypothyroidism is a rare cause of polyneuropathy. More commonly, hypothyroidism is associated with entrapment neuropathy, especially carpal tunnel syndrome (see below, under *Median Nerve*). Polyneuropathy may be mistakenly diagnosed in patients with proximal limb weakness caused by hypothyroid myopathy or in patients with delayed relaxation of tendon reflexes, a classic manifestation of hypothyroidism that is independent of neuropathy. Other neurological manifestations of hypothyroidism such as acute confusional state (see Chapter 1), dementia (see Chapter 2), and cerebellar degeneration (see Chapter 4) are discussed elsewhere.

Acromegaly also frequently produces carpal tunnel syndrome and, less often, polyneuropathy. Since many acromegalic patients are also diabetic, it may be difficult to determine which disorder is primarily responsible for polyneuropathy in a given patient.

Uremia

A symmetrical sensorimotor polyneuropathy may occur in uremia. It tends to affect the legs more than the arms and is more marked distally than proximally. The extent of any disturbance in peripheral nerve function appears to relate to the severity of im-

paired renal function. The neuropathy itself may improve markedly with renal transplantation. Carpal tunnel syndrome (see below) has also been described in patients with renal disease and may develop distal to the arteriovenous fistulas placed in the forearm for access during hemodialysis.

Liver Disease

Primary biliary cirrhosis may lead to a sensory neuropathy that is probably of the axonal type. A predominantly demyelinative polyneuropathy can occur in patients with chronic liver disease. There does not appear to be any correlation between the neurological findings and the severity of the hepatic dysfunction.

Vitamin B$_{12}$ Deficiency

Vitamin B$_{12}$ deficiency is associated with many features that are characteristic of polyneuropathy, including symmetrical distal sensory and motor impairment and loss of tendon reflexes. Because controversy exists about the relative importance of polyneuropathy and myelopathy in producing this syndrome, however, vitamin B$_{12}$ deficiency is considered in more detail below in the section on myelopathies.

INFECTIVE & GRANULOMATOUS NEUROPATHIES

AIDS

Neuropathy is a common complication of HIV-1 infection (Table 7–6); involvement of peripheral nerves is seen at autopsy in about 40% of patients with AIDS.

Distal symmetrical **sensorimotor polyneuropathy** is the most common neuropathy associated with HIV-1 infection. Axons, rather than myelin, are primarily affected. The cause is unknown, and HIV-1 is rarely identified in the affected nerves. Sensory symptoms predominate and include pain and paresthesias that affect the feet especially. Weakness is a minor or late feature. Ankle and sometimes knee reflexes are absent. The course is typically progressive and no treatment is available, but pain may be controlled with tricyclic antidepressants, as described above for diabetic neuropathy.

Chronic inflammatory demyelinating polyneuropathy may occur early in HIV-1 infection and may be immune-mediated. It is characterized by proximal, and sometimes distal, weakness with less-pronounced sensory disturbances and areflexia or hyporeflexia. Some patients improve spontaneously or stabilize, and others may respond to plasmapheresis.

Lumbosacral polyradiculopathy occurs late in the course of HIV-1 infection, usually in patients with prior opportunistic infections. Cytomegalovirus infection is thought to be the cause. Clinical features usually develop over several weeks and include dif-

Table 7–6. Neuropathies associated with AIDS.

Type	Stage of HIV-1 Infection	Immune Status	Distribution
Sensorimotor polyneuropathy	Early or late	Competent or suppressed	Symmetrical, distal, lower > upper limbs
Chronic inflammatory demyelinating polyneuropathy	Early	Competent	Proximal > distal limbs
Lumbosacral polyradiculopathy	Late	Suppressed	Proximal lower limbs, sphincters
Mononeuropathy multiplex	Early or late	Competent or suppressed	Cranial (eg, facial), peripheral (eg, peroneal)
Mononeuropathy simplex	Early	Competent	Cranial (eg, facial), peripheral (eg, peroneal)

fuse, progressive leg weakness, back pain, painful paresthesias of the feet and perineum, lower extremity areflexia, and early urinary retention. The course may be fulminant, with ascending paralysis leading to respiratory failure. CSF findings include mononuclear or polymorphonuclear pleocytosis, elevated protein, and decreased glucose. Patients may respond to ganciclovir, 2.5 mg/kg intravenously every eight hours for ten days, then 7.5 mg/kg/d five days per week.

Mononeuropathy multiplex affects multiple cranial and peripheral nerves, resulting in focal weakness and sensory loss. Nerve infarcts are the likely cause. In early HIV-1 infection, mononeuropathy multiplex may be a self-limited disorder restricted to a single limb, with spontaneous stabilization or improvement. Late in AIDS, multiple limbs may be affected in a progressive fashion.

Mononeuropathy simplex tends to occur acutely in early HIV-1 infection and improve spontaneously. A vascular cause is probable.

Leprosy

Leprosy is one of the most frequent causes of peripheral neuropathy worldwide. In turn, neuropathy is the most disabling manifestation of leprosy. *Mycobacterium leprae* affects the skin and peripheral nerves because its growth is facilitated by the cooler temperatures present at the body surface.

In **tuberculoid leprosy,** the immune response is adequate to confine the infection to one or more small patches of skin and their associated cutaneous and subcutaneous nerves. This produces a hypopigmented macule or papule over which sensation is impaired, with pain and temperature appreciation most affected. Anhidrosis occurs as a result of local involvement of autonomic fibers. Sensory deficits occur most often in the distribution of the digital, sural, radial, and posterior auricular nerves, while motor findings usually relate to involvement of the ulnar or peroneal nerve. Involved nerves are often enlarged.

Lepromatous leprosy is a more widespread disorder that results in a symmetrical, primarily sensory polyneuropathy that disproportionately affects pain and temperature sense. Its distribution is distinctive

in that exposed areas of the body—especially the ears; nose; cheeks; dorsal surfaces of the hands, forearms, and feet; and lateral aspects of the legs—are preferentially involved. Unlike most polyneuropathies, that caused by leprosy tends to spare the tendon reflexes. Associated findings include resorption of the digits, trophic ulcers, and cyanosis and anhidrosis of the hands and feet. Treatment is with dapsone, 50–100 mg/d orally, administered for 18 months in cases of tuberculoid leprosy and 10 years in lepromatous leprosy.

Diphtheria

Corynebacterium diphtheriae infects tissues of the upper respiratory tract and produces a toxin that causes demyelination of peripheral nerves. Within about one month after infection, patients may develop a cranial motor neuropathy with prominent impairment of ocular accommodation. Blurred vision is the usual presenting complaint. Extraocular muscles and the face, palate, pharynx, and diaphragm may also be affected, but the pupillary light reflex is preserved. Recovery typically occurs after several weeks. A more delayed syndrome that commonly has its onset two or three months following the primary infection takes the form of a symmetrical distal sensorimotor polyneuropathy. Most patients recover completely. Diphtheritic neuropathy is discussed in more detail in Chapter 6.

Sarcoidosis

Sarcoidosis can produce mononeuropathy or, rarely, polyneuropathy. The mononeuropathy commonly involves cranial nerves, especially the facial nerve, in which case the resulting syndrome may be indistinguishable from idiopathic facial paralysis (Bell's palsy). X-rays of the lungs and bones and determination of serum levels of angiotensin-converting enzyme are helpful in establishing the diagnosis. Treatment with prednisone, 60 mg/d orally, followed by tapering doses, may speed recovery.

NEUROPATHIES IN VASCULITIS & COLLAGEN VASCULAR DISEASE

Systemic vasculitides and collagen vascular diseases can produce polyneuropathy, mononeuropathy simplex, mononeuropathy multiplex, or entrapment neuropathy (Table 7–7).

Systemic necrotizing vasculitis includes polyarteritis nodosa and allergic angiitis and granulomatosis (Churg-Strauss syndrome). Neuropathy occurs in about 50% of patients, most often as mononeuropathy multiplex, which may manifest itself with the acute onset of pain in one or more cranial or peripheral nerves. Distal symmetrical sensorimotor polyneuropathy is less common. Treatment should begin as soon as the diagnosis is made; it includes prednisone, 60–100 mg/d orally, and cyclophosphamide, 2–3 mg/d orally. Plasmapheresis may also be helpful.

Wegener's granulomatosis is associated with mononeuropathy multiplex or polyneuropathy in up to 30% of cases. Treatment is the same as for systemic necrotizing vasculitis.

Giant cell arteritis is considered in detail in Chapter 3. Mononeuropathy affecting cranial nerves innervating the extraocular muscles can occur.

Rheumatoid arthritis produces entrapment neuropathy (most commonly involving the median nerve) in about 45% of patients and distal symmetrical sensorimotor polyneuropathy in about 30%. Mononeuropathy multiplex is a frequent feature in cases complicated by necrotizing vasculitis.

Systemic lupus erythematosus is discussed in Chapter 1 as a cause of acute confusional states. Neuropathy occurs in up to 20% of patients. The most common pattern is a distal, symmetrical sensorimotor polyneuropathy. An ascending, predominantly motor polyneuropathy (Guillain-Barré syndrome, see above) can also occur, as may mononeuropathy simplex or multiplex, which often affects the ulnar, radial, sciatic or peroneal nerve.

Sjögren's syndrome involves the peripheral nerves in about 20% of cases. Distal symmetrical sensorimotor polyneuropathy is most common, entrapment neuropathy (affecting especially the median nerve) is also frequent, and mononeuropathy multiplex can occur.

Progressive systemic sclerosis (scleroderma) and **mixed connective tissue disease** may produce cranial mononeuropathy, which most often involves the trigeminal (V) nerve.

NEOPLASTIC & PARAPROTEINEMIC NEUROPATHIES

Compression & Infiltration by Tumor

Nerve compression is a common complication of multiple myeloma, lymphoma, and carcinoma. Tumorous invasion of the epineurium may occur with leukemia, lymphoma, and carcinoma of the breast or pancreas.

Paraneoplastic Syndromes

Carcinoma (especially oat-cell carcinoma of the lung) and lymphoma may be associated with neuropathies that are thought to be immunologically mediated, based on the detection of autoantibodies to neuronal antigens in several cases.

Sensory or sensorimotor polyneuropathy occurs with both carcinoma and lymphoma. This can be either an acute or chronic disorder; it is sometimes asymmetrical and may be accompanied by prominent pain.

Carcinoma can also cause **sensory neuronopathy,** a polyneuropathy that primarily affects the cell bodies of sensory neurons in the dorsal root ganglion. This rare condition usually affects women and may be the presenting manifestation of cancer. All sensory modalities are affected, and pain may be a symptom. Motor involvement is late, and autonomic dysfunction is uncommon.

Lymphoma may be complicated by **motor neuronopathy,** a disorder of anterior horn cells, which is discussed in Chapter 6. Hodgkin's disease and an-

Table 7–7. Neuropathies associated with vasculitis and collagen vascular disease.

Disease	Polyneuropathy	Mononeuropathy Simplex or Multiplex[1]	Entrapment Neuropathy[1]
Vasculitis			
Systemic necrotizing vasculitis[2]	+	+	–
Wegener's granulomatosis	+	+	–
Giant cell arteritis	–	+ (III, VI, IV)	–
Collagen vascular disease			
Rheumatoid arthritis	+	+	+ (M, U, R)
Systemic lupus erythematosus	+	+	–
Sjögren's syndrome	+	+ (V, III, VI)	+ (M)
Progressive systemic sclerosis	–	+ (V)	–
Mixed connective-tissue disease	+	+(V)	–

[1]Commonly affected nerves = III, oculomotor; IV, trochlear; V, trigeminal; VI, abducens; M, median; U, ulnar; R, radial.
[2]Includes polyarteritis nodosa and Churg-Strauss syndrome.
+ = Present; – = Absent.

gioimmunoblastic lymphadenopathy are sometimes associated with Guillain-Barré syndrome.

Paraproteinemias

Polyneuropathy is a common complication of **multiple myeloma.** Patients affected by lytic myeloma are usually men. The clinical picture is of a distal symmetrical sensorimotor polyneuropathy. All sensory modalities are affected, pain is a frequent feature, and the reflexes are depressed. The disorder is usually progressive and leads to death within two years. **Sclerotic myeloma** may be accompanied by a chronic demyelinating polyneuropathy. Motor involvement predominates, but vibration and position sense may also be impaired, and the reflexes are depressed. Pain is less common than in the neuropathy of lytic myeloma, and symptoms may improve with treatment of the underlying cancer.

A sensorimotor polyneuropathy similar to that observed with lytic myeloma may also occur in **Waldenström's macroglobulinemia** or **benign monoclonal gammopathy.**

Amyloidosis

Nonhereditary amyloidosis occurs as an isolated disorder (primary generalized amyloidosis) or in patients with multiple myeloma and may be associated with polyneuropathy. Polyneuropathy is also a feature of hereditary amyloidosis. Amyloid neuropathies are considered below in the section on hereditary neuropathies.

DRUG-INDUCED & TOXIC NEUROPATHIES

Alcoholism

Polyneuropathy is one of the most common neurological complications of chronic alcoholism; it can occur alone or in combination with other alcohol-related neurological disorders, such as Wernicke's encephalopathy (see Chapter 1) or the Korsakoff amnestic syndrome (see Chapter 2). Controversy exists concerning the relative contributions of direct neurotoxicity of alcohol and associated nutritional (especially thiamine) deficiency in producing polyneuropathy.

Alcoholic polyneuropathy is typically a symmetrical distal sensorimotor neuropathy. The legs are particularly likely to be affected, resulting in defective perception of vibration and touch and depressed or absent ankle reflexes. In some cases, distal weakness is also pronounced and autonomic dysfunction may occur. When pain is a prominent feature, it may respond to the same treatment described above for painful diabetic neuropathy.

Abstinence from alcohol and thiamine repletion can halt the progression of symptoms.

Other Drugs

Dapsone, a drug used to treat leprosy, can produce a primarily motor polyneuropathy that is reversible.

Hydralazine, an antihypertensive drug, is associated on rare occasions with a predominantly sensory polyneuropathy that has been attributed to drug-induced pyridoxine deficiency and that resolves after the drug is discontinued.

Isoniazid is a widely used antituberculous agent that interferes with pyridoxine metabolism and produces a polyneuropathy that principally affects the sensory neurons. High doses, hereditary variations in drug metabolism, and malnutrition predispose to this complication. Spontaneous recovery is the rule when administration of the drug is halted. Isoniazid-induced neuropathy can be prevented by concurrent administration of pyridoxine, 100 mg/d orally.

Phenytoin is often mentioned as a cause of polyneuropathy, but evidence for phenytoin treatment as a cause of symptomatic neuropathy is sparse.

Pyridoxine (vitamin B_6) toxicity has been implicated as the cause of a sensory neuronopathy that disproportionately impairs vibration and position sense. This disorder occurs in patients taking at least 200 mg of pyridoxine daily—about 100 times the minimum daily requirement. Sensory ataxia, Romberg's sign, Lhermitte's sign, and ankle areflexia are common findings. Pain is less common, and motor involvement is unusual. Symptoms are usually reversible over months to years if the abuse ceases, but an irreversible syndrome has also been reported following intravenous administration of high doses of pyridoxine.

Vincristine produces a polyneuropathy in most patients who receive the drug for treatment of (usually hematological) cancer. The earliest manifestations are distal sensory symptoms and loss of reflexes. Motor deficits may predominate later in the course, however. Constipation is a common finding and may be due to autonomic involvement. Discontinuing the drug or administering it at a reduced dosage often leads to improvement.

Toxins

Organic compounds implicated as causes of polyneuropathy include hexacarbons present in solvents and glues (eg, *n*-hexane, methyl *n*-butyl ketone) and organophosphates used as plasticizers or insecticides (eg, triorthocresylphosphate). Sensory involvement is most striking in *n*-hexane neuropathy, whereas neuropathy caused by triorthocresylphosphate primarily affects motor nerves. Organophosphate neuropathy is discussed in more detail in Chapter 6.

Heavy metals may also be responsible for polyneuropathy. Neuropathy caused by lead, arsenic, and thallium is discussed in Chapter 6. Gold, which is used to treat rheumatoid arthritis, may cause a symmetrical polyneuropathy, and cisplatin (a platinum analogue with anticancer activity) may produce a sensory neuropathy.

Eosinophilia-myalgia syndrome was first identified in 1989 in patients taking L-tryptophan who developed disabling myalgias with blood eosinophil counts above $1,000/\mu L$. About 85% of patients are women. The cause appears to be 1,1'-ethylidenebis [tryptophan], a contaminant in certain commercial preparations of L-tryptophan, which have since been withdrawn. Symptoms include myalgia, arthralgia, dyspnea, cough, rash, fever, and sclerodermiform skin changes. Neurological findings include weakness of distal and proximal limb and bulbar muscles, distal sensory loss, and areflexia. Eosinophilia, leukocytosis, and elevated liver enzymes are typical. Nerve conduction studies and electromyography may show evidence of polyneuropathy, myopathy, or both. Inflammation is prominent in skin biopsy specimens, but less so in nerve and muscle, which show primarily axonal degeneration and muscle fiber atrophy. Treatment is discontinuation of L-tryptophan and administration of corticosteroids, non-steroidal anti-inflammatory drugs, and analgesics. Most patients improve or recover fully, but deaths have been reported.

HEREDITARY NEUROPATHIES

Idiopathic

Hereditary motor and sensory neuropathies (HMSN) include the hypertrophic (HMSN type I) and neuronal (HMSN type II) forms of **Charcot-Marie-Tooth disease** as well as **Dejerine-Sottas disease** (HMSN type III). **HMSN type I** is a slowly progressive demyelinating neuropathy that occurs either sporadically or with a dominant or recessive mode of inheritance. The nerves may be palpably enlarged. **HMSN type II,** which is less common, affects the anterior horn cells and thus resembles progressive spinal muscular atrophy (see Chapter 6). **HMSN type III** is a slowly progressive demyelinating disorder that usually has a recessive mode of inheritance and progresses from its onset in infancy or childhood to cause severe disability by the third decade of life. The nerves are typically enlarged.

Hereditary sensory neuropathies (HSN) also take a variety of forms. In **HSN type I,** there is a dominant inheritance, a gradually progressive course from onset in early adulthood, and symmetrical loss of distal pain and temperature perception, with relative preservation of light touch. Perforating ulcers over pressure points and painless infections of the extremities are common. The tendon reflexes are depressed, but there is little, if any, motor disturbance. In **HSN type II,** inheritance is recessive, onset is in infancy or early childhood, all sensory modalities are affected, and tendon reflexes are lost. **HSN type III (Riley-Day syndrome, familial dysautonomia)** is a recessive disorder that commences in infancy and is characterized by conspicuous autonomic dysfunction (absent tearing, labile temperature and blood pressure), accompanied by absent taste sensation, impaired pain and temperature sensation, and areflexia. **HSN type IV** is associated with congenital insensitivity to pain and absent sweating.

Polyneuropathy can occur in both the hereditary and nonhereditary forms of **amyloidosis.** Because small-diameter sensory and autonomic nerve fibers are especially likely to be involved, pain and temperature sensation and autonomic functions are prominently affected. Clinical presentation is commonly with distal paresthesias, dysesthesias, and numbness; postural hypotension; impaired thermoregulatory sweating; and disturbances of bladder, bowel, or sexual function. Distal weakness and wasting eventually occur. The tendon reflexes are often preserved until a relatively late stage. Entrapment neuropathy—especially carpal tunnel syndrome—may develop as a consequence of amyloid deposits. There is no specific treatment.

Friedreich's ataxia usually has a recessive mode of inheritance but occasionally occurs with dominant inheritance. The defective gene in classic recessive cases has been localized to chromosome 9. An ataxic gait develops, followed by clumsiness of the hands and other signs of cerebellar dysfunction. Involvement of peripheral sensory fibers leads to sensory deficits of the limbs, with depressed or absent tendon reflexes. There may also be leg weakness and extensor plantar responses from central motor involvement. This condition is considered in detail in Chapter 4.

Metabolic

In **acute intermittent porphyria,** which is transmitted by recessive inheritance, the initial neurological manifestation is often a polyneuropathy that (usually) involves motor more than sensory fibers. Sensory symptoms and signs may be predominantly proximal or distal. The peripheral nerves may also be affected in **variegate porphyria.** Neuropathy caused by porphyria is considered in greater detail in Chapter 6.

Two recessive lipidoses are associated with polyneuropathy with a typical onset in infancy or childhood. These are **metachromatic leukodystrophy,** which results from deficiency of the enzyme arylsulfatase A, and **Krabbe's disease,** which is due to galactocerebroside β-galactosidase deficiency. Both are inherited in an autosomal recessive fashion.

Lipoprotein deficiencies that cause polyneuropathy include **abetalipoproteinemia,** which is associated with acanthocytosis, malabsorption, retinitis pigmentosa, and cerebellar ataxia; and **Tangier disease,** which produces cataract, orange discoloration of the tonsils, and hepatosplenomegaly. These are autosomal recessive conditions.

Refsum's disease is an autosomal recessive disorder related to impaired metabolism of phytanic acid. It produces polyneuropathy, cerebellar ataxia, retinitis pigmentosa, and ichthyosis. It can be treated by restricting dietary intake of phytol.

Fabry's disease is an X-linked recessive deficiency of the enzyme α-galactosidase-A. It results in a painful sensory and autonomic neuropathy, angiokeratomas, renal disease, and an increased incidence of stroke.

ENTRAPMENT NEUROPATHIES

Certain peripheral nerves are particularly susceptible to mechanical injury at vulnerable sites. The term **entrapment neuropathy** is used when the nerve is compressed, stretched, or angulated by adjacent anatomical structures to such an extent that dysfunction occurs. There are numerous entrapment neuropathies, and in many the initial or most conspicuous clinical complaints are of sensory symptoms or pain. Some of the more common syndromes are described below.

ENTRAPMENT SYNDROMES OF UPPER LIMBS

Median Nerve Compression

Compression of the median nerve can occur in the carpal tunnel at the wrist. **Carpal tunnel syndrome** is common during pregnancy and can occur as a complication of trauma, degenerative arthritis, tenosynovitis, myxedema, and acromegaly. Early symptoms are pain and paresthesias confined to a median nerve distribution in the hand, ie, involving primarily the thumb, index, and middle fingers and the lateral half of the ring finger (see Appendix C). There may be pain in the forearm and, in occasional patients, even in the upper arm, shoulder, and neck. Symptoms are often particularly troublesome at night and may awaken the patient from sleep. As the neuropathy advances, weakness and atrophy may eventually develop in the thenar muscles. Examination reveals impaired cutaneous sensation in the median nerve distribution in the hand and, with motor involvement, weakness and wasting of the abductor pollicis brevis and opponens pollicis muscles (see Appendix C). There may be a positive **Tinel sign** (percussion of the nerve at the wrist causes paresthesias in its distribution) or a positive response to **Phalen's maneuver** (flexion of the wrist for one minute exacerbates or reproduces symptoms). The diagnosis can generally be confirmed by electrophysiological studies, showing sensory or motor conduction velocity to be slowed at the wrist; there may be signs of chronic partial denervation in median-supplied muscles of the hand.

If the symptoms fail to respond to local cortico steroid injections or simple maneuvers such as wearing a nocturnal wrist splint, surgical decompression of the carpal tunnel may be necessary.

Interdigital Neuropathy

Interdigital neuropathy may lead to pain in one or two fingers, and examination reveals hyperpathia or impaired cutaneous sensation in the appropriate distribution of the affected nerve or nerves. Such a neuropathy may result from entrapment in the intermetacarpal tunnel of the hand, direct trauma, tenosynovitis, or arthritis.

Treatment by local infiltration with corticosteroids is sometimes helpful, but in severe cases neurolysis may be necessary.

Ulnar Nerve Dysfunction

Ulnar nerve dysfunction at the **elbow** leads to paresthesias, hypesthesia, and nocturnal pain in the little finger and ulnar border of the hand. Pain may also occur about the elbow. Symptoms are often intensified by elbow flexion or use of the arm. Examination may reveal sensory loss on the ulnar aspect of the hand (see Appendix C) and weakness of the adductor pollicis, the deep flexor muscles of the fourth and fifth digits, and the intrinsic hand muscles (see Appendix C). The lesion may result from external pressure, from entrapment within the cubital tunnel, or from cubitus valgus deformity causing chronic stretch injury of the nerve. Electrodiagnostic studies may be helpful in localizing the lesion.

Avoiding pressure on or repetitive flexion and extension of the elbow, combined in some instances with splinting the elbow in extension, is sometimes sufficient to arrest progression and alleviate symptoms. Surgical decompression or ulnar nerve transposition to the flexor surface of the arm may also be helpful, depending on the cause and severity of the lesion and the duration of symptoms.

An ulnar nerve lesion may develop in the **wrist** or **palm** of the hand in association with repetitive trauma, arthritis, or compression from ganglia or benign tumors. Involvement of the deep terminal branch in the palm leads to a motor deficit in ulnar-innervated hand muscles other than the hypothenar group, while a more proximal palmar lesion affects the latter muscles as well; there is no sensory deficit. With lesions at the wrist involving either the ulnar nerve itself or its deep and superficial branches, both sensory and motor changes occur in the hand. Sensation over the dorsal surface of the hand is unaffected, however, because the cutaneous branch to this region arises proximal to the wrist. Surgical treatment is helpful in relieving compression from a ganglion or benign tumor.

Radial Nerve Compression

The radial nerve may be compressed in the axilla by pressure from crutches or other causes; this is frequently seen in alcoholics and drug addicts who have fallen asleep with an arm draped over some hard surface. The resulting deficit is primarily motor, with weakness or paralysis occurring in the muscles supplied by the nerve (see Appendix C), but sensory changes may also occur, especially in a small region on the back of the hand between the thumb and index finger (see Appendix C).

Treatment involves preventing further compression of the nerve. Recovery usually occurs spontaneously and completely except when a very severe injury has resulted in axonal degeneration. Physical therapy and a wrist splint may be helpful until recovery occurs.

Thoracic Outlet Syndrome

In thoracic outlet syndrome, a cervical rib or band or other anatomical structure may compress the lower part of the brachial plexus. Symptoms include pain, paresthesias, and numbness in a C8–T1 distribution (see Figure 7–4). There may be diffuse weakness of the intrinsic hand muscles, often particularly involving the muscles in the thenar eminence and thereby simulating carpal tunnel syndrome. See the section on cervical rib syndrome in Chapter 6 for further details.

ENTRAPMENT SYNDROMES OF LOWER LIMBS

Peroneal Nerve Lesions

Peroneal nerve lesions can occur secondary to trauma or to pressure about the knee at the head of the fibula. The resulting weakness or paralysis of foot and toe extension—and foot eversion (see Appendix C)—is accompanied by impaired sensation over the dorsum of the foot and the lower anterior aspect of the leg (see Appendix C). The ankle reflex is preserved, as is foot inversion.

Treatment is purely supportive. It is important to protect the nerve from further injury or compression. Patients with foot drop may require a brace until recovery occurs. Recovery occurs spontaneously with time and is usually complete unless the injury was severe enough to cause marked axonal degeneration.

Tarsal Tunnel Syndrome

The posterior tibial nerve or its branches can be compressed between the floor and the ligamentous roof of the tarsal tunnel, which is located at the ankle immediately below and behind the medial malleolus. The usual complaint is of burning in the foot—especially at night—sometimes accompanied by weakness of the intrinsic foot muscles. The diagnosis can usually be confirmed electrophysiologically.

If treatment with local injection of steroids is not helpful, surgical decompression may be necessary.

Femoral Neuropathy

Isolated femoral neuropathy may occur in association with diabetes mellitus, vascular disease, bleeding diatheses (eg, hemophilia, treatment with anticoagulant drugs), or retroperitoneal neoplasms. The most conspicuous symptoms and signs relate to weakness of the quadriceps muscle, with reduced or absent knee jerk reflex, but there may also be sensory disturbances in the anterior and medial aspects of the thigh and the medial part of the lower leg.

Treatment is of the underlying cause.

Saphenous Nerve Injury

The saphenous nerve is the terminal sensory branch of the femoral nerve and supplies cutaneous sensation to the medial aspect of the leg about and below the knee (see Figure 7–4). Mechanical injury to the nerve can occur at several points along its course; patients then complain of pain or impaired sensation in the distribution of the nerve. Weakness in quadriceps function (ie, extension at the knee; see Appendix C) reflects femoral nerve involvement.

There is no specific treatment, but the nerve should be protected from further injury.

Lateral Femoral Cutaneous Nerve Dysfunction

The lateral femoral cutaneous nerve supplies sensation to the outer border of the thigh (see Appendix C). Its function can be impaired by excessive angulation or compression by neighboring anatomical structures, especially in pregnancy or other conditions that cause exaggerated lumbar lordosis. This leads to pain and paresthesias in the lateral thigh, and examination reveals impaired sensation in this region. This syndrome, known as **meralgia paresthetica,** is best treated with symptomatic measures, since its course is often self-limited.

Obturator Nerve Injury

Trauma to the obturator nerve—eg, by pelvic fracture or a surgical procedure—can lead to pain radiating from the groin down the inner aspect of the thigh. An obturator hernia or osteitis pubis may cause a similar disorder; there is accompanying weakness of the adductor thigh muscles (see Appendix C).

ROOT & PLEXUS LESIONS

COMPRESSIVE & TRAUMATIC LESIONS

The clinical disturbances resulting from acute intervertebral disk prolapse, cervical spondylosis, traumatic plexopathy, cervical rib syndrome, and neuralgic amyotrophy were discussed in Chapter 6. In addition to these conditions, patients with metastatic cancer may develop root or plexus lesions from compression by tumor or as a result of trauma induced by radiation therapy. Root lesions are typically compressive in nature and usually occur in the setting of neoplastic meningitis, which is discussed in Chapter 1. Tumors (especially lung and breast cancer) can also infiltrate the brachial plexus, causing severe arm pain and sometimes dysesthesia. Because involvement of the lower trunk of the plexus is most common, symptoms usually occur within the C8 and T1 dermatomes, and Horner's syndrome (see Chapter 5) is present in about 50% of cases. Radiation injury—rather than direct invasion by tumor—should be suspected as the cause when the upper trunk of the brachial plexus (C5 and C6 nerve roots) is involved, weakness is a prominent presenting symptom, arm swelling occurs, or symptoms develop within one year after completion of radiation therapy with a total dose of more than 6000 R. Lumbosacral plexopathy is usually seen in patients with colorectal, cervical, uterine, or ovarian carcinoma or sarcoma. Clinical features that suggest tumor invasion in this setting include early and severe pain, unilateral involvement, leg swelling, and a palpable rectal mass. Radiation injury is more commonly associated with early prominent leg weakness and bilateral symptoms.

TABES DORSALIS

This type of neurosyphilis, now rare, is characterized mainly by sensory symptoms and signs that indicate marked involvement of the posterior roots, especially in the lumbosacral region, with resulting degeneration in the posterior columns of the spinal cord. Common complaints are of unsteadiness, sudden lancinating somatic pains, and urinary incontinence. Visceral crises characterized by excruciating abdominal pain also occur. Examination reveals marked impairment of vibration and joint position sense in the legs, together with an ataxic gait and Romberg's sign. Deep pain sensation is impaired, but superficial sensation is generally preserved. The bladder is often palpably enlarged; because it is flaccid and insensitive, there is overflow incontinence. Tendon reflexes are lost, and the limbs are hypotonic. Sensory loss and hypotonicity may lead to the occur-

rence of hypertrophic (Charcot) joints. In many patients there are other signs of neurosyphilis, including Argyll Robertson pupils, optic atrophy, ptosis, a variable ophthalmoplegia, and, in some cases, pyramidal and mental changes from cerebral involvement (taboparesis), as discussed in Chapter 2. Treatment is of the underlying infection.

LYME DISEASE

Lyme disease, like syphilis, is a spirochetal infection that produces both central and peripheral nervous system disease. Central nervous system involvement is manifested by meningitis or meningoencephalitis, as discussed in Chapter 1. Lyme disease is also associated with inflammatory mono- or polyradiculopathy, brachial plexopathy (see Chapter 6), mononeuropathy (including facial palsy), and mononeuropathy multiplex. The radiculopathy results in pain, sensory loss, or dysesthesia in affected dermatomes; it also causes focal weakness. One or more cervical, thoracic, or lumbar nerve roots may be involved. Electromyography can confirm the presence of radiculopathy, and serological testing establishes Lyme disease as the cause. Treatment is with intravenous penicillin, as described in Chapter 1.

MYELOPATHIES

Myelopathies may present with pain or with a variety of sensory complaints and with motor disturbances. The clinical findings should suggest the level of the lesion, but further investigation is necessary to delineate it more fully and determine its nature. Compressive, ischemic, inflammatory, demyelinative, and traumatic myelopathies were discussed in Chapter 6.

SYRINGOMYELIA

Syringomyelia is cavitation of the spinal cord. Communicating syringomyelia—with communication between the central canal of the cord and the cavity—is a hydrodynamic disorder of the CSF pathways. In noncommunicating syringomyelia, there is cystic dilation of the cord, which is not in communication with the CSF pathways. The precise clinical disturbance that results depends upon the site of cavitation. Typically, there is a dissociated sensory loss at the level of the lesion; pinprick and temperature appreciation are impaired, but light touch sensation is preserved. The sensory loss may be reflected by the presence of painless skin ulcers, scars, edema, hyperhidrosis, neuropathic joints, resorption of the terminal phalanges, and other disturbances. Weakness and wasting of muscles occur at the level of the lesion because of the involvement of the anterior horns of the cord. A pyramidal deficit and sphincter disturbances sometimes occur below the level of the lesion because of gliosis or compression of the corticospinal pathways in the lateral columns of the cord. The tendon reflexes may be depressed at the level of the lesion—because of interruption of their afferent, central, or efferent pathways—and increased below it. Scoliosis is a common accompaniment of cord cavitation. Cavitation commonly occurs in the cervical region; this can cause a capelike distribution of sensory loss over one or both shoulders, diffuse pain in the neck, and radicular pain in the arms; involvement of the T1 segment frequently leads to ipsilateral Horner's syndrome. If the cavitation involves the lower brain stem **(syringobulbia),** there may also be ipsilateral tongue wasting, palatal weakness, vocal cord paralysis, dissociated trigeminal sensory loss, and other evidence of brain stem involvement.

Communicating syringomyelia is often associated with developmental anomalies of the brain stem and foramen magnum region (such as Arnold-Chiari malformation; see Chapter 4) or with chronic arachnoiditis of the basal cisterns. Arnold-Chiari malformation can lead to hydrocephalus, cerebellar ataxia, pyramidal and sensory deficits in the limbs, and abnormalities of the lower cranial nerves, alone or in any combination. Myelography, MRI, or CT scanning of the foramen magnum region confirms the diagnosis. Treatment is surgical.

Noncommunicating syringomyelia is often due to trauma, intramedullary tumors, or spinal arachnoiditis.

Treatment depends upon the underlying cause. Decompression of a distended syrinx may provide transient benefit. In the case of communicating syringomyelia associated with Arnold-Chiari malformation, removal of the posterior rim of the foramen magnum and amputation of the cerebellar tonsils are sometimes helpful. The cord cavity should be drained, and, if necessary, an outlet should be made for the fourth ventricle. Posttraumatic syringomyelia is treated by surgery if it is causing a progressive neurological deficit or intolerable pain.

SUBACUTE COMBINED DEGENERATION (Vitamin B_{12} Deficiency)

Vitamin B_{12} deficiency may result from impaired absorption by the gastrointestinal tract such as occurs in pernicious anemia or because of gastrointestinal surgery, sprue, or infection with fish tapeworm; it can also be caused by a strictly vegetarian diet. It may affect the spinal cord, giving rise to the syndrome of subacute combined degeneration. Onset is with distal

paresthesias and weakness in the extremities (involvement of the hands occurs relatively early), followed by the development of spastic paraparesis, with ataxia from the impairment of postural sensation in the legs. Lhermitte's sign may be present, and examination reveals a combined posterior column (vibration and joint position sense) and pyramidal deficit in the legs. Plantar responses are extensor, but tendon reflexes may be increased or depressed, depending on the site and severity of the involvement. Signs of cord involvement can be accompanied by centrocecal scotoma or optic atrophy from optic (II) nerve involvement, by behavioral or psychiatric changes (see Chapter 1), or by peripheral neuropathy. The neurological manifestations are often accompanied by macrocytic megaloblastic anemia, but this is not invariably present.

The serum vitamin B_{12} level is low in untreated cases. If malabsorption of vitamin B_{12} is the cause, the Schilling test is abnormal, and there is usually gastric achlorhydria with pernicious anemia. Hematological findings may be normal, however, especially if folic acid supplements have been given.

Treatment is with vitamin B_{12} given by intramuscular injection daily (50–1000 µg) for two weeks, then weekly (100 µg) for 2 months, and monthly (100 µg) thereafter. Note that folic acid supplements do not help the neurological disorder; in addition, they may mask associated anemia.

CEREBRAL DISEASE

Sensory symptoms may relate to diverse diseases involving the brain stem or cerebral hemispheres. The clinical features of the sensory deficit have been described earlier in this chapter and, together with the nature and extent of any accompanying neurological signs, should suggest the probable site of the lesion. The differential diagnosis of such lesions is considered separately in Chapter 10.

PAIN SYNDROMES

Pain from infective, inflammatory, or neoplastic processes is a feature of many visceral diseases and may be a conspicuous component of certain neurological or psychiatric diseases. It can also occur with no obvious cause.

In evaluating patients with pain, it is important to determine the level of the nervous system at which the pain arises and whether it has a primary neurological basis. In taking the history, attention should be focused on the mode of onset, duration, nature, severity, and location; any associated symptoms; and factors that precipitate or relieve the pain.

PERIPHERAL NERVE PAIN

Pain arising from peripheral nerve lesions is usually localized to the region that is affected pathologically or confined to the territory of the affected nerve. It may have a burning quality, and when mixed (motor and sensory) nerves are involved, there may be an accompanying motor deficit. Painful peripheral neuropathies include those caused by diabetes, polyarteritis, alcoholic-nutritional deficiency states, and the various entrapment neuropathies. Treatment of pain associated with peripheral neuropathies is discussed in the section on diabetic neuropathy above. The term **causalgia** correctly is used for the severe persistent pain, often burning in quality, that results from nerve trauma. Such pain often radiates to a more extensive territory than is supplied by the affected nerve and is associated with exquisite tenderness. Onset of pain may be at any time within the first six weeks or so after nerve injury. The cause is uncertain, but it has been attributed to ephaptic transmission between efferent sympathetic and afferent somatic fibers at the site of injury. Pain may be accompanied by increased sweating and vasoconstriction of the affected extremity, which is commonly kept covered up and still by the patient. **Reflex sympathetic dystrophy** is a more general term that denotes sympathetically mediated pain syndromes precipitated by a wide variety of tissue injuries, including soft tissue trauma, bone fractures, and myocardial infarction. Medical approaches to treatment include sympathetic blockade by injection of local anesthetics into the sympathetic chain or by regional infusion of reserpine or guanethidine. One such procedure may produce permanent cessation of pain—or repeated sympathetic blocks may be required. Surgical sympathectomy is beneficial in up to 75% of cases.

RADICULAR PAIN

Radicular pain is localized to the distribution of one or more nerve roots and is often exacerbated by coughing, sneezing, and other maneuvers that increase intraspinal pressure. It is also exacerbated by maneuvers that stretch the affected roots. Passive straight leg raising leads to stretching of the sacral and lower lumbar roots, as does passive flexion of the neck. Spinal movements that narrow the intervertebral foramina can aggravate root pain. Extension and lateral flexion of the head to the affected side may thus exacerbate cervical root symptoms. In addition to pain, root lesions can cause paresthesias and numbness in a dermatomal distribution (see Figure 7–4); they can also cause segmental

weakness, and reflex changes, depending upon the level affected. Useful modes of treatment include immobilization, non-steroidal anti-inflammatory drugs or other analgesics, and surgical decompression.

THALAMIC PAIN

Depending upon their extent and precise location, thalamic lesions may lead to pain in all or part of the contralateral half of the body. The pain is of a burning nature with a particularly unpleasant quality that patients have difficulty describing. It is aggravated by emotional stress and tends to develop during partial recovery from a sensory deficit caused by the underlying thalamic lesion. Mild cutaneous stimulation may produce very unpleasant and painful sensations. This combination of sensory loss, spontaneous pain, and perverted cutaneous sensation has come to be called **Dejerine-Roussy** syndrome. Similar pain can be produced by a lesion that involves the parietal lobe or the sensory pathways at any point in the cord (posterior columns or spinothalamic tract) or in the brain stem. Treatment with analgesics, anticonvulsants (carbamazepine or phenytoin), or antidepressants and phenothiazines in combination is occasionally helpful.

BACK & NECK PAIN

Spinal disease occurs most commonly in the neck or low back and can cause local or root pain or both. It can also lead to pain that is referred to other parts of the involved dermatomes. Pain from the lower lumbar spine, for example, is often referred to the buttocks. Conversely, pain may be referred to the back from the viscera, especially the pelvic organs. Local pain may lead to protective reflex muscle spasm, which in turn causes further pain and may result in abnormal posture, limitation of movement, and local spinal tenderness.

The history may provide clues to the underlying cause, and physical examination will define any neurological involvement.

Diagnostic studies that can help in evaluating patients include x-rays of the affected region and a complete blood count and erythrocyte sedimentation rate (especially if infective or inflammatory disorders or myeloma is suspected); determination of serum protein and protein electrophoresis; and measurement of serum calcium, phosphorus, alkaline and acid phosphatase, and uric acid. Electromyography may be helpful in determining the extent and severity of root involvement; it also provides a guide to prognosis. A CT scan or MRI of the spine and a myelogram may be necessary, especially if neoplasm is suspected, neurological deficits are progressive, pain persists despite conservative treatment measures, or there is evidence of cord involvement. At myelography, CSF can be obtained for laboratory examination.

1. LOW BACK PAIN

Low back pain is a common cause of time lost from work. It has many causes.

Trauma

Unaccustomed exertion or activity—or lifting heavy objects without adequate bracing of the spine —can cause musculoskeletal pain that improves with rest. Clinical examination commonly reveals spasm of the lumbar muscles and restricted spinal movements. Management includes local heat, bed rest on a firm mattress, non-steroidal anti-inflammatory drugs or other analgesics, and muscle-relaxant drugs, eg, diazepam, 2 mg three times daily, increased gradually until symptoms are relieved (or to the highest dose tolerated). Vertebral fractures that follow more severe injury and lead to local pain and tenderness can be visualized at radiography. If cord involvement is suspected—eg, because of leg weakness following injury—the patient must be immobilized until radiographed to determine whether fracture-dislocation of the vertebral column has occurred.

Prolapsed Lumbar Intervertebral Disk

This most commonly affects the L5–S1 or the L4–5 disk. The prolapse may relate to injury, but in many patients it commonly follows minor strain or normal activity. Protruded disk material may press on one or more nerve roots and thus produce radicular pain, a segmental motor or sensory deficit, or a sphincter disturbance in addition to a painful stiff back. The pain may be reproduced by percussion over the spine or sciatic nerve, by passive straight leg raising, or by extension of the knee while the hip is flexed. The presence of bilateral symptoms and signs suggests that disk material has protruded centrally, and this is more likely to be associated with sphincter involvement than is lateral protrusion. An L5 radiculopathy causes weak dorsiflexion of the foot and toes, while an S1 root lesion leads to a depressed ankle jerk and weakness of eversion and plantar flexion of the foot. In either case, spinal movements are restricted, there is local tenderness, and Lasègue's sign (reproducing the patient's pain on stretching the sciatic nerve by straight leg raising) is positive. The L4 root is occasionally affected, but involvement of a higher lumbar root should arouse suspicion of other causes of root compression. Pelvic and rectal examination and plain x-rays of the spine help to exclude other diseases, such as local tumors or metastatic neoplastic deposits. Symptoms often resolve with simple analgesics, diazepam, and bed rest on a firm mattress for two to four weeks, followed by gradual mobilization.

Persisting pain, an increasing neurological deficit, or any evidence of sphincter dysfunction should lead to myelography, MRI or CT scanning, and surgical treatment if indicated by the results of these procedures.

Lumbar Osteoarthropathy

This tends to occur in later life and may cause low back pain that is increased by activity. Radiological abnormalities vary in severity. In patients with mild symptoms, a surgical corset is helpful, while in more severe cases operative treatment may be necessary. Even minor changes may cause root or cord dysfunction in patients with a congenitally narrowed spinal canal, leading to the syndrome of **intermittent claudication of the cord** or **cauda equina.** This is characterized by pain—sometimes accompanied by weakness or radicular sensory disturbances in the legs—that occurs with activity or with certain postures and is relieved by rest. In such circumstances, spinal decompression is indicated.

Ankylosing Spondylitis

Backache and stiffness, followed by progressive limitation of movement, characterize this disorder, which occurs predominantly in young men. Characteristic early radiological findings consist of sclerosis and narrowing of the sacroiliac joints. Treatment is with non-steroidal anti-inflammatory agents, especially indomethacin or aspirin. Physical therapy, including postural exercises, is also important.

Neoplastic Disease

Extradural malignant tumors are an important cause of back pain and should be suspected if there is persistent pain that worsens despite bed rest. They may eventually lead to cord compression or a cauda equina syndrome, depending upon the level of involvement. There may initially be no change on plain radiographs of the spine, but a bone scan is sometimes revealing. Benign osteogenic tumors also produce back pain, and plain x-rays then show a lytic lesion; treatment is by excision.

Infections

Tuberculous and pyogenic infections of the vertebrae or intervertebral disks can cause progressive low back pain and local tenderness. While there are sometimes no systemic signs of infection, the peripheral white cell count and sedimentation rate are raised. X-rays may show disk space narrowing and a soft tissue mass, but they are frequently normal initially.

The osteomyelitis requires long-term antimicrobial therapy; surgical debridement and drainage may also be needed. Spinal epidural abscess (see Chapter 6) similarly presents with localized pain and tenderness, sometimes associated with osteomyelitis. Cord compression may occur with the onset of a rapidly progressive flaccid paraplegia. MRI, CT scanning, or myelography and operative treatment are undertaken urgently if there is evidence of cord compression. In early cases without neurological involvement, treatment with antibiotics alone may be sufficient.

Osteoporosis

Low back pain is a common complaint in patients with osteoporosis, and vertebral fractures may occur spontaneously or after trivial trauma. Pain may be helped by a brace to support the back. It is important that patients keep active and take a diet containing adequate amounts of calcium, vitamin D, and protein. Estrogen therapy may be helpful in postmenopausal women. In special circumstances, calcitonin, sodium fluoride, or phosphate supplements are helpful.

Paget's Disease of the Spine

Paget's disease, which is characterized by excessive bone destruction and repair, is of unknown cause but may have a familial basis. Pain is commonly the first symptom. Vertebral involvement may also lead to evidence of cord or root compression. The serum calcium and phosphorus levels are normal, but the alkaline phosphatase is markedly increased. Urinary hydroxyproline and calcium are increased when the disease is active. X-rays show expansion and increased density of the involved bones, and fissure fractures may be evident in the long bones.

Treatment includes prescription of a high-protein diet with vitamin C supplements. Calcium intake should be high in active patients and restricted in immobilized patients. Vitamin D supplements—50,000 units three times a week—and anabolic hormones may also be helpful. In active, progressive disease, treatment with calcitonin, diphosphonates, or mithramycin reduces osteoclastic activity.

Congenital Anomalies

Minor spinal anomalies can cause pain because of altered mechanics or alignment or because reduction in the size of the spinal canal renders the cord or roots more liable to compression by degenerative or other changes. Children or young adults with congenital defects in spinal fusion (**spinal dysraphism**) occasionally present with pain, a neurological deficit in one or both legs, or sphincter disturbances.

Treatment is of the underlying disorder.

Arachnoiditis

Severe pain in the back and legs can result from inflammation and fibrosis of the arachnoid layer of the spinal meninges (arachnoiditis), which may be idiopathic or causally related to previous surgery, infection, myelography, or long-standing disk disease. There is no adequate treatment, but operation may be possible if the arachnoiditis is localized. This condition is considered in more detail in Chapter 6.

Referred Pain

Disease of the hip joints may cause pain in the back and thighs that is enhanced by activity; examination reveals limitation of movement at the joint with a positive **Patrick sign** (hip pain on rotation of the hip), and x-rays show degenerative changes. Aortic aneurysms, cardiac ischemia, visceral and genitourinary disease (especially pelvic disorders in women), and retroperitoneal masses also cause back pain. There are often other symptoms and signs that suggest the underlying disorder. Moreover, there is no localized spinal tenderness or restriction of motility.

Treatment is of the underlying cause.

Nonspecific Chronic Back Pain

In many patients whose chronic back pain poses a difficult management problem, there are no objective clinical signs or obvious causes for pain despite detailed investigations. In some cases, the pain may have a postural basis; in others, it may be a somatic manifestation of a psychiatric disorder. Pain that initially had an organic basis is often enhanced or perpetuated by nonorganic factors and leads to disability out of proportion to the symptoms.

Treatment with tricyclic antidepressant drugs is sometimes helpful, and psychiatric evaluation may be worthwhile. Unnecessary surgical procedures must be avoided.

2. NECK PAIN

Congenital abnormalities of the cervical spine, such as hemivertebrae or fused vertebrae, basilar impression, and instability of the atlantoaxial joint, can cause neck pain. The traumatic, infective, and neoplastic disorders mentioned above as causes of low back pain can also affect the cervical spine and then produce pain in the neck. Rheumatoid arthritis may involve the spine, especially in the cervical region, leading to pain, stiffness, and reduced mobility; cord compression may result from displacement of vertebrae or atlantoaxial subluxation and can be life-threatening if not treated by fixation.

Acute Cervical Disk Protrusion

Patients may present with neck and radicular arm pain that are exacerbated by head movement. With lateral herniation of the disk, there may also be segmental motor, sensory, or reflex changes, usually at the C6 or C7 level, on the affected side. With more centrally directed herniations, spastic paraparesis and a sensory disturbance in the legs, sometimes accompanied by impaired sphincter function, can occur as a result of cord involvement. The diagnosis is confirmed by myelography and CT scan or MRI.

In mild cases, bed rest or intermittent neck traction, followed by immobilization of the neck in a collar for several weeks, often helps. If these measures fail or if there is a significant neurological deficit, surgical treatment may be necessary.

Cervical Spondylosis

This is an important cause of pain in the neck and arms, sometimes accompanied by a segmental motor or sensory deficit in the arms or by spastic paraparesis. It is discussed in Chapter 6.

3. HERPES ZOSTER (Shingles)

This viral disorder becomes increasingly common with advancing age, causing an inflammatory reaction in one or more of the dorsal root or cranial nerve ganglia, in the affected root or nerve itself, and in the CSF. There seems to be spontaneous reactivation of varicella virus that remained latent in sensory ganglia after previous infection. Herpes zoster is common in patients with lymphoma, especially following regional radiotherapy. The initial complaint is of a burning or shooting pain in the involved dermatome, followed within two to five days by the development of a vesicular erythematous rash. The pain may diminish in intensity as the rash develops. The rash becomes crusted and scaly after a few days and then fades, leaving small anesthetic scars. The pain and dysesthesias may last for several weeks or, in some instances, may persist for many months (**post-herpetic neuralgia**) before subsiding, especially in the elderly. Pain is exacerbated by touching the involved area. Superficial sensation is often impaired in the affected dermatome, and focal weakness and atrophy can also occur. Signs are usually limited to one dermatome, but more are occasionally involved. Mild pleocytosis and an increased protein concentration sometimes occur in the CSF. The most commonly involved sites are the thoracic dermatomes, but involvement of the first division of the fifth cranial nerve, also common, is especially distressing and may lead to corneal scarring and anesthesia. Facial (VII) nerve palsy occurring in association with a herpetic eruption that involves the ear, palate, pharynx, or neck is called **Ramsay Hunt syndrome.**

There is no specific treatment. Analgesics provide symptomatic relief. Corticosteroids or acyclovir may reduce the duration and severity of the acute eruption. Corticosteroids—but not acyclovir—may also reduce the likelihood that postherpetic neuralgia will occur. Although postherpetic neuralgia can be very distressing, it sometimes responds to treatment with carbamazepine, up to 1200 mg/d; phenytoin, 300 mg/d; or amitriptyline, 10–100 mg at bedtime. Attempts at relieving postherpetic neuralgia by peripheral nerve section are generally unrewarding.

REFERENCES

General

Aminoff MJ: *Electromyography in Clinical Practice,* 2nd ed. Churchill Livingstone, 1987.

Davidoff RA: The dorsal columns. *Neurology* 1989; 39:1377–1385.

Layzer RB: *Neuromuscular Manifestations of Systemic Disease.* Vol 25 of: *Contemporary Neurology Series.* Davis, 1984.

Polyneuropathies

Asbury AK, Cornblath DR: Assessment of current diagnostic criteria for Guillain-Barré syndrome. *Ann Neurol* 1990;27(Suppl):S21–S24.

Barohn RJ et al: Chronic inflammatory demyelinating polyradiculoneuropathy: clinical characteristics, course, and recommendations for diagnostic criteria. *Arch Neurol* 1989;46:878–884.

Brown MJ, Asbury AK: Diabetic neuropathy. *Ann Neurol* 1984;15:2–12.

Browne SG: Leprosy: Clinical aspects of nerve involvement. Pages 1–16 in: *Topics on Tropical Neurology.* Hornabrook RW (editor). Vol 12 of: *Contemporary Neurology Series.* Davis, 1975.

Charness ME, Simon RP, Greenberg DA: Ethanol and the nervous system. *N Engl J Med* 1989;321:442–454.

Cornblath DR, McArthur JC: Predominatly sensory neuropathy in patients with AIDS and AIDS-related complex. *Neurology* 1988;38:794–796.

Dyck PJ et al: Chronic inflammatory polyradiculoneuropathy. *Mayo Clin Proc* 1975;50:621–637.

Lotti M, Becker CE, Aminoff MJ: Organophosphate polyneuropathy: Pathogenesis and prevention. *Neurology* 1984;34:658–662.

McKhann GM: Guillain-Barré syndrome: Clinical and therapeutic observations. *Ann Neurol* 1990;27 (Suppl):S13–S16.

Miller RG, Storey JR, Greco CM: Ganciclovir in the treatment of progressive AIDS-related polyradiculopathy. *Neurology* 1990;40:569–574.

Parry GJ: Peripheral neuropathies associated with human immunodeficiency virus infection. *Ann Neurol* 1988; 23(Suppl):S49–S53.

Parry GJ, Bredesen DE: Sensory neuropathy with low-dose pyridoxine. *Neurology* 1985;**35:**1466–1468.

Ropper AH: The Guillain-Barré syndrome. *N Engl J Med* 1992;326:1130–1136.

Schaumburg HH, Berger AR, Thomas PK: *Disorders of Peripheral Nerves,* 2nd ed. Vol 36 of: *Contemporary Neurology Series.* Davis, 1992.

Shannon KM, Goetz CG: Connective tissue diseases and the nervous system. Pages 389–411 in: *Neurology and General Medicine.* Aminoff MJ (editor). Churchill Livingstone, 1989.

Smith BE, Dyck PJ: Peripheral neuropathy in the eosinophilia-myalgia syndrome associated with L-tryptophan ingestion. *Neurology* 1990;40:1035–1040.

Entrapment Neuropathies

Dawson DM, Hallett M, Millender LH: *Entrapment Neuropathies,* 2nd ed. Little, Brown, 1990.

Spinner RJ, Bachman JW, Amadio PC: The many faces of carpal tunnel syndrome. *Mayo Clin Proc* 1989;64:829–836.

Root and Plexus Lesions

Jaeckle KA, Young DF, Foley KM: The natural history of lumbosacral plexopathy in cancer. *Neurology* 1985;35:8–15.

Kori SH, Foley KM, Posner JB: Brachial plexus lesions in patients with cancer: 100 cases. *Neurology* 1981;31:45–50.

Pachner AR: Lyme disease. *Trends Neurosci* 1989;12:177–181.

Steere AC: Lyme disease. *N Engl J Med* 1989;321:586–596.

Thomas JE, Cascino TL, Earle JD: Differential diagnosis between radiation and tumor plexopathy of the pelvis. *Neurology* 1985;35:1–7.

Myelopathies

Lindenbaum J et al: Neuropsychiatric disorders caused by cobalamin deficiency in the absence of anemia or macrocytosis. *N Engl J Med* 1988;318:1720–1728.

Pain Syndromes

Frymoyer JW: Back pain and sciatica. *N Engl J Med* 1988;318:291–300.

Portenoy RK, Duma C, Foley KM: Acute herpetic and

8

Movement Disorders

Movement disorders (sometimes called **extra-pyramidal disorders**) impair the regulation of voluntary motor activity without directly affecting strength, sensation, or cerebellar function. They include hyperkinetic disorders associated with abnormal, involuntary movements and hypokinetic disorders characterized by poverty of movement. Movement disorders result from dysfunction of deep subcortical gray matter structures termed the **basal ganglia.** While there is no universally accepted anatomical definition of the basal ganglia, for clinical purposes they may be considered to comprise the caudate nucleus, putamen, globus pallidus, subthalamic nucleus, and substantia nigra. The putamen and globus pallidus are collectively termed the **lentiform**

nucleus; the combination of lentiform nucleus and caudate nucleus is designated the **corpus striatum.**

The basic circuitry of the basal ganglia consists of three interacting neuronal loops (Figure 8–1). The first is a corticocortical loop that passes from the cerebral cortex, through the caudate and putamen, the internal segment of globus pallidus, and the thalamus, and then back to the cerebral cortex. The second is a nigrostriatal loop connecting the substantia nigra with the caudate and putamen. The third, a striopallidal loop, projects from the caudate and putamen to the external segment of globus pallidus, then to the subthalamic nucleus, and finally to the internal segment of globus pallidus. In some movement disorders (eg, Parkinson's disease), a discrete site of pathology

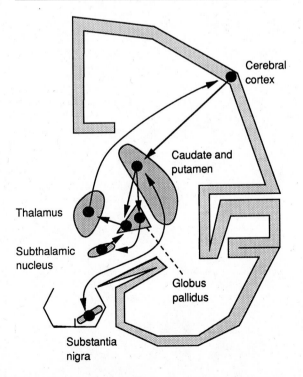

Figure 8–1. Basic neuronal circuitry of the basal ganglia.

within these pathways can be identified; in other cases (eg, essential tremor), the precise anatomical abnormality is unknown.

TYPES OF ABNORMAL MOVEMENTS

Categorizing an abnormal movement is generally the first step toward arriving at the neurological diagnosis. Abnormal movements can be classified as tremor, chorea, athetosis or dystonia, ballismus, myoclonus, or tics. Such movements can arise for a variety of reasons. In many disorders, abnormal movements are the sole clinical features.

TREMOR

A tremor is a rhythmic oscillatory movement best characterized by its relationship to voluntary motor activity—ie, according to whether it occurs at rest, during maintenance of a particular posture, or during movement. The major causes of tremor are listed in Table 8–1. Tremor is enhanced by emotional stress and disappears during sleep. Tremor that occurs when the limb is at rest is generally referred to as **static tremor,** or **rest tremor.** If present during sustained posture, it is called a **postural tremor;** while this tremor may continue during movement, movement does not increase its severity. When present during movement but not at rest, it is generally called

Table 8–1. Causes of tremor.

Postural tremor
  Physiological tremor
  Enhanced physiological tremor
    Anxiety or fear
    Excessive physical activity or sleep deprivation
    Sedative drug or alcohol withdrawal
    Drug toxicity (eg, lithium, bronchodilators, tricyclic antidepressants)
    Heavy metal poisoning (eg, mercury, lead arsenic)
    Carbon monoxide poisoning
    Thyrotoxicosis
    Familial (autosomal dominant) or idiopathic (benign essential) tremor
    Cerebellar disorders
    Wilson's disease
Intention tremor
  Brain stem or cerebellar disease
  Drug toxicity (eg, alcohol, anticonvulsants, sedatives)
  Wilson's disease
Rest tremor
  Parkinsonism
  Wilson's disease
  Heavy metal poisoning (eg, mercury)

an **intention tremor.** Both postural and intention tremors are also called **action tremors.**

Postural Tremor

A. Physiological Tremor: An 8- to 12-Hz tremor of the outstretched hands is a normal finding. Its physiological basis is uncertain.

B. Enhanced Physiological Tremor: Physiological tremor may be enhanced by fear or anxiety. A more conspicuous postural tremor may also be found following excessive physical activity or sleep deprivation. It can complicate treatment with certain drugs (notably lithium, tricyclic antidepressants, and bronchodilators) and is often conspicuous in patients with alcoholism or in alcohol or drug withdrawal states. It is common in thyrotoxicosis, and it can also result from poisoning with a number of substances, including mercury, lead, arsenic, and carbon monoxide.

There is no specific medical therapy.

C. Other Causes: The most common type of abnormal postural tremor is **benign essential tremor,** which often has a familial basis. Postural tremor may also be conspicuous in patients with Wilson's disease or cerebellar disorders.

Asterixis

Asterixis may be associated with postural tremor, but is itself more properly considered a form of myoclonus (see below) than of tremor. It is seen most commonly in patients with metabolic encephalopathy such as occurs with hepatic or renal failure.

To detect asterixis, the examiner asks the patient to hold the arm outstretched with fingers and wrists extended. Episodic cessation of muscular activity causes sudden flexion at the wrist followed by a return to extension, so that the hands flap in a regular or, more often, an irregular rhythm. The asterixis resolves with clearing of the metabolic encephalopathy.

Intention Tremor

Intention tremor occurs during activity. If the patient is asked to touch his or her nose with a finger, for example, the arm exhibits tremor during movement, often more marked as the target is reached. This form of tremor is sometimes mistaken for limb ataxia, but the latter has no rhythmic oscillatory component.

Intention tremor results from a lesion affecting the superior cerebellar peduncle. Because it is often very coarse, it can lead to severe functional disability. No satisfactory medical treatment exists, but stereotactic surgery of the ventrolateral nucleus of the thalamus is sometimes helpful when patients are severely incapacitated.

Intention tremor can also occur—together with other signs of cerebellar involvement—as a manifestation of toxicity of certain sedative or anticonvulsant drugs (such as phenytoin) or alcohol; it is seen in patients with Wilson's disease.

Rest Tremor

A. Parkinsonism: Rest tremor usually has a frequency of 4–6 Hz and is characteristic of parkinsonism whether the disorder is idiopathic or secondary (ie, postencephalitic, toxic, or drug-induced in origin). The rate of the tremor, its relationship to activity, and the presence of rigidity or hypokinesia usually distinguish the tremor of parkinsonism from other forms. Tremor in the hands may appear as a "pill-rolling" maneuver—rhythmic, opposing circular movements of the thumb and index finger. There may be alternating flexion and extension of the fingers or hand, or alternating pronation and supination of the forearm; in the feet, rhythmic alternating flexion and extension are common. Parkinsonism is discussed in more detail below.

B. Other Causes: Less common causes of rest tremor include Wilson's disease and poisoning with heavy metals such as mercury.

CHOREA

The word **chorea** denotes rapid irregular muscle jerks that occur involuntarily and unpredictably in different parts of the body. In florid cases, the often forceful involuntary movements of the limbs and head and the accompanying facial grimacing and tongue movements are unmistakable. Voluntary movements may be distorted by the superimposed involuntary ones. In mild cases, however, patients may exhibit no more than a persistent restlessness and clumsiness. Power is generally full, but there may be difficulty in maintaining muscular contraction such that, for example, hand grip is relaxed intermittently (milkmaid grasp). The gait becomes irregular and unsteady, with the patient suddenly dipping or lurching to one side or the other (dancing gait). Speech often becomes irregular in volume and tempo and may be explosive in character. In some patients, athetotic movements or dystonic posturing may also be prominent. Chorea disappears during sleep.

Classification & Pathology

The pathological basis of chorea is unclear, but in some cases it is associated with cell loss in the caudate nucleus and putamen, and it can be provoked by dopaminergic agonist drugs. The important causes of chorea are shown in Table 8–2 and are discussed later in this chapter. When chorea is due to a treatable medical disorder, such as polycythemia vera or thyrotoxicosis, adequate treatment of the primary disorder abolishes the dyskinesia.

HEMIBALLISMUS

Hemiballismus is unilateral chorea that is especially violent because the proximal muscles of the limbs are involved. It is due most often to vascular

Table 8–2. Causes of chorea.

Hereditary
  Huntington's disease
  Benign hereditary chorea
  Wilson's disease
  Paroxysmal choreoathetosis
  Familial chorea with associated acanthocytosis
Static encephalopathy (cerebral palsy) acquired antenatally or perinatally (eg, from anoxia, hemorrhage, trauma, kernicterus)
Sydenham's chorea
Chorea gravidarum
Drug toxicity
  Levodopa and other dopaminergic drugs
  Antipsychotic drugs
  Lithium
  Phenytoin
  Oral contraceptives
Miscellaneous medical disorders
  Thyrotoxicosis, hypoparathyroidism, or Addison's disease
  Hypocalcemia, hypomagnesemia, or hypernatremia
  Polycythemia vera
  Hepatic cirrhosis
  Systemic lupus erythematosus
  Encephalitis lethargica
Cerebrovascular disorders
  Vasculitis
  Ischemic or hemorrhagic stroke
  Subdural hematoma
Structural lesions of the subthalamic nucleus

disease in the contralateral subthalamic nucleus and commonly resolves spontaneously in the weeks following its onset. It is sometimes due to other types of structural disease; in the past, it was an occasional complication of thalamotomy. Pharmacological treatment is similar to that for chorea (see below).

DYSTONIA & ATHETOSIS

The term **athetosis** generally denotes abnormal movements that are slow, sinuous, and writhing in character. When the movements are so sustained that they are better regarded as abnormal postures, the term **dystonia** is used, and many now use the terms interchangeably. The abnormal movements and postures may be generalized or restricted in distribution. In the latter circumstance, one or more of the limbs may be affected (**segmental dystonia**) or the disturbance may be restricted to localized muscle groups (**focal dystonia**).

Factors Influencing Dystonia

The abnormal movements are not present during sleep. They are generally enhanced by emotional stress and by voluntary activity. In some cases, abnormal movements or postures occur only during voluntary activity and sometimes only during specific activities such as writing, speaking, or chewing.

Etiology

Table 8–3 lists some of the conditions in which

Table 8–3. Causes of dystonia and athetosis.

Static perinatal encephalopathy (cerebral palsy)
Wilson's disease
Huntington's disease
Parkinson's disease
Drugs
   Levodopa
   Antipsychotic drugs
   Others (see text)
Encephalitis lethargica
Ischemic anoxia
Focal intracranial disease
Progressive supranuclear palsy
Idiopathic torsion dystonia
   Hereditary
   Sporadic
Formes frustes of idiopathic torsion dystonia

these movement disorders are encountered. Perinatal anoxia, birth trauma, and kernicterus are the most common causes. In these circumstances, abnormal movements usually develop before age five years. Careful questioning usually discloses a history of abnormal early development and often of seizures. Examination may reveal signs of mental retardation or a pyramidal deficit in addition to the movement disorder.

Torsion dystonia may occur as a manifestation of Wilson's disease or Huntington's disease or as a sequela of previous encephalitis lethargica.

Dystonic movements and postures are the cardinal features of the disorder known as idiopathic torsion dystonia (discussed at length below).

Acute dystonic posturing may result from treatment with dopamine receptor antagonist drugs (discussed on p 224).

Lateralized dystonia may occasionally relate to focal intracranial disease, but the clinical context in which it occurs usually identifies the underlying cause.

MYOCLONUS

Myoclonic jerks are sudden, rapid, twitchlike muscle contractions. They can be classified according to their distribution, relationship to precipitating stimuli, or etiology. **Generalized myoclonus** has a widespread distribution, while **focal** or **segmental myoclonus** is restricted to a particular part of the body. Myoclonus can be spontaneous, or it can be brought on by sensory stimulation, arousal, or the initiation of movement **(action myoclonus).** Myoclonus may occur as a normal phenomenon **(physiological myoclonus)** in healthy persons, as an isolated abnormality **(essential myoclonus)** or as a manifestation of epilepsy **(epileptic myoclonus).** It can also occur as a feature of a variety of degenerative, infectious, and metabolic disorders **(symptomatic myoclonus).**

Generalized Myoclonus

The causes of generalized myoclonus are summa-

rized in Table 8–4. Physiological myoclonus includes the myoclonus that occurs upon falling asleep or awakening **(nocturnal myoclonus),** as well as hiccup. Essential myoclonus is a benign condition that occurs in the absence of other neurological abnormalities and is sometimes inherited. Epileptic myoclonus may be impossible to differentiate clinically from nonepileptic forms. It may be possible to distinguish the two types electrophysiologically, however, by the duration of the electromyographic burst associated with the jerking, by demonstrating an electroencephalographic correlate with a consistent temporal relationship to the jerks, or by determining whether muscles involved in the same jerk are activated synchronously.

Segmental Myoclonus

Segmental myoclonus can arise from lesions affecting the cerebral cortex, brain stem, or spinal cord. For example, involvement of the dentatorubro-olivary pathway by stroke, multiple sclerosis, tumors, or other disorders can produce **palatal myoclonus,** which may be associated with an audible click or synchronous movements of ocular, facial, or other bulbar muscles. Segmental myoclonus can result from many of the same disturbances that produce symptomatic generalized myoclonus (Table 8–4). Metabolic disorders such as hyperosmolar nonketotic hyperglycemia can cause **epilepsia partialis continua,** in which a repetitive focal epileptic discharge occurs from the contralateral sensorimotor cortex and leads to segmental myoclonus. Segmental myoclonus is usually unaffected by external stimuli and persists during sleep.

Table 8–4. Causes of generalized myoclonus.

Physiological myoclonus
   Nocturnal myoclonus
   Hiccup
Essential myoclonus
Epileptic myoclonus
Symptomatic myoclonus
   Degenerative disorders
      Dentatorubrothalamic atrophy (Ramsay Hunt syndrome)
      Storage diseases (eg, Lafora body disease)
      Wilson's disease
      Huntington's disease
      Alzheimer's disease
   Infectious disorders
      Creutzfeldt-Jakob disease
      AIDS dementia complex
      Subacute sclerosing panencephalitis
   Metabolic disorders
      Drug intoxications (eg, penicillin, antidepressants, anticonvulsants)
      Drug withdrawal (ethanol, sedatives)
      Hypoglycemia
      Hyperosmolar nonketotic hyperglycemia
      Hyponatremia
      Hepatic encephalopathy
      Uremia
      Hypoxia

Treatment

Although myoclonus can be difficult to treat, it sometimes responds to anticonvulsant drugs such as valproic acid, 250–500 mg orally three times daily, or to benzodiazepines such as clonazepam, 0.5 mg orally three times daily, gradually increased to as much as 12 mg/d. Postanoxic action myoclonus has recently been found to be remarkably responsive to 5-hydroxytryptophan, the metabolic precursor of the neurotransmitter 5-hydroxytryptamine (serotonin). The dosage of 5-hydroxytryptophan is increased gradually to a maximum of 1–1.5 mg/d orally and may be combined with carbidopa (maximum, 400 mg/d orally) to inhibit metabolism in peripheral tissues.

TICS

Tics are sudden, recurrent, quick, coordinated abnormal movements that can usually be imitated without difficulty. The same movement occurs again and again and can be suppressed voluntarily for short periods, although doing so may cause anxiety. Tics tend to worsen with stress, diminish during voluntary activity or mental concentration, and disappear during sleep.

Classification

Tics can be classified into four groups depending upon whether they are simple or multiple and transient or chronic.

Transient simple tics are very common in children, usually terminate spontaneously within one year (often within a few weeks), and generally require no treatment.

Chronic simple tics can develop at any age but often begin in childhood, and treatment is unnecessary in most cases. The benign nature of the disorder must be explained to the patient.

Persistent simple or multiple tics of childhood or adolescence generally begin before age 15 years. There may be single or multiple motor tics—and often vocal tics–but complete remission occurs by the end of adolescence.

The syndrome of **chronic multiple motor and vocal tics** is generally referred to as **Gilles de la Tourette's syndrome,** after the French physician who was one of the first to describe its clinical features. It is discussed in detail below.

CLINICAL EVALUATION OF PATIENTS

HISTORY

Age at Onset

The age at onset of a movement disorder may suggest the underlying cause. For example, onset in infancy or early childhood suggests birth trauma, kernicterus, cerebral anoxia, or an inherited disorder; abnormal facial movements developing in childhood are more likely to represent tics than involuntary movements of another sort; and tremor presenting in early adult life is more likely to be of the benign essential variety than due to Parkinson's disease.

The age at onset can also influence the prognosis. In **idiopathic torsion dystonia,** for example, progression to severe disability is much more common when symptoms develop in childhood than when they develop in later life. Conversely, **tardive dyskinesia** is more likely to be permanent and irreversible when it develops in the elderly than when it develops in the adolescent years.

Mode of Onset

Abrupt onset of dystonic posturing in a child or young adult should raise the possibility of a drug-induced reaction; a more gradual onset of dystonic movements and postures in an adolescent suggests the possibility of a chronic disorder such as idiopathic torsion dystonia or Wilson's disease. Similarly, the abrupt onset of severe chorea or ballismus suggests a vascular cause, and abrupt onset of severe parkinsonism suggests a neurotoxic cause; more gradual, insidious onset suggests a degenerative cause.

Course

The manner in which the disorder progresses from its onset may also be helpful diagnostically. For example, Sydenham's chorea usually resolves within about six months after onset and should, therefore, not be confused with other varieties of chorea that occur in childhood.

Medical History

A. Drug History: It is important to obtain an accurate account of all drugs that have been taken by the patient over the years, since many of the movement disorders are iatrogenic. The phenothiazine and butyrophenone drugs may lead to the development of abnormal movements either while patients are taking them or after their use has been discontinued, and the dyskinesia may be irreversible. Reversible dyskinesia may develop in patients taking certain other drugs, including oral contraceptives, levodopa, and phenytoin. Several drugs, especially lithium, tricyclic antidepressants, valproic acid, and bronchodilators, can cause tremor.

B. General Medical Background:

1. Chorea may be symptomatic of the disease in patients with a history of rheumatic fever, thyroid disease, systemic lupus erythematosus, polycythemia, hypoparathyroidism, or cirrhosis of the liver.

2. Movement disorders, including tremor, chorea, hemiballismus, dystonia, and myoclonus, have been described in patients with AIDS. Opportunistic infections such as cerebral toxoplasmosis appear to be the cause in some cases, but infection with HIV-1 may also have a direct pathogenetic role.

3. A history of birth trauma or perinatal distress may suggest the cause of a movement disorder that develops during childhood.

4. Encephalitis lethargica is no longer encountered clinically; it was epidemic in the 1920s, however, and was often followed by a wide variety of movement disorders, including parkinsonism. It is therefore important to inquire about this disease when elderly patients are being evaluated.

Family History

Some movement disorders have an inherited basis (Table 8–5), and it is essential that a complete family history be obtained, supplemented if possible by personal scrutiny of close relatives. Any possibility of consanguinity should be noted.

EXAMINATION

Clinical examination will indicate the nature of the abnormal movements, the extent of neurological involvement, and the presence of coexisting disease; these in turn may suggest the diagnosis.

The mental status examination may suggest psychiatric disease, raising the possibility that the abnormal movements are related to the psychiatric disorder or to its treatment with psychoactive drugs—or that the patient has a disorder characterized by both abnormal movements and behavioral disturbances, such as Huntington's disease or Wilson's disease.

Focal motor or sensory deficits raise the possibility of a structural space-occupying lesion, as does papilledema. Kayser-Fleischer rings suggest Wilson's disease. Signs of vascular, hepatic, or metabolic disease may suggest other causes for a movement disorder, such as acquired hepatocerebral degeneration or vasculitis.

INVESTIGATIVE STUDIES

Several investigations may be of diagnostic help.

Blood & Urine Tests

Serum and urine copper and serum ceruloplasmin levels are important in diagnosing Wilson's disease.

Complete blood count and sedimentation rate are helpful in excluding polycythemia, vasculitis, or systemic lupus erythematosus, any of which can occasionally lead to a movement disorder.

Blood chemistries may reveal hepatic dysfunction related to Wilson's disease or acquired hepatocerebral degeneration; hyperthyroidism or hypocalcemia as a cause of chorea; or a variety of metabolic disorders associated with myoclonus.

Serological tests are helpful for diagnosing movement disorders caused by systemic lupus erythematosus. Neurosyphilis can be manifested clinically in a variety of ways and should always be excluded by appropriate serological tests in patients with neurological disease of uncertain etiology.

Electroencephalography

An EEG is sometimes helpful in diagnosing patients with myoclonus; otherwise, it is of limited usefulness.

Imaging

Radiological studies are occasionally helpful in evaluating patients with movement disorders. In some patients, intracranial calcification may be found by skull x-rays or CT scans; the significance of this finding, however, is not clear. CT scans or MRI may also reveal a tumor associated with focal dyskinesia, caudate atrophy due to Huntington's disease, or basal ganglia abnormalities associated with Wilson's disease.

Genetic Studies

Recombinant DNA technology has been used to generate probes for genes that determine certain in-

Table 8–5. Inheritable movement disorders.

Disorder	Mode of Inheritance[1]	Location of Gene Defect[2]
Huntington's disease	AD	4p16.3
Idiopathic torsion dystonia	AD	9q32–34
	AR	Unknown
	XLR	Xq21.3
Wilson's disease	AR	13q14–21
Benign (essential) familial tumor	AD	Unknown
Benign hereditary chorea	AD, AR	Unknown
Familial chorea-acanthocytosis	AR	Unknown
Paroxysmal dystonic choreoathetosis	AD	Unknown

[1]AD, autosomal dominant; AR, autosomal recessive; XLR, X-linked recessive.

[2]Initial number or letter indicates chromosome; p indicates short arm, q indicates long arm of chromosome; final number indicates location on long or short arm.

heritable movement disorders. In this manner, the gene responsible for Huntington's disease has been localized to the terminal band of the short arm of chromosome 4, and the gene for Wilson's disease to the long arm of chromosome 13. Genetic markers are potentially of diagnostic value in such disorders. Their use may be limited, however, by the genetic heterogeneity of some diseases, imprecise gene localization by certain probes, ethical concerns about adverse psychological reactions to the presymptomatic diagnosis of fatal disorders, and the potential for misuse of such information by prospective employers, insurance companies, and government agencies.

DISEASES & SYNDROMES MANIFESTED BY ABNORMAL MOVEMENTS

The more common and well-defined diseases or syndromes characterized by abnormal movements are discussed here with the principles of their treatment.

FAMILIAL, OR BENIGN, ESSENTIAL TREMOR

A postural tremor may be prominent in otherwise normal subjects. Although the pathophysiological basis of this disorder is uncertain, it often has a familial basis with an autosomal dominant mode of inheritance.

Symptoms may develop in the teenage or early adult years but often do not appear until later. The tremor usually involves one or both hands or the head and voice, while the legs tend to be spared. Examination usually reveals no other abnormalities. Although the tremor may become more conspicuous with time, it generally leads to little disability other than cosmetic and social embarrassment. In occasional cases, tremor interferes with the ability to perform fine or delicate tasks with the hands; handwriting is sometimes severely impaired. Speech is affected when the laryngeal muscles are involved. Patients commonly report that a small quantity of alcohol provides remarkable but transient relief; the mechanism is not known.

If treatment is warranted, propranolol, 40–120 mg orally twice daily, can be prescribed—but it will need to be taken for an indefinite period. Alternatively, if tremor is particularly disabling under certain predictable circumstances, it can be treated with a single oral dose of 40–120 mg of propranolol taken in anticipation of the precipitating circumstances. Primidone

has also been effective, but patients with essential tremor are often very sensitive to this drug, so that it must be introduced more gradually than when it is used to treat epilepsy. Patients are therefore started on 50 mg/d and the daily dose increased by 50 mg every 2 weeks until benefit occurs or side effects limit further increments. A dose of 100 or 150 mg three times a day is often effective.

PARKINSONISM

Parkinsonism occurs in all ethnic groups; in the United States and western Europe it has a prevalence of 1–2/1000 population, with an approximately equal sex distribution. It is characterized by tremor, hypokinesia, rigidity, and abnormal gait and posture.

Etiology

A. Idiopathic: A very common variety of parkinsonism occurs without obvious cause; this idiopathic form is called **Parkinson's disease** or **paralysis agitans.**

B. Encephalitis Lethargica: In the first half of the 20th century, parkinsonism often developed in patients with a history of von Economo's encephalitis. Since this type of infection is not now encountered, cases of **postencephalitic parkinsonism** are becoming increasingly rare.

C. Drug- or Toxin-Induced Parkinsonism:

1. Therapeutic drugs–Many drugs, such as phenothiazines, butyrophenones, metoclopramide, reserpine, and tetrabenazine, can cause a reversible parkinsonian syndrome (see p 224).

2. Toxic substances–Toxins such as manganese dust or carbon disulfide can also lead to parkinsonism, and the disorder may appear as a sequela of severe carbon monoxide poisoning.

3. MPTP (1-Methyl-4-phenyl-1,2,5,6-tetrahydropyridine)–A drug-induced form of parkinsonism has been described in individuals who synthesized and self-administered a meperidine analogue, MPTP (Figure 8–2). This compound is metabolized to a toxin that selectively destroys dopaminergic neurons in the substantia nigra and adrenergic neurons in the locus ceruleus and induces a severe form of parkinsonism in humans and in subhuman primates. The ability of this drug to reproduce neurochemical, pathological, and clinical features of Parkinson's disease suggests that an environmental toxin could be responsible for the idiopathic disorder. MPTP-induced parkinsonism may provide a model that could assist in development of new drugs for treatment of this disease.

D. Parkinsonism Associated with Other Neurological Diseases: Parkinsonism that occurs in association with symptoms and signs of other neurological disorders is considered briefly under *Differential Diagnosis* (below).

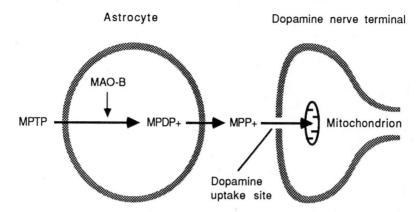

Figure 8–2. Proposed mechanism of MPTP-induced parkinsonism. MPTP enters brain astrocytes and is converted to MPDP$^+$ through the action of monoamine oxidase type B (MAO-B). MPDP$^+$ is then metabolized extracellularly to MPP$^+$, which is taken up through dopamine uptake sites on dopamine nerve terminals and concentrated in mitochondria. The resulting disturbance of mitochondrial function can lead to neuronal death.

Pathology

In idiopathic parkinsonism, pathological examination shows loss of pigmentation and cells in the **substantia nigra** and other brain stem centers, cell loss in the globus pallidus and putamen, and the presence of eosinophilic intraneural inclusion granules (**Lewy bodies**) in the basal ganglia, brain stem, spinal cord, and sympathetic ganglia. These inclusion bodies are not seen in postencephalitic parkinsonism; instead there may be nonspecific neurofibrillary degeneration in a number of diencephalic structures as well as changes in the substantia nigra.

Pathogenesis

Both dopamine and acetylcholine are present in the corpus striatum, where they act as neurotransmitters (Figure 8–3). In idiopathic parkinsonism, it is generally believed that the normal balance between these two antagonistic neurotransmitters is disturbed because of dopamine depletion in the dopaminergic nigrostriatal system (Figure 8–4). Other neurotransmitters, such as norepinephrine, are also depleted in the brains of patients with parkinsonism, but the clinical relevance of this deficiency is less clear.

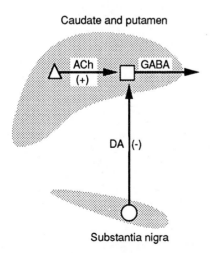

Figure 8–3. Simplified neurochemical anatomy of the basal ganglia. Dopamine (DA) neurons exert a net inhibitory effect and acetylcholine (ACh) neurons a net excitatory effect on the GABAergic output from the striatum.

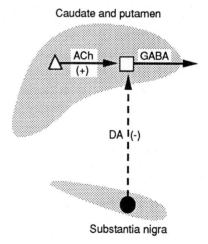

Figure 8–4. Neurochemical pathology of basal ganglia in Parkinson's disease. Dopamine (DA) neurons degenerate (black circle and dashed line), upsetting the normal balance between dopaminergic inhibition and cholinergic (ACh) excitation of striatal output (GABA) neurons. The net effect is to increase GABAergic output from the striatum.

Clinical Findings

A. Tremor: The 4- to 6-Hz tremor of parkinsonism is characteristically most conspicuous at rest; it increases at times of emotional stress and often improves during voluntary activity. It commonly begins in the hand or foot, where it takes the form of rhythmic flexion-extension of the fingers or of the hand or foot—or of rhythmic pronation-supination of the forearm. It frequently involves the face in the area of the mouth as well. Although it may ultimately be present in all of the limbs, it is not uncommon for the tremor to be confined to one limb—or to the two limbs on one side—for months or years before it becomes more generalized.

B. Rigidity: Rigidity, or increased tone—ie, increased resistance to passive movement—is a characteristic clinical feature of parkinsonism. The disturbance in tone is responsible for the flexed posture of many patients with parkinsonism. The resistance is typically uniform throughout the range of movement at a particular joint and affects agonist and antagonist muscles alike—in contrast to the findings in spasticity, where the increase in tone is often greatest at the beginning of the passive movement (clasp-knife phenomenon) and more marked in some muscles than in others. In some instances, the rigidity in parkinsonism is described as **cogwheel rigidity** because of ratchetlike interruptions of passive movement that may be due, in part, to the presence of tremor.

C. Hypokinesia: The most disabling feature of this disorder is hypokinesia (sometimes called bradykinesia or akinesia)—a slowness of voluntary movement and a reduction in automatic movement, such as swinging the arms while walking. The patient's face is relatively immobile **(masklike facies),** with widened palpebral fissures, infrequent blinking, a certain fixity of facial expression, and a smile that develops and fades slowly. The voice is of low volume **(hypophonia)** and tends to be poorly modulated. Fine or rapidly alternating movements are impaired, but power is not diminished if time is allowed for it to develop. The handwriting is small, tremulous, and hard to read.

D. Abnormal Gait and Posture: The patient generally finds it difficult to get up from bed or an easy chair and tends to adopt a flexed posture on standing (Figure 8–5). It is often difficult to start walking, so that the patient may lean farther and farther forward while walking in place before being able to advance. The gait itself is characterized by small, shuffling steps and absence of the arm swing that normally accompanies locomotion; there is generally some unsteadiness on turning, and there may be difficulty in stopping. In advanced cases, the patient tends to walk with increasing speed to prevent a fall **(festinating gait)** because of the altered center of gravity that results from the abnormal posture.

E. Other Clinical Features: There is often mild **blepharoclonus** (fluttering of the closed eyelids) and

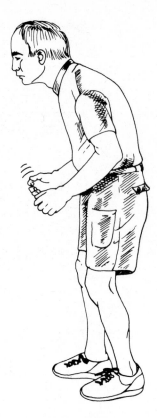

Figure 8–5. Typical flexed posture of a patient with parkinsonism.

occasionally **blepharospasm** (involuntary closure of the eyelids). The patient may drool, perhaps because of impairment of swallowing. There is typically no alteration in the tendon reflexes, and the plantar responses are flexor. Repetitive tapping (about twice per second) over the bridge of the nose produces a sustained blink response **(Myerson's sign);** the response is not sustained in normal subjects.

Differential Diagnosis

The diagnosis may be difficult to make in mild cases.

Depression may be accompanied by a somewhat expressionless face, poorly modulated voice, and reduction in voluntary activity; it can thus simulate parkinsonism. Moreover, the two diseases often coexist in the same patient. A trial of antidepressant drug treatment may be helpful if diagnostic uncertainty cannot be resolved by the presence of more widespread neurological signs indicative of parkinsonism.

Essential (benign, familial) tremor has been considered separately (see above). An early age at onset, a family history of tremor, a beneficial effect of alcohol on the tremor, and a lack of other neurological signs distinguish this disorder from parkinsonism. Furthermore, essential tremor commonly affects the head (causing a nod or head shake); parkinsonism typically affects the face and lips rather than the head.

Wilson's disease can also lead to a parkinsonian syndrome, but other varieties of abnormal movements are usually present as well. Moreover, the early age at onset and the presence of Kayser-Fleischer rings should distinguish Wilson's disease from Parkinson's disease, as should the abnormalities in serum and urinary copper and serum ceruloplasmin that occur in Wilson's disease.

Huntington's disease may occasionally be mistaken for parkinsonism when it presents with rigidity and akinesia, but a family history of Huntington's disease or an accompanying dementia, if present, should suggest the correct diagnosis.

Shy-Drager syndrome is a degenerative disorder characterized by parkinsonian features, autonomic insufficiency (leading to postural hypotension, anhidrosis, disturbance of sphincter control, impotence, etc), and signs of more widespread neurological involvement (pyramidal or lower motor neuron signs and often a cerebellar deficit). There is no treatment for the motor deficit, but the postural hypotension may respond to a liberal salt diet, fludrocortisone, 0.1–1 mg/d; indomethacin, 25–50 mg three times daily; wearing waist-high elastic hosiery; and sleeping with the head up at night.

Striatonigral degeneration is a rare disorder that is associated with neuronal loss in the putamen, globus pallidus, and caudate nucleus, and presents with bradykinesia and rigidity. Antiparkinsonian drugs are typically ineffective. Striatonigral degeneration may be associated with olivopontocerebellar degeneration (see Chapter 4), in which case the term **multiple system atrophy** or Shy-Drager syndrome is applied.

Progressive supranuclear palsy is a disorder in which there may be bradykinesia and rigidity, but its characteristic features are loss of voluntary control of eye movements (especially vertical gaze), dementia, pseudobulbar palsy, dysarthria, and axial dystonia. The disorder responds poorly, if at all, to antiparkinsonian drugs.

Creutzfeldt-Jakob disease may be accompanied by parkinsonian features, but dementia is usually present, myoclonic jerking is common, and ataxia is sometimes prominent; there may be pyramidal signs and visual disturbances, and the electroencephalographic findings of periodic discharges are usually characteristic.

Normal-pressure hydrocephalus leads to a gait disturbance (often mistakenly attributed to parkinsonism), urinary incontinence, and dementia. CT scanning reveals dilation of the ventricular system of the brain without cortical atrophy. The disorder may follow head injury, intracranial hemorrhage, or meningoencephalitis, but the cause is often obscure. Surgical shunting procedures to bypass any obstruction to the flow of cerebrospinal fluid (CSF) are often beneficial.

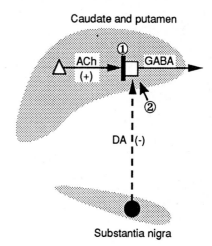

Figure 8–6. Therapeutic approaches in Parkinson's disease. The balance between dopaminergic (DA) and cholinergic (ACh) influences on striatal output (GABA) neurons can be restored by (1) blockade of cholinergic transmission with muscarinic anticholinergic drugs or (2) enhancement of dopaminergic transmission with the dopamine precursor levodopa, dopamine-receptor-agonist drugs (eg, bromocriptine), or amantadine (which stimulates the release of dopamine from surviving nerve terminals).

Treatment

Early parkinsonism requires no drug treatment, but it is important to discuss with the patient the nature of the disorder and the availability of medical treatment if symptoms become more severe. Treatment, when indicated, is directed toward restoring the dopaminergic:cholinergic balance in the striatum by blocking the effect of acetylcholine with anticholinergic drugs or by enhancing dopaminergic transmission (Figure 8–6).

A. Anticholinergic Drugs: Muscarinic anticholinergic drugs are more helpful in alleviating tremor and rigidity than hypokinesia but are generally less effective than dopaminergic drugs (see below). A number of preparations are available, and individual patients tend to favor different drugs. Among the most commonly prescribed drugs are trihexyphenidyl, benztropine, procyclidine, and orphenadrine (Table 8–6). Common side effects include dryness of the mouth, constipation, urinary retention, and defective pupillary accommodation; these are caused by muscarinic receptor blockade in parasympathetic end organs. Confusion, especially in the elderly, is due to antimuscarinic effects in the brain. Treatment is started with a small dose of one of the anticholinergics; the dosage is then gradually increased until benefit occurs or side effects limit further increments. If treatment is not helpful, the drug is withdrawn and another anticholinergic preparation is tried.

Table 8–6. Anticholinergic drugs used in the treatment of parkinsonism.[1]

	Usual Oral Daily Dose (mg)
Benztropine mesylate (Cogentin)	1–6
Biperiden (Akineton)	2–12
Chlorphenoxamine (Phenoxene)	150–400
Ethopropazine (Parsidol)	150–300
Orphenadrine (Disipal, Norflex)	150–400
Procyclidine (Kemadrin)	7.5–30
Trihexyphenidyl (Artane)	6–20

[1]Reproduced, with permission, from Aminoff MJ: Pharmacologic management of parkinsonian and other movement disorders. In: *Basic & Clinical Pharmacology,* 3rd ed. Katzung BG (editor). Appleton & Lange, 1987.

B. Amantadine: Amantadine can be given for mild parkinsonism either alone or in combination with an anticholinergic agent. Its precise mode of action is unclear, but it may potentiate the release of dopamine. Its advantages are that it improves all the clinical features of parkinsonism, its side effects (restlessness, confusion, skin rashes, edema, disturbances of cardiac rhythm) are relatively uncommon, its effects are exerted rapidly, and it is given in a standard dose of 100 mg orally twice daily. Unfortunately, however, many patients fail to respond to this drug, or its benefit is short-lived.

C. Levodopa: Levodopa, which is converted in the body to dopamine (Figure 8–7), ameliorates all the major clinical features of parkinsonism and, unlike the anticholinergic drugs, is often particularly helpful against hypokinesia. There is controversy about the best time to introduce dopaminergic therapy. Some feel that in many patients levodopa loses its efficacy with time—and accordingly that the drug should be reserved for patients with definite disability. The weight of present evidence suggests that any

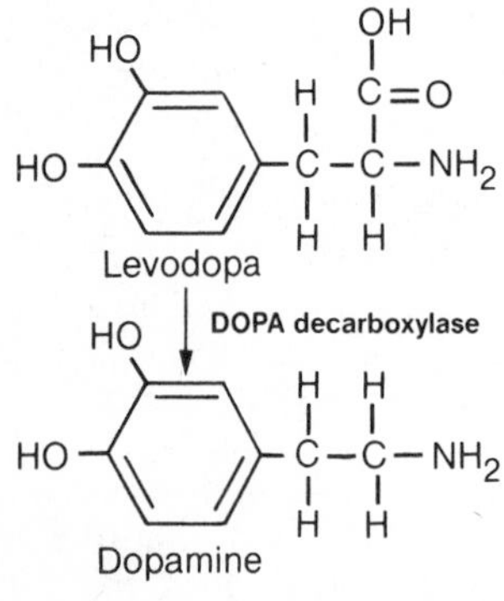

Figure 8–7. Metabolism of levodopa to dopamine. (Reproduced, with permission, from: *Basic & Clinical Pharmacology,* 3rd ed. Katzung BG [editor]. Appleton & Lange, 1987.)

decline in therapeutic response relates to disease duration and progression rather than to duration of treatment, however, and argues for early treatment with dopaminergic drugs, which may be most effective before the disease is far advanced. Furthermore, the mortality rate of patients with Parkinson's disease may be reduced if dopaminergic therapy is introduced within three years after onset of symptoms rather than at a later stage.

The most common side effects of levodopa are nausea, vomiting, hypotension, abnormal movements, restlessness, and confusion. Cardiac arrhythmias occur occasionally. A late complication of levodopa therapy is the **on-off phenomenon,** in which abrupt but transient fluctuations in the severity of parkinsonism occur at frequent intervals during the day, apparently without any relationship to the last dose of levodopa. This sometimes disabling problem is unaffected by concomitant administration of carbidopa. It can be controlled only partly by varying the dosing intervals, administering levodopa one hour before meals, restricting dietary protein intake, or providing treatment with bromocriptine.

Carbidopa is a drug that inhibits dopa decarboxylase, the enzyme responsible for the breakdown of levodopa to its active metabolite, dopamine (see Figure 8–7), but does not cross the blood-brain barrier. Accordingly, if levodopa is given in combination with carbidopa, the breakdown of levodopa is limited outside the central nervous system. The daily dose of levodopa required for benefit and the incidence of nausea, vomiting, hypotension, and cardiac irregularities can be reduced if levodopa is taken in combination with carbidopa. Carbidopa is generally combined with levodopa in a fixed proportion (1:10 or 1:4) as **Sinemet.** Treatment is started with a small dose, such as Sinemet 10/100 (mg) or Sinemet 25/100 (mg) orally three times daily, and is gradually increased, depending on the response. Most patients ultimately require Sinemet 25/250 (mg) three or four times daily.

D. Bromocriptine: Bromocriptine is an ergot derivative that directly stimulates dopamine D_2 receptors. It is perhaps slightly less effective than levodopa in relieving the symptoms of parkinsonism but is less likely to cause dyskinesias or the on-off phenomenon. In consequence, it has been recommended that when dopaminergic therapy is to be introduced, the patient be started on Sinemet 25/100 three times daily, with bromocriptine then added and gradually increased. The starting dose is 1.25 mg/d for one week and 2.5 mg/d for the next week, after which the daily dose is increased by 2.5-mg increments every two weeks, depending on the response and the development of side effects. Maintenance doses are usually between 2.5 and 10 mg orally three times daily. Side effects are similar to those associated with levodopa therapy, but psychiatric effects such as delusions or hallucinations are especially common, and bromocriptine is therefore contraindicated in patients with a history of psychotic disorders. Relative contraindications to its use are recent myocardial infarction, severe peripheral vascular disease, and active peptic ulceration.

E. Pergolide: Like bromocriptine, pergolide is an ergot derivative and dopamine receptor agonist; unlike bromocriptine, it activates both D_1 and D_2 receptors. Its indications, side effects, and contraindications are similar to those described above for bromocriptine, and it is unclear whether either compound is clinically superior to the other. The starting dose is 0.05 mg orally daily for two days, increased by 0.1–0.15 mg/d every three days for 12 days and by 0.25 mg/d every 3 days thereafter. The average maintenance dose is 1 mg orally three times daily.

F. Selegiline: Selegiline (also called eldepryl or deprenyl) is a monoamine oxidase type B inhibitor and therefore inhibits the metabolic breakdown of dopamine (Figure 8–8). It thus enhances the antiparkinsonian effect of levodopa and may reduce mild on-off fluctuations in responsiveness. Some clinical studies suggest that selegiline may also delay the progression of Parkinson's disease. The dose is 5 mg orally twice daily, usually given early in the day to avoid insomnia.

G. Surgery: Surgical treatment of parkinsonism by thalamotomy is rarely required, since pharmacological treatment is usually effective. Nevertheless, surgery is sometimes helpful in relatively young patients with predominantly unilateral tremor and rigidity that have failed to respond to medication. Diffuse vascular disease is a contraindication to this approach.

Autologous or fetal adrenal medullary tissue or

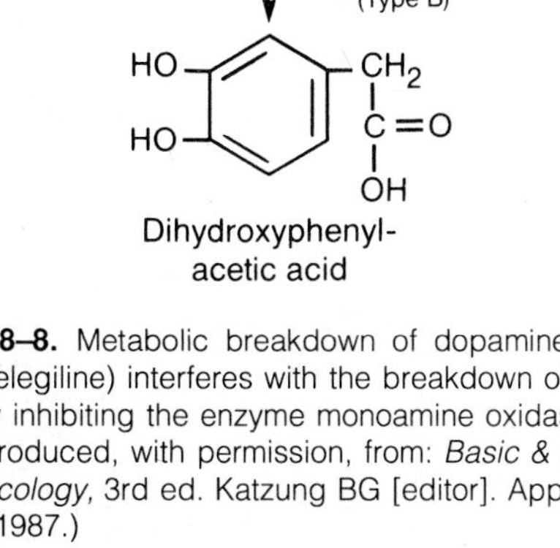

Figure 8–8. Metabolic breakdown of dopamine. Deprenyl (selegiline) interferes with the breakdown of dopamine by inhibiting the enzyme monoamine oxidase type B. (Reproduced, with permission, from: *Basic & Clinical Pharmacology*, 3rd ed. Katzung BG [editor]. Appleton & Lange, 1987.)

fetal substantia nigra has been transplanted to the caudate nucleus, in the belief that the transplanted tissue can continue to synthesize and release dopamine. Results from preliminary studies have been contradictory, and this approach is highly controversial. The precise mechanism of benefit, if it occurs, is unclear.

H. Physical Therapy and Aids for Daily Living: Physical therapy and speech therapy are beneficial to many patients with parkinsonism, and the quality of life can often be improved by providing simple aids to daily living. Such aids may include extra rails or banisters placed strategically about the home for additional support, table cutlery with large handles, nonslip rubber table mats, devices to amplify the voice, and chairs that will gently eject the occupant at the push of a button.

PROGRESSIVE SUPRANUCLEAR PALSY

Progressive supranuclear palsy is an idiopathic degenerative disorder that primarily affects subcortical gray matter regions of the brain. The principal neuropathological finding is neuronal degeneration with the presence of neurofibrillary tangles in the midbrain, pons, basal ganglia, and dentate nuclei of the cerebellum. Associated neurochemical abnormalities include decreased concentrations of dopamine and its metabolite, homovanillic acid, in the caudate nucleus and putamen. The classic clinical features are supranuclear ophthalmoplegia, pseudobulbar palsy, axial dystonia with or without extrapyramidal rigidity of the limbs, and dementia. Men are affected twice as often as women, and the disorder has its onset between ages 45 and 75 years.

Clinical Findings

Supranuclear ophthalmoplegia is characterized by early and prominent failure of voluntary vertical gaze, with later paralysis of horizontal gaze; oculocephalic and oculovestibular reflexes are preserved. In addition, the neck often assumes an extended posture (**axial dystonia in extension**), with resistance to passive flexion. Rigidity of the limbs and bradykinesia may mimic Parkinson's disease, but tremor is rare. A coexisting **pseudobulbar palsy** produces facial weakness, dysarthria, dysphagia, and often exaggerated jaw jerk and gag reflexes; there may also be exaggerated and inappropriate emotional responses (**pseudobulbar affect**). Hyperreflexia, extensor plantar responses, and cerebellar signs are sometimes seen. The **dementia** of progressive supranuclear palsy is characterized by forgetfulness, slowed thought processes, alterations of mood and personality, and impaired calculation and abstraction. Focal cortical dysfunction is rare.

Differential Diagnosis

Parkinson's disease differs in that voluntary downward and horizontal gaze are not usually lost, axial posture tends to be characterized by flexion rather than extension, tremor is common, the course is less fulminant, and antiparkinsonian medications are more often effective.

Treatment

Dopaminergic preparations are occasionally of benefit for rigidity and bradykinesia. Anticholinergics such as amitriptyline, 50–75 mg orally at bedtime, or benztropine, 6–10 mg/d orally, have been reported to improve speech, gait, and pathological laughing or crying, and methysergide, 8–12 mg/d orally, may ameliorate dysphagia. There is no treatment for the dementia.

Prognosis

The disorder typically follows a progressive course, with death from aspiration or inanition within 2–12 (usually 4–7) years.

HUNTINGTON'S DISEASE

Huntington's disease, characterized by a gradual onset and subsequent progression of chorea and dementia, is a hereditary disorder of the nervous system that has been traced to a single gene defect on the short arm of chromosome 4. It is inherited in an autosomal dominant manner, so that the offspring of an affected patient have a 50% chance of developing the disorder. In the few homozygous cases that have been identified, the clinical features are identical to those seen in heterozygotes. Huntington's disease occurs throughout the world and in all ethnic groups. Its prevalence rate is about 5 per 100,000 population. Symptoms usually do not appear until adulthood (typically between 30 and 50 years of age), by which time these patients have often started families of their own; thus, the disease continues from one generation to the next.

Pathogenesis

The manner in which the Huntington gene produces its devastating consequences is unknown. Postmortem examination of patients with the disease reveals cell loss, particularly in the cerebral cortex and corpus striatum (Figure 8–9). In the latter region, medium-sized spiny neurons that contain γ-aminobutyric acid (GABA) and enkephalin and project to the external segment of the globus pallidus are affected earliest, but other classes of neurons are eventually involved as well. Biochemical studies have shown that the concentration of the inhibitory neurotransmitter GABA, its biosynthetic enzyme glutamic acid decarboxylase (GAD), and acetylcholine and its biosynthetic enzyme choline acetyltransferase are all reduced in the basal ganglia of patients with Huntington's disease. The concentration of dopamine is normal or slightly increased. Changes in the concentrations of neuropeptides in the basal ganglia have also been found, including decreased substance P, methionine enkephalin, dynorphin, and

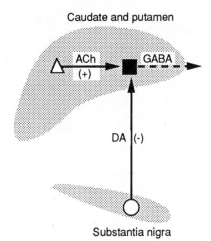

Figure 8–9. Neurochemical pathology of the basal ganglia in Huntington's disease. GABAergic neurons with cell bodies in the striatum degenerate (black square and dashed line), decreasing GABAergic output from the striatum.

cholecystokinin, and increased somatostatin and neuropeptide Y. Neurons containing NADPH diaphorase activity are spared. Positron emission tomography has shown reduced glucose utilization in an anatomically normal caudate nucleus.

Clinical Findings

Symptoms usually begin in the fourth or fifth decade, and the disease is progressive, with an average life span after onset of about 15 years.

A. Initial Symptoms: Either abnormal movements or intellectual changes may be the initial symptom, but ultimately both are present.

1. Dementia–The earliest mental changes often consist of irritability, moodiness, and antisocial behavior, but a more obvious dementia subsequently develops.

2. Chorea–Movement disturbance may be characterized initially by no more than an apparent fidgetiness or restlessness, but grossly abnormal choreiform movements are eventually seen.

3. Atypical forms–Especially in cases developing during childhood—but occasionally in adult-onset cases as well—the clinical picture is dominated by progressive rigidity and akinesia, with little or no chorea. This is known as the **Westphal variant,** and the correct diagnosis is suggested by the accompanying dementia and positive family history.

Epilepsy and cerebellar ataxia are frequent features of the juvenile form but not of adult cases.

B. Family History: In cases where a positive family history cannot be obtained, it must be remembered that the early death of a parent may make the history incomplete and that relatives often conceal the familial nature of the disorder. In addition, a certain degree of eccentric behavior, clumsiness, or restlessness may be regarded as normal by lay people and medical personnel unfamiliar with the disorder. The family history cannot therefore be regarded as negative until all close relatives of the patient have been examined by the physician personally. Nevertheless, apparently sporadic cases are occasionally encountered.

C. Imaging: CT scanning or MRI often demonstrates atrophy of the cerebral cortex and caudate nucleus in established cases.

Differential Diagnosis

Conditions that should be considered in the differential diagnosis of Huntington's disease are listed in Table 8–2. Drug-induced chorea, which is most common, can usually be identified from the history. Laboratory studies can exclude most medical disorders associated with chorea. Other hereditary disorders in which chorea is a conspicuous feature are described below.

Benign hereditary chorea is a recently recognized disorder that is inherited in either an autosomal dominant or recessive manner and is characterized by choreiform movements that develop in early childhood, do not progress during adult life, and are not associated with dementia.

Familial chorea sometimes occurs in association with circulating acanthocytes (spiny red blood cells), but examination of a wet blood film will clearly distinguish this disorder. Other clinical features of **chorea-acanthocytosis** include orolingual ticlike dyskinesias, vocalizations, mild intellectual decline, seizures, peripheral neuropathy, and muscle atrophy. Parkinsonian features are sometimes present. Unlike certain other disorders associated with circulating acanthocytes, there is no disturbance of beta-lipoprotein concentration into the peripheral blood.

Paroxysmal choreoathetosis may occur on a familial basis, but the intermittent nature of the symptoms and their relationship to movement or emotional stress usually distinguish this disorder from Huntington's disease.

The age at onset of symptoms usually distinguishes Huntington's disease from certain rare inherited childhood disorders characterized by choreoathetosis.

Wilson's disease can be distinguished from Huntington's disease by the mode of inheritance, the presence of Kayser-Fleischer rings, and abnormal serum copper and ceruloplasmin levels.

When the early symptoms constitute progressive intellectual failure, it may not be possible to distinguish Huntington's disease from other varieties of dementia unless the family history is characteristic or the movement disorder becomes noticeable.

Treatment & Prognosis

There is no cure for Huntington's disease, which, as a rule, terminates fatally 10–20 years after clinical onset. There is no treatment for the dementia, but the movement disorder may respond to drugs that interfere with dopaminergic inhibition of striatal output neurons. These include dopamine D_2-receptor-blocking drugs such as haloperidol, 0.5–4 mg orally four times daily, or chlorpromazine, 25–50 mg orally three times daily; and drugs that deplete dopamine from nerve terminals, such as reserpine, 0.5–5 mg/d orally, or tetrabenazine (investigational in the United States), 12.5 mg to 50 mg orally three times daily. Drugs that potentiate GABAergic or cholinergic neurotransmission are generally ineffective.

Prevention

Patients should be advised of the risk of transmitting the disease, and living offspring should receive genetic counseling. The use of genetic markers for detection of presymptomatic Huntington's disease and the problems associated with this approach are discussed on p 213.

SYDENHAM'S CHOREA

This disorder occurs principally in children and adolescents as a complication of a previous group A hemolytic streptococcal infection. The underlying pathological feature is probably arteritis. In about 30% of cases, it appears two or three months after an episode of rheumatic fever or polyarthritis, but in other patients no such history can be obtained. There is usually no recent history of sore throat and no fever. The disorder may have an acute or insidious onset, usually subsiding within the following four to six months. It may recur during pregnancy, however, or in patients taking oral contraceptive preparations.

Sydenham's chorea is characterized by abnormal choreiform movements that are sometimes unilateral and, when mild, may be mistaken for restlessness or fidgetiness. There may be accompanying behavioral changes, with the child becoming irritable or disobedient. In 30% of cases there is evidence of cardiac involvement, but the sedimentation rate and antistreptolysin O titer are usually normal.

The traditional treatment is bed rest, sedation, and prophylactic antibiotic therapy even if there are no other signs of acute rheumatism. A course of intramuscular penicillin is generally recommended, and continuous prophylactic oral penicillin daily until about age 20 years is also frequently advised to prevent streptococcal infections.

The prognosis is essentially that of the cardiac complications.

IDIOPATHIC TORSION DYSTONIA

This disorder is characterized by dystonic movements and postures and an absence of other neurological signs. The birth and developmental histories are normal. Before the diagnosis can be made, other possible causes of dystonia must be excluded on clinical grounds and by laboratory investigations.

Idiopathic torsion dystonia may be inherited as an autosomal dominant, autosomal recessive, or X-linked recessive disorder, and the defective genes have been localized in some cases (Table 8–5). Other cases seem to occur on a sporadic basis. Changes in the concentrations of norepinephrine, serotonin, and dopamine have been demonstrated in a variety of brain regions, but their role in the pathogenesis of dystonia is uncertain. Onset may be in childhood or later life, and this disorder remains as a lifelong affliction. The diagnosis is made on clinical grounds.

Clinical Findings

A. History: When onset is in childhood, a family history is usually obtainable. Symptoms generally commence in the legs. Progression is likely, and it leads to severe disability from generalized dystonia.

With onset in adult life, a positive family history is not likely to be obtained. The initial symptoms are usually in the arms or axial structures. Generalized dystonia may ultimately develop in about 20% of patients with adult-onset dystonia, but severe disability does not usually occur.

B. Examination: The disorder is characterized by abnormal movements and postures. For example, the neck may be twisted to one side (**torticollis),** the arm held in a hyperpronated position with the wrist flexed and fingers extended, the leg held extended with the foot plantar-flexed and inverted, or the trunk held in a flexed or extended position. There is often facial grimacing, and other characteristic facial abnormalities may also be encountered, including **blepharospasm** (spontaneous, involuntary forced closure of the eyelids for a variable period of time) and **oromandibular dystonia.** This consists of spasms of the muscles about the mouth, causing, for example, involuntary opening or closing of the mouth; pouting, pursing, or retraction of the lips; retraction of the platysma muscle; and roving or protruding movements of the tongue.

Differential Diagnosis

It is important to exclude other causes of dystonia (Table 8–3) before a diagnosis of idiopathic torsion dystonia is made. A normal developmental history prior to the onset of abnormal movements, together with the absence of other neurological signs and normal results of laboratory investigations, is important in this regard.

Treatment

The abnormal movements may be helped, at least in part, by drugs. Anticholinergic drugs given in the highest doses that can be tolerated (typically, trihexyphenidyl, 40–50 mg/d orally in divided doses) may be the most effective. Diazepam is occasionally helpful. Phenothiazines, haloperidol, or tetrabenazine (not available in the United States) may be worthwhile; however, at effective doses, these drugs usually lead to a mild parkinsonian syndrome. Other drugs that are occasionally helpful are levodopa, baclofen, and carbamazepine. Stereotactic thalamotomy is sometimes helpful for patients with predominantly unilateral dystonia that particularly involves the limbs.

Course & Prognosis

If all cases are considered together, about one-third of patients eventually become so severely disabled that they are confined to chair or bed, while another one-third are affected only mildly. In general, severe disability is more likely to occur when the disorder commences in childhood.

FOCAL TORSION DYSTONIA

A number of the dystonic features of idiopathic torsion dystonia may also occur as isolated phenomena. They are probably best regarded as focal dystonias that occur as formes frustes of idiopathic torsion dystonia in patients with a positive family history or that represent a focal manifestation of its adult-onset form when there is no family history.

Both **blepharospasm** and **oromandibular dystonia** can occur as isolated focal dystonias.

Spasmodic torticollis usually begins in the fourth or fifth decade and is characterized by a tendency for the neck to twist to one side. This often occurs episodically in early stages, but eventually the neck is held continuously to one side. Although the disorder is usually lifelong once it develops, spontaneous remission does occur occasionally, especially in the first 18 months after onset. Medical treatment is generally unsatisfactory. A trial of the drugs used in treating idiopathic torsion dystonia is worthwhile, since some patients do obtain undoubted benefit. Selective section of the spinal accessory nerve (cranial nerve XI) and the upper cervical nerve roots is sometimes helpful for patients in whom the neck is markedly deviated to the side, but recurrence of the abnormal posture is frequent. Local injection of botulinum toxin into the overactive muscles may also produce benefit for up to several months; it can be repeated as needed. It is the most effective treatment available for this disorder.

Writer's cramp is characterized by dystonic posturing of the hand and forearm when the hand is used for writing and sometimes other tasks such as playing the piano or using a screwdriver or table cutlery. Drug treatment is usually unrewarding, and it is often necessary for patients to learn to use the other hand for these tasks. Injections of botulinum toxin into the involved muscles are sometimes helpful.

WILSON'S DISEASE

Wilson's disease is an autosomal recessive disorder of copper metabolism that produces neurological and hepatic dysfunction. The gene defect has been localized to the long arm of chromosome 13. While the precise nature of the biochemical abnormality in Wilson's disease is unknown, its pathogenesis appears to involve decreased binding of copper to the transport protein **ceruloplasmin.** As a result, large amounts of unbound copper enter the circulation and are subsequently deposited in tissues, including the brain, liver, kidney, and cornea.

Clinical Findings

A. Mode of Presentation: Wilson's disease usually presents in childhood or young adult life. The average age at onset is about 11 years for patients presenting with hepatic dysfunction and 19 years for those with initial neurological manifestations, but the disease may begin as late as the sixth decade. Hepatic and neurological presentations are about equally common, and most patients, if untreated, eventually develop both types of involvement. Rare presentations include joint disease, fever, hemolytic anemia, and behavioral disturbances.

B. Nonneurological Findings: Ocular and hepatic abnormalities are the most prominent non-neurological manifestations of Wilson's disease. The most common ocular finding is **Kayser-Fleischer rings** (Figure 8–10): bilateral brown corneal rings that result from copper deposition in Descemet's membrane. The rings are present in virtually all patients with neurological involvement but may be detectable only by slit lamp examination. Hepatic involvement leads to chronic cirrhosis, which may be complicated by splenomegaly, esophageal varices with hematemesis, or fulminant hepatic failure. Splenomegaly may cause hemolytic anemia and thrombocytopenia.

C. Neurological Findings: Neurological findings in Wilson's disease reflect the disproportionate involvement of the caudate nucleus, putamen, cerebral cortex, and cerebellum. Neurological signs include resting or postural tremor, choreiform movements of the limbs, facial grimacing, rigidity, hypokinesia, dysarthria, dysphagia, abnormal (flexed) postures, and ataxia. Seizures may also occur. Psychological disorders in Wilson's disease include dementia, characterized by mental slowness, poor concentration, and memory impairment; disorders of affect, behavior, or personality; and (rarely) psychosis with hallucinations. There is a tendency for a dystonic or parkinsonian picture with hyperreflexia and extensor plantar responses to predominate when the disease begins before age 20 years—and for older pa-

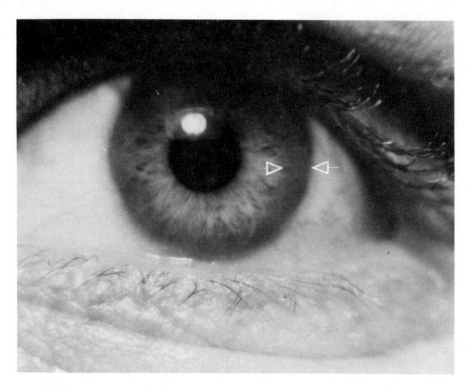

Figure 8–10. Kayser-Fleischer ring in Wilson's disease. This corneal ring (between arrows) was golden brown and contrasted clearly against a gray-blue iris. Note that the darkness of the ring increases as the outer border (limbus) of the cornea is approached (right arrow). (Photo courtesy of WF Hoyt.)

tients to exhibit wild tremor, chorea, or ballismus. Symptoms may progress rapidly, especially in younger patients, but are more often gradual in development with periods of remission and exacerbation.

Differential Diagnosis

When Wilson's disease presents as a neurological disorder, other conditions that must be considered in the differential diagnosis include multiple sclerosis and juvenile-onset Huntington's disease.

Investigative Studies

Investigation may reveal abnormal liver function blood tests and aminoaciduria as a result of renal tubular damage. The levels of serum copper and ceruloplasmin (an α_2-globulin to which 90% of the circulating copper is bound) are low, and 24-hour urinary copper excretion is generally increased. Liver biopsy reveals a huge excess of copper; it also usually reveals cirrhosis. Brain CT scanning or MRI may show cerebrocortical atrophy and abnormalities in the basal ganglia.

Treatment

Wilson's disease is treated with penicillamine, a copper-chelating agent that promotes extraction of copper from tissue deposition sites. Treatment should be started as early as possible and customarily employs 1.5–2 g/d of orally administered penicillamine. The response to treatment may take several months and can be monitored by serial slit lamp examinations and blood chemistries. Side effects of penicillamine include nausea, nephrotic syndrome, myasthenia gravis, arthropathy, pemphigus, diverse blood dyscrasias, and a lupuslike syndrome. Restriction of dietary copper and administration of zinc sulfate (200 mg/d orally) can decrease copper absorption. Treatment must be continued for the lifetime of the patient, and most patients treated early can expect a complete or nearly complete recovery.

Siblings of affected patients should be screened for presymptomatic Wilson's disease with neurological and slit lamp examinations and determination of serum ceruloplasmin levels. If no abnormalities are found, serum copper and urinary copper excretion should be assayed and liver biopsy performed if necessary. If these investigations reveal preclinical Wilson's disease, therapy should be instituted as described above for symptomatic disease.

DRUG-INDUCED MOVEMENT DISORDERS

Parkinsonism

Parkinsonism frequently complicates treatment with dopamine-depleting agents such as reserpine or antipsychotic dopamine-receptor antagonists such as phenothiazines or butyrophenones. In the case of antipsychotic drugs, the risk of this complication is greatest when agents are used that are potent D_2-receptor antagonists with little anticholinergic effect, such as piperazine phenothiazines, butyrophenones, and thioxanthenes (Table 8–7). In addition, women and elderly patients appear to be at somewhat increased risk. Tremor is relatively uncommon, while hypokinesia tends to be symmetrical and the most conspicuous neurological feature of parkinsonism. These points, together with the history of drug ingestion, often point to the iatrogenic nature of the disorder. Signs usually develop within three months after starting the offending drug and disappear over weeks or months following discontinuance.

Depending on the severity of symptoms and the necessity for continuing antipsychotic drug therapy, several strategies are available for treating drug-induced parkinsonism. These include discontinuing the antipsychotic drug, substituting a drug with greater anticholinergic potency, or adding an anticholinergic drug such as trihexyphenidyl or benztropine (Figure 8–11). Levodopa is of no help if the neuroleptic drugs are continued; it may be helpful if these drugs are discontinued but may aggravate the psychotic disorder for which they were originally prescribed.

Acute Dystonia or Dyskinesia

Acute dystonia or dyskinesia (such as blepharospasm, torticollis, or facial grimacing) is an occasional complication of dopamine receptor antagonist

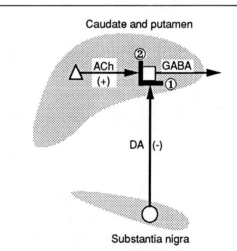

Figure 8–11. Mechanisms and treatment of drug-induced parkinsonism. Symptoms result from pharmacological blockade of dopamine receptors by antipsychotic drugs (1), which mimics the degeneration of nigrostriatal dopamine (DA) neurons seen in idiopathic parkinsonism. Symptoms may be relieved by the administration of muscarinic anticholinergic drugs (2) or by substituting an antipsychotic drug with anticholinergic properties. These measures restore the normal balance between dopaminergic and cholinergic (ACh) transmission in the striatum.

Table 8–7. Receptor-blocking properties of antipsychotic drugs.[1]

	Receptor			
	Dopamine D_2[2]	Muscarinic Cholinergic[3]	Histamine H_1[4]	α_1-Adrenergic[5]
Phenothiazines				
Piperidine				
Thioridazine (Mellaril)	+++	+++	+++	++++
Alkylamine				
Chlorpromazine (Thorazine)	+++	+++	++++	++++
Piperazine				
Trifluoperazine (Stelazine)	++++	++	+++	+++
Perphenazine (Trilafon)	++++	+	++++	++++
Fluphenazine (Prolixin)	+++++	+	+++	++++
Butyrophenones				
Haloperidol (Haldol)	++++	+	+	++++
Thioxanthines				
Thiothixene (Navane)	+++++	+	++++	+++
Indole compounds				
Molindone (Moban)	++	+	+	+
Dibenzoxazepines				
Loxapine (Loxitane)	+++	++	++++	+++
Dibenzodiazepines				
Clozapine (Clozaril)	++	+++	++++	++++

Antagonists range in potency from most potent (+++++) to least potent (+).

[1]Adapted from Black JL, Richelson E: Antipsychotic drugs: Prediction of side-effect profiles based on neuroreceptor data derived from human brain tissue. *Mayo Clin Proc* 1987;**62:**369–372.

[2]Blockade of dopamine D_2 receptors causes extrapyramidal side effects.

[3]Muscarinic cholinergic-receptor blockade attenuates extrapyramidal side effects and causes dry eyes, dry mouth, and urinary retention.

[4]Histamine H_1-receptor blockade produces sedation.

[5]α_1-adrenergic-receptor blockade causes hypotension.

treatment, generally occurring within 1 week after introduction of such medication and often within 48 hours. Men and younger patients show increased susceptibility to this complication. The pathophysiological basis of the disturbance is unclear, but intravenous treatment with an anticholinergic drug (eg, benztropine, 2 mg or diphenhydramine 50 mg) usually alleviates it.

Akathisia

Akathisia is a state of motor restlessness characterized by an inability to sit or stand still, which is relieved by moving about. It is a very common movement disorder induced by chronic treatment with antipsychotic drugs and occurs more often in women than in men. Akathisia is treated in the same manner as drug-induced parkinsonism.

Tardive Dyskinesia

Tardive dyskinesia may develop after long-term treatment with antipsychotic (dopamine-receptor-antagonist) drugs. It is commonly encountered in chronically institutionalized psychiatric patients, and the risk of developing tardive dyskinesia appears to increase with advancing age. The manner in which chronic drug treatment promotes a movement disorder is unknown.

Drug-induced supersensitivity of striatal dopamine receptors has been proposed but is unlikely to be responsible for several reasons. Supersensitivity always accompanies chronic antipsychotic drug treatment, whereas tardive dyskinesia does not. Supersensitivity may occur early in the course of treatment, while tardive dyskinesia does not develop for at least three months. In addition supersensitivity is invariably reversible when drugs are discontinued; tardive dyskinesia is not. The clinical features of tardive dyskinesia, particularly its persistent nature, are more suggestive of an underlying structural abnormality. Such an abnormality may involve γ-aminobutyric acid (GABA) neurons, because GABA and its synthesizing enzyme, glutamic acid decarboxylase, are depleted in the basal ganglia following chronic treatment of animals with antipsychotic drugs and GABA levels in CSF are decreased in patients with tardive dyskinesia. No consistent pathological features have been found in the brains of patients with tardive dyskinesia, although inferior olive atrophy, degeneration of the substantia nigra, and swelling of large neurons in the caudate nucleus have been described in some cases. The clinical disorder is characterized by abnormal choreoathetoid movements that are often especially conspicuous about the face and mouth in adults and tend to be more obvious in the limbs in children.

The onset of dyskinesia is generally not until months—or years—after the start of treatment with the responsible agent. Tardive dyskinesia may be impossible to distinguish from such disorders as Huntington's disease or idiopathic torsion dystonia unless a history of drug exposure is obtained.

Tardive dyskinesia is easier to prevent than to cure. Accordingly, antipsychotic drugs should be prescribed only on clear indication, and their long-term use should be monitored, with periodic drug holidays to determine whether the need for treatment continues. Drug holidays may also help to unmask incipient dyskinesias—which, curiously, tend to worsen when the drug is withdrawn. Antipsychotic medication should be stopped if possible when dyskinesia appears during a drug holiday, for in such circumstances the abnormal movements occasionally will remit.

Treating the established disorder is generally unsatisfactory, though it sometimes resolves spontaneously, especially in children or young adults. Antidopaminergic agents such as haloperidol or phenothiazines suppress the abnormal movements, but their use for this purpose is not recommended since they may aggravate the underlying disorder. Treatment with reserpine, 0.25 mg gradually increased to 2–4 mg/d orally, or tetrabenazine (not available in the United States), 12.5 mg gradually increased to as much as 200 mg/d orally daily may be helpful. Both these drugs deplete monoamine neurotransmitters, including dopamine. A number of other pharmacological approaches have been suggested, but there are conflicting reports regarding their utility.

A variety of other late and often persistent movement disorders may appear during the course of antipsychotic drug treatment. **Tardive dystonia** is usually segmental (affecting two or more contiguous body parts, such as the face and neck or arm and trunk) in nature. It is less often focal; when this is the case, the head and neck are particularly apt to be affected, producing blepharospasm, torticollis, or oromandibular dystonia. Generalized dystonia is least common and tends to occur in younger patients. Treatment is with tetrabenazine (if available) as described for tardive dyskinesia or with anticholinergic drugs as described above for idiopathic torsion dystonia. **Tardive akathisia** can also occur; it is treated in the same manner as drug-induced parkinsonism. **Tardive tic,** a drug-induced disorder resembling Gilles de la Tourette's syndrome (see below), is characterized by multifocal motor and vocal tics and can be similarly treated with clonidine (as described below) if symptoms do not remit spontaneously.

Neuroleptic Malignant Syndrome

This rare complication of treatment with antipsychotic drugs (neuroleptics) is manifested by rigidity, fever, altered mental status, and autonomic dysfunction. Haloperidol is implicated most often, but the syndrome can complicate treatment with any antipsy-

chotic drug; whether concomitant treatment with lithium or anticholinergic drugs increases the risk is uncertain. Symptoms typically develop over one to three days and can occur at any time during the course of treatment. The differential diagnosis includes infection, which must be excluded in any febrile patient. Neuroleptic malignant syndrome resembles malignant hyperthermia (see Chapter 6), but the latter disorder develops over minutes to hours rather than days, and is associated with the administration of inhalational anesthetics or neuromuscular blocking agents rather than antipsychotics. Treatment of neuroleptic malignant syndrome includes cessation of antipsychotic drugs, lithium, and anticholinergics; reduction of body temperature with antipyretics and artificial cooling; and rehydration. Dantrolene (see Chapter 6) may be beneficial, as may bromocriptine, levodopa preparations, or amantadine. The mortality rate is as high as 20%.

Other Drug-Induced Movement Disorders

Levodopa produces a wide variety of abnormal movements as a dose-related phenomenon in patients with parkinsonism. They can be reversed by withdrawing the medication or reducing the dose. Chorea may also develop in patients receiving bromocriptine, anticholinergic drugs, phenytoin, carbamazepine, amphetamines, lithium, and oral contraceptives; it resolves with discontinuance of the responsible drug. Dystonia has resulted from administration of bromocriptine, lithium, carbamazepine, and metoclopramide; and postural tremor from administration of theophylline, caffeine, lithium, thyroid hormone, tricyclic antidepressants, valproic acid, and isoproterenol.

GILLES DE LA TOURETTE'S SYNDROME

Gilles de la Tourette's syndrome, characterized by chronic—typically lifelong—multiple motor and verbal tics, is of unknown cause and does not relate to social class, ethnic group, perinatal abnormalities, birth trauma, or birth order. Symptoms begin before 21 years of age, and the course is one of remission and relapse. Most cases are sporadic, although there is occasionally a family history, and partial expression of the trait may occur in siblings or offspring of patients. Males are affected more commonly than females. The prevalence in the United States has been estimated to be 0.05%.

The pathophysiology is obscure. Dopaminergic excess in the brains of patients with Gilles de la Tourette's syndrome has been postulated, mainly because of the beneficial effects that dopamine-blocking drugs can have on the tics. The administration of dopamine receptor agonists often fails to produce the exacerbation of symptoms that might be anticipated from this hypothesis, however.

No structural basis for the clinical disorder has been recognized. Only a few cases have come to autopsy, and the findings are conflicting.

Clinical Findings

Symptoms usually commence between ages 2 and 15 years. The first signs consist of motor tics in 80% of cases and vocal tics in 20%; there may be either a single tic or multiple tics. When the initial sign is a motor tic, it most commonly involves the face, taking the form of sniffing, blinking, forced eye closure, etc. It is generally not possible to make the diagnosis at this stage.

All patients ultimately develop a number of different motor tics and involuntary vocal tics, the latter commonly consisting of grunts, barks, hisses, throat-clearing or coughing, and the like, and sometimes taking the form of verbal utterances including **coprolalia** (vulgar or obscene speech). There may also be **echolalia** (parroting the speech of others), **echopraxia** (imitation of others' movements), and **palilalia** (repetition of words or phrases). The tics vary over time in severity, character, and the muscle groups involved. In 40–50% of cases, some of the tics involve self-mutilation with such activities as severe nail-biting or hair-pulling, picking at the nose, or biting the lips or tongue. Sensory tics, consisting of pressure, tickling, and warm or cold sensations, also occur. Behavioral disorders, including obsessive compulsive disorder and attention deficit hyperactivity disorder, are common in patients with Gilles de la Tourette's syndrome, but their precise relationship to the tic disorder is uncertain.

Physical examination usually reveals no other abnormalities, but there is a higher than expected incidence of left-handedness or ambidexterity. In about 50% of cases, the EEG shows minor nonspecific abnormalities of no diagnostic relevance.

Differential Diagnosis

The differential diagnosis includes the various movement disorders that can present in childhood. Other disorders characterized by tics (see *Tics,* above) are distinguished by resolution of the tics by early adulthood or by the restricted number of tics.

Wilson's disease can simulate Gilles de la Tourette's syndrome; it must be excluded because it responds well to medical treatment. In addition to a movement disorder, Wilson's disease produces hepatic involvement, Kayser-Fleischer corneal rings, and abnormalities of serum copper and ceruloplasmin, which are absent in Gilles de la Tourette's syndrome.

Sydenham's chorea can be difficult to recognize if there is no recent history of rheumatic fever or polyarthritis and no clinical evidence of cardiac involvement, but this disorder is a self-limiting one, usually clearing in three to six months.

Bobble-head syndrome which can be difficult to distinguish from Gilles de la Tourette's syndrome, is characterized by rapid, rhythmic bobbing of the head in children with progressive hydrocephalus.

Complications

Gilles de la Tourette's syndrome is often unrecognized for years, the tics being attributed to psychiatric illness or mistaken for some other form of abnormal movement. Indeed, in many cases the correct diagnosis is finally made by the family rather than the physician. In consequence, patients are often subjected to unnecessary and expensive treatment before the true nature of the disorder is recognized. Psychiatric disturbances, sometimes culminating in suicide, may occur because of the cosmetic and social embarrassment produced by the tics.

Drug therapy can lead to a number of side effects, as discussed below.

Treatment

Treatment is symptomatic and, if effective, must be continued indefinitely.

Clonidine has been reported to ameliorate motor or vocal tics in roughly 50% of children so treated. It may act by reducing activity in noradrenergic neurons arising in the locus ceruleus. It is started in a dose of 2–3 μg/kg/d, increasing after two weeks to 4 μg/kg/d and then, if necessary, to 5 μg/kg/d. It may cause an initial transient fall in blood pressure. The most frequent side effect is sedation. Other adverse reactions include reduced or excessive salivation and diarrhea.

Haloperidol is often effective. It is started at a low daily dose (0.25 mg), which is gradually increased by 0.25 mg every four or five days until there is maximum benefit with a minimum of side effects or until side effects limit further increments. A total daily dose of 2–8 mg is usually optimal, but higher doses are sometimes necessary. Side effects include extrapyramidal movement disorders, sedation, dryness of the mouth, blurred vision, and gastrointestinal disturbances. Pimozide, another dopaminergic-receptor antagonist, may be helpful in patients who are either unresponsive to or cannot tolerate haloperidol, but the long-term safety of pimozide is unknown. Treatment is started with 1 mg/d and the dose increased by 2 mg every ten days; most patients require 7–16 mg/d.

Phenothiazines such as fluphenazine may help, but patients who are unresponsive to haloperidol usually fail with these drugs as well.

Patients occasionally respond favorably to clonazepam or carbamazepine, but diazepam, barbiturates, tricyclic antidepressants, phenytoin, and cholinergic agonists (such as deanol) are usually not helpful.

ACQUIRED HEPATOCEREBRAL DEGENERATION

Acquired hepatocerebral degeneration produces a neurological disorder associated with extrapyramidal, cerebellar, and pyramidal signs as well as dementia. Extrapyramidal signs include rigidity, rest tremor, chorea, athetosis, and dystonia. This condition is discussed in Chapter 2.

RESTLESS LEGS SYNDROME

Restless legs syndrome is characterized by an unpleasant creeping discomfort that is perceived as arising deep within the legs and occasionally in the arms as well. Such symptoms tend to occur when patients are relaxed, especially while lying down or sitting, and lead to a need to move about. They are often particularly troublesome at night and may delay the onset of sleep. A sleep disorder associated with periodic movements during sleep may also occur and can be documented by polysomnographic recording. The cause is unknown, although the disorder seems especially common among pregnant women and is not uncommon among uremic or diabetic patients with neuropathy. Most patients, however, have no obvious predisposing cause. Symptoms sometimes resolve following correction of coexisting iron-deficiency anemia, and they may respond to treatment with drugs such as levodopa, bromocriptine, diazepam, or clonazepam.

REFERENCES

General

Albin RL, Young AB, Penney JB: The functional anatomy of basal ganglia disorders. *Trends in Neurosci* 1989;12:366–375.

Campanella G, Roy M, Barbeau A: Drugs affecting movement disorders. *Annu Rev Pharmacol Toxicol* 1987;27:113–136.

Nath A, Jankovic J, Pettigrew LC: Movement disorders and AIDS. *Neurology* 1987;37:37–41.

Special Issue: Basal Ganglia Research. *Trends in Neurosci* 1990;13(7). [Entire issue.]

Familial, or Benign, Essential Tremor

Cleeves L, Findley LJ, Koller W: Lack of association between essential tremor and Parkinson's disease. *Ann Neurol* 1988;24:23–26.

Findley LJ, Koller WC: Essential tremor: a review. *Neurology* 1987;37:1194–1197.

Jankovic J, Fahn S: Physiologic and pathologic tremors: diagnosis, mechanism and management. *Ann Intern Med* 1980;93:460–465.

Parkinsonism

Ballard PA, Tetrud JW, Langston JW: Permanent human parkinsonism due to 1-methyl-4-phenyl-1,2,3,6-tetrahydropyridine (MPTP): Seven cases. *Neurology* 1985;35:949–956.

Goetz CG et al: Multicenter study of autologous adrenal medullary transplantation to the corpus striatum in patients with advanced Parkinson's disease. *N Engl J Med* 1989;320:337–341.

Klawans HL (editor): Emerging strategies in Parkinson's disease. *Neurology* 1990;40 (Suppl 3):1–76. [Entire issue.]

Scigliano G et al: Mortality associated with early and late levodopa therapy initiation in Parkinson's disease. *Neurology* 1990;40:265–269.

Progressive Supranuclear Palsy

Maher ER, Lees AJ: The clinical features and natural history of the Steele-Richardson-Olszewski syndrome (progressive supranuclear palsy). *Neurology* 1986;36:1005–1008.

Huntington's Disease

Gusella JF et al: A polymorphic DNA marker genetically linked to Huntington's disease. *Nature* 1983;306:234–238.

Martin JB, Gusella JF: Huntington's disease: Pathogenesis and management. *N Engl J Med* 1986;315:1267–1276.

Mazziotta JC et al: Reduced cerebral glucose metabolism in asymptomatic subjects at risk for Huntington's disease. *N Engl J Med* 1987;316:357–362.

Sydenham's Chorea

Nausieda PA et al: Sydenham chorea: An update. *Neurology* 1980;30:331–334.

Idiopathic and Focal Torsion Dystonia

Fahn S: High dosage anticholinergic therapy in dystonia. *Neurology* 1983;33:1255–1261.

Hornykiewicz O et al: Brain neurotransmitters in dystonia musculorum deformans. *N Engl J Med* 1986;315:347–353.

McGeer EG, McGeer PL: The dystonias. *Can J Neurol Sci* 1988;15:447–483.

Report of the Therapeutics and Technology Assessment Subcommittee of the American Academy of Neurology: Assessment: The clinical usefulness of botulinum toxin-A in treating neurological disorders. *Neurology* 1990;40:1332–1336.

Wilson's Disease

Dobyns WB, Goldstein NP, Gordon H: Clinical spectrum of Wilson's disease (hepatolenticular degeneration). *Mayo Clin Proc* 1979;54:35–42.

Drug-Induced Movement Disorders

Ball R: Drug-induced akathisia: a review. *J Roy Soc Med* 1985;78:748–752.

Black JL, Richelson E: Antipsychotic drugs: Prediction

of side-effect profiles based on neuroreceptor data derived from human brain tissue. *Mayo Clin Proc* 1987;62:369–372.

Burke RE: Tardive dyskinesia: Current clinical issues. *Neurology* 1984;34:1348–1353.

Jeste DV, Wisniewski AA, Wyatt RJ: Neuroleptic-associated tardive syndromes. *Psychiatr Clin North Am* 1986;9:183–192.

Smego RA Jr, Durack DT: The neuroleptic malignant syndrome. *Arch Intern Med* 1982;142:1183–1185.

Stephen PJ, Williamson J: Drug-induced parkinsonism in the elderly. *Lancet* 1984;2:1082–1083.

Gilles de la Tourette's Syndrome

Kurlan R.: Tourette's syndrome: Current concepts. *Neurology* 1989;39:1625–1630.

Nee LE et al: Gilles de la Tourette syndrome: Clinical and family study of 50 cases. *Ann Neurol* 1980;7:41–49.

9 Seizures & Syncope

EPISODIC LOSS OF CONSCIOUSNESS

Consciousness is lost when the function of both cerebral hemispheres or of the brain stem reticular activating system is compromised. Episodic dysfunction of these anatomical regions produces transient, and often recurrent, loss of consciousness.

There are two major causes of episodic loss of consciousness.

Seizures
These are disorders characterized by excessive or oversynchronized discharges of cerebral neurons.

Syncope
This loss of consciousness is due to a reduced supply of blood to the cerebral hemispheres or brain stem. It can result from pancerebral hypoperfusion caused by vasovagal reflexes, orthostatic hypotension, or decreased cardiac output or from selective hypoperfusion of the brain stem resulting from vertebrobasilar ischemia.

It is important to distinguish seizures from syncope because they have different causes, diagnostic approaches, and treatment.

APPROACH TO DIAGNOSIS

The initial step in evaluating a patient who has suffered a lapse of consciousness is to determine whether the setting in which the event occurred—or associated symptoms or signs—suggests that it was a direct result of a disease requiring prompt attention, such as hypoglycemia, meningitis, head trauma, cardiac arrhythmia, or acute pulmonary embolism. The number of spells and their similarity or dissimilarity should be established. If all spells are identical, then a single pathophysiological process can be assumed, and the following major differential features should be ascertained.

Phenomena at Onset of Spell
A detailed inquiry should always be made about prodromal and initial symptoms. The often brief, stereotyped premonitory symptoms (**aura**) at the onset of some seizures may localize the central nervous system abnormality responsible for the seizures.

A. An unambiguous description of a sudden onset of unconsciousness without prodromal features is highly suggestive of seizure.

B. Focal sensory or motor phenomena (eg, involuntary jerking of one hand, hemifacial paresthesias, forced head turning) suggest a seizure originating in the contralateral frontoparietal cortex.

C. A sensation of fear, olfactory or gustatory hallucinations, or visceral or déjà vu sensations is commonly associated with seizures originating in the temporal lobe.

D. Progressive lightheadedness, dimming of vision, and faintness, which indicate diffuse central nervous system dysfunction, are associated with decreased cerebral blood flow from any cause (simple faints, cardiac arrhythmias, orthostatic hypotension).

Events During the Spell

A. Generalized tonic-clonic (grand mal, or major motor) seizures are characterized by loss of consciousness, accompanied initially by tonic stiffening and subsequently by clonic (jerking) movements of the extremities.

B. Cerebral hypoperfusion usually produces flaccid unresponsiveness.

C. Cerebral hypoperfusion can also result in stiffening or jerking movements, especially if the patient is prevented from falling or otherwise assuming a recumbent posture. Such circulatory events are self-limited and do not require anticonvulsant treatment. Loss of consciousness rarely lasts more than 15 seconds and is not followed by postictal confusion unless prolonged brain ischemia has occurred.

Posture When Loss of Consciousness Occurs

Orthostatic hypotension and simple faints occur in the upright or sitting position. Episodes also (or only) occurring in the lying position suggest seizure or cardiac arrhythmia as a likely cause, although syncope induced by strong emotional stimuli may be responsible.

Relationship to Physical Exertion

Syncope associated with exertion is usually due to cardiac outflow obstruction (eg, aortic stenosis, hypertrophic obstructive cardiomyopathy, atrial myxoma) or arrhythmias.

Phenomena Following the Spell

A. A period of confusion, disorientation, or agitation (**postictal state**) commonly follows a generalized tonic-clonic seizure. The period of confusion is usually brief—lasting only for minutes. While such behavior is often strikingly evident to witnesses, it may not be recalled by the patient.

B. Prolonged alteration of consciousness (**prolonged postictal state**) may follow status epilepticus. It may also occur after a single seizure in patients with diffuse structural cerebral disease (eg, dementia, encephalitis) or metabolic encephalopathy.

C. Recovery from a simple faint is characterized by a prompt return to consciousness with full lucidity.

SEIZURES

A seizure is a transient disturbance of cerebral function caused by an abnormal neuronal discharge. **Epilepsy,** a group of disorders characterized by recurrent seizures, is a common cause of episodic loss of consciousness; idiopathic epilepsy affects 0.2–0.4% of the general population.

An actively convulsing patient or a reported seizure in a known epileptic usually poses no diagnostic difficulty. Since most seizures occur outside the hospital unobserved by medical personnel, however, the diagnosis must usually be established retrospectively. The two historical features most suggestive of a seizure are the aura associated with seizures of focal onset and the postictal confusional state that follows generalized tonic-clonic seizures (see below). Neither urinary incontinence nor the occurrence of a few tonic or jerking movements is significant in distinguishing seizures from other causes of transient loss of consciousness, since either can occur also with loss of consciousness from cerebral hypoperfusion.

ETIOLOGY

Seizures can result from either primary central nervous system dysfunction or an underlying metabolic derangement or systemic disease. This distinction is critical, since therapy must be directed at the underlying disorder as well as at seizure control. A list of common neurological and systemic disorders that induce seizures is presented in Table 9–1. The age of the patient may help in establishing the cause of seizures (Figure 9–1).

Primary Neurological Disorders

A. Benign febrile convulsions of childhood are seizures that occur in children three months to five years old, usually during the first day of a febrile illness, and in the absence of central nervous system infection (meningitis or encephalitis). There may be a family history of benign febrile convulsions or other

Table 9–1. Common causes of seizures of new onset.

Primary neurological disorders
Benign febrile convulsions of childhood
Idiopathic epilepsy
Head trauma
Stroke or vascular malformations
Mass lesions
Meningitis or encephalitis
Systemic disorders
Hypoglycemia
Hyponatremia
Hyperosmolar states
Hypocalcemia
Uremia
Hepatic encephalopathy
Porphyria
Drug overdose
Drug withdrawal
Global cerebral ischemia
Hypertensive encephalopathy
Eclampsia
Hyperthermia

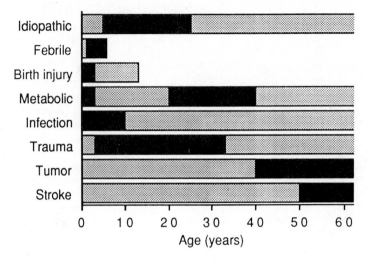

Figure 9–1. Causes of seizures as a function of age at onset. Bars show the range of ages at which seizures from a given cause typically begin; darker shading indicates peak incidence.

types of seizures. Benign febrile convulsions usually last for less than 15 minutes and lack focal features. About two-thirds of patients experience a single seizure and fewer than one-tenth have more than three. The differential diagnosis includes meningitis and encephalitis (Chapter 1) and brain abscess (Chapter 11); if present, these should be treated as described elsewhere in this volume. Since benign febrile convulsions are usually self-limited, treatment is often unnecessary; prolonged convulsions (>15 minutes) can be treated with diazepam, 0.3 mg/kg intramuscularly or intravenously or 0.6 mg/kg rectally. The probability of developing a chronic seizure disorder is 2–6%, and is highest in patients with persistent neurological abnormalities; prolonged, focal, or multiple seizures; or a family history of nonfebrile seizures. Long-term administration of phenobarbital to reduce the risk of subsequent afebrile seizures is controversial, since the efficacy of such prophylactic therapy is disputed, and cognitive impairment is a common side effect of treatment.

B. Idiopathic epilepsy for which no specific cause can be established accounts for more than 75% of seizure disorders. Idiopathic epilepsy usually begins between the ages of 5 and 25 years, with more than 75% of patients having their first seizure before age 18 years. Less frequently, idiopathic epilepsy begins in later life, although in this age group seizures are also commonly associated with strokes, tumors, trauma, and systemic or metabolic disorders (see Figure 9–1). Not all patients with a single idiopathic seizure go on to develop recurrent seizures: Recurrence rates vary from about 30% to as high as 70% in different series, and may be higher in patients with electroencephalographic abnormalities such as a generalized spike and wave pattern, postictal Todd's

paralysis (see below), persistent neurological abnormalities, status epilepticus, or a family history of afebrile seizures.

C. Head trauma is a common cause of epilepsy, especially when it occurs perinatally or is associated with a depressed skull fracture or intracerebral or subdural hematoma. Seizures that occur within the first week after nonpenetrating head injuries are not predictive of a chronic seizure disorder, however. Although patients with serious head injuries are often treated prophylactically with anticonvulsant drugs, this practice has been questioned, since a reduction in the incidence of posttraumatic seizures has not been consistently observed beyond one week of treatment.

D. Stroke affecting the cerebral cortex produces seizures in 5–15% of patients and can occur following thrombotic or embolic infarction or intracerebral hemorrhage (see Chapter 10). As with head trauma, early seizures are not necessarily indicative of chronic epilepsy, and long-term anticonvulsant therapy is not required. Even without rupturing, **vascular malformations** may be associated with seizures, presumably as a result of their irritative effects on adjacent brain tissue.

E. Mass lesions, such as brain tumors (see Chapter 3) or abscesses (see Chapter 11), can present with seizures or produce them later in the course. Glioblastomas, astrocytomas, and meningiomas are the most common tumors associated with seizures, reflecting their high prevalence among tumors that affect the cerebral hemispheres.

F. Meningitis or **encephalitis** caused by bacterial (eg, *Haemophilus influenzae*), tuberculous, viral (eg, herpes simplex), fungal, or parasitic (eg, cysticercosis) infections can also cause seizures (see Chapter 1). Seizures in patients with AIDS are most often associated with AIDS dementia complex, toxoplasmosis, or cryptococcal meningitis.

Systemic Disorders

Metabolic and other systemic disorders, including drug-overdose and drug-withdrawal syndromes, may be associated with seizures that abate with correction of the underlying abnormality. In these cases, the patient is not considered to have epilepsy.

A. Hypoglycemia can produce seizures, especially with serum glucose levels of 20–30 mg/dL, but neurological manifestations of hypoglycemia are also related to the rate at which serum glucose levels fall. Hypoglycemia is discussed in detail in Chapter 1.

B. Hyponatremia may be associated with seizures at serum sodium levels below 120 meg/L or at higher levels following rapid decline. Hyponatremia is considered further in Chapter 1.

C. Hyperosmolar states, including both hyperosmolar nonketotic hyperglycemia (see Chapter 1) and hypernatremia, may lead to seizures when serum osmolality rises above about 330 mosm/L.

D. Hypocalcemia with serum calcium levels in the range of 4.3–9.2 mg/dL can produce seizures with or without tetany (see Chapter 1).

E. Uremia can cause seizures, especially when it develops rapidly, but this tendency correlates poorly with absolute serum urea nitrogen levels (see Chapter 1).

F. Hepatic encephalopathy is sometimes accompanied by generalized or multifocal seizures (see Chapter 1).

G. Porphyria is a disorder of heme biosynthesis that produces both neuropathy (discussed in Chapter 6) and seizures. The latter may be difficult to treat because most anticonvulsants can exacerbate the disorder. As a result, seizures caused by porphyria are treated with bromides, 1–2 g orally three times daily. Therapeutic serum levels are typically 10–20 meq/L and must be closely monitored because toxicity (manifested by rash, gastrointestinal symptoms, psychiatric disturbances, or impaired consciousness) is common even within this range.

H. Drug overdose can exacerbate epilepsy or cause seizures in nonepileptic patients. Generalized tonic-clonic seizures are most common, but focal or multifocal partial seizures can also occur. The drugs most frequently associated with seizures are antidepressants, antipsychotics, cocaine, insulin, isoniazid, lidocaine, and methylxanthines (Table 9–2).

I. Drug withdrawal, especially withdrawal from ethanol or sedative drugs, may be accompanied by one or more generalized tonic-clonic seizures that usually resolve spontaneously. Alcohol withdrawal seizures occur within 48 hours after cessation or reduction of ethanol intake in 90% of cases, and are characterized by brief flurries of one to six attacks that resolve within 12 hours. Acute abstinence from sedative drugs can also produce seizures in patients

Table 9–2. Major categories of drugs reported to cause seizures.

Anticholinesterases (organophosphates, physostigmine)
Antidepressants
Antihistamines
Antipsychotics (phenothiazines, butyrophenones)
β-adrenergic receptor blockers (propranolol, oxprenolol)
Cyclosporine
Hypoglycemic agents (including insulin)
Hypo-osmolar parenteral solutions
Isoniazid
Local anesthetics (bupivacaine, lidocaine, procaine, etidocaine)
Methylxanthines (theophylline, aminophylline)
Narcotic analgesics (fentanyl, meperidine, pentazocine, propoxyphene)
Penicillins
Phencyclidine
Sympathomimetics (amphetamines, cocaine, ephedrine, phenylpropanolamine, terbutaline)

habituated to more than 600–800 mg/d of secobarbital or equivalent doses of other short-acting sedatives. Seizures from sedative drug withdrawal typically occur two to four days after abstinence, but may be delayed for up to one week. Focal seizures are rarely due to alcohol or sedative drug withdrawal alone; they suggest an additional focal cerebral lesion that requires evaluation.

J. Global cerebral ischemia from cardiac arrest, cardiac arrhythmias, or hypotension may produce, at onset, a few tonic or tonic-clonic movements that resemble seizures, but they probably reflect abnormal brain stem activity instead. Global ischemia may also be associated with spontaneous myoclonus (see Chapter 8) or, after consciousness returns, with myoclonus precipitated by movement (action myoclonus). Partial or generalized tonic-clonic seizures also occur; these may be manifested only by minor movements of the face or eyes and must be treated. Nonetheless, seizures following global cerebral ischemia do not necessarily indicate a poor outcome. Global cerebral ischemia is discussed in more detail in Chapter 10.

K. Hypertensive encephalopathy, which may be accompanied by generalized tonic-clonic or partial seizures, is considered in Chapter 1.

L. Eclampsia refers to the occurrence of seizures or coma in a pregnant woman with hypertension, proteinuria, and edema (**preeclampsia**). As in hypertensive encephalopathy in nonpregnant patients, cerebral edema, ischemia, and hemorrhage may contribute to neurological complications. Although magnesium sulfate has been widely used to treat eclamptic seizures, most neurologists recommend conventional anticonvulsants such as phenytoin.

M. Hyperthermia can result from infection, exposure (heat stroke), hypothalamic lesions, or drugs such as phencyclidine, as well as anticholinergics or neuroleptics (neuroleptic malignant syndrome; see Chapter 8) and inhalational anesthetics or neuromuscular blocking agents (malignant hyperthermia; see Chapter 6). Clinical features of severe hyperthermia (>42°C, or 107°F) include seizures, confusional states or coma, shock, and renal failure. Treatment is with antipyretics and artificial cooling to reduce body temperature immediately to 39°C (102°F) and anticonvulsants and more specific therapy (eg, antibiotics for infection, dantrolene for malignant hyperthermia) where indicated. Patients who survive may be left with ataxia as a result of the special vulnerability of cerebellar neurons to hyperthermia.

CLASSIFICATION & CLINICAL FINDINGS

Seizures are classified as follows:
    Generalized seizures
        Tonic-clonic (grand mal)
        Absence (petit mal)
        Other types (tonic, clonic, myoclonic)
    Partial seizures
        Simple partial
        Complex partial (temporal lobe, psychomotor)

Generalized Seizures

A. Generalized tonic-clonic seizures are attacks in which consciousness is lost, usually without aura or other warning. When a warning does occur, it usually consists of nonspecific symptoms.

1. Tonic phase–The initial manifestations are unconsciousness and tonic contractions of limb muscles for 10–30 seconds, producing extension of the extremities and arching of the body in apparent opisthotonos (Figure 9–2). Tonic contraction of the muscles of respiration may produce an expiration-induced vocalization (cry or moan) and cyanosis, and contraction of masticatory muscles may cause tongue trauma. The patient falls to the ground and may be injured.

2. Clonic phase–The tonic phase is followed by a clonic (alternating muscle contraction and relaxation) phase of symmetric limb jerking that persists for an additional 30–60 seconds—or longer. Ventilatory efforts return immediately after cessation of the tonic phase, and cyanosis clears. The mouth may froth with saliva. With time, the jerking becomes less frequent, until finally all movements cease and the

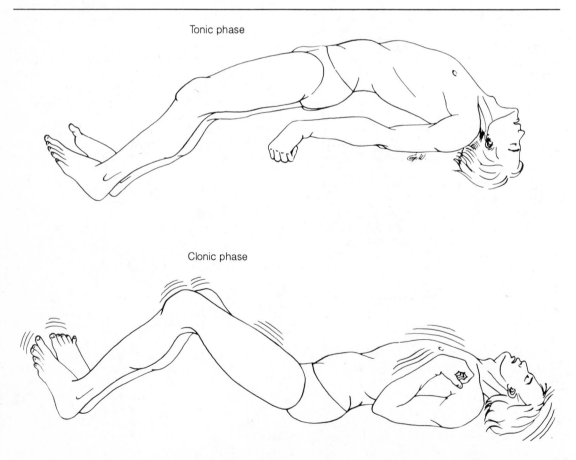

Tonic phase

Clonic phase

Figure 9–2. Generalized tonic-clonic seizure, illustrating the appearance of the patient in the tonic (stiffening) and clonic (shaking) phases.

muscles are flaccid. Sphincteric relaxation or detrusor muscle contraction may produce urinary incontinence. The patient then remains unconscious for a variable period that is seldom longer than 30 minutes.

3. Recovery–As the patient regains consciousness, there is postictal confusion and often headache. Full orientation commonly takes 10–30 minutes—or even longer in patients with status epilepticus (see below) or preexisting structural or metabolic brain disorders. Physical examination during the postictal state is usually otherwise normal in idiopathic epilepsy or seizures of metabolic origin, except that plantar responses may be transiently extensor (Babinski's sign). The pupils always react to light, even when the patient is unconscious. Transient unilateral weakness (hemiparesis) in the postictal period **(Todd's paralysis)** should be sought, because such a finding suggests a focal brain lesion as the cause and calls for further investigation.

4. Status epilepticus–In this condition, seizures fail to cease spontaneously or recur so frequently that full consciousness is not restored between successive episodes. Status epilepticus is a medical emergency because it can lead to permanent brain damage—from hyperpyrexia, circulatory collapse, or excitotoxic neuronal damage—if untreated.

B. Absence (petit mal) seizures are genetically transmitted seizures that always begin in childhood and usually do not persist after age 20 years. The spells are characterized by brief loss of consciousness (for five to ten seconds) without loss of postural tone. Subtle motor manifestations, such as eye blinking or a slight head turning, are common. Automatisms are rare. Full orientation immediately follows cessation of the seizure. There may be as many as several hundred spells daily, leading to impaired school performance and social interactions, so that children may be mistakenly thought to be mentally retarded before the diagnosis of petit mal epilepsy is made. The spells are characteristically inducible by hyperventilation. The EEG shows a characteristic 3-per-second spike-wave pattern (Figure 9–3). In most patients with normal intelligence and normal background activity on EEG, absence spells occur only during childhood; in other cases, however, the attacks continue into adult life, either alone or in association with other types of seizures.

C. Other types of generalized seizures include tonic seizures (not followed by a clonic phase), clonic seizures (not preceded by a tonic phase), and myoclonic seizures.

1. Tonic seizures are characterized by continuing muscle contraction that can lead to fixation of the limbs and to deviation of the head and eyes to one side; the accompanying arrest of ventilatory movements leads to cyanosis. Consciousness is lost, and there is no clonic phase to these seizures.

2. Clonic seizures are characterized by repetitive clonic jerking accompanied by loss of consciousness. There is no initial tonic component.

3. Myoclonic seizures are characterized by sudden, brief, shocklike contractions that may be localized to a few muscles or one or more extremities or that may have a more generalized distribution. Myoclonic seizures are associated with a variety of rare hereditary neurodegenerative disorders, including Unverricht-Lundborg disease, Lafora body disease, neuronal ceroid lipofuscinosis (late infantile, juvenile, and adult forms), sialidosis, and mitochondrial encephalomyopathy (myoclonus epilepsy with ragged red fibers on skeletal muscle biopsy). Not all myoclonic jerks have an epileptic basis, however, as discussed in Chapter 8.

Partial Seizures

A. Simple partial seizures begin with motor, sensory, or autonomic phenomena, depending on the cortical region affected. For example, clonic movements of a single muscle group in the face, a limb, or the pharynx may occur and may be self-limited; they may be recurrent or continuous or may spread to involve contiguous regions of the motor cortex **(jacksonian march).**

Autonomic symptoms may consist of pallor, flushing, sweating, piloerection, pupillary dilatation, vomiting, borborygmi, and incontinence. Psychic symptoms include dysphasia, distortions of memory (eg, déjà vu, the sensation that a new experience is being repeated), forced thinking or labored thought processes, cognitive deficits, affective disturbances (eg, fear, depression, an inappropriate sense of pleasure), hallucinations, or illusions. During simple partial seizures, consciousness is preserved unless the seizure discharge spreads to other areas of the brain, producing tonic-clonic seizures **(secondary generalization).** The **aura** is the portion of the seizure that precedes loss of consciousness and of which the patient retains some memory. The aura is sometimes the sole manifestation of the epileptic discharge.

In the postictal state, a focal neurological deficit such as hemiparesis **(Todd's paralysis)** that resolves over a period of 15–36 hours is a manifestation of an underlying focal brain lesion.

B. Complex partial seizures, formerly called temporal lobe or psychomotor seizures, consist of episodes in which consciousness is impaired but not lost. The seizure discharge usually arises from the temporal lobe or medial frontal lobe. The symptoms take many forms but are usually stereotyped for the individual patient. Epigastric sensations are most common, but affective (fear), cognitive (déjà vu), and sensory (olfactory hallucinations) symptoms also occur. Consciousness is then impaired. Seizures generally persist for less than 30 minutes (on the average, one to three minutes). The motor manifestations of complex partial seizures are characterized by coordinated involuntary motor activity, termed **automa-**

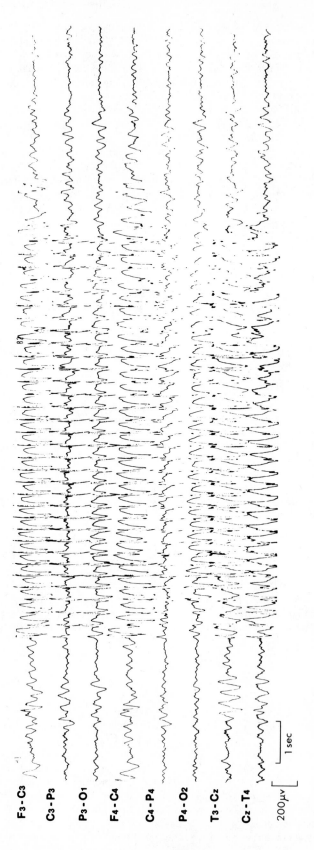

Figure 9–3. Electroencephalogram of a patient with typical absence (petit mal) seizures, showing a burst of generalized 3-Hz spike-and-wave activity (center of record) that is bilaterally symmetrical and bisynchronous. Odd-numbered leads indicate electrode placements over the left side of the head; even numbers, those over the right side.

tism, which takes the form of orobuccolingual movements in about 75% of patients and other facial or neck movements in about 50%. Sitting up or standing, fumbling with objects, and bilateral limb movements are less common. Secondary generalization may occur.

DIAGNOSIS

The diagnosis of seizures is based on clinical recognition of one of the seizure types described above. The EEG can be a helpful confirmatory test in distinguishing seizures from other causes of loss of consciousness (Figure 9–4). On the other hand, however, a normal or nonspecifically abnormal EEG never excludes the diagnosis of seizures. Specific electroencephalographic features that suggest epilepsy include abnormal spikes, polyspike discharges, and spike-wave complexes.

A standard diagnostic evaluation of patients with recent onset of seizures is presented in Table 9–3. Metabolic and toxic disorders (see Table 9–1) should be excluded, because they do not require anticonvulsants.

Seizures with a clearly focal onset or those that begin after age 25 years require prompt evaluation to exclude the presence of a structural brain lesion. CT or MRI is helpful for this purpose. If no cause is found, the decision to begin chronic anticonvulsant therapy should be based on the probability of recurrence. Following a single generalized tonic-clonic seizure, recurrence can be expected within three or four years in 30–70% of untreated adult patients.

SELECTION OF THERAPY

Therapy should be directed toward the cause of the seizures, if known. Seizures associated with metabolic and systemic disorders usually respond poorly to anticonvulsants but cease with correction of the underlying abnormality. Acute withdrawal from alcohol and other sedative drugs produces self-limited seizures that, in general, require no anticonvulsant drug therapy. Acute head trauma and other structural brain lesions that result in seizures must be rapidly diagnosed and treated, and the associated seizures controlled by anticonvulsant drug therapy. Idiopathic epilepsy is treated with anticonvulsant medications.

Anticonvulsant Drug Treatment

Commonly used anticonvulsant drugs and their dosages and methods of administration are listed in Table 9–4. There are four key principles of management:

Establish the diagnosis of epilepsy before start-

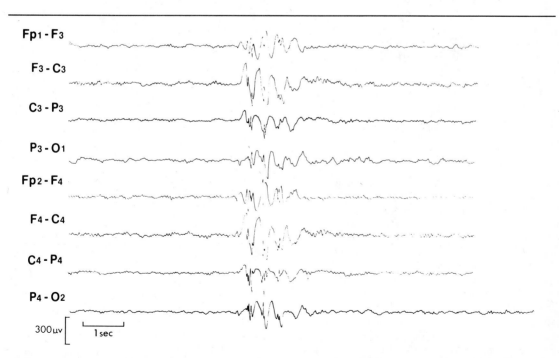

Figure 9–4. Electroencephalogram of a patient with idiopathic (primary generalized) epilepsy. A burst of generalized epileptiform activity (center) is seen on a relatively normal background. These findings, obtained at a time when the patient was not experiencing seizures, support the clinical diagnosis of epilepsy. Odd-numbered leads indicate electrode placements over the left side of the head; even numbers, those over the right side.

Table 9–3. Evaluation of a new seizure disorder in a stable patient.

History (including medications or drug exposure)
General physical examination
Complete neurological examination
Blood studies
    Fasting glucose
    Serum calcium
    Serum FTA
    Serum electrolytes
    Complete blood count
    Erythrocyte sedimentation rate
    Renal function studies
    Hepatic function studies
Electroencephalogram
CT brain scan or MRI (especially with abnormal examination, progressive disorder, or onset of seizures after 25 years of age)

ing drug therapy. Therapeutic trials of anticonvulsant drugs intended to establish or reject a diagnosis of epilepsy may yield incorrect diagnoses.

Choose the right drug for the seizure type. Absence seizures, for example, do not respond to most drugs used for complex partial or generalized tonic-clonic seizures.

Treat the seizures, rather than the serum drug levels. Control of seizures is achieved at different drug levels in different patients.

Evaluate one drug at a time. In most cases, seizures can be controlled with a single drug. Therefore, beginning therapy with multiple drugs may expose patients to increased drug toxicity without added therapeutic benefit.

Most patients with epilepsy fall into one of the following treatment categories.

A. New Seizures: Most epileptologists do not recommend chronic anticonvulsant drug treatment following a single seizure unless an underlying cause is found that is not correctable and is likely to produce recurrent seizures (eg, brain tumor). However, recurrent seizures do require anticonvulsant treatment, and if such therapy is to be administered, the oral loading schedules presented in Table 9–4 can be used. Note that starting a drug at its daily maintenance dose produces stable serum drug levels only after approximately five half-lives have elapsed. Therefore, loading doses should be given whenever possible to achieve therapeutic drug levels promptly in patients with frequent seizures. **Phenytoin** or **carbamazepine** is the current drug of first choice for treating generalized tonic-clonic or partial seizures in adults, and **phenobarbital** or **carbamazepine** is preferred for children. Some epileptologists also include **valproic acid** as a first-line drug for generalized tonic-clonic seizures. Phenobarbital is also very effective in treating generalized tonic-clonic seizures in adults, but it is less helpful for treatment of complex partial seizures.

Absence attacks of the petit mal variety are treated with **valproic acid** or **ethosuximide** (Table 9–4). The former has the advantage of also providing protection against tonic-clonic seizures but has caused fatalities from hepatic damage in children under ten (usually under two) years of age.

Myoclonic seizures are treated with **valproic acid** or **clonazepam** (Table 9–4).

B. Recurrent Seizures on Drug Therapy:

1. Determining serum levels of drugs–Blood levels of the anticonvulsant drugs the patient has been taking should be measured in samples taken just prior to a scheduled dose. No acute change in medication is indicated for a single seizure if there has been no interruption of drug therapy and anticonvulsant drug levels are in the therapeutic range. If the history or serum drug levels suggest that treatment has been interrupted, the prescribed drug should be started again as for new seizures.

2. Adding a second drug–A second anticonvulsant should be added only if seizures continue to occur after maximum therapeutic benefit has been achieved with the initial drug. This means not only that blood levels of the drug are in the therapeutic range but also that drug toxicity precludes further dosage increments. An anticonvulsant that has failed to alter seizure frequency should be discontinued gradually once therapeutic levels of the second drug have been achieved. If the first drug has produced partial control of the seizure disorder, however, it is often continued along with the second drug.

3. Treating refractory seizures: In some patients, disabling seizures persist despite trials of all major anticonvulsants, alone and in combination— and at the highest doses the patient can tolerate. When no treatable cause can be found, seizures are not due to a progressive neurodegenerative disease, and medical treatment has been unsuccessful for at least two years, evaluation for possible surgical therapy should be considered. Presurgical evaluation begins with a detailed history and neurological examination to explore the cause of seizures and their site of origin within the brain and to document the adequacy of prior attempts at medical treatment. MRI and electrophysiological studies are performed to identify the epileptogenic zone within the brain. Several electrophysiological techniques can be used: **electroencephalography,** in which cerebral electrical activity is recorded from the scalp; **stereotactic depth electrode electroencephalography,** in which activity is recorded from electrodes inserted into the brain; and **electrocorticography,** which involves intraoperative recording from the surface of the brain. When an epileptogenic zone can be identified in this manner and its removal is not expected to produce undue neurological impairment, surgical excision may be indicated. Patients with complex partial seizures arising from a single temporal lobe are the most frequent surgical candidates; unilateral anterior temporal lobec-

Table 9–4. Summary of anticonvulsant drug therapy.

| Drug | Dosage | | | Serum Half-Life (Normal Renal and Hepatic Function) | Therapeutic Serum Levels | Symptoms of Acute Overdose | Indications |
	Intravenous Loading	Oral Loading or Initial	Maintenance				
Phenytoin (Dilantin)	1000–1500 mg (15–18 mg/kg) directly into a large vein at a rate not exceeding 50 mg/min. Continuous electrocardiographic monitoring is mandatory. Cannot be infused in dextrose solutions.	Loading: 1000 mg in two or four divided doses over 12–24 hours.	300–400 mg/d in a single dose or divided doses.	Oral: 18–24 hours; IV: 12 hours. (Kinetics are dose-dependent and may vary widely.)	10–20 µg/mL	Ataxia, nystagmus, somnolence. (Nystagmus on extreme lateral gaze suggests therapeutic drug level.)	Generalized tonic-clonic and partial seizures.
Carbamazepine (Tegretol)	No intravenous preparation.	200 mg twice a day; increase by 200 mg/d to maintenance dose.	600–1200 mg/d in three or four doses.	12–18 hours.	4–12 µg/mL	Nausea, ataxia.	Generalized tonic-clonic and partial seizures.
Phenobarbital (Luminal)	700 mg (10 mg/kg) over 20 minutes. Ventilatory support equipment must be available at bedside.	Loading: 180 mg twice a day for three days.	90–180 mg/d in a single dose.	3–5 days.	20–40 µg/mL	Ataxia, somnolence.	Generalized tonic-clonic and partial seizures.
Primidone (Mysoline)	No intravenous preparation.	Slowly increase from 125 mg/d to maintenance dose over one month.	250 mg three or four times a day.	6–12 hours.	5–15 µg/mL	Somnolence, ataxia.	Second-line maintenance drug for generalized tonic-clonic and partial seizures.
Valproic acid (Depakote, Depakene)	No intravenous preparation.	Same as maintenance dose.	750–2000 mg/d in three doses.	6–18 hours.	50–150 µg/mL	Drowsiness and nausea at onset.	Generalized tonic-clonic, myoclonic, light-induced, and absence seizures.
Ethosuximide (Zarontin)	No intravenous preparation.	15 mg/kg/d, then increase by 25 mg/d at weekly intervals to maintenance dose.	15–40 mg/kg/d in two doses.	24–36 hours (children); 60 hours (adult).	40–100 µg/mL	Nausea, anorexia at onset of therapy.	Absence seizures.
Clonazepam (Klonopin)	No intravenous preparation.	Children: 0.01–0.03 mg/kg/d in two or three divided doses. Adults: 0.5 mg three times daily.	Children: 0.1–0.2 mg/kg/d; Adults: 1.5–20 mg/d; in two or three divided doses.	20–40 hours.	0.02–0.10 µg/mL	Drowsiness, ataxia, behavioral change; increased seizure frequency with discontinuance (therefore reduce by 0.25 mg/wk).	Myoclonic seizures.

tomy abolishes seizures in about 50% of these patients and significantly reduces their frequency in another 25%. Hemispherectomy and corpus callosum section are also sometimes used to treat intractable epilepsy.

C. Multiple Seizures or Status Epilepticus:

1. Early management–

a. Immediate attention should be given to ensuring that the airway is patent and the patient positioned to prevent aspiration of stomach contents.

b. The laboratory studies listed in Table 9–5 should be ordered without delay.

c. Dextrose, 50 mL of 50% solution, should be given intravenously.

d. If fever or meningeal signs are present, immediate lumbar puncture is mandatory, and a gram-stained smear of spinal fluid should be examined to exclude bacterial meningitis. Patients without these signs should also undergo lumbar puncture if the cause of the seizures has not been determined (eg, by their cessation upon administration of dextrose), unless signs of increased intracranial pressure or of focal brain dysfunction are present. It should be noted that **postictal pleocytosis** is detectable in CSF in approximately 2% of patients with single generalized tonic-clonic seizures (and about 15% of those with status epilepticus) in the absence of infection. The white blood cell count may be as high as 80/μL, with either polymorphonuclear or mononuclear predominance. Serum protein content may be slightly elevated, but glucose concentration is normal, and Gram's stain is

negative. The postictal pleocytosis resolves in two to five days.

2. Drug therapy to control seizures–Every effort must be made to establish a precise etiological diagnosis so that treatment of the underlying disorder can be started. Because generalized seizure activity per se damages the brain if it persists for more than one or two hours, drug therapy to terminate seizures should be instituted immediately. An outline for rapid pharmacological control of acute multiple seizures is presented in Table 9–6.

3. Management of hyperthermia–The metabolic consequences of status epilepticus are related to increased motor activity and high levels of circulating catecholamines; they include hyperthermia (to 42–43 °C [108–109 °F]), lactic acidosis (to pH < 7.00), and peripheral blood leukocytosis (to 60,000 cells/μL). These derangements typically resolve over a few hours after cessation of the seizures. Only hyperthermia, which is known to increase the risk of brain damage from status epilepticus, requires specific attention.

Hyperthermia must be treated with a cooling blanket and, if necessary, the induction of motor paralysis with neuromuscular blocking agent such as curare. Lactic acidosis resolves spontaneously over one hour and should not be treated. Infection should, of course, be excluded.

Discontinuance of Anticonvulsants

Patients (usually children) with epilepsy who are seizure-free on medication for two to five years may wish to discontinue anticonvulsant drugs. In patients with normal intelligence and a normal neurological examination, the risk of seizure recurrence may be as low as 25%. Risk factors for recurrence include slowing or spikes (maximum risk with both present) on electroencephalography. When anticonvulsants are to be withdrawn, one drug is eliminated at a time by tapering the dose slowly over two to three months. Recurrence of seizures has been reported in approximately 20% of children and 40% of adults following medication withdrawal, in which case prior medication should be reinstituted at the previously effective levels.

Table 9–5. Emergency evaluation of serial seizures, or status epilepticus.

Treatment with anticonvulsants should be instituted immediately (Table 9–6), while the following measures are taken.
Vital signs:
    Blood pressure: exclude hypertensive encephalopathy and shock.
    Temperature: exclude hyperthermia.
    Pulse: exclude life-threatening cardiac arrhythmia.
Draw venous blood for serum glucose, calcium, electrolytes, hepatic and renal function blood studies, complete blood count, erythrocyte sedimentation rate, and toxicology.
Insert intravenous line.
Administer glucose (50 mL of 50% dextrose) intravenously.
Obtain any available history.
Rapid physical examination, especially for:
    Signs of trauma.
    Signs of meningeal irritation or systemic infection.
    Papilledema.
    Focal neurological signs.
    Evidence of metastatic, hepatic, or renal disease.
Arterial blood gases.
Lumbar puncture, unless the cause of seizures has already been determined or signs of increased intracranial pressure or focal neurological signs are present.
Electrocardiogram.
Calculate serum osmolality: 2 (serum sodium concentration) + serum glucose/20 + Serum urea nitrogen/3 (normal range: 270–290).
Urine sample for toxicology, if indicated.

COMPLICATIONS OF EPILEPSY & ANTICONVULSANT THERAPY

Complications of Epilepsy

When the diagnosis of epilepsy is made, the patient should be warned against working around moving machinery or at heights and reminded of the risks of swimming alone. The issue of driving must also be addressed. Many state governments have notification requirements when a diagnosis of epilepsy is made.

Side Effects of Anticonvulsant Drugs

The side effects of anticonvulsant drug therapy are

Table 9–6. Drug treatment of status epilepticus in adults.

Drug	Dosage/Route	Advantages/Disadvantages/ Complications
Diazepam or Lorazepam[1]	10 mg IV over two minutes. 0.1 mg/kg IV at rate not greater than 2 mg/min.	Fast-acting. Effective half–life 15 minutes for diazepam and 14 hours for lorazepam. Abrupt respiratory depression or hypotension in 5%, especially when given in combination with other sedatives. Seizure recurrence in 50% of patients; therefore must add maintenance drug (phenytoin or phenobarbital).
	IMMEDIATELY PROCEED TO PHENYTOIN	
Phenytoin	1000–1500 mg (18 mg/kg) IV slowly at rate not greater than 50 mg/min (cannot be given in dextrose solution).	Little or no respiratory depression. Drug levels in the brain are therapeutic at completion of infusion. Effective as maintenance drug. Hypotension and cardiac arrhythmias can occur.
	IF SEIZURES CONTINUE FOLLOWING TOTAL DOSE, PROCEED IMMEDIATELY TO PHENOBARBITAL	
Phenobarbital	1000–1500 mg (18 mg/kg) IV slowly (50 mg/min).	Peak brain levels within 30 minutes. Effective as maintenance drug. Respiratory depression and hypotension common at higher doses. (Intubation and ventilatory support should be immediately available.)
	IF ABOVE IS INEFFECTIVE, PARALDEHYDE CAN BE USED	
Paraldehyde	PR: 5–10 mL diluted in 2 volumes of mineral oil. IV: 0.05–0.1 mL/kg diluted to 4% (vol/vol) in normal saline; IM: 0.1–0.25 mg/kg in ≤5 mL.	Decomposes with storage. Can cause metabolic acidosis, pulmonary hemorrhage, and cardiovascular depression. Respiratory depression may occur. Slow absorption when given PR (IM route gives peak levels in 15–20 minutes).
	IF ABOVE IS INEFFECTIVE, PROCEED IMMEDIATELY TO GENERAL ANESTHESIA	
Pentobarbital	15 mg/kg IV slowly, followed by 0.5–4 mg/kg/h.	Intubation and ventilatory support required. Hypotension is limiting factor. Pressors may be required to maintain blood pressure.

[1]Investigational in the United States.

summarized in Table 9–7. All anticonvulsant drugs may lead to blood dyscrasias, but carbamazepine and valproic acid have been associated with the highest incidence of hematological—and hepatic—toxicity. For this reason, a complete blood count and liver function tests should be obtained before initiating administration of these drugs and at intervals during the course of treatment. *The authors recommend performing these tests at two weeks, one month, three months, six months, and every six months thereafter.* Carbamazepine should be discontinued if the total neutrophil count falls below 1,500/ml or if aplastic anemia is suspected. Valproic acid should be terminated if symptoms of hepatotoxicity, such as nausea, vomiting, anorexia or jaundice occur.

Most anticonvulsant drugs (especially barbiturates) affect cognitive function to some degree, even in therapeutic doses.

Drug Interactions

A variety of drugs alter the absorption or metabolism of anticonvulsants when given concomitantly. The changes in anticonvulsant levels are summarized in Table 9–8.

Epilepsy & Anticonvulsant Therapy in Pregnancy

The incidence of stillbirth, microcephaly, mental retardation, and seizure disorders is increased in children born to epileptic mothers. Anticonvulsant therapy during pregnancy, however, is also associated with a greater than normal frequency of congenital malformations—especially cleft palate, cleft lip, and cardiac anomalies. Such malformations are about twice as common in the offspring of medicated as of unmedicated epileptic mothers, but since patients with more severe epilepsy are more likely to be treated, it is difficult to know whether epilepsy or its treatment is the more important risk factor.

Among commonly used anticonvulsants, valproic acid is associated with an increased incidence of neural tube defects. Phenobarbital, phenytoin, and carbamazepine pose some teratogenic risk, but the extent of the risk is controversial. Trimethadione, which is sometimes used to treat absence seizures, is clearly associated with fetal dysmorphism; it is not widely used.

When an epileptic patient who has been seizure-free for several years is contemplating pregnancy, an attempt should be made to withdraw anticonvulsants

Table 9–7. Side effects of anticonvulsant drugs.

Drug	Dose-Related	Idiosyncratic
Phenytoin	Diplopia Ataxia Gingival hyper- plasia Hirsutism Coarse facial features Polyneuropathy Osteomalacia Megaloblastic anemia	Skin rash Fever Lymphoid hyperpla- sia Hepatic dysfunction Blood dyscrasia
Carbamaze- pine	Diplopia Ataxia Gastrointestinal distress Sedation	Skin rash Blood dyscrasia Hepatic dysfunction
Phenobarbital or primidone	Sedation Insomnia Behavioral dis- turbance Diplopia Ataxia	Skin rash
Valproic acid	Gastrointestinal distress Tremor Sedation Weight gain Hair loss	Hepatic dysfunction Thrombocytopenia
Ethosuximide	Gastrointesti- nal distress Sedation Ataxia Headache	Skin rash Blood dyscrasia
Clonazepam	Sedation Diplopia Ataxia Behavioral dis- turbance Hypersalivation	. . .

Table 9–8. Some major anticonvulsant drug interactions.

Drug	Levels Increased by	Levels Decreased by
Phenytoin	Benzodiazepines Chloramphenicol Disulfiram Ethanol Isoniazid Phenylbutazone Sulfonamides Trimethoprim Warfarin	Carbamazepine Phenobarbital Pyridoxine
Carbamazepine	Erythromycin Isoniazid Propoxyphene Valproic acid	Phenobarbital Phenytoin
Phenobarbital	Methsuximide Primidone Valproic acid	. . .
Primidone	Isoniazid	Acetazolamide
Valproic acid	. . .	. . .
Ethosuximide	Valproic acid	. . .
Clonazepam	. . .	. . .

prior to conception. If anticonvulsant drugs are required, carbamazepine should be used for generalized tonic-clonic or partial seizures and ethosuximide for absence seizures. In contrast to generalized tonic-clonic seizures, partial and absence seizures present little risk to the fetus, and it may be possible to tolerate imperfect control of these seizures during pregnancy to avoid fetal drug exposure. Clonazepam can also be used; but phenytoin, phenobarbital, and primidone should be avoided if possible, and trimethadione and valproic acid should not be used. Every effort should be made to control the seizures with a single drug. Status epilepticus is treated as described above for nonpregnant patients.

Plasma levels of anticonvulsant drugs may decrease during pregnancy because of the patient's enhanced metabolism, and higher doses may be required to maintain control of seizures. It is therefore important to monitor drug levels closely in this setting.

PROGNOSIS

With appropriate anticonvulsant drug treatment, seizures can be well controlled, although not always eliminated, in most epileptic patients. Patients should be seen every few months to monitor seizure frequency, adverse drug effects, and compliance with treatment.

PSEUDOSEIZURES

Attacks that resemble seizures (psychogenic seizures, or pseudoseizures) may be manifestations of a psychiatric disturbance such as conversion disorder, somatization disorder, factitious disorder with physical symptoms, or malingering. In conversion or somatization disorder, the patient is unaware of the psychogenic nature of symptoms and the motivation for their production. In factitious disorder, the patient recognizes that the spells are self-induced, but not the reason for doing so. In malingering, there is conscious awareness of both the production of symptoms and the underlying motivation.

Pseudoseizures can usually be distinguished both clinically and by the electroencephalographic findings. In patients with pseudoseizures resembling tonic-clonic attacks, there may be warning and preparation before the attack; there is usually no tonic phase, and the clonic phase consists of wild thrashing movements during which the patient rarely comes to harm or is incontinent. In some instances, there are abnormal movements of all extremities without loss of consciousness; in others, there is shouting or obscene utterances during apparent loss of consciousness or goal-directed behavior if the airway is passively closed off. There is no postictal confusion or abnormal clinical signs following the attack. The EEG recorded during the episode does not show organized seizure activity, and postictal slowing does not occur.

It is important to appreciate that many patients with pseudoseizures also have genuine epileptic attacks that require anticonvulsant medications.

SYNCOPE

VASOVAGAL SYNCOPE
(Simple Faints)

Vasovagal disorders, which are exceedingly common, occur in all age groups and affect men and women equally. Precipitating factors include emotional stimulation, pain, the sight of blood, fatigue, medical instrumentation, blood loss, or prolonged motionless standing. Vagally mediated decreases in arterial blood pressure and heart rate combine to produce central nervous system hypoperfusion and subsequent syncope. Severe cerebral ischemia resulting in tonic-clonic movements can occur if the unconscious patient remains in an upright position during the episode (eg, fainting in a toilet stall).

Vasovagal episodes generally begin while the patient is in a standing or sitting position and only rarely in a horizontal position (eg, with phlebotomy or IUD insertion). A prodrome lasting ten seconds to a few minutes usually precedes syncope and can include lassitude, lightheadedness, nausea, pallor, diaphoresis, salivation, blurred vision, and tachycardia. The patient, who then loses consciousness and falls to the ground, is pale and diaphoretic and has dilated pupils. Bradycardia replaces tachycardia as consciousness is lost. During unconsciousness, abnormal movements may occur; these are mainly tonic or opisthotonic, but seizurelike tonic-clonic activity is occasionally seen. Urinary incontinence may also occur.

The patient recovers consciousness very rapidly (seconds to a few minutes) after assuming the horizontal position, but residual nervousness, dizziness, headache, nausea, pallor, diaphoresis, and an urge to defecate may be noted. A postictal confusional state with disorientation and agitation either is very brief (< 30 seconds) or does not occur. Syncope may recur, especially if the patient stands up within the next 30 minutes.

Reassurance and a recommendation to avoid precipitating factors are usually the only treatment necessary.

CARDIOVASCULAR SYNCOPE

A cardiovascular cause is suggested when syncope occurs with the patient in a recumbent position, during or following physical exertion, or in a patient with known heart disease. Loss of consciousness related to cardiac disease is most often due to an abrupt decrease in cardiac output with subsequent cerebral hypoperfusion. Such cardiac dysfunction can result from cardiac arrest, rhythm disturbances (either brady- or tachyarrhythmias), cardiac inflow or outflow obstruction, intracardiac right-to-left shunts, leaking or dissecting aortic aneurysms, or acute pulmonary embolus (Table 9–9).

1. CARDIAC ARREST

Cardiac arrest (ventricular fibrillation, or asystole) from any cause will cause loss of consciousness in three to five seconds if the patient is standing or, within 15 seconds if the patient is recumbent.

Table 9–9. Causes of syncope from cardiovascular diseases.

Cardiac arrest
Cardiac dysrhythmias
  Tachyarrythmias
    Supraventricular
      Paroxysmal atrial tachycardia
      Atrial flutter
      Atrial fibrillation
      Accelerated junctional tachycardia
    Ventricular
      Ventricular tachycardia
      Ventricular fibrillation
  Bradyarrhthmias
    Sinus bradycardia
    Sinus arrest
    Second- or third-degree heart block
    Implanted pacemaker failure or malfunction
  Mitral valve prolapse (click-murmur syndrome)
  Prolonged QT-interval syndromes
  Sick-sinus syndrome (tachycardia-bradycardia syndrome)
  Drug toxicity (especially digitalis, quinidine, procainamide, propranolol, phenothiazines, tricyclic antidepressants, potassium)
Cardiac inflow obstruction
  Left atrial myxoma or thrombus
  Tight mitral stenosis
  Constrictive pericarditis or cardiac tamponade
  Restrictive cardiomyopathies
  Tension pneumothorax
Cardiac outflow obstruction
  Aortic stenosis
  Pulmonary stenosis
  Hypertropic obstructive cardiomyopathy (asymmetric septal hypertrophy, idiopathic hypertrophic subaortic stenosis)

Dissecting aortic aneurysm
Severe pulmonary-vascular disease
  Pulmonary hypertension
  Acute pulmonary embolus

Seizurelike activity and urinary and fecal incontinence may be seen as the duration of cerebral hypoperfusion increases.

2. TACHYARRHYTHMIAS

Supraventricular Tachyarrhythmias

Supraventricular tachyarrhythmias (atrial or junctional tachycardia, atrial flutter, or atrial fibrillation) may be paroxysmal or chronic and can occur in all age groups—and in persons with or without clinical heart disease. Such rhythm disturbances may be spontaneous, or they may be secondary to metabolic abnormalities, hypoxia, drug overdose, and many systemic and cardiovascular disorders.

Heart rates faster than 160–200/min reduce cardiac output by decreasing the ventricular filling period or inducing myocardial ischemia. Prolonged tachycardia of 180–200 beats or more per minute will produce syncope in 50% of normal persons in the upright posture; in patients with underlying heart disease, a heart rate of 135/min may impair cardiac output enough to induce loss of consciousness. In addition, patients with sinus node dysfunction (**sick-sinus syndrome**) may develop profound sinus, junctional, or idioventricular bradycardias—or even asystole—upon termination of their tachyarrhythmias. This can cause syncope, atrial fibrillation, and other forms of atrioventricular dissociation and further reduce cardiac output by loss of coordinated atrial activity.

Routine ECGs, even if abnormal, are often not helpful in establishing a diagnosis, which is firmly established only when arrhythmias are demonstrated during a symptomatic episode. Continuous electrocardiographic monitoring or outpatient portable Holter monitoring may be required.

Ventricular Tachyarrhythmias

Ventricular tachyarrhythmias (ventricular tachycardia or multiform, frequent, or paired premature ventricular contractions) are found on prolonged electrocardiographic monitoring in some patients with syncope. These arrhythmias do not often coincide with syncopal symptoms. Frequent or repetitive premature ventricular contractions, however, are predictive of sudden death.

Mitral Valve Prolapse

Mitral valve prolapse (**click-murmur syndrome**) is a common disorder associated with supraventricular and ventricular arrhythmias. In one series, 25% of patients reported lightheadedness or dizziness, and 4% had syncope. The condition is twice as frequent in women as in men. Atypical chest pain that is characteristically nonexertional, left precordial, sharp in quality, and of variable duration is the most common complaint, followed by dyspnea and fatigue. Serious

ventricular arrhythmias and profound bradycardia may occur.

Auscultation of the heart may reveal midsystolic clicks, mid-to-late systolic murmurs that vary with specific maneuvers, or a classic mitral regurgitation murmur. The ECG may be entirely normal or may show nonspecific ST-T wave changes. Frequent premature ventricular contractions are often noted. The diagnosis can be established by echocardiography.

Prolonged QT Syndrome

The congenital prolonged QT-interval syndrome consists of paroxysmal ventricular arrhythmias (often torsade de pointes), syncope, and sudden death and is inherited either as an autosomal recessive condition associated with deafness or in an autosomal dominant form without deafness. Sporadic nonfamilial cases have also been reported. Drugs such as quinidine and electrolyte disturbances such as hypocalcemia or hypokalemia can also produce QT prolongation.

Symptoms generally begin in infancy, but patients may be asymptomatic until the second or third decade, especially in the dominantly inherited disorder. The ECG may occasionally show a normal QT_c interval at rest that becomes abnormally prolonged with exercise. Treatment with propranolol is often effective.

3. BRADYARRHYTHMIAS

Sinoatrial Node Disease

Sinoatrial node disease may present as profound sinus bradycardia, prolonged sinus pauses, or sinus arrest with the appearance of a slow atrial, junctional, or idioventricular escape rhythm. Patients with sinus node dysfunction may also develop profound bradycardia or asystole sufficient to produce syncope upon termination of a supraventricular tachycardia. Sinus node dysfunction may be idiopathic or the result of fibrosis, vascular occlusion, infiltrative processes, or drug therapy (especially propranolol).

All such patients should be promptly evaluated by a cardiologist, since a permanent pacemaker is necessary in many cases.

Complete Heart Block

Complete heart block (third-degree atrioventricular block) is the most common bradyarrhythmia that produces syncope. Permanent atrioventricular conduction abnormalities are easily noted on a routine ECG, but intermittent conduction abnormalities may not be present on a random tracing. Transient complete heart block is suggested as the cause of syncope by an ECG demonstrating bundle branch block with or without a prolonged PR interval. A normal PR interval on an ECG obtained after the episode does not exclude the diagnosis of transient complete heart block.

Patients with syncope and documented or suspected complete heart block should be promptly hospitalized. Patients with acute inferior myocardial infarctions are at high risk for atrioventricular block.

4. CARDIAC INFLOW OBSTRUCTION

Atrial or ventricular **myxomas** and atrial **thrombi** usually present with embolic events, but they may also produce a left ventricular inflow or outflow obstruction that results in a sudden decrease in cardiac output, followed by syncope. Physical examination of the patient with left atrial myxoma often suggests mitral stenosis, but a mitral regurgitation murmur is occasionally heard. Fever, petechiae, and an elevated sedimentation rate may also be present. A history of syncope occurring with change in position is classic but uncommon. Echocardiography can confirm the diagnosis. Surgical removal of the myxoma is indicated.

With **constrictive pericarditis** or **pericardial tamponade,** any maneuver or drug that decreases heart rate or venous return can result in suddenly inadequate cardiac output and syncope.

5. CARDIAC OUTFLOW OBSTRUCTION

Aortic Stenosis

Loss of consciousness from congenital or acquired severe aortic stenosis occurs in all age groups, usually following exercise, and is often associated with dyspnea, angina, and diaphoresis. Several pathophysiological processes have been hypothesized, including acute left ventricular failure resulting in coronary hypoperfusion, with subsequent ventricular fibrillation. Alternatively, abrupt increases in left ventricular pressure may stimulate baroreceptors, leading to reflexive peripheral vascular dilation.

Physical findings include a characteristic systolic murmur (often associated with a palpable thrill), a sustained and prolonged left ventricular lift, and a paradoxically split second heart sound. Calcification of the valve is usually evident on fluoroscopy in patients over age 35 years. Echocardiography can help confirm the diagnosis.

Symptomatic aortic stenosis associated with angina, congestive heart failure, or syncope requires valve replacement, and all such patients should be promptly hospitalized. The average survival following syncope from aortic stenosis is one-and-one-half to three years without treatment.

Pulmonary Stenosis

Severe pulmonary stenosis can produce syncope, especially following exertion. A hemodynamic process similar to that occurring in aortic stenosis is responsible.

Hypertrophic Obstructive Cardiomyopathy

Hypertrophic obstructive cardiomyopathy (asymmetric septal hypertrophy, hypertrophic cardiomyopathy, idiopathic hypertrophic subaortic stenosis [IHSS]) comprises a group of congenital cardiomyopathies inherited as autosomal dominant conditions of variable severity. Symptoms most often have their onset between the second and fourth decades; dyspnea is the most common presenting complaint (60% of patients), but syncope occurs in 30% and is the presenting complaint in 10%. Syncope characteristically develops during or following exercise, but orthostatic and posttussive episodes also occur. Loss of consciousness has been attributed to left ventricular outflow obstruction caused by abnormal movement of the anterior mitral leaflet against the septum in midsystole, by inflow obstruction from decreased ventricular compliance, or by transient arrhythmias.

Suggestive features on physical examination include a double apical and carotid impulse, a precordial thrill, a prominent fourth heart sound, and a left ventricular heave. The classic long systolic ejection murmur of IHSS is heard best at the lower left sternal border or apex, radiates poorly into the neck, and has a prominent midsystolic accentuation. Mitral valve prolapse is common, and a mitral regurgitation murmur may be noted. Unlike valvular aortic stenosis, the IHSS murmur increases under circumstances that reduce the volume of the ventricle or increase its contractility (eg, Valsalva's maneuver, amyl nitrite inhalation, or a premature ventricular contraction).

If IHSS is suspected, the diagnosis can be confirmed by echocardiography. Propranolol has been used successfully to control symptoms.

6. DISSECTING AORTIC ANEURYSM

Approximately 5–10% of patients with acute aortic dissections present with isolated syncope; other neurological abnormalities may or may not be present. In 15% of patients, the dissection is painless.

7. PULMONARY HYPERTENSION & PULMONARY EMBOLUS

Syncope, often exertional, may be the presenting symptom of pulmonary hypertension. Signs of right ventricular failure (parasternal heave, increased second heart sound, murmur of pulmonary insufficiency), electrocardiographic evidence of right ventricular hypertrophy, and tachypnea may be found. Unrecognized showers of pulmonary emboli can cause pulmonary hypertension, as can a host of systemic, cardiac, and primary pulmonary diseases. A history of exertional dyspnea is usual, and hypoxemia on blood gas analysis is present even at rest.

Syncope is the presenting symptom in about 20%

of patients experiencing a massive pulmonary embolus; it is uncommonly a result of small pulmonary emboli. Upon recovery from syncope, such patients often complain of pleuritic chest pain, dyspnea, and apprehension. Hypotension, tachycardia, tachypnea, and significant arterial hypoxia frequently accompany these large emboli.

CEREBROVASCULAR SYNCOPE

Cerebrovascular disease is an often suspected but actually uncommon cause of episodic unconsciousness.

1. BASILAR ARTERY INSUFFICIENCY

Basilar artery transient ischemic attacks usually occur after the sixth decade. The symptom complex of diplopia, vertigo, dysphagia, dysarthria, various sensory or motor symptoms, drop attacks, and occipital headaches suggests diffuse brain stem ischemia. Attacks are typically sudden in onset and brief in duration (seconds to minutes), but when consciousness is lost, recovery is frequently prolonged (30–60 minutes or longer). Isolated unconsciousness without other symptoms of brain stem ischemia is rarely due to basilar artery insufficiency. Two-thirds of patients have recurrent attacks, and strokes eventually occur in about one-fifth of all cases. Treatment is discussed in Chapter 10.

2. SUBCLAVIAN STEAL SYNDROME

The subclavian steal syndrome results from subclavian or innominate artery stenosis that causes retrograde blood flow in the vertebral artery, with subsequent brain stem hypoperfusion. The degree of subclavian artery stenosis that will produce symptoms is quite variable, and a minor (40%) stenosis may cause the syndrome in some patients. A difference between blood pressures measured in the two arms is nearly always found, the average difference being a 45-mm Hg decrease in systolic pressure in the arm supplied by the stenotic vessel. In one series of cases, while syncope was described in 18% of patients, vertigo, diplopia, limb paresis and paresthesias, and ataxia were more common manifestations. Stroke resulting from this condition is rare.

If this diagnosis is suspected, arteriography and subsequent surgical correction may be indicated.

3. MIGRAINE

Syncope occurs in 10% of migrainous patients, often upon rapid rising to a standing position, suggesting that loss of consciousness is due to orthostatic hypotension. In some patients, **basilar migraine** produces symptoms similar to those of basilar artery transient ischemic attacks. Antimigraine drug therapy (see Chapter 3) is often effective in preventing attacks.

4. TAKAYASU'S DISEASE

Takayasu's disease (aortic arch syndrome, pulseless disease) is a panarteritis of the great vessels that is most common in Asian women. Symptoms of central nervous system hypoperfusion such as impaired vision, confusion, or syncope are often prominent. In one reported series, syncope was noted in 75% of patients, particularly following exercise, standing, or head movement. Physical examination reveals decreased or absent brachial pulses with low blood pressures in both arms. The erythrocyte sedimentation rate is moderately elevated during the acute stage. Hospitalization for evaluation and initiation of corticosteroid treatment is indicated.

5. CAROTID SINUS SYNCOPE

Carotid sinus syncope is uncommon. Men are affected twice as often as women, and most affected individuals are over 60 years of age. Drugs known to predispose to carotid sinus syncope include propranolol, digitalis, and methyldopa. Classically, pressure on the carotid sinus by a tight collar, a neck mass, enlarged cervical lymph nodes, or a tumor causes vagal stimulation, which inhibits the cardiac sinoatrial and atrioventricular nodes and reduces sympathetic vascular tone. The resultant bradycardia or systemic hypotension may then produce syncope; pure cardioinhibitory or vasodepressor syncope also occurs. The bradycardia can be abolished or prevented by administration of atropine.

Carotid sinus syncope may be mistakenly diagnosed when symptoms result from compression of a normal carotid artery contralateral to an occluded internal carotid. Under these circumstances, unilateral compression transiently interrupts the entire anterior cerebral circulation. Performing carotid sinus massage in an attempt to diagnose carotid sinus syncope in patients with carotid atherosclerotic disease produces a risk of distal embolization of atheromatous material.

MISCELLANEOUS CAUSES OF SYNCOPE

1. ORTHOSTATIC HYPOTENSION

Orthostatic hypotension occurs more often in men than in women and is most common in the sixth and seventh decades. It may, however, appear even in teenagers. Loss of consciousness usually occurs upon rapidly rising to a standing position, standing motionless for a prolonged period (especially following exercise), and standing after prolonged recumbency (especially in elderly patients).

Numerous conditions can produce orthostatic hypotension (Table 9–10), which generally results from either reduced blood volume or autonomic nervous system dysfunction. The latter may be due to sympathetic drugs, autonomic neuropathy, or central nervous system disorders affecting sympathetic pathways in the hypothalamus, brain stem, or spinal cord. Two neurogenic causes of orthostatic hypotension deserve special consideration. **Idiopathic orthostatic hypotension** is associated mainly with the degeneration of postganglionic sympathetic neurons without other neuropathological changes. In **Shy-Drager syndrome,** orthostatic hypotension appears to be related to degeneration of preganglionic sympathetic neurons; this occurs in combination with par-

kinsonian, pyramidal, cerebellar, or lower motor neuron signs.

The diagnosis of orthostatic hypotension is established by demonstrating a drop in blood pressure of at least 30 mm Hg systolic or 10 mm Hg diastolic when the patient changes from the lying to the standing position. In equivocal cases, tilt-table testing may be necessary. A detailed general physical and neurological examination and laboratory studies (hematocrit, stool occult blood, serum glucose and electrolytes, FTA, nerve conduction studies) should be directed toward establishing the cause of the disorder.

Any medication that might be responsible should be discontinued if possible, and the patient should be instructed to stand up gradually, to elevate the head of the bed on blocks, and to use waist-high elasticized support hosiery. Other therapy is dictated by the specific cause of hypotension. The potent mineralocorticoid fludrocortisone has been effective in idiopathic cases and in diabetic patients in doses beginning with 0.1 mg/d orally and increased gradually, as necessary, up to 1 mg/d orally. Its mode of action is unclear, but its benefit may relate to increased responsiveness to circulating norepinephrine, as well as to an increased plasma volume. Side effects include recumbent hypertension.

2. HYPERVENTILATION SYNCOPE

Hyperventilation is a frequent cause of faintness or dizziness but rarely culminates in syncope. Common symptoms include lightheadedness, shortness of breath, circumoral numbness and tingling, and muscular twitching. Pathophysiologically, **hypocapnia** produces cerebral vasoconstriction and results in central nervous system hypoperfusion. Patients are usually between 20 and 40 years of age, and women are affected far more frequently than men. The disorder is usually benign, with anxiety a prominent precipitant, but serious cardiopulmonary causes of hyperventilation or subjective dyspnea must be excluded. Symptoms commonly occur in the lying position, which can be diagnostically helpful. Patients often report prolonged unconsciousness, but upon close questioning proves this rarely to be true. Hyperventilation at the examiner's request often reproduces the symptoms.

3. COUGH SYNCOPE

Cough syncope occurs chiefly in middle-aged men with chronic obstructive pulmonary disease but has also been reported in children. Coughing need not be prolonged and immediately precedes unconsciousness, which may occur while the patient is supine. Prodromal symptoms are absent, and the duration of unconsciousness is brief—often only a few seconds.

Table 9–10. Causes of orthostatic hypotension.

Hypovolemia or hemorrhage
Addison's disease
Drug-induced hypotension
  Antidepressants
  Antihypertensives
  Bromocriptine
  Diuretics
  Levodopa
  Monoamine oxidase inhibitors
  Nitroglycerin
  Phenothiazines
Polyneuropathies
  Amyloid neuropathy
  Diabetic neuropathy
  Guillain-Barré syndrome
  Porphyric neuropathy
  Vincristine neuropathy
Other neurological disorders
  Idiopathic orthostatic hypotension
  Multiple sclerosis
  Parkinsonism
  Posterior fossa tumor
  Shy-Drager syndrome
  Spinal cord injury with paraplegia
  Surgical sympathectomy
  Syringomyelia/syringobulbia
  Tabes dorsalis
  Wernicke's encephalopathy
Cardiovascular disorders
Prolonged bed rest

Full recovery of consciousness occurs immediately. A history of similar episodes is common, and symptoms may be reproduced by having the patient cough on request. The cause may be a decrease in cerebral blood flow from increased intracranial pressure, which results from transmission of increased intrathoracic pressure to the intracranial compartment via the spinal fluid or venous connections.

The condition is usually benign, and there is no specific treatment except for antitussive drugs such as dextromethorphan.

4. MICTURITION SYNCOPE

Micturition syncope occurs almost exclusively in men, probably because of the standing position for urination. Episodes can occur immediately before, during, or after micturition. They are more likely to occur at night following the prolonged recumbency of sleep and are due to peripheral pooling of blood plus a vagally induced bradycardia. Urination in a sitting position usually eliminates the symptoms.

5. GLOSSOPHARYNGEAL NEURALGIA

Glossopharyngeal neuralgia is a rare syndrome of intermittent, agonizing paroxysmal pain localized to the tonsillar pillar or occasionally to the external auditory meatus. The pain is triggered by contact with or movement of the tonsillar pillars, especially during swallowing or talking. Syncope occurs as a consequence of the activation of a glossopharyngeal-vagal reflex arc, producing a transient bradyarrhythmia with resultant cerebral hypoperfusion.

Carbamazepine, 400–1000 mg/d orally, will prevent pain and bradycardia in most patients.

6. PSYCHOGENIC SYNCOPE

Psychogenic syncope is a diagnosis of exclusion and is often made erroneously. Suggestive features are lack of any prodrome, possible secondary gain, bizarre postures and movements, lack of pallor, and a prolonged period of apparent unresponsiveness. Psychogenic spells rarely occur when the patient is alone and they rarely are associated with incontinence or result in injury. Most patients are young or have a well-documented history of conversion disorder. Without such a history, diagnosis after the third decade is suspect.

The EEG during psychogenic unconsciousness is normal, without the slowing that typically follows unconsciousness from a seizure. Caloric testing (see Chapter 11), which produces nystagmus in conscious, and tonic eye deviation in unconscious, patients, can distinguish psychogenic unresponsiveness from coma caused by a metabolic or structural lesion.

7. MÉNIÈRE'S DISEASE

Ménière's disease (see Chapter 4) is characterized by recurrent attacks of severe vertigo that persist for several hours and are associated with tinnitus and progressive hearing loss. A small percentage of patients experience loss of consciousness for a few seconds at the onset of an attack. Basilar artery transient ischemic attacks pose the most important differential diagnostic problem; however, signs or symptoms suggesting more diffuse brain stem involvement (especially visual field disturbances or diplopia) strongly support basilar artery insufficiency.

Dimenhydrinate, 50 mg orally three times daily, is often helpful in treatment. Other forms of treatment are discussed in Chapter 4.

REFERENCES

SEIZURES

General

Engel J Jr: *Seizures and Epilepsy*. Vol 31 of: *Contemporary Neurology Series*. Davis, 1989.

Hansotia P, Broste SK: The effect of epilepsy or diabetes mellitus on the risk of automobile accidents. *N Engl J Med* 1991;324:22–26.

Hauser WA et al: Seizure recurrence after a 1st unprovoked seizure: An extended follow-up. *Neurology* 1990;40:1163–1170.

Etiology

Alldredge BK, Lowenstein DH, Simon RP: Seizures associated with recreational drug abuse. *Neurology* 1989;39:1037–1039.

Charness ME, Simon RP, Greenberg DA: Ethanol and the nervous system. *N Engl J Med* 1989;321:442–454.

Fox MW, Harms RW, Davis DH: Selected neurological complications of pregnancy. *Mayo Clin Proc* 1990;65:1595–1618.

Holtzman DM, Kaku DA, So YT: New-onset seizures associated with human immunodeficiency virus infection: Causation and clinical features in 100 cases. *Am J Med* 1989;87:173–177.

Kilpatrick CJ et al: Epileptic seizures in acute stroke. *Arch Neurol* 1990;47:157–160.

Messing RO, Closson RG, Simon RP: Drug-induced seizures: A 10-year experience. *Neurology* 1984;34: 1582–1586.

Messing RO, Simon RP: Seizures as a manifestation of systemic disease. *Neurol Clin* 1986;4:563–584.

Olsen T, Hogerhaven H, Thage O: Epilepsy after stroke. *Neurology* 1987;37:1209–1211.

Pomeroy SL et al: Seizures and other neurological sequelae of bacterial meningitis in children. *N Engl J Med* 1990;323:1651–1657.

Classification & Clinical Findings

Aminoff MJ, Simon RP: Status epilepticus: Causes, clinical features and consequences in 98 patients. *Am J Med* 1980;69:657–666.

Berkovic SF et al: Progressive myoclonus epilepsies: Specific causes and diagnosis. *N Engl J Med* 1986; 315:296–305.

Daly DD: Ictal clinical manifestations of complex partial seizures. Pages 57–83 in: *Complex Partial Seizures and Their Treatment.* Penry JK, Daly DD (editors). Vol 11 of: Advances in Neurology. Raven, 1975.

Gomez MR, Klass DW: Epilepsies of infancy and childhood. *Ann Neurol* 1983;13:113–124.

Leppik IE (editor): Status epilepticus in perspective. *Neurology* 1990;40(Suppl 2):1–51. [Entire issue.]

So EL, Penry JK: Epilepsy in adults. *Ann Neurol* 1981;9:3–16.

Treatment

Callaghan N, Garrett A, Goggin T: Withdrawal of anticonvulsant drugs in patients free of seizures for two years. *N Engl J Med* 1988;318:942–946.

Cascino GD: Intractable partial epilepsy: Evaluation and treatment. *Mayo Clin Proc* 1990;65:1578–1586.

Dalessio DJ: Seizure disorders and pregnancy. *N Engl J Med* 1985;312:559–563.

Dodson WE: Level off. *Neurology* 1989;39:1009–1010.

Elwes RD et al: The prognosis for seizure control in newly diagnosed epilepsy. *N Engl J Med* 1984;311: 944–947.

Farwell JR et al: Phenobarbital for febrile seizures—Effects on intelligence and on seizure recurrence. *N Engl J Med* 1990;322:364–369.

Jones KL et al: Pattern of malformations in the children of women treated with carbamazepine during pregnancy. *N Engl J Med* 1989;320:1661–1666.

Mattson RH et al: Comparison of carbamazepine, phenytoin, and primidone in partial and secondarily generalized tonic-clonic seizures. *N Engl J Med* 1985;313:145–151.

Scheuer ML, Pedley TA: The evaluation and treatment of seizures. *N Engl J Med* 1990;323:1468–1474.

Temkin NR et al: A randomized, double-blind study of phenytoin for the prevention of post-traumatic seizures. *N Engl J Med* 1990;323:497–502.

Pseudoseizures

King DW et al: Pseudoseizures: Diagnostic evaluation. *Neurology* 1982;32:18–23.

SYNCOPE

General

Kapoor WN: Diagnostic evaluation of syncope. *Am J Med* 1991;90:91–106.

Manolis AS et al: Syncope: Current diagnostic evaluation and management. *Ann Intern Med* 1990;112: 850–863.

Vasovagal

Lin JT et al: Convulsive syncope in blood donors. *Ann Neurol* 1982;11:525–528.

Cardiovascular

Aminoff MJ et al: Electrocerebral accompaniments of syncope associated with malignant ventricular arrhythmias. *Ann Intern Med* 1988;108:791–796.

Fujimura O et al: The diagnostic sensitivity of electrophysiologic testing in patients with syncope caused by transient bradycardia. *N Engl J Med* 1989;321:1703–1707.

Kapoor WN et al: Prolonged electrocardiographic monitoring in patients with syncope. *Am J Med* 1987;82: 20–28.

Markel ML, Waller BF, Armstrong WF: Cardiac myxoma: A review. *Medicine* 1987;66:114–125.

Richards AM et al: Syncope in aortic valvular stenosis. *Lancet* 1984;2:1113–1116.

Simpson RJ Jr et al: Vagal syncope during recurrent pulmonary embolism. *JAMA* 1983;249:390–393.

Cerebrovascular

Hennerici M, Klemm C, Rautenberg W: The subclavian steal phenomenon: A common vascular disorder with rare neurological deficits. *Neurology* 1988;38:669–673.

Sugrue DD, Wood DL, McGoon MD: Carotid sinus hypersensitivity and syncope. *Mayo Clin Proc* 1984;59: 637–640.

Miscellaneous Causes

Haslam RHA, Freigang B: Cough syncope mimicking epilepsy in asthmatic children. *Can J Neurol Sci* 1985;12:45–47.

Lagerlund TD et al: An electroencephalographic study of glossopharyngeal neuralgia with syncope. *Arch Neurol* 1988;45:472–475.

Lipsitz LA: Orthostatic hypotension in the elderly. *N Engl J Med* 1989;321:952–957.

Perkin GD, Joseph R: Neurological manifestations of the hyperventilation syndrome. *J Roy Soc Med* 1986;79: 448–450.

Stroke is the third most common cause of death in the United States and the most common disabling neurological disorder. Its incidence increases with age and is somewhat higher in men than in women and in blacks than in whites. Risk factors for stroke include systolic or diastolic hypertension, hypercholesterolemia, cigarette smoking, heavy alcohol consumption, and oral contraceptive use. Despite its importance as a leading cause of disability and death, the incidence of stroke has decreased in recent decades, largely because of improved treatment of hypertension.

APPROACH TO DIAGNOSIS

Stroke is a syndrome characterized by the acute onset of a neurological deficit that persists for at least 24 hours, reflects focal involvement of the central nervous system, and is the result of a disturbance of the cerebral circulation. The acute onset and subsequent duration of symptoms are documented by the history. The site of central nervous system involvement is suggested by the nature of the symptoms. It is delineated more precisely by the neurological examination and confirmed by imaging studies (CT or MRI). A vascular etiology may be inferred from the acute onset of symptoms and often from the presence of symptoms and signs that reflect involvement of the territory of a particular cerebral blood vessel. When this is confirmed by imaging studies, further investigations can be undertaken to identify a specific cause.

Acute Onset

Strokes begin abruptly. Neurological deficits may be maximal at onset, as is common in embolic stroke, or may progress over seconds to hours (or occasionally days), which is characteristic of progressive arterial thrombosis or recurrent emboli. A stroke that is actively progressing as a direct consequence of the underlying vascular disorder (but not because of associated cerebral edema) or has done so in recent minutes is termed **stroke in evolution** or **progressing stroke**. Focal cerebral deficits that develop slowly (over weeks to months) are unlikely to be due to stroke and are more suggestive of tumor or inflammatory or degenerative disease.

Duration of Deficits

By definition, stroke produces neurological deficits that persist for at least 24 hours. When symptoms and signs resolve completely after briefer periods (usually within 30 minutes), the term **transient ischemic attack (TIA)** is used. Recurrent TIAs with identical clinical features are usually caused by thrombosis or embolism arising within the cerebral circulation. TIAs that differ in character from event to event suggest recurrent emboli from a cardiac source. Although TIAs do not themselves produce lasting neurological dysfunction, they are important to recognize because about one-third of patients with TIAs will go on to have a stroke within five years—and because this risk may be reduced with treatment.

In some cases, deficits last for longer than 24

hours, but resolve completely or almost completely within a few days; the term **reversible ischemic neurological deficit (RIND)** is sometimes used to describe these events.

As their names imply, TIAs and RINDs are uniquely associated with cerebral ischemia, as opposed to hemorrhage.

Focal Involvement

Stroke produces focal symptoms and signs that correlate with the area of the brain supplied by the affected blood vessel. In ischemic stroke, occlusion of a blood vessel interrupts the flow of blood to a specific region of the brain, interfering with neurological functions dependent on that region and producing a more or less stereotyped pattern of deficits. Hemorrhage produces a less predictable pattern of focal involvement because complications such as increased intracranial pressure, cerebral edema, compression of brain tissue and blood vessels, or dispersion of blood through the subarachnoid space or cerebral ventricles can impair brain function at sites remote from the hemorrhage.

Cerebrovascular disorders can also affect the brain in more diffuse fashion and produce global cerebral dysfunction, but the term *stroke* should not be applied in these cases. These disorders include **global cerebral ischemia** (usually from cardiac arrest) and **subarachnoid hemorrhage** (discussed in Chapter 3).

In most cases of stroke, the history and neurological examination provide enough information to localize the lesion to one side of the brain (eg, to the side opposite a hemiparesis or hemisensory deficit; to the left side if aphasia is present) and to the anterior or posterior cerebral circulation.

A. Anterior Circulation: The anterior cerebral circulation, which supplies most of the cerebral cortex and subcortical white matter, basal ganglia, and internal capsule, consists of the internal carotid artery and its branches: the anterior choroidal, anterior cerebral, and middle cerebral arteries. The middle cerebral artery in turn gives rise to deep, penetrating lenticulostriate branches (Figure 10–1). The specific territory of each of these vessels is shown in Table 10–1. Anterior circulation strokes are commonly associated with symptoms and signs that indicate hemispheric dysfunction (Table 10–2), such as aphasia, apraxia, or agnosia. They also produce hemiparesis, hemisensory disturbances, and visual field defects, which can also occur with posterior circulation strokes.

B. Posterior Circulation: The posterior cerebral circulation supplies the brain stem, cerebellum, and thalamus, and portions of the occipital and temporal lobes. It consists of the paired vertebral arteries, the basilar artery, and their branches: the posterior inferior cerebellar, anterior inferior cerebellar, superior cerebellar, and posterior cerebral arteries (Figure 10–1). The posterior cerebral artery also gives off thalamoperforate and thalamogeniculate branches. Areas supplied by these arteries are listed in Table 10–1. Posterior circulation strokes produce symptoms and signs of brain stem dysfunction (Table 10–2), including coma, drop attacks (sudden collapse

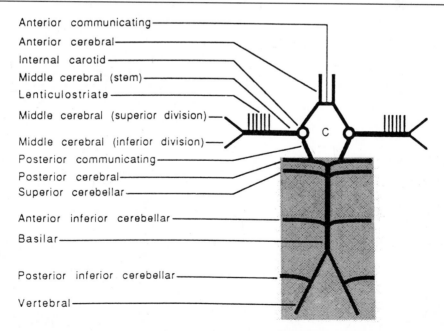

Figure 10–1. Arteries of the anterior (unshaded) and posterior (shaded) cerebral circulation in relation to the circle of Willis (C).

Table 10–1. Territories of the principal cerebral arteries.

Artery	Territory
Anterior circulation	
Internal carotid	
Anterior choroidal	Hippocampus, globus pallidus, lower internal capsule
Anterior cerebral	Medial frontal and parietal cortex and subjacent white matter, anterior corpus callosum
Middle cerebral	Lateral frontal, parietal, occipital and temporal cortex and subjacent white matter
Lenticulostriate branches	Caudate nucleus, putamen, upper internal capsule
Posterior circulation	
Vertebral	
Posterior inferior cerebellar	Medulla, lower cerebellum
Basilar	
Anterior inferior cerebellar	Lower and midpons, midcerebellum
Superior cerebellar	Upper pons, lower midbrain, upper cerebellum
Posterior cerebral	Medial occipital and temporal cortex and subjacent white matter, posterior corpus callosum, upper midbrain
Thalamoperforate branches	Thalamus
Thalamogeniculate branches	Thalamus

without loss of consciousness), vertigo, nausea and vomiting, cranial nerve palsies, ataxia, and crossed sensorimotor deficits that affect the face on one side of the body and the limbs on the other. Hemiparesis, hemisensory disturbances, and visual field deficits also occur, but are not specific to posterior circulation strokes.

Vascular Origin

Although other pathological processes such as hypoglycemia or other metabolic disturbances, trauma, and seizures can produce focal central neurological deficits that begin abruptly and last for at least 24 hours, the term *stroke* is used only when such events are caused by cerebrovascular disease. The underlying pathological process in stroke can be either ischemia or hemorrhage, usually from an arterial lesion. In recent series, ischemia accounted for about two-thirds and hemorrhage for about one-third of strokes. It may not be possible to distinguish between ischemia and hemorrhage from the history and neuro-

Table 10–2. Symptoms and signs of anterior and posterior circulation ischemia.[1]

Symptom or Sign	Incidence (%)[2]	
	Anterior	Posterior
Headache	25	3
Altered consciousness	5	16
Aphasia[3]	20	0
Visual field defect	14	22
Diplopia[3]	0	7
Vertigo[3]	0	48
Dysarthria	3	11
Drop attacks[3]	0	16
Hemi- or monoparesis	38	12
Hemisensory deficit	33	9

[1]Modified from Hutchinson EC, Acheson EJ: *Strokes: Natural History, Pathology and Surgical Treatment.* Saunders, 1975.
[2]Most patients have multiple symptoms and signs.
[3]Most useful distinguishing features.

logical examination, but CT or MRI permits a definitive diagnosis.

A. Ischemia: Ischemia causes stroke by depriving the cerebral tissue of oxygen and glucose and preventing the removal of metabolic products. The brain is particularly sensitive to ischemia because of its high metabolic activity and low energy reserves. Neuronal energy depletion disrupts normal transmembrane ion gradients, leading to the accumulation of potassium in the extracellular space, release of excitotoxic neurotransmitters (eg, glutamate), and influx of calcium through voltage-gated and receptor-gated channels. The resulting intracellular calcium overload surpasses the ability of the neuron to sequester or extrude calcium and activates calcium-dependent proteases, phospholipases and endonucleases. These enzymes and their metabolic products (eg, arachidonic acid, lysophospholipids, oxygen free radicals) cause the breakdown of plasma membranes and cytoskeletal elements, leading to cell death.

If the blood flow to ischemic brain tissue is restored before neurons are irreversibly injured, the clinical symptoms and signs are transient. Prolonged interruption of blood flow, however, leads to irreversible ischemic injury (**infarction**) and persistent neurological deficits.

Two pathogenetic mechanisms can produce ischemic stroke—thrombosis and embolism. While about two-thirds of ischemic strokes are attributed to thrombosis and about one-third to embolism, the distinction is often difficult or impossible to make on clinical grounds.

1. Thrombosis produces stroke by occluding large cerebral arteries (especially the internal carotid, middle cerebral, or basilar), small penetrating arteries (this causes lacunar stroke), cerebral veins, or venous sinuses. Symptoms typically evolve over minutes to hours, and thrombotic strokes are often preceded by transient ischemic attacks.

2. Embolism produces stroke when cerebral arteries are occluded by the distal passage of thrombus from the heart or large cerebral arteries. Emboli in the anterior cerebral circulation most often occlude the middle cerebral artery or its branches, since about 85% of the hemispheric blood flow is carried by this vessel. Emboli in the posterior cerebral circulation usually lodge at the apex of the basilar artery or in the posterior cerebral arteries. Embolic strokes characteristically produce neurological deficits that are maximal at onset.

B. Hemorrhage: Hemorrhage may interfere with cerebral function through a variety of mechanisms, including destruction or compression of brain tissue and compression of vascular structures, leading to secondary ischemia and edema. Intracranial hemorrhage is classified by its location as intracerebral, subarachnoid, subdural, or epidural, all of which—except subdural hemorrhage—are usually caused by arterial bleeding.

1. Intracerebral hemorrhage causes symptoms by compressing adjacent tissue (which can then produce local ischemia) and, to a lesser extent, by destroying tissue. Unlike ischemic stroke, intracerebral hemorrhage tends to cause more severe headache and depression of consciousness as well as neurological deficits that do not correspond to the distribution of any single blood vessel.

2. Subarachnoid hemorrhage leads to cerebral dysfunction by elevating intracranial pressure as well as by still poorly understood toxic effects of subarachnoid blood on brain tissue. In addition, subarachnoid hemorrhage may be complicated by vasospasm, leading to ischemia, and by extension of blood into brain tissue producing an intracerebral hematoma. Subarachnoid hemorrhage typically presents with headache rather than focal neurological deficits; it is discussed in Chapter 3.

3. Subdural or epidural hemorrhage produces a mass lesion that can compress the underlying brain. These hemorrhages are often traumatic in origin, and usually present with headache or altered consciousness. Because their recognition is most critical in the setting of coma, subdural and epidural hemorrhage are discussed in Chapter 11.

FOCAL CEREBRAL ISCHEMIA

Etiology

A variety of disorders of the blood, blood vessels, and heart can lead to focal cerebral ischemia (Table 10–3).

A. Vascular Disorders:

1. Atherosclerosis–In most cases, atherosclerosis of the large extracranial arteries in the neck and

Table 10–3 Conditions associated with focal cerebral ischemia.

Vascular disorders
  Atherosclerosis
  Fibromuscular dysplasia
  Inflammatory disorders
    Giant cell arteritis
    Systemic lupus erythematosus
    Polyarteritis nodosa
    Granulomatous angiitis
    Syphilitic arteritis
    AIDS
  Carotid or veterbral artery dissection
  Lacunar infarction
  Drug abuse
  Migraine
  Multiple progressive intracranial occlusions (moyamoya syndrome)
  Venous or sinus thrombosis
Cardiac disorders
  Mural thrombus
  Rheumatic heart disease
  Arrhythmias
  Endocarditis
  Mitral valve prolapse
  Paradoxic embolus
  Atrial myxoma
  Prosthetic heart valves
Hematologic disorders
  Thrombocytosis
  Polycythemia
  Sickle cell disease
  Leukocytosis
  Hypercoagulable states

at the base of the brain is the underlying cause of focal cerebral ischemia. The sites of predilection (Figure 10–2) are the origin of the common carotid artery, the internal carotid artery just above the common carotid bifurcation and within the cavernous sinus, the origin of the middle cerebral artery, the vertebral artery at its origin and just above where it enters the skull, and the basilar artery.

The pathogenesis of atherosclerosis is incompletely understood, but injury to vascular endothelial cells is thought to be an early step. Endothelial cells may be injured by the accumulation of cholesterol esters derived from circulating low-density lipoproteins or by other mechanical, biochemical, or inflammatory mechanisms. Blood monocytes adhere to the sites of endothelial injury or denudation and subsequently migrate subendothelially, where they are transformed into tissue macrophages and accumulate lipids. The resulting lesion is called a **fatty streak.** The release of growth and chemotactic factors from endothelial cells and monocytic macrophages stimulates the proliferation and migration of intimal smooth muscle cells, and leads to formation of a **fibrous plaque.** Further endothelial injury or denudation ensues, promoting the adherence of platelets, which also release growth and chemotactic factors. The resulting atheromatous lesion (Figure 10–3) may

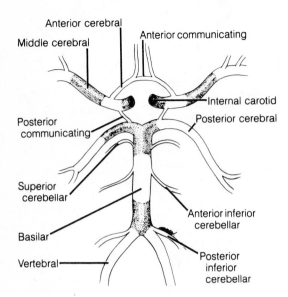

Figure 10–2. Sites of predilection (shaded areas) for atherosclerosis in the intracranial arterial circulation.

enlarge to occlude the vessel lumen, or it may provide a source of atheromatous or platelet emboli. Ulcerated atheromas may be especially likely sources of emboli.

The most important risk factor for atherosclerosis leading to stroke is systolic or diastolic hypertension. In one study of more than 5000 symptom-free men and women aged from 30 to 60 years followed prospectively for 18 years, the likelihood of hypertensive subjects developing stroke was seven times that of the nonhypertensives. Furthermore, the incidence of all the major cardiac and cerebrovascular sequelae of hypertension increased in direct proportion to the blood pressure even in the nonhypertensive range, without any identifiable critical or safe value. A blood pressure of 160 mm Hg systolic or 95 mm Hg diastolic observed during any clinic visit tripled the risk of stroke, suggesting that such patients should receive antihypertensive treatment.

Atherosclerosis can also occur in the absence of hypertension. In such cases, other factors such as diabetes, elevated serum cholesterol and triglycerides, cigarette smoking, hereditary predisposition, and the use of oral contraceptives may be implicated. Genetic disorders associated with accelerated atherosclerosis include homocystinuria and dyslipoproteinemias.

2. Fibromuscular dysplasia–This is a segmental nonatherosclerotic condition of large arteries characterized by segmental thinning of the media and fragmentation of the elastic lamina, alternating with rings of fibrous and muscular hyperplasia within the media (Figure 10–4). Extracranial vessels are involved more often than intracranial ones, and the cervical portion of the internal carotid is involved more than is the vertebral artery. Lesions are often bilateral, and women are more often affected than men. Transitory or fixed cerebral ischemic deficits may occur, although complete occlusion of involved arteries is rare, suggesting that symptoms may be due to the embolization of vascular thrombi. There is a characteristic string-of-beads appearance on angiography, indicating the presence of saccular dilations of involved arteries. The disorder is associated with saccular aneurysms of the cerebral arteries, which can in turn produce subarachnoid hemorrhage. Cerebral ischemic complications of fibromuscular dysplasia may be reduced by treatment with aspirin or by graduated intraluminal dilation of the affected extracranial vessels in symptomatic cases.

3. Inflammatory disorders–

a. Giant cell arteritis (see Chapter 3), also called temporal arteritis or cranial arteritis, sometimes produces signs of cerebral ischemia. Inflammatory changes affect the branches of the external carotid,

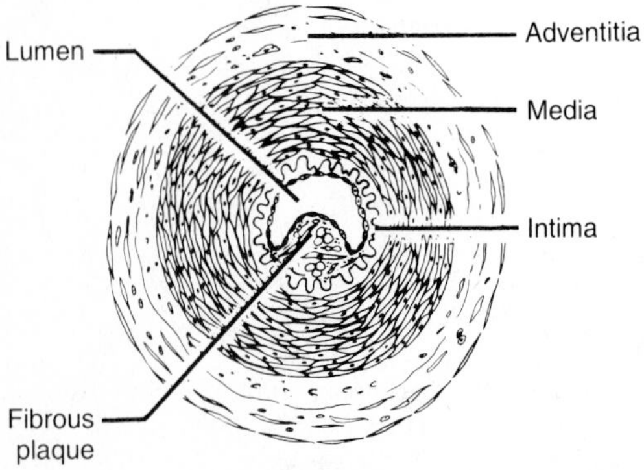

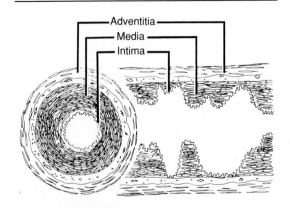

Figure 10–3. Arterial lesion in atherosclerosis. A fibrous plaque arising from the intimal surface encroaches on the arterial lumen and can occlude the vessel or provide a source of emboli.

Figure 10–4. Arterial lesion in fibromuscular dysplasia. The usual underlying lesion is hyperplasia of the media, which leads to multifocal stenosis of affected vessels.

cervical internal carotid, posterior ciliary, extracranial vertebral, and intracranial arteries. Inflammatory changes in the arterial wall may stimulate platelet adhesion and aggregation on damaged surfaces, leading to thrombosis or distal embolism. Although it is an uncommon cause of cerebral ischemic symptoms, giant cell arteritis should be considered in patients with transient monocular blindness or transient cerebral ischemic attacks—especially elderly patients—because the disorder is responsive to corticosteroid therapy and its complications (especially permanent blindness) may thus be avoided.

b. Systemic lupus erythematosus is associated with a vasculopathy that involves small cerebral vessels and leads to multiple microinfarctions. Inflammatory changes characteristic of true vasculitis are absent. There is no correlation between cerebral microinfarcts and verrucous (Libman-Sacks) endocarditis; cardiac emboli therefore appear to play little or no role in the genesis of cerebral symptoms.

c. Polyarteritis nodosa is a segmental vasculitis of small and medium-sized arteries that affects multiple organs. Transient symptoms of cerebral ischemia, including typical spells of transient monocular blindness, can occur.

d. Granulomatous angiitis (also called primary angiitis of the central nervous system) is an idiopathic inflammatory disease that affects small arteries and veins in the central nervous system and can cause transient or progressive multifocal lesions. Clinical features include headache, hemiparesis and other focal neurological abnormalities, and cognitive disturbances. The CSF usually shows pleocytosis and elevated protein, but the erythrocyte sedimentation rate is typically normal. The diagnosis should be suspected in any patient with multifocal central nervous system dysfunction and cerebrospinal fluid pleocytosis. Angiography demonstrates focal and segmental narrowing of small arteries and veins, and a meningeal biopsy is diagnostic. Treatment with corticosteroids, alone or in combination with cyclophosphamide, may be beneficial.

e. Syphilitic arteritis is uncommon but is being seen with increasing frequency in the male homosexual and other at-risk populations. It generally occurs within five years after the initial infection and reflects the underlying meningeal inflammatory process. It is important to recognize and treat the disorder at this early stage to prevent the later development of tertiary parenchymal neurosyphilis (general paresis or tabes dorsalis). Medium-sized penetrating vessels are typically involved (Figure 10–5), producing punctate areas of infarction in the deep white matter of the cerebral hemisphere, that can be seen on CT scan or MRI.

f. AIDS is associated with an increased incidence of transient ischemic attacks and ischemic stroke. The reason for this association is unclear, but the toxic effects of HIV-1 on blood vessels or the deposition of immune complexes may be involved. In some cases, ischemic neurological complications of AIDS are associated with endocarditis or with opportunistic infections of the central nervous system, such as toxoplasmosis or cryptococcal meningitis.

4. Carotid or vertebral artery dissection– Dissection of the carotid or vertebral artery is associated with hemorrhage into the vessel wall, which can occlude the vessel or predispose to thrombus formation and embolization. Posttraumatic carotid dissections present little difficulty in diagnosis. Certain patients, however—usually young men—suffer cerebral infarction after apparently spontaneous carotid artery dissection. Internal carotid artery dissections usually originate near the carotid bifurcation and can extend to the base of the skull. The underlying pathological process is usually **cystic medial necrosis.** Prodromal transient hemispheric ischemia or monocular blindness sometimes precedes a devastating stroke. Carotid dissection may be accompanied by pain in the jaw or neck, visual abnormalities akin to those that occur in migraine, or Horner's syndrome.

Dissection of the vertebral or basilar artery is less common. The clinical features of this disorder include headache, posterior neck pain, and the sudden onset of signs of brain stem dysfunction.

The treatment of carotid or vertebral artery dissection is controversial. Approaches include no treatment, removal of the intramural hematoma, and measures to prevent embolization from the site of dissection (aspirin, anticoagulants, or occlusion of the vessel distal to the dissection).

5. Lacunar infarction–Lacunar infarction of the brain results from the occlusion of small penetrating branches of the major cerebral arteries, especially those that supply the basal ganglia, thalamus, internal capsule, and pons. Lacunar infarcts are believed to be caused by either atherosclerosis or degenerative changes in arterial walls (including lipohyalinosis and fibrinoid necrosis) that are related to long-standing hypertension. Both hypertension and diabetes appear to predispose to this type of stroke (see p 266).

6. Drug abuse–Recreational use of cocaine hydrochloride, alkaloidal (crack) cocaine, amphetamines, or heroin appears to be a common risk factor for stroke in patients less than 35 years old. Patients who take these agents intravenously may develop infective endocarditis (see below) leading to embolic stroke. Stroke also occurs in drug users without endocarditis, however, including those who take drugs only intranasally or by smoke or vapor inhalation, and often has its onset within hours of drug use. Mechanisms that have been proposed to explain these events include drug-induced vasospasm, vasculitis, and the rupture of preexisting aneurysms or vascular malformations. Cocaine hydrochloride is most often associated with intracerebral hemorrhage but can also cause subarachnoid hemorrhage or ischemic stroke. Stroke from crack cocaine is most commonly is-

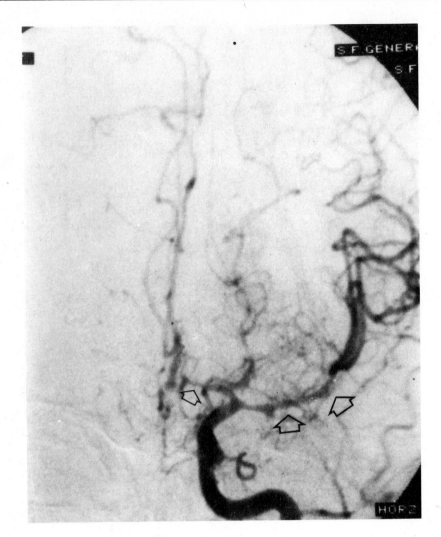

Figure 10–5. Left carotid angiogram (AP projection) in syphilitic arteritis showing marked narrowing of the proximal middle cerebral artery (arrows at right) and anterior cerebral artery (arrow at left). (Reproduced, with permission, from Lowenstein DH, Mills C, Simon RP: Acute syphilitic transverse myelitis: Unusual presentation of meningovascular syphilis. *Genitourin Med* 1987;63:333–338.)

chemic in origin, but intracerebral or subarachnoid hemorrhage also occurs. Amphetamines can produce vasculitis, with necrosis of the vessel wall leading to intracerebral hemorrhage; ischemic stroke and subarachnoid hemorrhage are less·frequent. Heroin is associated primarily with embolic stroke resulting from endocarditis.

7. Multiple progressive intracranial arterial occlusions (moyamoya)–This syndrome has two essential features: bilateral narrowing or occlusion of the distal internal carotid arteries and the adjacent anterior and middle cerebral artery trunks; and the presence of a fine network of collateral channels at the base of the brain. The term *moyamoya* derives from a Japanese word meaning *smoke* or *haze,* which characterizes the angiographic appearance of these fine collaterals (Figure 10–6). These same features have

been noted in patients from all ethnic groups and in patients with atherosclerosis, sickle cell anemia, or a history of basilar meningitis. The term therefore denotes an angiographic pattern of collateral vessels rather than a clinical or pathological syndrome. Children tend to present with ischemic strokes; adults present with intracerebral, subdural, or subarachnoid hemorrhage. Transient episodes of cerebral ischemia are infrequent.

8. Migraine–Stroke is a rare complication of migraine, which is considered in detail in Chapter 3. Migrainous stroke typically occurs during an attack of classic migraine. The anterior (especially middle cerebral artery) and posterior (especially posterior cerebral artery) cerebral circulations are affected about equally often. Stroke tends to occur in the same vascular territory affected by previous migraine attacks,

A

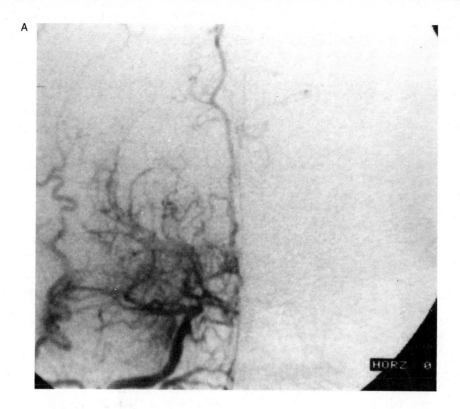

B

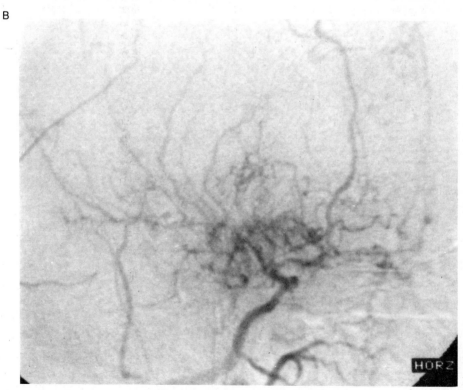

Figure 10–6. Right carotid angiogram in moyamoya. The middle cerebral artery and its branches are replaced by a diffuse capillary pattern that has the appearance of a puff of smoke. **A:** AP view. **B:** lateral view.

and investigative studies usually show no associated cardiac or cerebrovascular abnormality, suggesting that migraine itself is the cause of stroke.

9. Venous or sinus thrombosis–This uncommon cause of stroke is typically associated with a predisposing condition such as otitis or sinusitis, pregnancy or a postpartum state, dehydration, or coagulopathy. Clinical features include headache, papilledema, impaired consciousness, seizures, and focal neurological deficits. CSF pressure is typically increased, and in cases of septic thrombosis, pleocytosis may occur. When the site of thrombosis is the superior sagittal sinus, a CT scan with contrast sometimes shows a filling defect corresponding to the clot. The diagnosis is confirmed by cerebral angiography. In patients presenting with headache and papilledema, venous or sinus thrombosis must be differentiated from intracranial mass lesions and idiopathic pseudotumor cerebri. The radiological studies mentioned above are useful in this regard. Septic thromboses are treated with antibiotics. Anticoagulation has been used for aseptic thrombosis, but its efficacy has not been proved, and it may be precipitate intracranial hemorrhage.

B. Cardiac Disorders:

1. Mural thrombus–Mural thrombus complicating myocardial infarction or cardiomyopathy is a recognized source of cerebral embolism. The risk of stroke in the first weeks after myocardial infarction is related to the size of the cardiac lesion. More extensive myocardial damage may increase the tendency for mural thrombi to form; it may exacerbate the generalized hypercoagulable state that accompanies the infarct—or it may do both. Accordingly, patients with large transmural myocardial infarcts require anticoagulation therapy to substantially reduce the incidence of early thromboembolic events, including stroke.

2. Rheumatic heart disease–The incidence of focal cerebral ischemia is increased in patients with rheumatic heart disease—particularly those with mitral stenosis and atrial fibrillation—presumably as a result of embolization. In other cases, symptoms are temporally related to exertion, suggesting hypoperfusion as the cause.

3. Arrhythmias–Atrial fibrillation (especially when associated with rheumatic heart disease) and the bradycardia-tachycardia (sick-sinus) syndrome are well-recognized causes of embolic stroke. Other cardiac arrhythmias are more likely to produce pancerebral hypoperfusion with diffuse rather than focal symptoms (eg, syncope, dimming of vision, nonspecific lightheadedness, generalized seizures) unless severe carotid artery stenosis is also present.

4. Endocarditis–

a. Infective (bacterial or fungal) endocarditis is a cause of transient cerebral ischemia and embolic cerebral infarction during the active phase of infection and during the first few months following antibiotic cure. At autopsy, cerebral emboli are identified in 30% and systemic emboli in 60% of such patients. The middle cerebral artery is the most common site of cerebral embolization. Intracerebral or subarachnoid hemorrhage can also occur as a result of bleeding into an infarct or rupture of a mycotic aneurysm. Infective endocarditis is seen most often in intravenous drug users and patients with valvular heart disease or prosthetic valves. Streptococci and staphylococci are the most common causes, but gram-negative bacilli (eg, *Pseudomonas*) and fungi (especially *Candida* and *Aspergillus*) are also frequent pathogens in intravenous drug users and prosthetic valve recipients.

Signs of infective endocarditis include heart murmurs, petechiae, subungual splinter hemorrhages, retinal Roth's spots (red spots with white centers), Osler's nodes (painful red or purple digital nodules), Janeway's lesions (red macules on the palms or soles), and clubbing of the fingers or toes. The diagnosis is usually made by culturing the responsible organism from the blood. Treatment is with antibiotics; valve replacement is sometimes required. Anticoagulation should be avoided because of the risk of intracranial hemorrhage.

b. Nonbacterial (marantic) endocarditis is most frequent in patients with cancer and is responsible for the vast majority of ischemic strokes in this population. The tumors most often associated with this type of stroke are adenocarcinomas of the lung or gastrointestinal tract. Vegetations are present on the mitral or aortic valves; associated murmurs are rare. Identification of valvular vegetations by 2-D echocardiography may be diagnostic, but failure to demonstrate vegetations does not exclude the diagnosis. Anticoagulation with heparin may be useful in patients with treatable tumors or with other treatable causes of marantic endocarditis, such as sepsis.

5. Mitral valve prolapse–Myxomatous degeneration of the mitral valve (mitral valve prolapse) causes mitral regurgitation and predisposes to infective endocarditis, fatal cardiac arrhythmias, and cerebral ischemic events. In asymptomatic patients, the prevalence of mitral valve prolapse by M-mode echocardiography (Figure 10–7) is between 5% and 10% but reaches 40% in young patients with symptoms of cerebral ischemia. While there appears to be a genuine association of mitral valve prolapse with cerebral ischemia, the degree to which the disorder increases the risk of stroke is apparently small, and massive strokes related to mitral valve prolapse are rare.

6. Paradoxical embolus–Congenital cardiac anomalies associated with a pathological communication between the right and left sides of the heart, such as **atrial septal defect** or **patent foramen ovale,** permit the passage of embolic material from the systemic venous circulation to the brain. Under these circumstances, venous thrombi can give rise to embolic stroke.

7. Atrial myxoma–This rare disorder can lead to

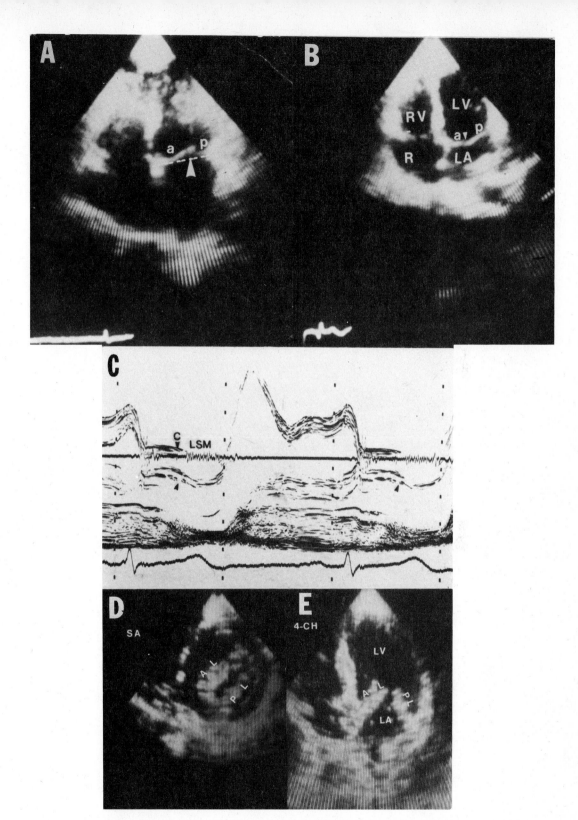

Figure 10–7. Echocardiogram in mitral valve prolapse. **A:** Normal echocardiogram shows the anterior (a) and posterior (p) leaflets of the mitral valve, which close above the plane of the mitral annulus (dashed line). **B:** In mitral valve prolapse, the posterior leaflet of the mitral valve (p) is much longer than normal and closes across the plane of the mitral annulus (arrowhead) to enter the left atrium (LA). **C:** The M-mode echocardiogram, shown with superimposed phonocardiogram (upper thick line) and electrocardiogram (lower thick line) tracings, demonstrates mitral valve prolapse (arrowheads) associated with a midsystolic click (C) and late systolic murmur (LSM). In a subgroup of patients with malignant mitral valve prolapse, who are especially prone to develop mitral regurgitation and endocarditis (but not stroke), short axis (**D**) and four-chamber view (**E**) echocardiograms show thickened anterior (AL) and posterior (PL) leaflets of the mitral valve. (Courtesy of N Schiller.)

either embolization (producing stroke) or cardiac outflow obstruction (producing syncope). Embolic events occur in one-fourth to one-half of patients with nonhereditary left atrial myxoma; some cases, however, are familial. Hemorrhagic strokes may occur. Diagnosis is by echocardiography (Figure 10–8). This disorder is discussed in Chapter 9.

8. Prosthetic heart valves–Patients with prosthetic heart valves are at particular risk for cerebral emboli and are generally treated with anticoagulants on a long-term basis.

C. Hematological Disorders:

1. Thrombocytosis–Thrombocytosis occurs in myeloproliferative disorders, in other systemic malignant neoplastic diseases or infections, and following splenectomy. Thrombocytosis may predispose to focal cerebral ischemia, particularly when the platelet count exceeds 1,000,000/μL. While hyperaggregability of platelets has also been described in association with focal cerebral ischemia, it is uncertain whether this is primary and causal or a result of the cerebrovascular disorder.

2. Polycythemia–The occurrence of neurological signs and symptoms in patients with polycythemia has long been recognized. In addition to nonspecific signs such as headache, dizziness, and blurred vision, patients may have focal neurological symptoms that often respond to venesection. Hematocrits above 46% may be associated with reduced cerebral blood flow, but there is a poor correlation between blood viscosity measured in vitro and the risk of stroke. This risk increases with hematocrits of more than 50%, however, and rises dramatically above 60%.

3. Sickle cell disease–Sickle cell (**hemoglobin SS**) disease is a cause of thrombotic cerebral infarcts in affected children and adolescents. Most such infarcts are due to the occlusion of large arteries, but small-vessel occlusion also occurs. This diagnosis should be considered in any young black patient with focal symptoms of cerebral ischemia. In patients with sickle cell disease who must undergo angiography, the level of hemoglobin SS should be reduced by exchange transfusion to less than 20%, since radiological contrast media may induce sickling.

4. Leukocytosis–Transient cerebral ischemia has been reported in association with leukocytosis, usually in patients with leukemia and white blood cell counts in excess of 150,000/μL.

5. Hypercoagulable states–Hyperviscosity of the serum from paraproteinemia (especially macroglobulinemia) is an infrequent cause of focal cerebral ischemia. Stasis of blood in these conditions can lead to cerebral infarction or diffuse encephalopathy.

Many conditions, such as pregnancy, estrogen therapy or the use of oral contraceptives, postpartum and postoperative states, and cancer, are accompanied by coagulation abnormalities. Patients with such coagulopathies may exhibit symptoms of cerebral thrombosis or embolism.

Antiphospholipid antibodies, including lupus anticoagulants and anticardiolipin antibodies, may be associated with an increased incidence of ischemic stroke. The mechanism by which antiphospholipid antibodies promote thrombosis is uncertain.

Stroke has also been reported in patients with hereditary coagulopathies, including heparin cofactor II deficiency, protein C deficiency, defective release of plasminogen activator, and factor XII deficiency.

Pathology

A. Infarction in Major-Cerebral-Artery Distribution: On gross inspection at autopsy, a recent in-

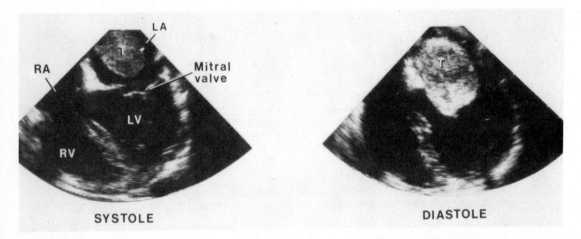

Figure 10–8. Echocardiogram in atrial myxoma. Transesophageal echocardiograms obtained in systole and diastole show the right atrium (RA), left atrium (LA), right ventricle (RV), and left ventricle (LV). The tumor mass (T) is located in the left atrium during systole (left) and herniates through the mitral valve during diastole (right), nearly obstructing the mitral valve inflow orifice. (Courtesy of N Schiller.)

farct is a swollen, softened area of brain that usually affects both gray and white matter. Microscopy shows acute ischemic changes in neurons (shrinkage, microvacuolization, dark staining), destruction of glial cells, necrosis of small blood vessels, disruption of nerve axons and myelin, and accumulation of interstitial fluid from vasogenic edema. In some cases, perivascular hemorrhages are observed in the infarcted area.

Cerebral infarcts are typically associated with cerebral edema, which is maximal during the first four or five days after onset. Most deaths that occur within a week after massive cerebral infarction are attributable to cerebral edema, with swelling of the affected hemisphere causing herniation of the ipsilateral cingulate gyrus across the midline beneath the free edge of the dural falx, followed by downward displacement of the brain through the tentorial incisure.

B. Lacunar Infarction: In contrast to infarcts associated with major cerebral blood vessels, smaller lacunar infarcts result from lipohyalinosis of small resistance vessels, usually in patients with chronic hypertension. Lacunar infarcts—often multiple—are found in about 10% of brains at autopsy. The pathological appearance is of small cavities ranging in size from 0.5 to 15 mm in diameter.

Clinicoanatomical Correlation

A rational clinical approach to cerebral ischemia depends on the ability to identify the neuroanatomic basis of clinical deficits.

A. Anterior Cerebral Artery:

1. Anatomy–The anterior cerebral artery supplies the parasagittal cerebral cortex (Figures 10–9 and 10–10), which includes portions of motor and sensory cortex related to the contralateral leg and the so-called bladder inhibitory or micturition center.

2. Clinical syndrome of anterior cerebral artery occlusion–Anterior cerebral artery strokes are uncommon, perhaps because emboli from the extracranial vessels or the heart are more apt to enter the larger-caliber middle cerebral artery, which receives the bulk of cerebral blood flow. There is a contralateral paralysis and sensory loss affecting the leg. Voluntary control of micturition may be impaired because of failure to inhibit reflex bladder contractions, resulting in precipitate micturition.

B. Middle Cerebral Artery:

1. Anatomy–The middle cerebral artery supplies most of the remainder of the cerebral hemisphere and deep subcortical structures (Figures 10–9 and 10–10). The cortical branches of the middle cerebral artery include the **superior division,** which supplies the entire motor and sensory cortical representation of the face, hand, and arm; and the **expressive language (Broca's) area** of the dominant hemisphere (Figure 10–11). The **inferior division** supplies the visual radiations, the region of visual

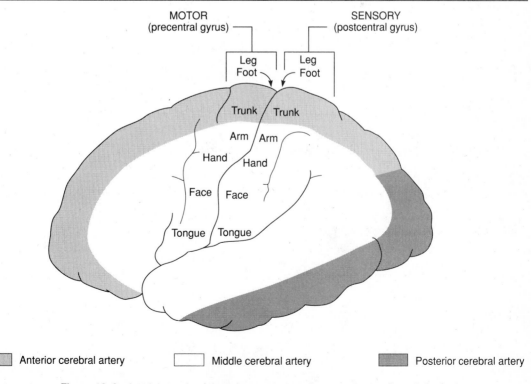

Figure 10–9. Arterial supply of the primary motor and sensory cortex (lateral view).

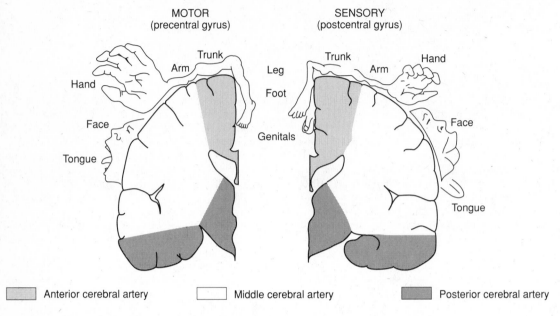

Figure 10–10. Arterial supply of the primary motor and sensory cortex (coronal view).

cortex related to macular vision, and the **receptive language (Wernicke's) area** of the dominant hemisphere. **Lenticulostriate** branches of the most proximal portion (stem) of the middle cerebral artery supply the basal ganglia as well as motor fibers related to the face, hand, arm, and leg as they descend in the genu and the posterior limb of the internal capsule.

2. Clinical syndrome of middle cerebral artery occlusion–The middle cerebral artery is the vessel most commonly involved in ischemic stroke. Depending on the site of involvement, several clinical syndromes can occur (Figure 10–11).

a. Superior division stroke results in contralateral hemiparesis that affects the face, hand, and arm but spares the leg; contralateral hemisensory deficit in the same distribution; but no homonymous hemianopia. If the dominant hemisphere is involved, these features are combined with Broca's (expressive) aphasia, which is characterized by impairment of language expression with intact comprehension.

b. Inferior division stroke is less common in isolation and results in contralateral homonymous hemianopia that may be denser inferiorly; marked impairment of cortical sensory functions, such as graphesthesia and stereognosis on the contralateral side of the body; and disorders of spatial thought, including a lack of awareness that a deficit exists (anosognosia), neglect of and failure to recognize the contralateral limbs, neglect of the contralateral side of external space, dressing apraxia, and constructional apraxia. If the dominant hemisphere is involved, Wernicke's (receptive) aphasia occurs and is manifested by impaired comprehension and fluent but often nonsensical speech. With involvement of

the nondominant hemisphere, an acute confusional state may occur.

c. Occlusion at the bifurcation or trifurcation of the middle cerebral artery involves a lesion situated at the point where the artery splits into two (superior and inferior) or three (superior, middle, and inferior) major divisions. This severe stroke syndrome combines the features of superior and inferior division stroke. Its clinical features include contralateral hemiparesis and hemisensory deficit involving the face and arm far more than the leg; homonymous hemianopia; and, if the dominant hemisphere is affected, global (combined expressive and receptive) aphasia.

d. Occlusion of the stem of the middle cerebral artery occurs proximal to the origin of the lenticulostriate branches. Since the entire territory of the artery is affected, this is the most devastating of middle cerebral artery strokes. The resulting clinical syndrome is similar to that seen following occlusion at the trifurcation except that, in addition, infarction of motor fibers in the internal capsule causes paralysis of the contralateral leg. The result is a contralateral hemiplegia and sensory loss affecting the face, hand, arm, and leg.

C. Internal Carotid Artery:

1. Anatomy–The internal carotid artery arises where the common carotid artery divides into internal and external carotid branches in the neck. In addition to its anterior cerebral and middle cerebral branches discussed above, the internal carotid artery also gives rise to the ophthalmic artery, which supplies the retina. The severity of internal carotid artery strokes is highly variable, depending on the adequacy of collat-

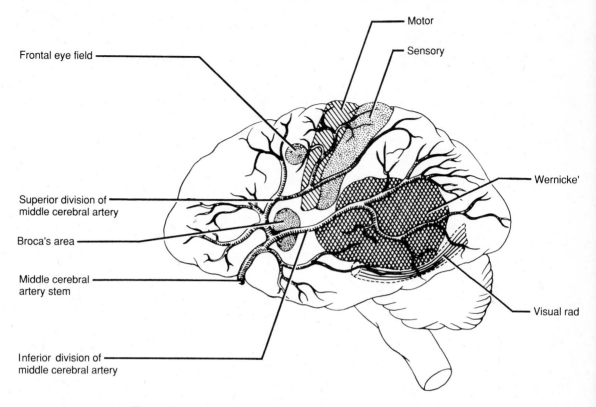

Figure 10–11. Anatomical basis of middle cerebral artery syndromes.

eral circulation, which tends to develop in compensation for a slowly evolving occlusion.

2. Clinical syndrome of internal carotid artery occlusion–Intra- or extracranial internal carotid artery occlusion is responsible for about one-fifth of ischemic strokes. In approximately 15% of cases, progressive atherosclerotic occlusion of the internal carotid artery is preceded by premonitory TIAs or by **transient monocular blindness** caused by ipsilateral retinal artery ischemia.

Carotid artery occlusion may be asymptomatic. Symptomatic occlusion results in a syndrome similar to that of middle cerebral artery stroke (contralateral hemiplegia, hemisensory deficit, and homonymous hemianopia; aphasia is also present with dominant hemisphere involvement).

D. Posterior Cerebral Artery:

1. Anatomy–The paired posterior cerebral arteries arise from the tip of the basilar artery (Figure 10–12) and supply the occipital cerebral cortex, medial temporal lobes, thalamus, and rostral midbrain. Emboli carried up the basilar artery tend to lodge at its apex, where they can occlude one or both posterior cerebral arteries. These emboli can subsequently break up and produce signs of asymmetric or patchy posterior cerebral artery infarction.

2. Clinical syndrome of posterior cerebral

artery occlusion–Occlusion of a posterior cerebral artery produces homonymous hemianopia affecting the contralateral visual field. Macular vision may be spared, however, because of the dual (middle and posterior cerebral artery) blood supply to the portion of the visual cortex representing the macula (see Figure 5–4). In contrast to visual field defects from infarction in the middle cerebral artery territory, those caused by posterior cerebral artery occlusion may be denser superiorly. With occlusions near the origin of the posterior cerebral artery at the level of the midbrain, ocular abnormalities can include vertical gaze palsy, oculomotor (III) nerve palsy, internuclear ophthalmoplegia, and vertical skew deviation of the eyes. When posterior cerebral artery occlusion affects the occipital lobe of the dominant (usually left) hemisphere, patients may exhibit anomic aphasia (difficulty in naming objects), alexia without agraphia (inability to read, with no impairment of writing), or visual agnosia. The last is a failure to identify objects presented in the left side of the visual field caused by a lesion of the corpus callosum that disconnects the right visual cortex from language areas of the left hemisphere. Bilateral posterior cerebral artery infarction may result in **cortical blindness,** memory impairment (from temporal lobe involvement), or the inability to recognize familiar faces (**prosopagno-**

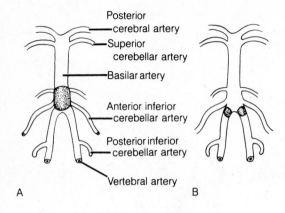

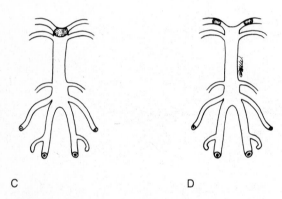

Figure 10–12. Sites of thrombotic and embolic occlusions in the vertebrobasilar circulation. **A:** Thrombotic occlusion of the basilar artery. **B:** Thrombotic occlusion of both vertebral arteries. **C:** Embolic occlusion at the apex of the basilar artery. **D:** Embolic occlusion of both posterior cerebral arteries.

sia), as well as a variety of exotic visual and behavioral syndromes.

E. Basilar Artery:

1. Anatomy–The basilar artery usually arises from the junction of the paired vertebral arteries (Figure 10–12), though in some cases only a single vertebral artery is present. The basilar artery courses over the ventral surface of the brain stem to terminate at the level of the midbrain, where it bifurcates to form the posterior cerebral arteries (see above). Branches of the basilar artery supply the occipital and medial temporal lobes, the medial thalamus, the posterior limb of the internal capsule, and the entire brain stem and cerebellum.

2. Clinical syndromes of basilar artery occlusion–

a. Thrombosis–Thrombotic occlusion of the basilar artery (Figure 10–12A)—a serious event that is often incompatible with survival—produces bilateral neurological signs referable to involvement of multiple branch arteries (Figure 10–13). Occlusion of both vertebral arteries (Figure 10–12B) or of a lone unpaired vertebral artery produces a similar syndrome. Temporary occlusion of one or both vertebral arteries can also occur in relation to rotation of the head in patients with cervical spondylosis, leading to transient symptoms and signs of brain stem dysfunction.

Major stenosis or occlusion of the subclavian artery before it has given rise to the vertebral artery can lead to the **subclavian steal syndrome,** in which blood passes from the vertebral artery into the distal subclavian artery with physical activity of the ipsilateral arm. The syndrome is a manifestation of generalized atherosclerosis and is not predictive of stroke in the vertebrobasilar system. Patients are usually asymptomatic, and stroke, when it occurs, is typically due to coexisting carotid lesions.

Basilar thrombosis usually affects the proximal portion of the basilar artery (Figure 10–12A), which supplies the pons. Involvement of the dorsal portion (tegmentum) of the pons produces unilateral or bilateral abducens (VI) nerve palsy; horizontal eye movements are impaired, but vertical nystagmus and ocular bobbing may be present. The pupils are constricted as a result of the involvement of descending sympathetic pupillodilator fibers in the pons, but they may remain reactive. Hemiplegia or quadriplegia is usually present, and coma is common. Although the syndrome of basilar occlusion in unconscious patients may be confused with pontine hemorrhage, a CT or MRI brain scan will differentiate the two.

In some patients with basilar occlusion, the ventral portion of the pons (basis pontis) is infarcted and the tegmentum is spared. Such patients remain conscious but quadriplegic. The term **locked-in syndrome** has been applied to this state. Locked-in patients may be able to signify that they are conscious by opening their eyes or moving their eyes vertically on command. In other cases, a conventional EEG with stimulation may be needed to distinguish the locked-in state (in which the EEG is normal) from coma (see Chapter 11).

b. Embolism–Emboli small enough to pass through the vertebral arteries into the larger basilar artery are usually arrested at the top of the basilar artery, where it bifurcates into the posterior cerebral arteries (Figure 10–12C). The resulting reduction in blood flow to the ascending reticular formation of the midbrain and thalamus produces immediate loss or impairment of consciousness. Unilateral or bilateral oculomotor (III) nerve palsies are characteristic. Hemiplegia or quadriplegia with decerebrate or decorticate posturing occurs because of the involvement of the cerebral peduncles in the midbrain. Thus,

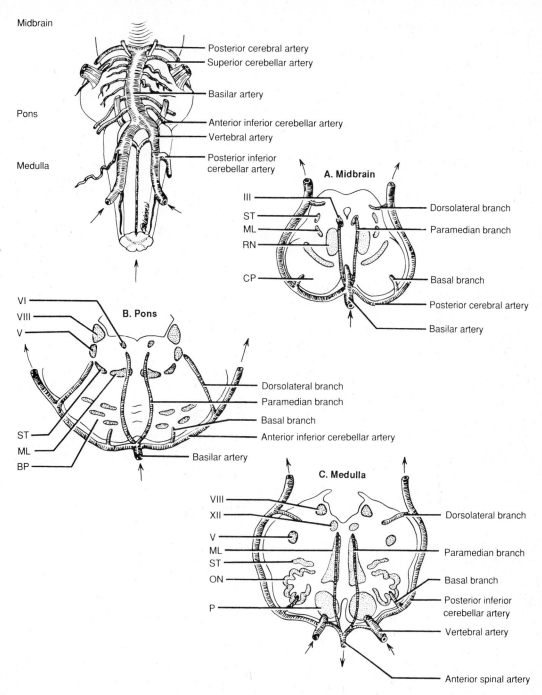

Figure 10–13. Arterial supply of the brain stem. **A:** Midbrain. The basilar artery gives off paramedian branches that supply the oculomotor (III) nerve nucleus and the red nucleus (RN). A larger branch, the posterior cerebral artery, courses laterally around the midbrain, giving off a basal branch that supplies the cerebral peduncle (CP) and a dorsolateral branch supplying the spinothalamic tract (ST), medial lemniscus (ML), and superior cerebellar peduncle. The posterior cerebral artery continues (upper arrows) to supply the thalamus, occipital lobe, and medial temporal lobe. **B:** Pons. Paramedian branches of the basilar artery supply the abducens (VI) nucleus and the medial lemniscus (ML). The anterior inferior cerebellar artery gives off a basal branch to the descending motor pathways in the basis pontis (BP) and a dorsolateral branch to the trigeminal (V) nucleus, the vestibular (VIII) nucleus, and the spinothalamic tract (ST), before passing to the cerebellum (upper arrows). **C:** Medulla. Paramedian branches of the vertebral arteries supply descending motor pathways in the pyramid (P), the medial lemniscus (ML), and the hypoglossal (XII) nucleus. Another vertebral branch, the posterior inferior cerebellar artery, gives off a basal branch to the olivary nuclei (ON) and a dorsolateral branch that supplies the trigeminal (V) nucleus, the vestibular (VIII) nucleus, and the spinothalamic tract (ST), on its way to the cerebellum (upper arrows).

the **top of the basilar syndrome** may be confused with midbrain failure caused by transtentorial uncal herniation. Less commonly, an embolus may lodge more proximally in an atheromatous narrowed portion of the basilar artery, producing a syndrome indistinguishable from basilar thrombosis.

Smaller emboli may occlude the rostral basilar artery transiently before fragmenting and passing into one or both posterior cerebral arteries (Figure 10–12D). In such cases, portions of the midbrain, thalamus, and temporal and occipital lobes can be infarcted. If conscious, these patients display a variety of visual (homonymous hemianopia, cortical blindness), visuomotor (impaired convergence, paralysis of upward or downward gaze, diplopia), and behavioral (especially confusion) abnormalities without prominent motor dysfunction. Sluggish pupillary responses are a helpful sign of midbrain involvement.

F. Long Circumferential Vertebrobasilar Branches:

1. Anatomy–The long circumferential branches arising from the vertebral and basilar arteries are the posterior inferior cerebellar, the anterior inferior cerebellar, and the superior cerebellar arteries (Figure 10–13). These vessels supply the dorsolateral brain stem, including dorsolaterally situated cranial nerve nuclei (V, VII, VIII) and pathways entering and leaving the cerebellum in the cerebellar peduncles.

2. Clinical syndrome of long circumferential artery occlusion–occlusion of one of the circumferential branches produces infarction in the dorsolateral area of the medulla or pons.

a. Posterior inferior cerebellar artery occlusion results in the **lateral medullary (Wallenberg's) syndrome** (see Figure 4–9). This syndrome varies in its presentation with the extent of infarction, but it can include ipsilateral cerebellar ataxia, Horner's syndrome, and facial sensory deficit; contralateral impaired pain and temperature sensation; and nystagmus, vertigo, nausea, vomiting, dysphagia, dysarthria, and hiccup. The motor system is characteristically spared because of its ventral location in the brain stem.

b. Anterior inferior cerebellar artery occlusion leads to infarction of the lateral portion of the caudal pons and produces a syndrome with many of the same features. Horner's syndrome, dysphagia, dysarthria, and hiccup do not occur, however, but ipsilateral facial weakness, gaze palsy, deafness, and tinnitus are common findings.

c. The syndrome of lateral rostral pontine infarction from **superior cerebellar artery occlusion** resembles that associated with anterior inferior cerebellar artery lesions, but impaired optokinetic nystagmus or skew deviation of the eyes may occur. Auditory function is unaffected, and the contralateral sensory disturbance may involve touch, vibration, and position sense as well as pain and temperature sense.

G. Long Penetrating Paramedian Vertebrobasilar Branches–

1. Anatomy–Long penetrating paramedian arteries supply the medial brain stem from its ventral surface to the floor of the fourth ventricle. Structures located in this region include the medial portion of the cerebral peduncle, sensory pathways, the red nucleus, the reticular formation, and the midline cranial nerve nuclei (III, IV, VI, XII).

2. Clinical syndrome of long penetrating paramedian artery occlusion–Occlusion of a long penetrating artery causes paramedian infarction of the brain stem and results in contralateral hemiparesis if the cerebral peduncle is affected. Associated cranial nerve involvement depends on the level of the brain stem at which occlusion occurs: Occlusion in the **midbrain** results in ipsilateral third nerve palsy, which may be associated with contralateral tremor or ataxia from involvement of pathways connecting the red nucleus and cerebellum. Ipsilateral sixth and seventh nerve palsies are seen in the **pons,** and 12th nerve involvement can occur in the **medulla.**

If the lesion appears patchy or involves both sides of the brain stem (as manifested by coma or quadriparesis), the differential diagnosis includes occlusion of a main trunk vessel (both vertebral arteries or the basilar artery); intramedullary lesions such as hemorrhage, pontine glioma, or multiple sclerosis; and compression of the brain stem by a cerebellar mass (hemorrhage, infarct, or tumor).

H. Short Basal Vertebrobasilar Branches:

1. Anatomy–Short branches arising from the long circumferential arteries (discussed above) penetrate the ventral brain stem to supply the brain stem motor pathways.

2. Clinical syndrome of basal brain stem infarction–The most striking finding is contralateral hemiparesis caused by corticospinal tract involvement in the cerebral peduncle or basis pontis. Cranial nerves (eg, III, VI, VII) that emerge from the ventral surface of the brain stem may be affected as well, giving rise to ipsilateral cranial nerve palsies.

I. Lacunar Infarction: Small penetrating arteries located deep in the brain may become occluded as a result of changes in the vessel wall induced by chronic hypertension. The resulting lacunar infarcts are most common in deep nuclei of the brain (putamen, 37%; thalamus, 14%; caudate nucleus, 10%), the pons (16%), and the posterior limb of the internal capsule (10%) (Figure 10–14). They occur in lesser numbers in the deep cerebral white matter, the anterior limb of the internal capsule, and the cerebellum. Because of their small size and their frequent location in relatively silent areas of the brain, many lacunar infarctions are not recognized clinically. In as many as three-fourths of autopsy-proved cases, there is no history of stroke or clear evidence of neurological deficit on antemortem examinations.

In many cases, the isolated nature of the neurolog-

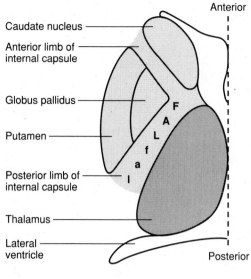

Caudate nucleus

Anterior limb of internal capsule

Globus pallidus

Putamen

Posterior limb of internal capsule

Thalamus

Lateral ventricle

Anterior

Posterior

☐ Anterior circulation (lenticulostriate branches of middle cerebral artery; anterior choroidal artery)

■ Posterior circulation (thalamoperforate and thalamogeniculate branches of posterior cerebral artery)

Figure 10–14. Arterial supply of deep cerebral structures frequently involved in lacunar infarction. Descending motor fibers to the face (F), arm (A), and leg (L) and ascending sensory fibers from face (f), arm (a), and leg (l) are shown in the posterior limb of the internal capsule.

ical deficit makes the clinical picture of lacunar infarction distinctive. The onset of lacunar stroke may be gradual, developing over several hours or days. Headache is absent or minor, and the level of consciousness is unchanged.

Recognition of lacunar stroke syndromes is important because the prognosis for complete or nearly complete recovery is good. In addition, the likelihood of future lacunar strokes can be reduced by treating the hypertension that is usually associated with and causally related to them. Because the arteries involved are small, angiography is normal (for that reason, it is not required). The CSF is also normal, and it is possible that a CT brain scan or MRI will not disclose the lesion. CT scanning or MRI should be performed to exclude other causes of stroke, however. Anticoagulation is not indicated since there is no evidence that it confers any benefit in this context. Aspirin is also of uncertain benefit, but it is often given because of the low risk of serious complications. Although a wide variety of deficits can be produced, there are four classic and distinctive lacunar syndromes.

1. Pure motor hemiparesis–This consists of hemiparesis affecting the face, arm, and leg to a roughly equal extent, without an associated disturbance of sensation, vision, or language. When lacunar in origin, it is usually due to a lesion in the contralateral internal capsule or pons. Pure motor hemiparesis may also be caused by internal carotid or middle cerebral artery occlusion, subdural hematoma, or intracerebral mass lesions.

2. Pure sensory stroke–This is characterized by hemisensory loss, which may be associated with paresthesia, and results from lacunar infarction in the contralateral thalamus. It may be mimicked by occlusion of the posterior cerebral artery or by a small hemorrhage in the thalamus or midbrain.

3. Ataxic hemiparesis–In this syndrome (sometimes called **ipsilateral ataxia and crural [leg] paresis),** pure motor hemiparesis is combined with ataxia of the hemiparetic side and usually predominantly affects the leg. Symptoms result from a lesion in the contralateral pons, internal capsule, or subcortical white matter.

4. Dysarthria–clumsy hand syndrome–This consists of dysarthria, facial weakness, dysphagia, and mild weakness and clumsiness of the hand on the side of facial involvement. When the syndrome is caused by a lacunar infarct, the lesion is in the contralateral pons or internal capsule. Infarcts or small intracerebral hemorrhages at a variety of locations can produce a similar syndrome, however. In contrast to the lacunar syndromes described above, premonitory TIAs are unusual.

Clinical Findings

A. History:

1. Predisposing factors–In patients with cerebrovascular disorders, possible risk factors such as TIAs, hypertension, and diabetes should be sought. In women, the use of oral contraceptives has been associated with cerebral arterial and venous occlusive disease, especially in the presence of such hypertension and cigarette smoking. The presence of such medical conditions as ischemic or valvular heart disease or cardiac arrhythmias must also be ascertained. A variety of systemic disorders involving the blood or blood vessels (Table 10–3) also increase the risk of stroke. Antihypertensive drugs can precipitate cerebrovascular symptoms if the blood pressure is lowered excessively in patients with nearly total cerebrovascular occlusion and poor collateral circulation.

2. Onset and course–The history must address whether the clinical picture is that of TIA, stroke in evolution, or completed stroke. In some cases, it may also be possible to evaluate whether a stroke is likely to be thrombotic or embolic in origin from the clinical history.

a. Features suggesting thrombotic stroke– Patients with thrombotic vascular occlusion often present with stepwise incremental neurological deficits; the occlusion may be preceded by a series of

TIAs. TIAs, for example, precede infarction in 25–50% of patients with occlusive atherosclerotic disease of the extracranial internal carotid arteries. In approximately one-third of such patients, however, the onset of infarction is abrupt, suggesting that embolization from the distal extracranial artery to the intracranial artery may be the cause of stroke.

b. Features suggesting embolic stroke–Cerebral embolism typically causes neurological deficits that occur abruptly with no warning and are maximal at onset. In many patients, a cardiac origin of emboli is suggested by signs of multifocal cerebral infarction, cardiac valvular disease, cardiomegaly, arrhythmias, or endocarditis.

3. Associated symptoms–

a. Seizures accompany the onset of stroke in a small number of cases; in other instances, they follow the stroke by weeks to years. The presence of seizures does not definitively distinguish embolic from thrombotic strokes, but seizure at the onset of stroke may be more common with embolus. If patients with vertebrobasilar stroke or an additional condition predisposing to seizures are not considered, the incidence of epilepsy after stroke is about 10%. The risk of epilepsy increases to about 25% with cortical strokes and to 50% when cortical strokes are associated with a persistent motor deficit.

b. Headache occurs in about 25% of patients with ischemic stroke, possibly because of the acute dilation of collateral vessels.

B. Physical Examination:

1. General physical examination–The general physical examination of a patient with a cerebrovascular disorder should focus on searching for an underlying systemic cause, especially a treatable one.

a. The blood pressure should be measured to ascertain whether hypertension—a known risk factor for stroke—is present.

b. Comparison of blood pressure and pulse on the two sides can reveal differences related to atherosclerotic disease of the aortic arch or coarctation of the aorta.

c. Ophthalmoscopic examination of the retina can provide evidence of embolization in the anterior circulation in the form of visible embolic material in retinal blood vessels.

d. Examination of the neck may reveal the absence of carotid pulses or the presence of carotid bruits. Reduced carotid artery pulsation in the neck is a poor indicator of internal carotid artery disease, however. Although carotid bruits have been associated with cerebrovascular disease, significant carotid stenosis can occur without an audible bruit; conversely, a loud bruit can occur without stenosis.

e. A careful cardiac examination is essential in order to detect arrhythmias or murmurs related to valvular disease, either of which may predispose to embolization from heart to brain.

f. Palpation of the temporal arteries is useful in the diagnosis of giant cell arteritis, in which these vessels may be tender, nodular, or pulseless.

2. Neurological examination–Patients with cerebrovascular disorders may or may not have abnormal neurological findings on examination. A normal examination is expected, for example, after a TIA has resolved. Where deficits are found, the goal of the neurological examination is to define the anatomical site of the lesion, which may suggest the cause or optimal management of the stroke. Thus, clear evidence that the anterior circulation is involved may lead to angiographic evaluation in contemplation of possible surgical correction of an internal carotid lesion. Establishing that the symptoms are referable to the vertebrobasilar circulation or to a lacunar infarction is likely to dictate a different course of action.

a. Cognitive deficits that indicate cortical lesions in the anterior circulation should be sought. For example, if aphasia is present, the underlying disorder cannot be in the posterior circulation and is unlikely to represent lacunar infarction. The same is true for nondominant hemisphere lesions producing parietal lobe syndromes such as unilateral neglect or constructional apraxia (see discussion of inferior division middle cerebral artery stroke, above).

b. The presence of visual field abnormalities similarly excludes lacunar infarction. Hemianopia may occur, however, with involvement of either the anterior or posterior cerebral arteries. Isolated hemianopia suggests posterior cerebral artery infarction.

c. Ocular palsies, nystagmus, or internuclear ophthalmoplegia assign the underlying lesion to the brain stem and thus to the posterior circulation.

d. Hemiparesis can be due to lesions in cerebral cortical regions supplied by the anterior circulation, descending motor pathways in the brain stem supplied by the vertebrobasilar system, or lacunae at subcortical (corona radiata, internal capsule) or brain stem sites. However, hemiparesis affecting the face, hand, and arm more than the leg is characteristic of lesions within the distribution of the middle cerebral artery. Hemiparesis that is nonselective with respect to the face, arm, and leg is consistent with occlusion of the internal carotid artery or the stem of the middle cerebral artery, lacunar infarction in the internal capsule or basal ganglia, or brain stem disease. A crossed hemiparesis—ie, one that involves the face on one side and the rest of the body on the other—means that the abnormality must lie between the level of the facial nerve nucleus in the pons and the decussation of the pyramids in the medulla.

e. Cortical sensory deficits such as astereognosis and agraphesthesia with preserved primary sensory modalities imply a cerebral cortical deficit within the territory of the middle cerebral artery. Isolated hemisensory deficits without associated motor involvement are usually lacunar in origin. Crossed sensory deficits result from brain stem lesions in the medulla, as seen in the lateral medullary plate syndrome.

f. Hemiataxia usually points to a lesion in the ipsilateral brain stem or cerebellum but can also be produced by lacunae in the internal capsule.

Investigative Studies

A. Blood Tests: These should be obtained routinely to detect treatable causes of stroke and to exclude conditions that can mimic stroke. The recommended studies are listed below.

1. Complete blood count to investigate such possible causes of stroke as thrombocytosis, thrombocytopenia, polycythemia, anemia (including sickle cell disease), and leukocytosis (eg, leukemia).

2. Erythrocyte sedimentation rate to detect elevations indicative of giant cell arteritis or other vasculitides.

3. Serological assay for syphilis—treponemal assay in blood, such as the FTA or MHA-TP, or the CSF VDRL test.

4. Serum glucose to document hypoglycemia or hyperosmolar nonketotic hyperglycemia, which can present with focal neurological signs and thereby masquerade as stroke.

5. Serum cholesterol and lipids to detect elevations that can represent risk factors for stroke.

B. Electrocardiography: An ECG should be obtained routinely to detect unrecognized myocardial infarction or cardiac arrythmias, such as atrial fibrillation, which predispose to embolic stroke.

C. CT Scan or MRI: A CT scan or MRI should be obtained routinely to distinguish between infarction and hemorrhage as the cause of stroke, to exclude other lesions (eg, tumor, abscess) that can mimic stroke, and to localize the lesion. MRI may be superior to CT for demonstrating early ischemic infarcts, showing ischemic strokes in the brain stem or cerebellum, and detecting thrombotic occlusion of venous sinuses.

D. Lumbar Puncture: This should be performed in selected cases to exclude subarachnoid hemorrhage (manifested by xanthochromia and red blood cells) or to document meningovascular syphilis (reactive VDRL) as the cause of stroke.

E. Cerebral Angiography: Angiography is used to identify operable extracranial carotid lesions in patients with anterior circulation TIAs who are good surgical candidates. Angiography is also useful in the diagnosis of certain vascular disorders associated with stroke, including vasculitis, fibromuscular dysplasia, and carotid or vertebral artery dissection. Transfemoral arch aortography with selective catheterization of the carotid (and, if indicated, vertebral) arteries is the procedure of choice.

F. Noninvasive Cerebrovascular Studies: Doppler ultrasonography can detect stenosis or occlusion of the internal carotid artery, but it lacks the sensitivity of angiography. In cases where the likelihood of finding operable symptomatic carotid stenosis is insufficient to justify the risk of angiography, or where

the risk is especially high because of coexisting illness or the lack of angiographic expertise, the finding of normal carotid blood flow or complete occlusion by Doppler studies can obviate the need for angiography.

G. Echocardiography: Echocardiography may be useful for demonstrating the cardiac lesions responsible for embolic stroke in patients with clinically evident cardiac disease, such as atrial fibrillation.

H. Electroencephalography: The EEG is rarely useful in evaluating stroke. It may, however, help differentiate between a seizure disorder and TIAs or between lacunar and cortical infarcts in the occasional patient in whom these possibilities cannot otherwise be distinguished.

Differential Diagnosis

In patients presenting with focal central nervous system dysfunction of sudden onset, ischemic stroke must be distinguished from structural and metabolic processes that can mimic it. An underlying process other than focal cerebral ischemia should be suspected when the resulting neurological deficit does not conform to the distribution of any single cerebral artery. In addition, strokes do not typically impair consciousness in the absence of profound focal deficits, while other cerebral disorders may do so.

Vascular disorders mistaken for ischemic stroke include intracerebral hemorrhage, subdural or epidural hematoma, and subarachnoid hemorrhage from rupture of an aneurysm or vascular malformation. These conditions can often be distinguished by a history of trauma or of excruciating headache at onset, a more marked depression of consciousness, or by the presence of neck stiffness on examination. They can be excluded by CT scan or MRI.

Other structural brain lesions such as tumor or abscess can also produce focal cerebral symptoms of acute onset. Brain abscess is suggested by concurrent fever, and both abscess and tumor can usually be diagnosed by CT scan or MRI.

Metabolic disturbances, particularly hypoglycemia and hyperosmolar nonketotic hyperglycemia, may present in strokelike fashion. The serum glucose level should therefore be determined in all patients with apparent stroke.

Treatment

A. Asymptomatic Carotid Bruit: Epidemiological studies have confirmed an association between asymptomatic carotid bruits and systemic vascular disease, which in turn is associated with TIA and stroke. The risk of stroke is not localized to the vessel over which the bruit is heard; however, neither is it any greater than the risk of stroke from endarterectomy. Therefore, there is no rationale for performing prophylactic endarterectomy in the setting of an asymptomatic carotid bruit.

B. Transient Ischemic Attack: Because TIAs

can indicate an impending stroke and because it may be possible to prevent such an event by appropriate treatment, TIAs must be accurately and promptly diagnosed and treatment instituted (Figure 10–15). Evidence for the efficacy of several commonly used treatments is equivocal at best, however, while evidence that such interventions can be dangerous is clear. The potential risks and benefits of a proposed therapy must therefore be evaluated carefully for each patient.

1. Antiplatelet therapy–Of the various treatments proposed for stroke prophylaxis in patients with noncardiogenic TIAs, the use of antiplatelet agents has been subjected to the most careful scrutiny. The rationale for this approach is that embolism from platelet-fibrin thrombi on arterial surfaces may be responsible for many cases of TIA and stroke. Antiplatelet agents inhibit platelet function by irreversibly inhibiting the enzyme cyclo-oxygenase, which catalyzes the synthesis of thromboxane A$_2$, an eicosanoid with procoagulant and platelet-aggregating properties.

Aspirin, when administered to patients with TIAs or minor stroke (defined as little or no neurological deficit after one week) has been shown to reduce the incidence of subsequent TIAs, stroke, or death in several studies. Although most studies have focused on noncardiogenic TIA or stroke, it now appears that aspirin is also beneficial for preventing recurrent cerebral ischemia caused by cardiac emboli. Doses between 300 and 1300 mg orally daily (1–4 tablets) appear to be equally effective, and daily oral administration of 325 mg of aspirin is probably used most often. A sex-related difference in benefit favoring men has been observed, but only inconsistently. Administration of low-dose aspirin (325 mg orally every other day) to men age 40 and older *without* a history of TIA or stroke does not reduce the risk of stroke, although it decreases the incidence of myocardial infarction. Adverse effects of aspirin include dyspepsia, nausea, abdominal pain, diarrhea, skin rash, peptic ulcer, gastritis, and gastrointestinal bleeding.

Ticlopidine (250 mg orally twice daily), an investigational antiplatelet agent, may be somewhat more effective than aspirin in preventing stroke and reduc-

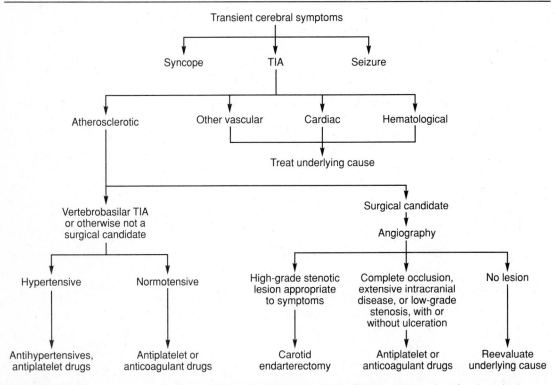

Figure 10–15. Clinical screening of patients with transient ischemic attacks. Patients with transient, focal cerebral symptoms suggesting TIA should be separated from those with syncope or seizures (see Chapter 9). The cause of TIA (see Table 10–3) should then be identified, based on the history, examination, and laboratory data, and appropriate treatment should be instituted. If atherosclerosis is the likely cause, carotid and vertebrobasilar ischemia should be distinguished, based on symptoms (Table 10–2). Patients with vertebrobasilar TIA and those with carotid TIAs who are not surgical candidates are treated with antiplatelet drugs (usually aspirin) or anticoagulants, while those with carotid TIAs who are surgical candidates should undergo angiography. Carotid endarterectomy is indicated for high-grade (70–90%) stenosis of the extracranial internal carotid artery ipsilateral to the involved hemisphere. Hypertensive patients should be treated with antihypertensive drugs.

ing mortality in patients with TIAs or mild stroke. However, ticlopidine is more expensive than aspirin and appears to be associated with such side effects as diarrhea, skin rash, and occasional cases of severe but reversible neutropenia.

Other antiplatelet drugs such as **sulfinpyrazone** and **dipyridamole** are commonly used to treat thrombotic vascular disease. These drugs are more expensive than aspirin, however, and there is no convincing evidence that they are more effective in preventing TIA or stroke or that a combination of aspirin and one of these compounds is more effective than aspirin alone.

2. Anticoagulation–Anticoagulation is indicated for patients with TIAs caused by cardiac embolus. The value of anticoagulation is less certain for TIAs from arterial thrombosis. Several studies have analyzed the effect of anticoagulation with heparin or warfarin (or both) in patients with TIAs. Some appear to demonstrate a reduction in the incidence of subsequent stroke—which in at least one case was most pronounced for patients with vertebrobasilar TIAs. Other studies have failed to show a beneficial effect of anticoagulation, and many series have been poorly controlled. Where anticoagulation has been of apparent value, the effect was noted only within the first two or three months after the TIA. Therefore, anticoagulants should be used only for a limited time, such as two or three months, in patients with noncardiogenic TIAs who have failed to respond to aspirin therapy.

Heparin is the drug of choice for acute anticoagulation, while warfarin is used for long-term therapy. Heparin is usually administered as an intravenous bolus (loading dose) of 5000–10,000 units, followed by continuous intravenous infusion (maintenance) at 1000–2000 units/h. The partial thromboplastin time (PTT) is measured at least daily, and the maintenance dose of heparin is adjusted to maintain the PTT at about twice the pretreatment value.

Warfarin (the usual maintenance dose is 5–15 mg/d orally) can be started simultaneously with heparin therapy. About two days after the prothrombin time (PT) reaches roughly one and one-half times the pretreatment value (typically about five days), heparin can be discontinued. The PT should be measured at least every two weeks and the dose of warfarin adjusted accordingly. Warfarin therapy is commonly continued for about three months following a TIA. Even in studies that appear to show a beneficial effect of anticoagulation in reducing the risk of stroke following TIA, this effect does not continue beyond about three months, while the risk of complications persists.

Enthusiasm for the use of anticoagulant therapy should be tempered by an appreciation of its potential hazards. The risk of intracranial hemorrhage is greatest in hypertensive patients and those over 65 years of age.

3. Carotid endarterectomy–Carotid endarterectomy, in which thrombus is removed surgically from a stenotic common or internal carotid artery in the neck, has been widely used for many years in an attempt to prevent stroke in patients with TIAs. Well-controlled studies demonstrating its effectiveness have been reported only recently, however. These indicate that endarterectomy plus aspirin is superior to aspirin alone for preventing stroke in patients with TIAs and high-grade (70–99%) carotid stenosis.

The best results of endarterectomy have been in patients with typical hemispheric carotid TIAs who have demonstrable atherosclerotic high-grade stenosis in the extracranial internal carotid artery on the side appropriate to the symptoms. It should be noted this operation has no place in the treatment of vertebrobasilar TIAs or those related to intracranial arterial disease or complete carotid occlusion. The value of carotid endarterectomy for minimally stenotic but ulcerated carotid lesions is uncertain. The operative mortality rate for carotid endarterectomy has ranged from 1% to 5% or more.

4. Extracranial-intracranial bypass–Many patients with TIAs referable to the carotid circulation have stenoses in intracranial portions of the artery not accessible through the neck, or they exhibit tandem lesions in both the extracranial and intracranial cerebral circulations. Because carotid endarterectomy does not correct these problems, an alternative approach was suggested involving anastomosis of the extracranial (temporal artery) and intracranial (middle cerebral artery) circulations distal to the stenosis; this bypass procedure is ineffective.

In experienced hands, carotid endarterectomy can be a safe procedure that reduces the risk of subsequent TIAs or stroke in patients with carotid TIAs. Angiography should be used with these patients to define surgically accessible high-grade stenotic lesions.

5. Conclusions–Medical treatment with aspirin should be instituted with both nonsurgical and postoperative patients. For patients who continue to have TIAs despite aspirin treatment, a three-month course of warfarin should be substituted unless there are contraindications such as active peptic ulcer disease or severe hypertension. The prothrombin time should be maintained at one and one-half times the control value. In addition to the above measures, such contributory risk factors as hypertension and cardiac disease should be treated and cigarette smoking discontinued.

C. Stroke in Evolution: The optimal treatment for stroke in evolution is uncertain. Since the onset of aspirin's antiplatelet effect is delayed by several hours after oral administration, aspirin is not likely to prevent worsening of an ongoing stroke. Endarterectomy also involves considerable delay in treatment, and even though emergency endarterectomies are performed successfully at some centers, their usefulness has not been established.

The most widely used treatment is **anticoagula-**

tion with heparin and subsequent administration of warfarin as previously described for TIAs, although the efficacy of this approach has not been proved.

Recent advances in treating acute myocardial infarction suggest that **thrombolytic agents** such as streptokinase or tissue plasminogen activator might be of value for stroke in evolution, but these possibilities require further study.

D. Completed Stroke:

1. Antiplatelet agents—As noted above in discussing the treatment of TIAs, some but not all studies have shown a decrease in the incidence of subsequent stroke when aspirin is administered chronically following a stroke. The regimen is as described in the section on treatment of TIA.

2. Anticoagulation—In contrast to existing evidence that anticoagulation may be of value in the treatment of TIAs and stroke in evolution, such therapy is not useful in most cases of completed stroke. An exception is where a persistent source of cardiac embolus is present; anticoagulation is then indicated to prevent subsequent embolic strokes, although it does not affect the course of the stroke that has already occurred. Recent evidence indicates that while immediate anticoagulation of such patients may result in hemorrhage into the infarct, this rarely affects the ultimate outcome adversely unless the infarct is massive. The risk of hemorrhage is more than offset by the particularly high risk of recurrent embolization soon after an embolic stroke, and anticoagulation should not be delayed in this setting. Heparin and warfarin are administered as described in the section on treatment of TIA.

3. Surgery—The indications for surgical treatment of completed stroke are extremely limited. When patients deteriorate as a consequence of brain stem compression following cerebellar infarction, however, posterior fossa decompression with evacuation of infarcted cerebellar tissue can be lifesaving.

4. Antihypertensive agents—Although hypertension contributes to the pathogenesis of stroke and many patients with acute stroke have elevated blood pressures, attempts to reduce the blood pressure in stroke patients can have disastrous results, since the blood supply to ischemic but as yet uninfarcted brain tissue may be further compromised. Therefore, such attempts should not be made. In the usual course of events, the blood pressure declines spontaneously over a period of hours to a few days.

5. Antiedema agents—Antiedema agents such as mannitol and corticosteroids have not been shown to be of benefit for cytotoxic edema (cellular swelling) associated with cerebral infarction.

6. Neuroprotective agents—A variety of drugs with diverse pharmacological actions have been proposed as neuroprotective agents that might reduce ischemic brain injury by decreasing cerebral metabolism or interfering with the cytotoxic mechanisms triggered by ischemia. These include barbiturates and the opioid antagonist naloxone, neither of which appears to be beneficial in stroke.

Drugs that block voltage-gated or excitatory amino acid receptor-gated calcium channels have potential value in the treatment of stroke because cellular calcium overload may be an important mediator of irreversible ischemic neuronal injury. The voltage-gated calcium channel antagonist nimodipine (30 mg orally every six hours for four weeks) has been reported to improve neurological outcome and reduce mortality following ischemic stroke; it is undergoing further investigation. Clinical trials with excitatory amino acid antagonists in stroke are also under way.

Prognosis

Outcome following stroke is influenced by a number of factors, the most important being the nature and severity of the resulting neurological deficit. The patient's age, the cause of stroke, and coexisting medical disorders also affect prognosis. Overall, somewhat less than 80% of patients with stroke survive for at least one month, and ten-year survival rates in the neighborhood of 35% have been cited. The latter figure is not surprising, considering the advanced age at which stroke commonly occurs. Of patients who survive the acute period, about one-half to two-thirds regain independent function, while approximately 15% require institutional care.

INTRACEREBRAL HEMORRHAGE

Hypertensive Hemorrhage

Hypertension is the most common underlying cause of nontraumatic intracerebral hemorrhage.

A. Pathophysiology:

1. Cerebral autoregulation—Autoregulation of cerebral blood flow (Figure 10–16), which is achieved by changes in the caliber of small resistance cerebral arteries, maintains constant cerebral blood flow as systemic blood pressure rises and falls. The range of autoregulated blood pressures is variable.

In normotensive individuals, the lowest mean blood pressure at which autoregulation is effective is approximately 60 mm Hg. Below this level, changes in the caliber of cerebral arteries cannot compensate for decreased perfusion pressure; cerebral blood flow therefore declines, producing symptoms of hypoxia, such as lightheadedness, confusion, and dimming of vision. These symptoms are followed by somnolence and loss of consciousness if the mean blood pressure falls below 35–40 mm Hg. In contrast, at blood pressures above the upper limit of the range of autoregulation (150–200 mm Hg), cerebral blood flow is in-

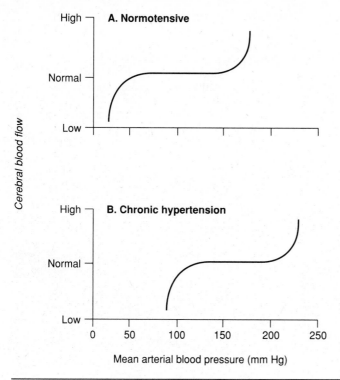

A. Normotensive

High —

Normal —

Low —

Cerebral blood flow

B. Chronic hypertension

High —

Normal —

Low —

0   50   100   150   200   250

Mean arterial blood pressure (mm Hg)

Figure 10–16. Cerebrovascular autoregulation. *A:* Cerebral blood flow is maintained in the normal range over a wide range of blood pressures. At very low pressures, cerebral hypoperfusion occurs, producing syncope. Pressures that rise beyond the autoregulatory range can cause hypertensive encephalopathy. *B:* Structural changes in cerebral arteries shift the autoregulatory range to higher blood pressures. Hypoperfusion and syncope can occur at normal pressures, and pressures associated with hypertensive encephalopathy are increased.

creased, which can produce hypertensive encephalopathy.

In chronically hypertensive individuals, the lower limit of the autoregulatory range is higher (Figure 10–16), which may be due to damage to small arterial walls. As a result, cerebral blood flow declines when the mean arterial blood pressure falls below about 120 mm Hg. The clinical relevance of this observation is that blood pressure should be reduced rarely, if ever—and never to hypotensive levels—in patients with stroke.

2. Chronic hypertension–Chronic hypertension appears to promote structural changes in the walls of penetrating arteries, predisposing them to intracerebral hemorrhage. In 1888, Charcot and Bouchard found minute aneurysms on the small intraparenchymal arteries of hypertensive patients and postulated that aneurysmal rupture led to intracerebral hemorrhage. Subsequently, Ross Russell showed microaneurysms of small resistance arteries in cerebral sites at which hypertensive hemorrhages occur most commonly. Some aneurysms were surrounded by small areas of hemorrhage, and the aneurysmal walls often showed changes of lipohyalinosis or fibrinoid necrosis. These processes are characterized by destruction of the vessel wall with deposition of fibrinoid material, focal aneurysmal expansion of the involved vessel, thrombotic occlusion, and extravasation of red cells. There is now general agreement that massive cerebral hemorrhage often follows the

rupture of either a microaneurysmal or lipohyalinotic segment of a small resistance artery and that the underlying lesion is caused by chronic hypertension.

3. Acute hypertension–In addition to structural changes in the cerebral arterial wall produced by chronic hypertension, acute elevation of blood pressure appears to play a role in the pathogenesis of intracerebral hemorrhage. Although most patients with intracerebral hemorrhage are hypertensive following the event, many have no prior history of hypertension and lack such signs of hypertensive end-organ disease as left ventricular hypertrophy, retinopathy, or nephropathy. It has therefore been suggested that a sudden increase in blood pressure may itself be sufficient to cause intracerebral hemorrhage, as with amphetamine or cocaine abuse. Acute elevation of blood pressure may also be the immediate precipitating cause of intracerebral hemorrhage in chronically hypertensive patients with Charcot-Bouchard aneurysms.

B. Pathology: Most hypertensive hemorrhages originate in certain areas of predilection, corresponding to long, narrow, penetrating arterial branches along which Charcot-Bouchard aneurysms are found at autopsy (Figure 10–17). These include the caudate and putaminal branches of the middle cerebral arteries (42%); branches of the basilar artery supplying the pons (16%); thalamic branches of the posterior cerebral arteries (15%); branches of the superior cerebellar arteries supplying the dentate nuclei and the

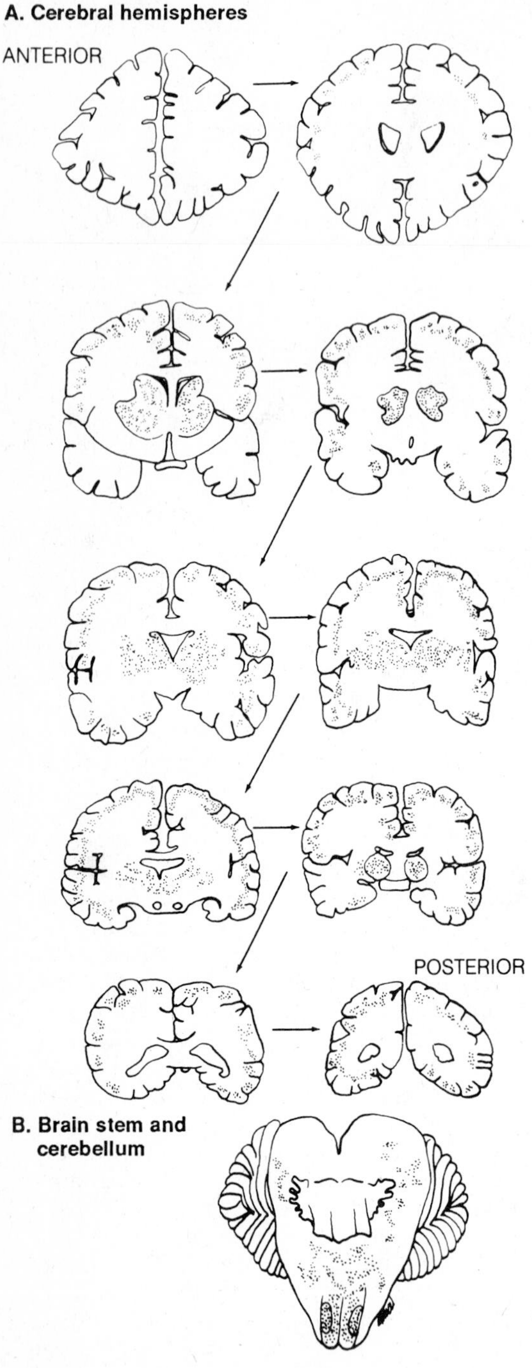

A. Cerebral hemispheres

ANTERIOR

POSTERIOR

B. Brain stem and cerebellum

Figure 10–17. Distribution of Charcot-Bouchard aneurysms (stippling) underlying hypertensive intracerebral hemorrhage.

deep white matter of the cerebellum (12%); and some white matter branches of the cerebral arteries (10%), especially in the parieto-occipital and temporal lobes.

C. Clinical Findings: Hypertensive hemorrhage occurs without warning, most commonly while the

patient is awake. Headache is present in 50% of patients and may be severe; vomiting is common. Blood pressure is elevated after the hemorrhage has occurred. Thus, normal or low blood pressure in a patient with stroke makes the diagnosis of hypertensive hemorrhage unlikely, as does onset before 50 years of age.

Following the hemorrhage, edema surrounding the area of hemorrhage produces clinical worsening over a period of minutes to days. The duration of active bleeding, however, is brief. Once the deficit stabilizes, improvement occurs slowly. Since the deficit is caused principally by hemorrhage and edema, which compress rather than destroy brain tissue, considerable return of neurological function can occur.

Massive hypertensive hemorrhages may rupture through brain tissue into the ventricles, producing bloody CSF; direct rupture through the cortical mantle is unusual. A fatal outcome is most often due to herniation caused by the combined mass effect of the hematoma and the surrounding edema.

Clinical features vary with the site of hemorrhage (Table 10–4).

1. Deep cerebral hemorrhage—The two most common sites of hypertensive hemorrhage are the **putamen** and the **thalamus,** which are separated by the posterior limb of the internal capsule. This segment of the internal capsule is traversed by descending motor fibers and ascending sensory fibers, including the optic radiations (Figure 10–18). Pressure on these fibers from an expanding lateral (putaminal) or medial (thalamic) hematoma produces a contralateral sensorimotor deficit. In general, putaminal hemorrhage leads to a more severe motor deficit and thalamic hemorrhage to a more marked sensory disturbance. Homonymous hemianopia may occur as a transient phenomenon after thalamic hemorrhage and is often a persistent finding in putaminal hemorrhage. In large thalamic hemorrhages, the eyes may deviate downward, as in staring at the tip of the nose, because of impingement on the midbrain center for upward gaze. Aphasia may occur if hemorrhage at either site exerts pressure on the cortical language areas. A separate aphasic syndrome has been described with localized hemorrhage into the thalamus; it carries an excellent prognosis for full recovery.

2. Lobar hemorrhage—Hypertensive hemorrhages also occur in subcortical white matter underlying the frontal, parietal, temporal, and occipital lobes. Symptoms and signs vary according to the location; they can include headache, vomiting, hemiparesis, hemisensory deficits, aphasia, and visual field abnormalities. Seizures are more frequent than with hemorrhages in other locations, while coma is less so.

3. Pontine hemorrhage—With bleeding into the pons, coma occurs within seconds to minutes and usually leads to death within 48 hours. Ocular findings typically include pinpoint pupils. Horizontal eye movements are absent or impaired, but vertical eye

Table 10–4. Clinical features of hypertensive intracerebral hemorrhage.

Location	Coma	Pupils	Eye Movements	Sensorimotor Disturbance	Hemianopia	Seizures
Putamen	Common	Normal	Ipsilateral deviation	Hemiparesis	Common	Uncommon
Thalamus	Common	Small, sluggish	Downward and medial deviation may occur	Hemisensory deficit	May occur transiently	Uncommon
Lobar	Uncommon	Normal	Normal or ipsilateral deviation	Hemiparesis or hemisensory deficit	Common	Common
Pons	Early	Pinpoint	Absent horizontal	Quadriparesis	None	None
Cerebellum	Delayed	Small, reactive	Impaired late	Gait ataxia	None	None

movements may be preserved. In some patients, there may be ocular bobbing, a bilateral downbeating excursion of the eyes at about five-second intervals. Patients are commonly quadriparetic and exhibit decerebrate posturing. Hyperthermia is sometimes present. The hemorrhage usually ruptures into the fourth ventricle, and rostral extension of the hemorrhage into the midbrain with resultant midposition fixed pupils is common. In contrast to the classic pre-

sentation of pontine hemorrhage described above, small hemorrhages that spare the reticular activating system—and that are associated with less severe deficits and excellent recovery—also occur.

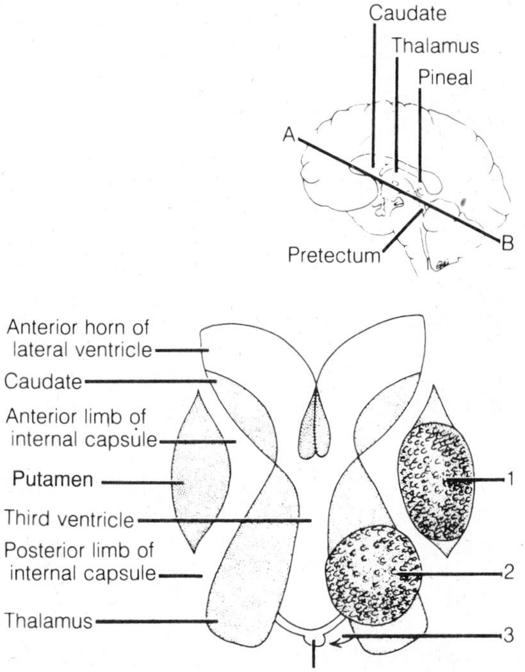

4. Cerebellar hemorrhage–The distinctive symptoms of cerebellar hemorrhage (headache, dizziness, vomiting, and the inability to stand or walk) begin suddenly, within minutes after onset of bleeding. While patients may initially be alert or only mildly confused, large hemorrhages lead to coma within 12 hours in 75% of patients and within 24 hours in 90%. When coma is present at the onset, the clinical picture is indistinguishable from that of pontine hemorrhage.

Common ocular findings include impairment of gaze to the side of the lesion or forced deviation away from the lesion caused by pressure on the pontine lateral gaze center. Skew deviation may also occur, in which case the eye ipsilateral to the lesion is depressed. The pupils are small and reactive. Ipsilateral facial weakness of lower motor neuron type occurs in about 50% of cases, but strength in the limbs is normal. Limb ataxia is usually slight or absent. Plantar responses are flexor early in the course but become extensor as the brain stem becomes compromised and the patient deteriorates. Impairment of voluntary or reflex upward gaze indicates upward transtentorial herniation of the cerebellar vermis and midbrain, leading to compression of the pretectum. It implies a poor prognosis.

D. Differential Diagnosis: Putaminal, thalamic, and lobar hypertensive hemorrhages may be difficult to distinguish from cerebral infarctions. To some extent, the presence of severe headache, nausea and vomiting, and impairment of consciousness are useful clues that a hemorrhage may have occurred; the CT scan or MRI identifies the underlying disorder definitively.

Brain stem stroke or cerebellar infarction can mimic cerebellar hemorrhage. When cerebellar hemorrhage is a possibility, CT scan or MRI is the most useful diagnostic procedure, since hematomas can be quickly and accurately localized. If neither CT nor MRI is available, vertebral angiography should be

Figure 10–18. Anatomical relationships in deep cerebral hemorrhage. *Top:* Plane of section. *Bottom:* Putaminal (1) and thalamic (2) hemorrhages can compress or transect the adjacent posterior limb of the internal capsule. Thalmic hemorrhages can also extend into the ventricles or compress the hypothalamus or midbrain upgaze center (3).

performed. The angiogram shows a cerebellar mass effect in about 85% of cases, but the procedure is time-consuming. Bloody CSF will confirm the diagnosis of hemorrhage, but a clear tap does not exclude the possibility of an intracerebellar hematoma—and lumbar puncture may hasten the process of herniation. Lumbar puncture is therefore not advocated if a cerebellar hemorrhage is suspected.

Like cerebellar hemorrhage, acute peripheral vestibulopathy also produces nausea, vomiting, and gait ataxia. Severe headache, impaired consciousness, elevated blood pressure, or later age at onset, however, strongly favors cerebellar hemorrhage.

E. Treatment:

1. Surgical measures–

a. Cerebellar decompression–The most important therapeutic intervention in hypertensive hemorrhage is surgical decompression for cerebellar hematomas. Unless this step is taken promptly, there may be a fatal outcome or unexpected deterioration. Note that this procedure may also reverse the neurological deficit. Since surgical results are much better for responsive than unresponsive patients, surgery should be performed early in the course when the patient is still conscious.

b. Cerebral decompression–Surgery can be useful when a superficial hemorrhage in the cerebral white matter is large enough to cause a mass effect with shift of midline structures and incipient herniation. The prognosis is directly related to the level of consciousness before the operation, and surgery is usually fruitless in an already comatose patient.

c. Contraindications to surgery–Surgery is not indicated for pontine or deep cerebral hypertensive hemorrhages, since in most cases spontaneous decompression occurs with rupture into the ventricles—and the areas in question are accessible only at the expense of normal overlying brain.

2. Medical measures–The use of antihypertensive agents in acute intracerebral hemorrhage is controversial. Attempts to lower systemic blood pressure may compromise cerebral blood flow and lead to infarction, but continued hypertension may exacerbate cerebral edema. On this basis, it seems reasonable to lower blood pressure to diastolic levels of approximately 100 mm Hg following intracerebral hemorrhage, but this must be done with great care because the cerebral vasculature may be unusually sensitive to antihypertensive agents. The use of nitroglycerin paste ($\frac{1}{2}$–1 inch topically) has an advantage in that if the blood pressure declines excessively, the drug can be wiped off the skin and its effect rapidly terminated. If volume overload is considered to contribute to the hypertension, the judicious use of a diuretic such as furosemide (from 10 mg intravenously in patients unused to the drug to 40 mg intravenously in patients accustomed to receiving it) can be helpful.

There is no other effective medical treatment for intracerebral hemorrhage. Rebleeding at the site of a hypertensive intracerebral hemorrhage is uncommon, and antifibrinolytic agents are not indicated. Corticosteroids are commonly prescribed to reduce vasogenic edema in patients with intracerebral hemorrhage, but the evidence of their benefit is poor. Antiedema agents (see p. 272) have provided only temporary benefit.

Other Causes of Intracerebral Hemorrhage

A. Trauma: Intracerebral hemorrhage is a frequent consequence of closed-head trauma. Such hemorrhages may occur under the skull at the site of impact or directly opposite the site of impact (contrecoup injury). The most common locations are the frontal and temporal poles. The appearance of traumatic hemorrhages on CT scans may be delayed for as much as 24 hours after injury; MRI permits earlier detection.

B. Vascular Malformations: Bleeding from cerebral angiomas and aneurysms can lead to both intracerebral and subarachnoid hemorrhage. Angiomas may come to medical attention because of seizures, in which case anticonvulsants are the treatment of choice, or because of bleeding. In the latter instance, surgical removal is indicated to prevent rebleeding— provided the malformation is surgically accessible. Aneurysms usually present with intracranial hemorrhage but occasionally with compressive focal deficits such as third nerve palsy. Their treatment is considered in Chapter 3.

C. Hemorrhage into Cerebral Infarcts: Some cases of cerebral infarction, especially when embolic in origin, are accompanied by hemorrhage into the infarct.

D. Amphetamine or Cocaine Abuse: Intravenous, intranasal, and oral amphetamine or cocaine use can result in intracerebral hemorrhage, which typically occurs within minutes to hours after the drug is administered. Most such hemorrhages are located in subcortical white matter and may be related to either acute elevation of blood pressure, leading to spontaneous hemorrhage or rupture of a vascular anomaly, or drug-induced arteritis.

E. Cerebral Amyloid Angiopathy: Cerebral amyloid (congophilic) angiopathy is a rare cause of intracerebral hemorrhage. Amyloid deposits are present in the walls of small cortical blood vessels and in the meninges. The disorder is most common in elderly patients (a mean age of 70 years) and typically produces lobar hemorrhages at multiple sites. Some cases are familial.

F. Acute Hemorrhagic Leukoencephalitis: This is a demyelinating and hemorrhagic disorder that characteristically follows a respiratory infection and has a fulminant course resulting in death within several days. Multiple small hemorrhages are found in the brain, and red blood cells may be present in CSF.

G. Hemorrhage into Tumors: Bleeding into

primary or metastatic brain tumors is an occasional cause of intracerebral hemorrhage. Tumors associated with hemorrhage include glioblastoma multiforme, melanoma, choriocarcinoma, renal cell carcinoma, and bronchogenic carcinoma. Bleeding into a tumor should be considered when a patient with known cancer experiences acute neurological deterioration; it may also be the presenting manifestation of cancer.

H. Coagulopathies: Intracerebral hemorrhage is a complication of disorders of both clotting factors and platelets, such as hemophilia (factor VIII deficiency) and idiopathic thrombocytopenic purpura. Acute myelogenous leukemia with white blood cell counts greater than 150,000/μL may also predispose to intracerebral hemorrhage.

I. Anticoagulation: Patients receiving heparin or warfarin are at increased risk for developing spontaneous or traumatic intracerebral hemorrhage.

GLOBAL CEREBRAL ISCHEMIA

Etiology

Global cerebral ischemia occurs when the blood flow is inadequate to meet the metabolic requirements of the brain, as in cardiac arrest. The result is a spectrum of neurological disorders. The greater severity of neurological involvement in ischemia than in pure anoxia may be due to the fact that in the former condition, the delivery of glucose and removal of potentially toxic metabolites are also impaired.

Pathology

Neuropathological changes depend on the degree and duration of cerebral ischemia.

A. Distribution: Complete interruption of cerebral blood flow followed by reperfusion, such as occurs in cardiac arrest with resuscitation, produces damage that selectively affects metabolically vulnerable neurons of the cerebral cortex, basal ganglia, and cerebellum.

With less profound hypotension for prolonged periods, the damage is concentrated in the anatomically vulnerable border zones between the territories supplied by the major arteries of cerebral cortex, cerebellum, basal ganglia, and spinal cord. It is most severe in the watershed region between the territories supplied by the anterior, middle, and posterior cerebral arteries (Figure 10–19).

B. Modifying Factors: Reducing cerebral energy requirements, such as with deep anesthesia or hypothermia, can minimize or prevent brain damage from ischemic insults. Hyperglycemia or hypermetabolic states such as status epilepticus, on the other

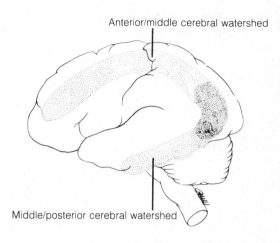

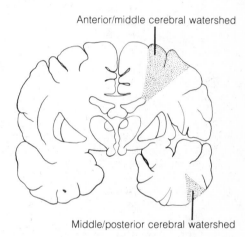

Figure 10–19. Distribution of watershed cerebral infarctions (stippled areas).

hand, can increase ischemic damage. Superimposed occlusive atherosclerotic disease of the craniocervical arteries may lead to asymmetries in the distribution of cerebral damage from panhypoperfusion.

Clinical Findings

A. Brief Ischemic Episodes: Reversible encephalopathies are common following brief episodes of systemic circulatory arrest. In such cases, coma persists for less than 12 hours. Transient confusion or amnesia may occur on awakening, but recovery is rapid and complete. Some patients show a severe anterograde and variable retrograde amnesia and a bland, unconcerned affect with or without confabulation. Recovery often occurs within seven to ten days but may be delayed by one month or longer. This syndrome may reflect reversible bilateral damage to the thalamus or hippocampus.

B. Prolonged Ischemic Episodes:

1. Focal cerebral dysfunction–Patients are usually comatose for at least 12 hours and may have lasting focal or multifocal motor, sensory, and cognitive deficits if they awaken. Full recovery may not occur or may require weeks to months. Some such patients are eventually capable of leading an independent existence, while those who are more severely disabled may require institutional care.

Focal neurological signs after cardiac arrest include partial or complete cortical blindness, weakness of both arms (bibrachial paresis), and quadriparesis. Cortical blindness is usually transient but can rarely be permanent. It probably results from disproportionate ischemia of the occipital poles because of their location in the border zone between the middle and posterior cerebral arteries (Figure 10–19). Bibrachial paresis (**man-in-a-barrel syndrome**) results from bilateral infarction of the motor cortex in the border zone between the anterior and middle cerebral arteries (Figure 10–19).

2. Persistent vegetative state–Some patients who are initially comatose following cardiac arrest survive and awaken but remain functionally decorticate and unaware of their surroundings. They typically regain spontaneous eye-opening, sleep-wake cycles, and roving eye movements and brain stem and spinal cord reflexes. The persistent vegetative state is thus distinct from coma and appears to be associated with destruction of the neocortex. A persistent vegetative state associated with an isoelectric (flat) electroencephalogram is termed **neocortical death.** Persistent vegetative states must be distinguished from brain death (see Chapter 11), in which both cerebral and brain stem function are absent.

3. Spinal cord syndromes–The spinal cord seems to be more resistant to transient ischemia than the brain, so that cord damage from hypoperfusion is usually accompanied by profound cerebral involvement. Hypoperfusion does occasionally lead to isolated spinal cord infarction, however. In such cases, the anterior and central structures of the spinal cord are more involved because of their location in the critical border zones between territories supplied by the anterior and posterior spinal arteries (see Figure 6–2). These watersheds, especially in the upper and lower levels of the thoracic cord, are vulnerable to profound drops in perfusion pressure. In the acute period, spinal stroke from hypotension produces a flaccid paraplegia and urinary retention. The sensory level in the thoracic region is characterized more by marked impairment of pain and temperature sensation than of light touch. With time, flaccid paralysis is replaced by spastic paraplegia with brisk tendon reflexes in the legs and extensor plantar responses.

Treatment

A. Established Measures: The clinical management of patients in coma caused by global cerebral ischemia involves immediate restoration of adequate cerebral circulation, elimination of cardiac dysrhythmias, maintenance of effective systemic blood pressure, and correction of acid-base or electrolyte abnormalities. Ventilatory assistance may be necessary if either medullary depression or injury to the chest wall prevents adequate ventilation, and supplemental oxygen can also be administered.

Beyond these measures, there are no other uniformly satisfactory methods of treatment. Attempts to prevent cerebral edema in this setting have not been successful, and treatment with corticosteroids, dehydrating agents, calcium channel antagonists, hypothermia, and hyperventilation have not improved the prognosis.

B. Experimental Measures: Although barbiturates have a protective effect in some experimental models of global cerebral ischemia, a similar benefit does not appear to occur in patients.

Excitatory-amino-acid-receptor antagonists may find application in the treatment of cerebral anoxic ischemia but are at present experimental. The rationale for considering the use of these drugs lies in existing evidence that ischemia or hypoxia may trigger the release of excitatory amino acid neurotransmitters, which may in turn interact with vulnerable neurons to promote cell death.

REFERENCES

GENERAL

Barnett HJM et al: *Stroke: Pathophysiology, Diagnosis and Management.* Churchill Livingstone, 1986.

Colditz GA et al: Cigarette smoking and risk of stroke in middle-aged women. *N Engl J Med* 1988;318:937–941.

Gill JS et al: Stroke and alcohol consumption. *N Engl J Med* 1986;315:1041–1046.

Iso H et al: Serum cholesterol levels and six-year mortality from stroke in 350,977 men screened for multiple risk factor intervention trial. *N Engl J Med* 1989;320:904–910.

Stampfer MJ et al: A prospective study of moderate alcohol consumption and the risk of coronary disease and stroke in women. *N Engl J Med* 1988;319:267–273.

Stampfer MJ et al: A prospective study of past use of oral contraceptive agents and risk of cardiovascular diseases. *N Engl J Med* 1988;319:1313–1317.

Welin L et al: Analysis of risk factors for stroke in a cohort of men born in 1913. *N Engl J Med* 1987;317:521–526.

FOCAL CEREBRAL ISCHEMIA

Adams HP Jr et al: Nonhemorrhagic cerebral infarction in young adults. *Arch Neurol* 1986;43:793–796.

Allen CM: Clinical diagnosis of the acute stroke syndrome. *Q J Med* 1983;52:515–523.

Choi DW, Rothman SM: The role of glutamate neurotoxicity in hypoxic-ischemic neuronal death. *Annu Rev Neurosci* 1990;13:171–182.

Gautier JC: Stroke-in-progression. *Stroke* 1985;16:729–733.

Helgason CM: Blood glucose and stroke. *Stroke* 1988;19:1049–1053.

Levy DE: How transient are transient ischemic attacks? *Neurology* 1988;38:674–677.

Powers WJ: Cerebral hemodynamics in ischemic cerebrovascular disease. *Ann Neurol* 1991;29:231–240.

Rolak LA, Gilmer W, Strittmatter WJ: Low yield in the diagnostic evaluation of transient ischemic attacks. *Neurology* 1990;40:747–748.

Werdelin L, Juhler M: The course of transient ischemic attacks. *Neurology* 1988;38:677–680.

Vascular Causes

Bougousslavsky J et al: Migraine stroke. *Neurology* 1988;38:223–227.

Bousser MG et al: Cerebral venous thrombosis: A review of 38 cases. *Stroke* 1985;16:199–213.

Calabrese LH, Mallek JA: Primary angiitis of the central nervous system: Report of 8 new cases, review of the literature, and proposal for diagnostic criteria. *Medicine* 1987;67:20–39.

Caselli RJ, Hunder GG, Whisnant JP: Neurological disease in biopsy-proven giant cell (temporal) arteritis. *Neurology* 1988;38:352–359.

Engstrom JW, Lowenstein DH, Bredesen DE: Cerebral infarctions and transient neurological deficits associated with acquired immunodeficiency syndrome. *Am J Med* 1989;86:528–532.

Fisher CM: Lacunar strokes and infarcts: A review. *Neurology* 1982;32:871–876.

Hart RG, Easton JD: Dissections of cervical and cerebral arteries. *Neurol Clin* 1983;1:155–182.

Hennerici M, Klemm C, Rautenberg W: The subclavian steal phenomenon: A common vascular disorder with rare neurological deficits. *Neurology* 1988;38:669–673.

Jordan KG: Modern neurosyphilis—A critical analysis. *West J Med* 1988;149:47–57.

Kaku DA, Lowenstein DH: Emergence of recreational drug abuse as a major risk factor for stroke in young adults. *Ann Intern Med* 1990;113:821–827.

Levine SR et al: Cerebrovascular complications of the use of the "crack" form of alkaloidal cocaine. *N Engl J Med* 1990;323:699–704.

Luscher TF et al: Arterial fibromuscular dysplasia. *Mayo Clin Proc* 1987;62:931–952.

Miller VT: Lacunar stroke: A reassessment. *Arch Neurol* 1983;40:129–134.

Ross R: The pathogenesis of atherosclerosis—An update. *N Engl J Med* 1986;314:488–500.

Yatsu FM, Fisher M.: Atherosclerosis: Current concepts on pathogenesis and interventional therapies. *Ann Neurol* 1989;26:3–12.

Cardiac Causes

Cerebral Embolism Task Force: Cardiogenic brain embolism: The second report of the Cerebral Embolism Task Force. *Arch Neurol* 1989;46:727–743.

Kittner SJ et al: Infarcts with a cardiac source of embolism in the NINCDS stroke data bank: Historical features. *Neurology* 1990;40:281–284.

Markel ML, Waller BF, Armstrong WF: Cardiac myxoma: A review. *Medicine* 1987;66:114–125.

Marks AR et al: Identification of high-risk and low-risk subgroups of patients with mitral-valve prolapse. *N Engl J Med* 1989;320:1031–1036.

Rogers LR et al: Cerebral infarction from non-bacterial thrombotic endocarditis: Clinical and pathological study including the effects of anticoagulation. *Am J Med* 1987;83:746–756.

Wipf JE, Lipsky BA: Atrial fibrillation: Thromboembolic risk and indications for anticoagulation. *Arch Intern Med* 1990;150:1598–1603.

Hematological Causes

Adams RJ et al: Cerebral infarction in sickle cell anemia: Mechanism based on CT and MRI. *Neurology* 1988;38:1012–1017.

Amico L, Caplan LR, Thomas C: Cerebrovascular complications of mucinous cancers. *Neurology* 1989;39:522–526.

Levine SR, Welch KMA: Antiphospholipid antibodies. *Ann Neurol* 1989;26:386–389.

Longstreth WT Jr, Swanson PD: Oral contraceptives and stroke. *Stroke* 1984;15:747–750.

General Medical Treatment

Grotta JC: Current medical and surgical therapy for cerebrovascular disease. *N Engl J Med* 1987;317:1505–1516.

Scheinberg P: Controversies in the management of cerebral vascular disease. *Neurology* 1988;38:1609–1616.

Wallace JD, Levy LL: Blood pressure after stroke. *JAMA* 1981;246:2177–2180.

Antiplatelet Agents

Antiplatelet Trialists' Collaboration: Secondary prevention of vascular disease by prolonged antiplatelet treatment. *Br Med J* 1988;296:320–331.

Hass WK et al: A randomized trial comparing ticlopidine hydrochloride with aspirin for the prevention of stroke in high-risk patients. *N Engl J Med* 1989;321:501–507.

Petersen P et al: Placebo-controlled, randomised trial of warfarin and aspirin for prevention of thromboembolic complications in chronic atrial fibrillation: The Copenhagen AFASAK study. *Lancet* 1989;1:175–179.

Steering Committee of the Physicians' Health Study Research Group: Final report on the aspirin component of the ongoing physicians' health study. *N Engl J Med* 1989;321:129–135.

Stroke Prevention in Atrial Fibrillation Study Group Investigators: Preliminary report of the stroke prevention in atrial fibrillation study. *N Engl J Med* 1990;322:863–868.

UK-TIA Study Group: United Kingdom transient ischaemic attack (UK-TIA) aspirin trial: interim results. *Br Med J* 1988;296:316–320.

Anticoagulation

Boston Area Anticoagulation Trial for Atrial Fibrillation Investigators: The effect of low-dose warfarin on the risk of stroke in patients with nonrheumatic atrial fibrillation. *N Engl J Med* 1990;323:1505–1511.

Miller VT, Hart RG: Heparin anticoagulation in acute brain ischemia. *Stroke* 1987;22:7–11.

Petersen P et al: Placebo-controlled, randomised trial of warfarin and aspirin for prevention of thromboembolic complications in chronic atrial fibrillation: The Copenhagen AFASAK study. *Lancet* 1989;1:175–179.

Petty GW: Complications of long-term anticoagulation. *Ann Neurol* 1988;23:570–574.

Phillips SJ: An alternative view of heparin anticoagulation in acute focal brain ischemia. *Stroke* 1989;20:295–298.

Stroke Prevention in Atrial Fibrillation Study Group Investigators: Preliminary report of the stroke prevention in atrial fibrillation study. *N Engl J Med* 1990;322:863–868.

Wipf JE, Lipsky BA: Atrial fibrillation: Thromboembolic risk and indications for anticoagulation. *Arch Intern Med* 1990;150:1598–1603.

Yatsu FM et al: Anticoagulation of embolic strokes of cardiac origin: An update. *Neurology* 1988;38:314–316.

Other Medical Treatment

Gelmers HJ et al: A controlled trial of nimodipine in acute ischemic stroke. *N Engl J Med* 1988;318:203–207.

Meldrum B: Protection against ischaemic neuronal damage by drugs acting on excitatory neurotransmission. *Cerebrovasc Brain Metab Rev* 1990;2:27–57.

Norris JW, Hachinski VC: High dose steroid treatment in cerebral infarction. *Br Med J* 1986;292:21–23.

Sloan MA: Thrombolysis and stroke: Past and future. *Arch Neurol* 1987;44:748–768.

Surgical Treatment

Cebul RD, Whisnant JP: Carotid endarterectomy. *Ann Int Med* 1989;111:660–670.

Chambers BR, Norris JW: Outcome in patients with asymptomatic neck bruits. *N Engl J Med* 1986;315:860–865.

EC/IC Bypass Study Group: Failure of extracranial-intracranial arterial bypass to reduce the risk of ischemic stroke. *N Engl J Med* 1985;313:1191–1200.

European Carotid Surgery Trialists' Collaborative Group: MRC European Carotid Surgery Trial: Interim results for symptomatic patients with severe (70–99%) or with mild (0–29%) carotid stenosis. *Lancet* K91;337:1235–1243.

Grotta JC: Current medical and surgical therapy for cerebrovascular disease. *N Engl J Med* 1987;317:1505–1516.

North American Symptomatic Carotid Endarterectomy Trial Collaborators: Beneficial effect of carotid endarterectomy in symptomatic patients with high-grade carotid stenosis. *N Engl J Med* 1991;325:445–453.

Reed GL III et al: Stroke following coronary-artery bypass surgery: A case-controlled estimate of the risk from carotid bruits. *N Engl J Med* 1988;319:1246–1250.

Van Ruiswyk J, Noble H, Sigmann P: The natural history of carotid bruits in elderly persons. *Ann Intern Med* 1990;112:340–343.

Winslow CM et al: The appropriateness of carotid endarterectomy. *N Engl J Med* 1988;318:721–727.

Prognosis

Caronna JJ, Levy DE: Clinical predictors of outcome in ischemic stroke. *Neurol Clin* 1983;1:103–117.

Jongbloed L: Prediction of function after stroke: A critical review. *Stroke* 1986;17:765–776.

INTRACEREBRAL HEMORRHAGE

Caplan L: Intracerebral hemorrhage revisited. *Neurology* 1988;38:624–627.

Chen ST et al: Progression of hypertensive intracerebral hemorrhage. *Neurology* 1989;39:1509–1514.

Cuneo RA, Caronna JJ: The neurological complications of hypertension. *Med Clin No Am* 1977;61:565–580.

Kase CS et al: Lobar intracerebral hematomas: Clinical and CT analysis of 22 cases. *Neurology* 1982;32:1146–1150.

Paulson OB, Strandgaard S, Edvinsson L: Cerebral autoregulation. *Cerebrovasc Brain Metab Rev* 1990;2:161–192.

Poungvarin N et al: Effects of dexamethasone in primary supratentorial intracerebral hemorrhage. *N Engl J Med* 1987;316:1229–1233.

Sacco RL et al: Subarachnoid and intracerebral hemorrhage: Natural history, prognosis, and precursive factors in the Framingham Study. *Neurology* 1984;34:847–854.

Weisberg LA et al: Nontraumatic parenchymal brain hemorrhages. *Medicine* 1990;69:277–295.

GLOBAL CEREBRAL ISCHEMIA

Caronna JJ: Diagnosis, prognosis, and treatment of hypoxic coma. *Adv Neurol* 1979;26:1–15.

Levy DE et al: Predicting outcome from hypoxic-ischemic coma. *JAMA* 1985;253:1420–1426.

Coma

11

Coma is a state in which the patient makes no purposeful response to the environment and from which he or she cannot be aroused. The eyes are typically closed and do not open spontaneously. The patient does not speak, and there is no purposeful movement of the face or limbs. Verbal stimulation produces no response. Mechanical (eg, painful) stimulation may also produce no response, or may elicit nonpurposeful reflex movements mediated through spinal cord or brain stem pathways.

Coma results from a disturbance in the function of either the brain stem reticular activating system above the midpons, or both cerebral hemispheres

(Figure 11–1), since these are the brain regions that maintain consciousness.

APPROACH TO DIAGNOSIS

The approach to diagnosis of the comatose patient consists first of emergency measures to stabilize the patient and treat presumptively certain life-threatening disorders, followed by efforts to establish an etiologic diagnosis.

EMERGENCY MANAGEMENT

As summarized in Table 11–1, emergency management of the comatose patient includes the following steps:

1. Ensure patency of the airway and adequacy of ventilation and circulation. This is accomplished by rapid visual inspection and by measuring the vital signs. If the **airway** is obstructed, the obstruction should be cleared and the patient intubated. If there is

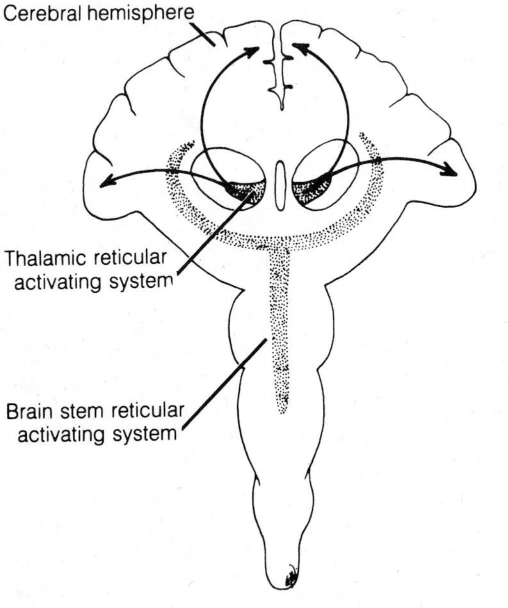

Figure 11–1. Anatomical basis of coma. Consciousness is maintained by the normal functioning of the brain stem reticular activating system and its bilateral projections to the thalamus and cerebral hemispheres. Coma results from lesions that affect either the reticular activating system or both hemispheres.

Cerebral hemisphere

Thalamic reticular activating system

Brain stem reticular activating system

Table 11-1. Emergency management of the comatose patient.

Immediately	Next	Later
Ensure adequacy of airway, ventilation, and circulation.	Obtain a history if possible.	ECG.
Draw blood for serum glucose, electrolytes, liver and renal function tests, PT, PTT, and CBC.	Perform detailed general physical and neurological examination	Correct hyper- or hypothermia.
Start IV and administer 25 g of dextrose, 100 mg of thiamine, and 0.4–1.2 mg of naloxone IV.	Order CT scan of head if history or findings suggest structural lesion.	Correct severe acid-base and electrolyte abnormalities.
Draw blood for arterial blood gas determinations.	Perform LP if meningitis or subarachnoid hemorrhage is suspected.	Chest x-ray.
Treat seizures (see Chapter 9).		Blood and urine toxicology studies.
		EEG.

evidence of trauma that may have affected the cervical spine, however, the neck should not be moved until this possibility has been excluded by x-rays of the cervical spine. In this case, if intubation is required, it should be performed by tracheostomy. Adequacy of **ventilation** can be established by the absence of cyanosis, a respiratory rate > 8/min, the presence of breath sounds on auscultation of the chest, and the results of arterial blood gas and pH studies (see below). If any of these suggest inadequate ventilation, the patient should be ventilated mechanically. Measurement of the pulse and blood pressure provides a rapid assessment of the status of the **circulation.** Circulatory embarrassment should be treated with intravenous fluid replacement, pressors, and antiarrhythmic drugs, as indicated.

2. Insert an intravenous catheter and withdraw blood for laboratory studies. These studies should include measurement of serum glucose and electrolytes, hepatic and renal function tests, prothrombin time, partial thromboplastin time, and a complete blood count. Extra tubes of blood should also be obtained for additional studies that may be useful in certain cases, such as drug screens, and for tests that become necessary as diagnostic evaluation proceeds.

3. Begin an intravenous infusion and administer dextrose, thiamine, and naloxone. Every comatose patient should be given 25 g of **dextrose** intravenously, typically as 50 mL of a 50% dextrose solution, to treat possible hypoglycemic coma. Since administration of dextrose alone may precipitate or worsen Wernicke's encephalopathy in thiamine-deficient patients, all comatose patients should also receive 100 mg of **thiamine** by the intravenous route. To treat possible opiate overdose, the opiate antagonist **naloxone,** 0.4–1.2 mg intravenously, should also be administered routinely to comatose patients.

4. Withdraw arterial blood for blood gas and pH determinations. In addition to assisting in the assessment of ventilatory status, these studies can provide clues to metabolic causes of coma (Table 11-2).

5. Institute treatment for seizures, if present. Persistent or recurrent seizures in a comatose patient should be considered to represent status epilepticus and treated accordingly, as described in Chapter 9 (see particularly Table 9-6).

After these measures have been taken, the history (if available) is obtained and general physical and neurological examinations are performed.

HISTORY AND EXAMINATION

History

The most crucial aspect of the history is the time over which coma develops. In the absence of precise details about the mode of onset, information about when the patient was last seen in an apparently normal state may assist in establishing the time course of the disease process.

A. A sudden onset of coma suggests a vascular origin, especially a brain stem stroke or subarachnoid hemorrhage.

B. Rapid progression from hemispheric signs, such

Table 11-2. Metabolic coma: Differential diagnosis by acid-base abnormalities.[1]

Respiratory acidosis
  Sedative drug intoxication
  Pulmonary encephalopathy
Respiratory alkalosis
  Hepatic encephalopathy
  Salicylate intoxication
  Sepsis

Metabolic acidosis
  Diabetic ketoacidosis
  Uremic encephalopathy
  Lactic acidosis
  Paraldehyde intoxication
  Methanol intoxication
  Ethylene glycol intoxication
  Isoniazid intoxication
  Salicylate intoxication
  Sepsis (terminal)
Metabolic alkalosis
  Coma unusual

[1]Adapted from Plum F, Posner JB: *The Diagnosis of Stupor and Coma,* 3rd ed. Vol 19 of: *Contemporary Neurology Series.* Davis, 1980.

as hemiparesis, hemisensory deficit, or aphasia, to coma within minutes to hours is characteristic of intracerebral hemorrhage.

C. A more protracted course leading to coma (days to a week or more) is seen with tumor, abscess, or chronic subdural hematoma.

D. Coma preceded by a confusional state or agitated delirium, without lateralizing signs or symptoms, is probably due to a metabolic derangement.

General Physical Examination

A. Signs of Trauma:

1. Inspection of the head may reveal signs of **basilar skull fracture,** including the following:

a. Raccoon eyes–Periorbital ecchymoses.

b. Battle's sign–Swelling and discoloration overlying the mastoid bone behind the ear.

c. Hemotympanum–Blood behind the tympanic membrane.

d. Cerebrospinal fluid rhinorrhea or otorrhea–Leakage of CSF from the nose or ear. CSF rhinorrhea must be distinguished from other causes of rhinorrhea, such as allergic rhinitis. It has been suggested that CSF can be distinguished from nasal mucus by the higher glucose content of CSF, but this is not always the case. The chloride level may be more useful, since CSF chloride concentrations are 15–20 meq/L higher than those in mucus.

2. Palpation of the head may demonstrate a **depressed skull fracture** or **swelling of soft tissues** at the site of trauma.

B. Blood Pressure: Elevation of blood pressure in a comatose patient may reflect long-standing hypertension, which predisposes to intracerebral hemorrhage or stroke. In the rare condition of hypertensive encephalopathy, the blood pressure is above 250/150 mm Hg in chronically hypertensive patients; it may be lower following acute elevation of blood pressure in previously normotensive patients (eg, in acute renal failure). Elevation of blood pressure may also be a consequence of the process causing the coma, as in intracerebral or subarachnoid hemorrhage or, rarely, brain stem stroke.

C. Temperature: Hypothermia can occur in coma caused by ethanol or sedative drug intoxication, hypoglycemia, Wernicke's encephalopathy, hepatic encephalopathy, and myxedema. Coma with hyperthermia is seen in heat stroke, status epilepticus, malignant hyperthermia related to inhalational anesthetics, anticholinergic drug intoxication, pontine hemorrhage, and certain hypothalamic lesions.

D. Signs of Meningeal Irritation: Signs of meningeal irritation (eg, nuchal rigidity) are of great importance in leading to the prompt diagnosis of meningitis or subarachnoid hemorrhage, but they are lost in deep coma.

E. Optic Fundi: Examination of the optic fundi may reveal papilledema or retinal hemorrhages compatible with chronic or acute hypertension or an elevation in intracranial pressure. Subhyaloid (superficial retinal) hemorrhages in an adult strongly suggest subarachnoid hemorrhage.

Neurological Examination

The neurological examination is the key to etiological diagnosis in the comatose patient. Pupillary size and reactivity, oculocephalic and oculovestibular reflexes, and the motor response to pain should be evaluated in detail (Figure 11–2).

A. Pupils:

1. Normal pupils–Normal pupils are 3–4 mm in diameter and equal bilaterally; they constrict briskly and symmetrically in response to light.

2. Thalamic pupils–Slightly smaller reactive pupils are present in the early stages of thalamic compression with early herniation, perhaps because of the interruption of the descending sympathetic pathways.

3. Fixed dilated pupils–Pupils greater than 7 mm in diameter and fixed (nonreactive to light) usually result from compression of the oculomotor (III) cranial nerve anywhere along its course from the midbrain to the orbit but may also be seen in anticholinergic or sympathomimetic drug intoxication. The most common cause of a fixed dilated pupil in a comatose patient is transtentorial herniation of the medial temporal lobe from a supratentorial mass.

4. Fixed midsized pupils–Pupils fixed at about 5 mm in diameter are the result of brain stem damage at the midbrain level.

5. Pinpoint pupils–Pinpoint pupils (1–1.5 mm in diameter) in a comatose patient usually indicate opioid overdose or focal damage at the pontine level. Under these conditions, the pupils may appear unreactive to light except, perhaps, with a magnifying glass. Pinpoint pupils are also caused by organophosphate poisoning, miotic eye drops, or neurosyphilis.

6. Asymmetric pupils–Asymmetry of pupillary size **(anisocoria)** with a difference of 1 mm or less in diameter is a normal finding in 20% of the population; the pupils constrict to a similar extent in response to light, and extraocular movements are not impaired. In contrast, a pupil that constricts less rapidly or to a lesser extent than its fellow usually implies a structural lesion affecting the midbrain or oculomotor nerve.

B. Extraocular Movements:

1. Pathways tested–The neuronal pathways to be tested begin at the pontomedullary junction (vestibular [VIII] nerve and nucleus), synapse in the caudal pons (horizontal gaze center and abducens [VI] nerve nucleus), ascend through the central core of the brain stem (medial longitudinal fasciculus), and arrive at the midbrain level (oculomotor [III] nucleus and nerve; see Figure 11–3).

2. Methods of testing–In the comatose patient, eye movements are tested by stimulating the vestibular system (semicircular canals of the middle ear) by

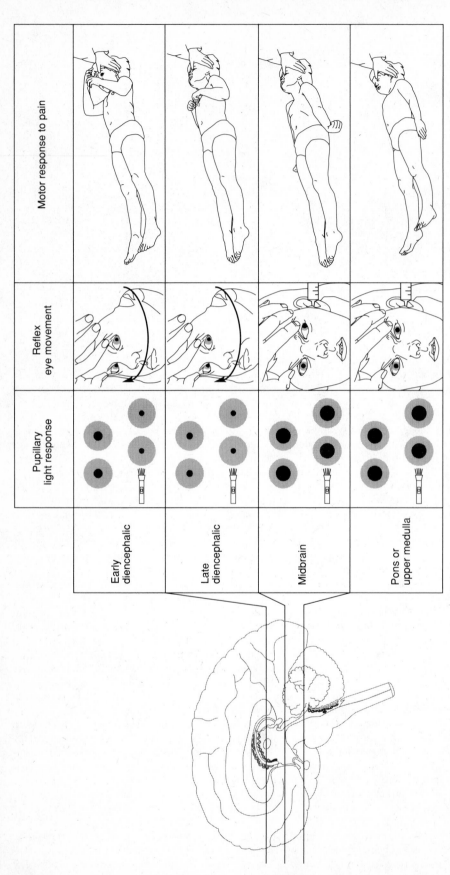

Figure 11–2. Neurological signs in coma with downward transtentorial herniation. In the **early diencephalic** phase, the pupils are small (about 2 mm in diameter) and reactive, reflex eye movements are intact, and the motor response to pain is purposeful or semipurposeful (localizing), and often asymmetrical. The **late diencephalic** phase is associated with similar findings, except that painful stimulation results in decorticate (flexor) posturing, which may also be asymmetrical. With **midbrain** involvement, the pupils are fixed and midsized (about 5 mm in diameter), reflex adduction of the eyes is impaired, and pain elicits decerebrate (extensor) posturing. Progression to involve the **pons or medulla** also produces fixed, midsized pupils, but these are accompanied by loss of reflex abduction as well as adduction of the eyes, and by no motor response or only leg flexion upon painful stimulation. Note that although a lesion restricted to the pons produces pinpoint pupils as a result of the destruction of descending sympathetic (pupillodilator) pathways, downward herniation to the pontine level is associated with midsized pupils. This happens because herniation also interrupts parasympathetic (pupilloconstrictor) fibers in the oculomotor (III) nerve.

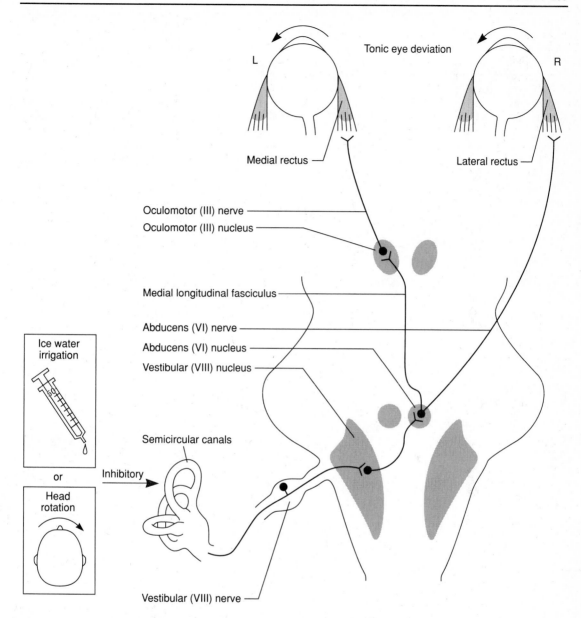

Figure 11–3. Brain stem pathways mediating conjugate horizontal eye movements. In a comatose patient with intact brain stem function, irrigation of the tympanic membrane with ice water inhibits the vestibulo-ocular pathways shown, resulting in tonic deviation of both eyes toward the irrigated side; head rotation causes eye deviation away from the direction of rotation.

means of passive head rotation (the **oculocephalic reflex,** or doll's-head maneuver) or by the stronger stimulus of ice-water irrigation against the tympanic membrane (**oculovestibular reflex,** or **cold-water calorics** testing). This latter maneuver is described in more detail in Chapter 4.

3. Normal movements–A comatose patient without brain stem disease will often demonstrate full conjugate horizontal eye movements during the doll's-head maneuver, and always exhibits tonic conjugate movement of both eyes to the side of the ice-

water irrigation during caloric testing. The presence of full reflex eye movements in the comatose patient attests to the integrity of the brain stem from the pontine to the midbrain level.

4. Abnormal movements–

a. With lesions of the oculomotor nerve or midbrain lesions involving the oculomotor nucleus (such as in the rostral-caudal herniation syndrome), oculovestibular testing will reveal failure of ocular adduction with unimpaired contralateral abduction.

b. Complete absence of response on oculovestibular testing in a comatose patient implies either a structural lesion of the brain stem at the level of the pons or a metabolic disorder with a particular predilection for brain stem involvement; this is usually caused by sedative drug intoxication.

c. Downward deviation of one or both eyes in response to unilateral cold-water irrigation is most suggestive of sedative drug intoxication.

C. Motor Response to Pain: The motor response to pain is tested by applying strong pressure on the supraorbital ridge, sternum, or nail beds. The response to such stimuli may be helpful in localizing the level of cerebral dysfunction in comatose patients or providing a guide to the depth of coma.

1. With cerebral dysfunction of only moderate severity, patients may localize the offending stimulus by reaching toward the site of stimulation. Although semipurposeful localizing responses to pain can sometimes be difficult to distinguish from the reflex responses described below, movements that involve limb abduction are virtually never reflexive in nature.

2. A **decorticate** response to pain (flexion of the arm at the elbow, adduction at the shoulder, and extension of the leg and ankle) is classically associated with lesions that involve the thalamus directly or large hemispheric masses that compress it from above.

3. A **decerebrate** response (extension at the elbow, internal rotation at the shoulder and forearm, and leg extension) tends to occur when midbrain function is compromised. Decerebrate posturing generally implies more severe brain dysfunction than decorticate posturing, but neither response localizes the site of disease precisely.

4. Bilateral symmetric posturing may be seen in both structural and metabolic disorders.

5. Unilateral or asymmetric posturing suggests structural disease in the contralateral cerebral hemisphere or brain stem.

6. In patients with pontine and medullary lesions, there is usually no response to pain, but occasionally some flexion at the knee is noted.

PATHOPHYSIOLOGICAL ASSESSMENT

The most important step in evaluating the comatose patient is to decide whether unconsciousness is the result of a structural brain lesion (for which emergency neurosurgical intervention may be critical) or a diffuse encephalopathy caused by metabolic disturbance, meningitis, or seizures (for which surgical procedures are unnecessary and medical treatment may be required). The most common diagnostic dilemma is to try to differentiate between a supratentorial (hemispheric) mass lesion and metabolic encephalopathy.

Supratentorial Structural Lesions

When coma is the result of a supratentorial mass lesion, the history and physical findings early in the

course usually point to a hemispheric disorder. Hemiparesis with hemisensory loss is typical. Aphasia occurs with dominant (usually left) hemispheric lesions, and agnosia (indifference to or denial of the deficit) with injury to the nondominant hemisphere. As the mass expands (commonly from associated edema), somnolence supervenes because of the compression of the contralateral hemisphere or downward pressure on the diencephalon. Stupor progresses to coma, but the findings often remain asymmetrical. As rostral-caudal compression progresses, the thalamus, midbrain, pons, and medulla become involved, and the neurological examination reveals dysfunction at successively lower anatomical levels (Figure 11–2). Such segmental involvement strongly supports the diagnosis of a supratentorial mass with downward transtentorial herniation (Figure 11–4) and dictates the need for neurosurgical intervention. Once the pontine level is reached, a fatal outcome is inevitable. Even at the fully developed midbrain level, chances of survival without severe neurological impairment decrease rapidly, especially in adults.

When supratentorial mass lesions produce herniation of the medial portion of the temporal lobe (the uncus) across the cerebellar tentorium (Figure 11–4), thus exerting direct pressure on the rostral brain stem, signs of oculomotor nerve and midbrain compression such as ipsilateral pupillary dilatation and impaired adduction of the eye **(uncal syndrome)** may precede loss of consciousness. As consciousness is lost with progressive uncal herniation, the fully developed

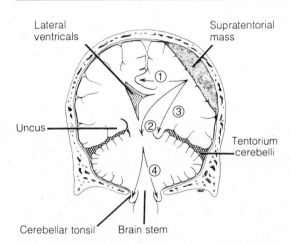

Figure 11–4. Anatomical basis of herniation syndromes. An expanding supratentorial mass lesion may cause brain tissue to be displaced into an adjacent intracranial compartment, resulting in (1) cingulate herniation under the falx, (2) downward transtentorial (central) herniation, (3) uncal herniation over the edge of the tentorium, or (4) cerebellar tonsillar herniation into the foramen magnum. Coma and ultimately death result when (2), (3), or (4) produces brain stem compression.

midbrain stage rapidly appears, with marked ipsilateral pupillary dilation and loss of reactivity to light. Neurosurgical treatment must be given early in the course of third nerve involvement if useful recovery is to be achieved.

Subtentorial Structural Lesions

Coma of sudden onset with focal brain stem signs strongly supports a diagnosis of subtentorial structural lesion. Pupillary function and extraocular movements are the most helpful features of the neurological examination, especially if the abnormalities are asymmetric. With focal midbrain lesions, pupillary function is lost: the pupils are midsized (about 5 mm in diameter) and nonreactive to light. Pinpoint pupils are found in pontine hemorrhage and less often in pontine infarction or pontine compression caused by cerebellar hemorrhage or infarction. Conjugate gaze deviation away from the side of the lesion and toward the hemiparesis—or disconjugate eye movements, such as internuclear ophthalmoplegia (selective impairment of eye adduction)—strongly suggests a subtentorial lesion. Motor responses are generally not helpful in separating subtentorial from supratentorial lesions. Ventilatory patterns associated with subtentorial lesions are abnormal but variable and may be ataxic or gasping (Figure 11–5). Since the fully developed syndrome of transtentorial herniation from a supratentorial mass is characterized by extensive brain stem dysfunction, its differentiation from a primary subtentorial process may be impossible except by history.

Diffuse Encephalopathies

Diffuse encephalopathies that result in coma (sometimes termed **metabolic coma**) include not only metabolic disorders such as hypoglycemia and drug intoxication but other processes that affect the brain diffusely, such as meningitis, subarachnoid hemorrhage, and seizures.

The clinical presentation is distinct from that of a mass lesion. There are usually no focal signs, such as hemiparesis, hemisensory loss, or aphasia, and no sudden loss of consciousness. Instead, the history reveals a period of progressive somnolence or toxic delirium followed by gradual descent into a stuporous and finally comatose state.

A symmetrical neurological examination supports a metabolic cause of coma. Hepatic encephalopathy, hypoglycemia, and hyperosmolar nonketotic hyperglycemia may be accompanied by focal signs—especially hemiparesis, which may alternate from side to side. Asterixis, myoclonus, and tremor are important clues that suggest metabolic disease. Decorticate or decerebrate posturing is seen occasionally with hepatic, uremic, anoxic, hypoglycemic, or sedative-drug-induced coma.

The finding of reactive pupils in the presence of otherwise impaired brain stem function is the hall-

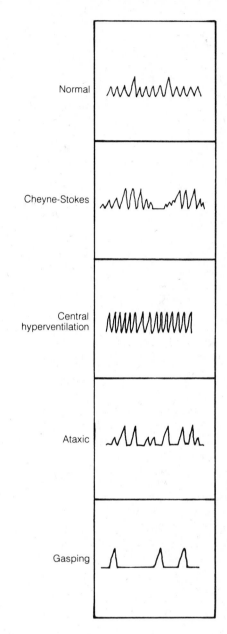

Figure 11–5. Ventilatory patterns in coma. Cheyne-Stokes respiration and central hyperventilation are seen with metabolic disturbances and with structural lesions at a variety of sites in the brain. They are therefore not useful for anatomical localization of disorders producing coma. Ataxic and gasping ventilatory patterns are most commonly seen with pontomedullary lesions.

mark of metabolic encephalopathy. Although coma with intact pupillary reactivity is also seen in the early stages of transtentorial herniation (Figure 11–2), this latter syndrome is associated with asymmetrical neurological findings. The few metabolic causes of coma that also impair pupillary reflexes include glutethimide overdose, massive barbiturate overdose with apnea and hypotension, acute anoxia, marked hypothermia, and anticholinergic poisoning (large pupils); and opioid overdose (pinpoint pupils). Even in these conditions, however, completely nonreactive pupils are uncommon.

The respiratory patterns in metabolic coma vary widely, and measurement of arterial blood gases and pH may provide a further basis for establishing an etiological diagnosis. Arterial blood gas abnormalities in coma are outlined in Table 11–2.

Summary

The relationship between neurological signs and the pathophysiological basis of coma is summarized in Table 11–3. Examining pupillary size and reactivity and testing reflex eye movements and the motor response to pain help determine whether brain function is disrupted at a discrete anatomic level (**structural lesion**) or in a diffuse manner (**metabolic coma**).

Supratentorial structural lesions compromise the brain in an orderly way, producing dysfunction at progressively lower anatomic levels. In patients with metabolic coma, such localization is not possible, and scattered, anatomically inconsistent findings are noted on examination. An impressive example of the anatomically discordant findings characteristic of metabolic encephalopathy is the retention of pupillary reactivity in the face of otherwise depressed brain stem functions: paralysis of eye movements, respiratory depression, flaccid muscle tone, and unresponsiveness to painful stimuli. The same degree of brain stem dysfunction produced by a supratentorial mass lesion would have to compromise the more rostrally situated midbrain structures that mediate pupillary reactivity before affecting the lower brain stem centers.

ETIOLOGY

SUPRATENTORIAL STRUCTURAL LESIONS

1. SUBDURAL HEMATOMA

Subdural hematoma is a correctable supratentorial mass lesion and must be considered in any comatose patient. It is more common in older patients, since cerebral atrophy makes bridging cortical veins more subject to laceration from shearing injury or to apparently spontaneous rupture.

Trauma is the most common cause, and in the acute stage following head injury, focal neurological deficits are often conspicuous. The severity of injury needed to produce a subdural hematoma becomes less with advancing age, so that in perhaps 25% of cases a history of trauma is denied by the patient.

The most common clinical findings are headache and altered consciousness, but symptoms and signs may be absent, nonspecific, or nonlocalizing, especially with chronic subdural hematomas that appear months or years after injury (Table 11–4). The classic history of waxing and waning signs and symptoms is too infrequent to be relied on for diagnosis. Hemiparesis, when present, is contralateral to the lesion in about 70% of cases. Pupillary dilation, when present, is ipsilateral in approximately 90%. The frequency of bilateral hematoma makes localization of the lesion even more difficult, as may coexisting cerebral contusion.

Diagnosis is made by CT scan or MRI (Figure 11–6), but if these are not available, bilateral carotid arteriography is necessary to establish the diagnosis. Lumbar puncture may precipitate herniation and is therefore contraindicated.

Table 11–3. Pathophysiological assessment of the comatose patient.

	Supratentorial Structural Lesion	Subtentorial Structural Lesion	Diffuse Encephalopathy
Pupil size and light reaction	Usually normal size (3–4 mm) and reactive; large (>7 mm) and unreactive after transtentorial herniation.	Midsized (about 5 mm) and unreactive with midbrain lesions; pinpoint (1–1.5 mm) and unreactive with pontine lesion.	Usually normal size (3–4 mm) and reactive; pinpoint (1–1.5 mm) and unreactive with opiates; large (>7 mm) and unreactive with anticholinergics.
Reflex eye movements	Normal.	Impaired adduction with midbrain lesion; impaired adduction and abduction with pontine lesion.	Usually normal; impaired by sedative drugs or Wernicke's encephalopathy.
Motor responses	Usually asymmetrical; may be symmetrical after transtentorial herniation.	Asymmetrical (unilateral lesion) or symmetrical (bilateral lesion).	Usually symmetrical; may be asymmetrical with hypoglycemia, hyperosmolar nonketotic hyperglycemia, or hepatic encephalopathy.

Table 11–4. Clinical features of subdural hematoma.[1]

	Acute[2] (82 Cases) (%)	Subacute[3] (91 Cases) (%)	Chronic[4] (216 Cases) (%)
Symptoms			
Depression of consciousness	100	88	47
Vomiting	24	31	30
Weakness	20	19	22
Confusion	12	41	37
Headache	11	44	81
Speech disturbance	6	8	6
Seizures	6	3	9
Vertigo	0	4	5
Visual disturbance	0	0	12
Signs			
Depression of consciousness	100	88	59
Pupillary inequality	57	27	20
Motor asymmetry	44	37	41
Confusion and memory loss	17	21	27
Aphasia	6	12	11
Papilledema	1	15	22
Hemianopia	0	4	3
Facial weakness	0	3	3

[1]Data from McKissock W: *Lancet* 1960;1:1365–1370.
[2]Within 3 days of trauma.
[3]4–20 days after trauma.
[4]More than 20 days after trauma.

Treatment of symptomatic subdural hematoma is by surgical evacuation.

2. EPIDURAL HEMATOMA

Epidural hematoma typically results from head trauma associated with a lateral skull fracture and tearing of the middle meningeal artery and vein. Patients may or may not lose consciousness initially. There is often a lucid interval of several hours before the onset of coma during which headache, vomiting, obtundation, seizures, and focal neurological signs may occur. The diagnosis is made by CT scan or MRI (Figure 11–6), which classically shows a radiodense biconvex lens-shaped mass compressing the cerebral hemisphere. Lumbar puncture is contraindicated. Prompt surgical evacuation of the hematoma is essential to prevent a fatal outcome.

3. CEREBRAL CONTUSION

Cerebral contusion caused by head trauma is associated with initial unconsciousness from which the patient recovers. Edema surrounding the contusion may cause the level of consciousness to fluctuate, and seizures and

A

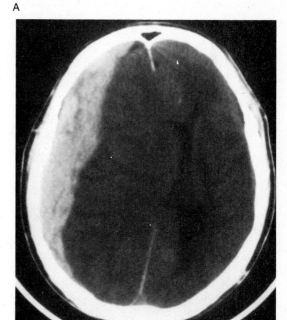

B

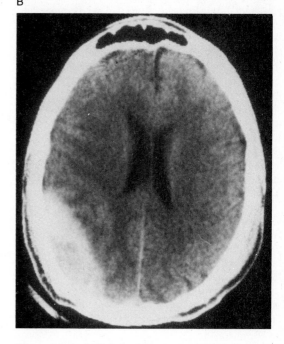

Figure 11–6. *A:* Subdural hematoma. Unenhanced CT scan showing a large, high-density crescentic mass over the right cerebral hemisphere, with shift of the lateral ventricles across the midline. ***B:*** Epidural hematoma. Unenhanced CT scan, showing a large, high-density lens-shaped mass in the right parietooccipital region. Fracture of the occipital bone was seen on bone windows.

focal neurological signs may develop. Patients must be carefully monitored for neurological deterioration related to progressive edema and herniation.

Lumbar puncture is unnecessary and potentially dangerous. The abnormalities usually found (xanthochromic fluid with an increased protein content) are nonspecific and cannot differentiate subdural hematoma from cerebral contusion without hematoma. CT scan or MRI is the diagnostic procedure of choice. In contrast to subdural and epidural hematomas, cerebral contusions are rarely operated upon.

4. INTRACEREBRAL HEMORRHAGE

Etiology

The most common cause of nontraumatic intracerebral hemorrhage is chronic hypertension. This and other causes are discussed in more detail in Chapter 10.

Clinical Findings

A. Symptoms: Hemorrhage usually occurs when the patient is awake and is not preceded by prodromal symptoms such as the transient ischemic attacks often associated with cerebral infarction. Headache occurs in many cases and can be moderate to severe. If present, headache may overlie the site of hemorrhage or be generalized. Nausea and vomiting are common. Hemiparesis is a frequent early symptom because of the proximity of common hemorrhage sites, such as the basal ganglia and thalamus, to the internal capsule. Seizures occur in about 10% of cases and are often focal. Altered consciousness is common and may progress steadily to stupor or coma over minutes to hours. Neurological deficits do not fluctuate spontaneously.

B. Physical Examination: Patients are nearly always hypertensive (blood pressure 170/90 mm Hg or higher) even in the late stages of transtentorial herniation. The funduscopic examination usually show vascular changes associated with chronic hypertension. Nuchal rigidity is common, as is conjugate deviation of the eyes toward the side of hemorrhage in the cerebral hemisphere—and thus away from the hemiparetic side.

C. Investigative Studies: CT brain scan without contrast or MRI confirms the diagnosis, showing the presence of intraparenchymal blood. Lumbar puncture is generally unnecessary and can be dangerous if intracranial pressure is markedly increased. The spinal fluid is bloody in 90% of cases. CSF red blood cell counts range from 2000 (rare) to 1 million/μL, and white blood cell counts are approximately 1/1000th as high. CSF pressure is in the range of 180–300 mm water; total protein content is as high as 100 mg/dL; and the CSF glucose level is normal. The peripheral blood may show an elevated white blood cell count of 15,000–20,000/μL. The EEG may show a focal slow wave disturbance on a diffusely slowed background, and electrocardiographic features suggestive of subendocardial ischemia (deep T wave inversions) may be seen.

Treatment

Treatment for intracerebral hemorrhage is limited, especially because the hemorrhage usually occurs over a brief period and then stops. Bleeding generally does not recur, but the patient's condition worsens because of cerebral edema.

A. Acute Management of Blood Pressure: Acute reduction of systemic blood pressure is usually ineffective in decreasing edema. In addition, it may result in dangerous hypoperfusion of ischemic brain adjacent to the hematoma, since autoregulation of the cerebral circulation is already impaired by the injury. Once the acute phase is over, the blood pressure should be controlled pharmacologically.

B. Surgical Treatment: Surgical evacuation of the clot would seem appropriate, but because the hematoma is usually deep within the brain, surgical results are disappointing. Operation may be useful, however, in the cases (approximately 10%) in which the hemorrhage is located superficially in the cerebral hemisphere and produces a mass effect.

C. Treatment of Cerebral Edema: Cerebral edema may be treated with steroids, mannitol, glycerol, or intravenous urea (Table 11–5), but such measures rarely alter the eventual outcome.

Prognosis

Many patients experience a rapid downhill course leading to death. Those who do survive may be left with a surprisingly mild deficit as the clot resolves over a period of weeks to months.

5. BRAIN ABSCESS

Brain abscess is an uncommon disorder, accounting for only 2% of intracranial masses.

Etiology

The common conditions predisposing to brain abscess, in approximate order of frequency, are bloodborne metastasis from distant systemic (especially pulmonary) infection; direct extension from parameningeal sites (otitis, cranial osteomyelitis, sinusitis); an unknown source; infection associated with recent or remote head trauma or craniotomy; and infection associated with cyanotic congenital heart disease.

The most common pathogenic agents are aerobic, anaerobic, and microaerophilic streptococci, *Staphylococcus aureus, Bacteroides,* and *Proteus* and other gram-negative bacilli. *Actinomyces, Nocardia,* and *Candida* are also found. Multiple organisms are present in many cases.

Table 11–5. Drug therapy for cerebral edema.

Drug	Dose	Route	Indications and Comments
Glucocorticoids Dexamethasone	10–100 mg, then 4 mg four times daily.	IV or orally.	Dexamethasone preferred for lowest mineralocorticoid effect. Antacid treatment indicated. Effective for edema associated with brain tumor or abscess, perhaps also intracerebral hemorrhage, but not infarction.
Prednisone	60 mg, then 25 mg four times daily.	Orally.	
Methylprednisone	60 mg, then 25 mg four times daily.	IV or orally.	
Hydrocortisone	300 mg, then 130 mg four times daily.	IV or orally.	
Osmotic diuretic agents Mannitol	1.5–2 g/kg over 30 minutes to 1 hour.	20% IV solution.	Effective acutely. Major dehydrating effect on normal tissue; osmotic effect short-lived, and more than two intravenous doses rarely effective. Side effects include osmotic diuresis, electrolyte imbalance, and (with glycerol) nausea and vomiting.
Urea	1–5 g/kg.	IV.	
Glycerol	1.5–4 g/kg/d.	Orally.	

Clinical Findings

The course is that of an expanding mass lesion, and its usual presentation is with headache and focal signs in a conscious patient. Coma may develop over days but rarely over hours. Common presenting signs and symptoms are shown in Table 11–6. Of importance is the fact that the common correlates of infection may be absent: The temperature is within normal limits in 40% of patients, and the peripheral white blood cell count is below 10,000/μL in 20% of patients.

Investigative Studies

The diagnosis is strongly supported by the finding of an avascular mass on angiography or a lesion with a contrast-enhanced rim on CT scan or MRI.

The EEG may show a high-voltage focal slow wave disturbance.

Examination of the CSF reveals an opening pressure greater than 200 mm water in 75% of patients; pleocytosis of 25–500 or more white cells/μL, depending on the proximity of the abscess to the ventricular surface and its degree of encapsulation; and elevation

Table 11–6. Brain abscess: Presenting features in 43 cases.[1]

Headache	72%
Lethargy	71%
Fever	60%
Nuchal rigidity	49%
Nausea, vomiting	35%
Seizures	35%
Ocular palsy	27%
Confusion	26%
Visual disturbance	21%
Weakness	21%
Dysarthria	12%
Stupor	12%
Papilledema	10%
Aphasia	9%
Hemiparesis	9%
Dizziness	7%

[1]Data from Chun CH et al: *Medicine* 1986;**65**:415–431.

of protein (45–500 mg/dL) in about 60% of patients. CSF cultures are usually negative. Marked clinical deterioration may follow lumbar puncture in patients with brain abscess, however, so lumbar puncture should not be performed if brain abscess is suspected.

Treatment

Treatment of pyogenic brain abscess can be with antibiotics alone or combined with surgical drainage. Surgical therapy should be strongly considered when there is a significant mass effect or the abscess is near the ventricular surface, because catastrophic rupture into the ventricular system may occur. Medical treatment alone is indicated for surgically inaccessible, multiple, or early abscesses. If the causal organism is unknown, broad coverage with antibiotics is indicated. A suggested regimen includes penicillin G, 2 million units intravenously every two hours, and chloramphenicol, 1–2 g intravenously every six hours. Some clinicians add metronidazole, 15 mg/kg administered intravenously over one hour, followed by 7.5 mg/kg intravenously or orally every six hours. If staphylococcal infection is suspected, oxacillin or nafcillin should be added at a dose of 3 g intravenously every six hours. Glucocorticoids (Table 11–5) may attenuate edema surrounding the abscess. Response to medical treatment is assessed by the clinical examination and by frequent CT scans or MRIs. When medically treated patients do not improve, needle aspiration of the abscess is indicated to identify the organisms present.

6. CEREBRAL INFARCTION (Stroke)

Embolic or thrombotic occlusion of one carotid artery does not cause coma directly except in rare instances. Cerebral edema following massive hemispheric infarction, however, can produce contralateral hemispheric compression or transtentorial herniation that will result in coma. Such cerebral swelling becomes maximal within 48–72 hours after the infarct. Thus, the history is of the strokelike onset of a focal neurological deficit, with progression over hours or days to stupor and coma. A cerebral hemorrhage is excluded by CT scan or MRI.

The use of corticosteroids and dehydrating agents to treat associated cerebral edema has produced no clear benefit. Cerebral infarction is discussed in more detail in Chapter 10.

7. BRAIN TUMOR

Clinical Findings

Primary or metastatic tumors of the central nervous system (see Chapter 3) rarely present with coma, although they can do so when hemorrhage into the tumor or tumor-induced seizures occur. More often, coma occurs late in the clinical course of brain tumor, and there is a history of headache, focal neurological deficits, and altered consciousness. Papilledema occurs in 25% of cases.

Investigative Studies

If brain tumor is suspected, a CT scan or MRI should be obtained. It may or may not be possible to determine the nature of the tumor by its radiographic appearance alone; in this case, biopsy may be required. Chest x-ray is useful, because lung carcinoma is the most common source of intracranial metastasis and because other tumors that metastasize to the brain commonly involve the lungs first.

Treatment

In contrast to its lack of therapeutic effect in cerebral infarction, corticosteroid treatment (Table 11–5) is often remarkably effective in reducing tumor-associated vasogenic brain edema and improving related neurological deficits. Specific approaches to the treatment of tumors include excision, radiotherapy, and chemotherapy, depending on the site and nature of the lesion.

SUBTENTORIAL STRUCTURAL LESIONS

1. BASILAR ARTERY THROMBOSIS OR EMBOLIC OCCLUSION

Clinical Findings

These relatively common vascular syndromes (discussed in more detail in Chapter 10) produce coma by impairing blood flow to the brain stem reticular activating system. Patients are typically middle-aged to elderly and often have a history of hypertension, atherosclerotic vascular disease, or transient ischemic attacks. Thrombosis usually affects the midportion,

and embolic occlusion the top, of the basilar artery. Virtually all patients present with some alteration of consciousness, and 50% of patients are comatose at presentation. Focal signs are present from the outset.

Pupillary abnormalities vary with the site of the lesion and include midsized fixed pupils with midbrain involvement and pinpoint pupils with pontine lesions. Vertically skewed deviation of the eyes is common, and horizontal eye movements may be absent or asymmetrical during doll's-head or caloric testing. Conjugate eye deviation, if present, is directed away from the side of the lesion and toward the hemiparesis. Vertical eye movements may be impaired or intact.

Symmetrical or asymmetrical long-tract signs, such as hemiparesis, hyperreflexia, and Babinski responses, may be present. There is no blood in the spinal fluid.

Treatment & Prognosis

Current opinion supports anticoagulation for progressive subtotal basilar artery thrombosis or cardiac emboli. The prognosis depends directly upon the degree of brain stem injury.

2. PONTINE HEMORRHAGE

Pontine hemorrhage is essentially restricted to hypertensive patients and is the least common of the hypertensive intracerebral hemorrhages (6% of cases). The apoplectic onset of coma is the hallmark of this syndrome. Physical examination reveals many of the findings noted in basilar artery infarction, but transient ischemic episodes are not encountered. Features especially suggestive of pontine involvement include ocular bobbing (spontaneous brisk, periodic, mainly conjugate downward movements of the eyes, with slower return to the primary position), pinpoint pupils, and loss of lateral eye movements. Hyperthermia (with temperature elevations to 39.5°C [103°F] or greater) occurs in most patients surviving for more than several hours. The diagnosis is made by CT scan or MRI. Spinal fluid is grossly bloody and under increased pressure, but lumbar puncture is not indicated. There is no effective treatment. Pontine hemorrhage is considered in greater detail in Chapter 10.

3. CEREBELLAR HEMORRHAGE OR INFARCTION

The clinical presentation of cerebellar hemorrhage or infarction ranges from sudden onset of coma, with rapid evolution to death, to a progressive syndrome developing over hours or even several days. Acute deterioration may occur without warning; this emphasizes the need for careful observation and early treatment of all patients. CT scan or MRI is helpful in confirming the diagnosis.

Surgical decompression may produce dramatic reduction of symptoms, and with proper surgical treatment, lethargic or even stuporous patients may survive with minimal or no residual deficits and intact intellect. If the patient is deeply comatose, however, the likelihood of useful survival is small. Additional discussion of these disorders can be found in Chapter 10.

4. POSTERIOR FOSSA SUBDURAL & EPIDURAL HEMATOMAS

These very uncommon lesions have similar clinical pictures and are important to recognize because they are treatable. The history is frequently of occipital trauma that precedes the onset of brain stem involvement by hours to many weeks. Physical findings are those of extra-axial (extrinsic) compression of the brain stem: ataxia, nystagmus, vertigo, vomiting, and progressive obtundation. Nuchal rigidity may be present, as may papilledema in more chronic cases. Skull x-rays or CT scans of the skull often reveal a fracture line crossing the transverse and sigmoid sinuses. The source of the hematoma is the traumatic tearing of these vessels. Examination of the CSF is not helpful.

Treatment is by surgical decompression.

DIFFUSE ENCEPHALOPATHIES

1. HYPOGLYCEMIA

Etiology

In most cases, the cause of hypoglycemic encephalopathy is insulin overdose. Other causes include alcoholism, severe liver disease, oral hypoglycemic agents, insulin-secreting neoplasms (insulinoma), and large retroperitoneal tumors.

Clinical Findings

As the blood glucose level falls, signs of sympathetic nervous system hyperactivity (tachycardia, sweating, and anxiety) may warn patients of impending hypoglycemia. These prodromal symptoms may be absent however, in patients with diabetic autonomic neuropathy. Neurological findings in hypoglycemia include seizures, focal signs that often alternate sides, delirium, stupor, and coma. Progressive hypothermia is common during coma. Table 1–11 summarizes the symptoms and signs observed in patients with hypoglycemia.

Investigative Studies

There is no precise correlation between blood levels of glucose and symptoms, so that levels of 30 mg/dL can result in coma in one patient, delirium in a second, and hemiparesis with preserved consciousness in a third. Coma, stupor, and confusion have been reported with blood glucose concentrations of 2–28, 8–59, and 9–60 mg/dL, respectively.

Treatment

Permanent brain damage can be avoided if glucose is rapidly administered, intravenously, orally, or by nasogastric tube. Because this condition is so easily treated and since a delay in instituting therapy may have tragic consequences, every patient presenting with a syndrome of altered consciousness (psychosis, acute confusional state, or coma) should have blood drawn for glucose determination and immediately receive 50 mL of 50% dextrose intravenously, without waiting for the result. This allows blood to be analyzed without delaying in therapy.

Prognosis

The duration of hypoglycemia that will result in permanent damage to the brain is variable. Hypoglycemic coma may be tolerated for 60–90 minutes, but once the stage of flaccidity with hyporeflexia has been reached, glucose must be administered within 15 minutes if recovery is to be expected. If the brain has not been irreparably damaged, full recovery should occur within seconds after intravenous administration of glucose and within 10 to 30 minutes after nasogastric administration. Rapid and complete recovery is the rule, but gradual improvement to full normality may take place over hours to several days. Any lingering signs or symptoms suggest irreversible brain damage from hypoglycemia or the presence of an additional neuropathological process.

2. GLOBAL CEREBRAL ISCHEMIA

Global cerebral ischemia produces encephalopathy that culminates in coma; it most often occurs following cardiac arrest. The pupils dilate rapidly, and there may be tonic, often opisthotonic, posturing with a few seizurelike tonic-clonic movements. Fecal incontinence is common. With prompt reestablishment of cerebral perfusion, recovery begins at the brain stem level with the return of reflex eye movements and pupillary function. Reflex motor activity (extensor or flexor posturing) then gives way to purposive movements, and consciousness is regained. The persistence of impaired brain stem function (fixed pupils) in adults following the return of cardiac function makes the outlook virtually hopeless. Incomplete recovery may occur, leading to the return of brain stem function and wakefulness (ie, eye opening with sleep-wake cycles) without higher-level intellectual functions. The condition of such patients—**awake but not aware**—has been termed **persistent vegetative state** (see below). Although such an outcome is possible following other major brain insults such as trauma, bihemispheric stroke, or subarachnoid hemorrhage, anoxia is the most common cause.

The prognosis in anoxic or ischemic encephalopathy is related to the rapidity with which central nervous system function returns. Patients without pupillary reactivity within one day—or those who fail to regain consciousness within four days—have a poor prognosis for functional recovery (Table 11–7).

3. DRUG INTOXICATION

Sedative-Hypnotic Drugs

Sedative-hypnotic drug overdose is the most common cause of coma in many series; barbiturates and benzodiazepines are the prototypical drugs. Coma is preceded by a period of intoxication marked by prominent nystagmus in all directions of gaze, dysarthria, and ataxia. Shortly after consciousness is lost, the neurological examination may briefly suggest an upper motor neuron lesion as hyperreflexia, ankle clonus, extensor plantar responses, and (rarely) decerebrate or decorticate posturing appear. With the single exception of glutethimide, which regularly produces midsized pupils nonreactive to light, the characteristic feature of sedative-hypnotic overdose is the absence of extraocular movements on oculocephalic testing, with preservation of the pupillary light reflex. Rarely, concentrations of barbiturates or other sedative drugs sufficient to produce severe hypotension and respiratory depression requiring pressors and ventilatory support can compromise pupillary reactivity, resulting in pupils 2–3 mm in diameter that are nonreactive to light. The EEG may be flat—and in overdose with long-acting barbiturates may remain isoelectric for at least 24 hours—yet full recovery will occur with support of cardiopulmonary function. Bullous skin eruptions and hypothermia are also characteristic of barbiturate-induced coma.

Treatment should be supportive, centered upon maintaining adequate ventilation and circulation. Barbiturates are dialyzable; however, with the shorter-acting barbiturates, morbidity and mortality rates are clearly lower in more conservatively managed patients. The use of benzodiazepine-receptor antagonists such as flumazenil to reverse sedative-hypnotic drug intoxication is experimental.

Ethanol

Ethanol overdose produces a similar syndrome, although nystagmus during wakefulness, early impairment of lateral eye movements, and progression to coma are not as common. Peripheral vasodilation is prominent, producing tachycardia, hypotension, and hypothermia. Stupor is typically associated with blood ethanol levels of 250–300 mg/dL and coma with levels of 300–400 mg/dL, but alcoholic patients who have developed tolerance to the drug may remain awake with considerably higher levels.

Opioids

Opioid overdose is characterized by pupillary constriction that is mimicked by miotic eye drops, pontine hemorrhage, Argyll Robertson pupils, and organophosphate poisoning. The diagnosis of opioid intoxication is confirmed by rapid pupillary dilation and awakening after intravenous administration of 0.4–1.2 mg of the narcotic antagonist naloxone. The duration of action of naloxone is typically one to four hours. Repeated doses may therefore be necessary, especially following intoxication with long-acting narcotics such as methadone.

4. HEPATIC ENCEPHALOPATHY

Clinical Findings

Hepatic encephalopathy (also discussed in Chapter 1) leading to coma can occur in patients with severe liver disease, especially those with portacaval shunting. Jaundice need not be present. Coma may be precipitated by an acute insult, especially gastrointestinal hemorrhage, and the production of ammonia by colonic bacteria may contribute to pathogenesis. Neuronal depression may result from an increase in inhibitory γ-aminobutyric acid (GABA)-mediated neurotransmission, perhaps from elevated levels of endogenous benzodiazepine receptor agonists in the brain. As in other metabolic encephalopathies, the patient presents with somnolence or delirium. Asterixis may be especially prominent. Muscle tone is often increased, hyperreflexia is common, and alternating hemiparesis and decorticate or decerebrate posturing have been described. Generalized and focal seizures occur but are infrequent.

Investigative Studies

A helpful diagnostic clue is the nearly invariable presence of hyperventilation with resultant respiratory alkalosis; serum bicarbonate levels are rarely depressed below 16 meq/L, however. The CSF is usually normal but may appear yellow (xanthochromic) in patients with serum bilirubin levels greater than 4–6 mg/dL. The diagnosis is confirmed by an ele-

Table 11–7. Prognostic signs in coma from global cerebral ischemia.[1]

Sign	Probability of Recovering Independent Function (%) Time Since Onset of Coma (Days)			
	0	1	3	7
No verbal response	13	8	5	6
No eye opening	11	6	4	0
Unreactive pupils	0	0	0	0
Absent corneal reflexes	4	0	0	0
No spontaneous eye movements	6	5	2	0
No caloric responses	5	6	6	0
Absent or reflex motor responses	12	11	6	2

[1]Data from Levy DE et al: Predicting outcome from hypoxic-ischemic coma. *JAMA* 1985;**253**:1420–1426.

vated CSF glutamine concentration. Coma is usually associated with concentrations above 50 mg/dL but may occur with values as low as 35 mg/dL. Hepatic encephalopathy is treated by controlling gastrointestinal bleeding or systemic infection, decreasing protein intake to less than 20 g/d, and decreasing intracolonic pH with lactulose (30 mg orally two to three times per day or titrated to produce two to four bowel movements daily). Abdominal cramping may occur during the first 48 hours of lactulose treatment. Production of ammonia by colonic bacteria may be reduced with neomycin, 6 g/d orally in three or four divided doses. Some patients may respond to treatment with the experimental benzodiazepine-receptor antagonist flumazenil.

5. HYPEROSMOLAR STATES

Coma with focal seizures is a common presentation of the hyperosmolar state, which is most often associated with nonketotic hyperglycemia. Hyperosmolar nonketotic hyperglycemia is discussed in Chapter 1.

6. HYPONATREMIA

Hyponatremia causes neurologic symptoms when serum sodium levels fall below 120 meq/L or when the serum sodium level falls rapidly. Delirium and seizures are common presenting features.

Hyponatremia is considered in detail in Chapter 1.

7. HYPOTHERMIA

All patients with temperatures below 26°C (79°F) are comatose; whereas mild hypothermia (temperatures > 32.2°C [90°F]) does not cause coma. Causes of coma associated with hypothermia include hypoglycemia, sedative drug intoxication, Wernicke's encephalopathy, and myxedema. Exposure can also produce hypothermia, such as may occur when a structural brain lesion causes acute coma out of doors or in another unheated area; therefore, such a lesion should not be excluded from consideration in the differential diagnosis of coma with hypothermia.

On physical examination, the patient is obviously cold to the touch but may not be shivering (it ceases at temperatures below 32.5°C [90.5°F]). A thermometer with a low recording capability should be used to measure the body temperature: standard hospital thermometers do not record values below 35°C (95°F). Neurological examination shows the patient to be unresponsive to pain, with diffusely increased muscle tone. Pupillary reactions may be sluggish or even absent.

The ECG may show prolonged PR, QRS, and QT intervals; bradycardia; and characteristic J point ele-vation (Osborn waves). Serum creatine phosphokinase (CPK) may be elevated in the absence of myocardial infarction, and high levels of serum amylase are common. Arterial blood gas values and pH must be corrected for temperature; otherwise, falsely high PO_2 and PCO_2 and false low pH values will be reported.

Treatment is aimed at the underlying disease and at restoration of normal body temperature. The optimal method and speed of rewarming are controversial, but passive rewarming with blankets in a warm room is an effective and simple treatment. Ventricular fibrillation may occur during rewarming. Since warming produces vasodilation and can lead to hypotension, intravenous fluids may be required.

Most patients who recover from hypothermia do so without neurological sequelae; except in myxedema, however, there is no direct correlation between recorded temperature and survival. Death, when it occurs, is caused by the underlying disease process responsible for hypothermia or by ventricular fibrillation, to which the human myocardium becomes especially susceptible at temperatures below 30°C (86°F); myocardial sensitivity is maximal below 21–24°C (70–75°F).

8. HYPERTHERMIA

At body temperatures over 42–43°C (107.6–109.4°F), the metabolic activity of the central nervous system is unable to provide for increased energy demands, and coma ensues. The cause of hyperthermia in most cases is exposure to elevated environmental temperatures—what is commonly known as heat stroke. Additional causes include status epilepticus, idiosyncratic reactions to halogenated inhalational anesthetics (malignant hyperthermia), anticholinergic drugs, hypothalamic damage, and delirium tremens. Patients surviving pontine hemorrhage for more than a few hours have centrally mediated temperature elevations ranging from 38.5 to 42.8°C (101.3–109°F). The neurological examination in hyperthermia reveals reactive pupils and a diffuse increase in muscle tone as well as coma.

Treatment is immediate reduction of body temperature to 39°C (102.2°F) by sponging the patient with ice water and alcohol and using an electric fan or cooling blanket. Care must be taken to prevent overhydration, since cooling results in vasoconstriction that may produce pulmonary edema in volume-expanded patients.

9. MENINGITIS & ENCEPHALITIS

Meningitis and encephalitis may be manifested by an acute confusional state or coma, which is characteristically associated with fever and headache. In meningitis, signs of meningeal irritation are also typically present and should be sought meticulously so that lumbar puncture and diagnosis are not delayed. These signs include resistance of the neck to full forward flexion, knee flexion during passive neck flexion, and flexion of the neck or contralateral knee during passive elevation of the extended straight leg. Meningeal signs may be absent in encephalitis without meningeal involvement and in meningitis occurring at the extremes of age—or in patients who are deeply comatose or immunosuppressed. The findings on examination are usually symmetric, but focal features may be seen in certain infections, such as herpes simplex encephalitis or bacterial meningitis complicated by vasculitis. CSF findings and treatment are considered in Chapter 1.

10. SUBARACHNOID HEMORRHAGE

In subarachnoid hemorrhage, discussed in detail in Chapter 3, symptoms are sudden in onset and almost always include headache that is typically, but not invariably, severe. Consciousness is frequently lost, either transiently or permanently, at onset. Decerebrate posturing or, rarely, seizures may occur at this time. Because bleeding is confined mainly to the subarachnoid space on the surface of the brain, prominent focal neurological signs other than oculomotor (III) nerve palsies are uncommon, although bilateral extensor plantar responses occur frequently. Examination of the optic fundi may show acute hemorrhages secondary to suddenly increased intracranial pressure or the more classic superficial subhyaloid hemorrhages. In coma-producing subarachnoid hemorrhage, the CSF is bloody and the CT brain scan shows blood in the subarachnoid space.

SEIZURE OR PROLONGED POSTICTAL STATE

Status epilepticus should always be considered in the differential diagnosis of coma. Motor activity may be restricted to repetitive movements of part of a single limb or one side of the face. Although these signs of seizure activity can be subtle, they must not escape notice: status epilepticus requires urgent treatment (see Chapter 9).

Coma may also be due to a prolonged postictal state, which is also discussed in Chapter 9.

DIFFERENTIAL DIAGNOSIS

Coma can be confused with a variety of psychiatric and neurological disorders.

PSYCHOGENIC UNRESPONSIVENESS

Psychogenic unresponsiveness is a diagnosis of exclusion that should be made only on the basis of compelling evidence. It may be a manifestation of schizophrenia (catatonic type), somatoform disorders (conversion disorder or somatization disorder), or malingering. The general physical examination reveals no abnormalities; neurological examination generally reveals symmetrically decreased muscle tone, normal reflexes, and a normal (flexor) response to plantar stimulation. The pupils are 2–3 mm in diameter or occasionally larger and respond briskly to light. Lateral eye movements on oculocephalic (doll's-head) testing may or may not be present, since visual fixation can suppress this reflex. The slow conjugate roving eye movements of metabolic coma cannot be imitated, however, and, if present, are incompatible with a diagnosis of psychogenic unresponsiveness. Likewise, the slow, often asymmetric and incomplete eye closure commonly seen after the eyes of a comatose patient are passively opened cannot be voluntarily reproduced. The patient with psychogenic unresponsiveness usually exhibits some voluntary muscle tone in the eyelids during passive eye opening. A helpful diagnostic test is irrigation of the tympanic membrane with cold water. Brisk nystagmus is the characteristic response in conscious patients, whereas no nystagmus occurs in coma. The EEG in psychogenic unresponsiveness is that of a normal awake person.

PERSISTENT VEGETATIVE STATE

Some patients who are comatose because of cerebral hypoxia or ischemia—or structural brain lesions—regain wakefulness but not awareness. This condition is termed *persistent vegetative state*. Such patients exhibit spontaneous eye opening and sleep-wake cycles, which distinguish them from patients in coma, as well as intact brain stem and autonomic function. However, they neither comprehend nor produce language, and they make no purposeful motor responses. This condition may persist for years.

LOCKED-IN SYNDROME

Because the portion of the reticular formation responsible for consciousness lies above the level of the midpons, functional transection of the brain stem below this level—by pontine infarct, or hemorrhage, central pontine myelinolysis, tumor, or encephalitis—can interrupt descending neural pathways to produce an akinetic and mute state, with preserved consciousness. Such patients appear comatose but are awake and alert although mute and quadriplegic. Decerebrate posturing or flexor spasms may be seen. The diagnosis is made by noting that voluntary eye opening, vertical eye movements, ocular convergence, or some combination of these movements is preserved. During the examination of any apparently comatose patient, the patient should be told to "open your eyes," "look up," "look down," and "look at the tip of your nose" to elicit such movements. The EEG is normal. Outcome is variable and related to the underlying cause. Mortality is approximately 70% when the cause is a vascular disturbance and about 40% in nonvascular cases, usually from pneumonia. Survivors may recover partially or completely over a period of weeks to months.

BRAIN DEATH

Current standards for the determination of brain death, developed by the President's Commission for the Study of Ethical Problems in Medicine and Biomedical and Behavioral Research (1981), are summarized below. Irreversible cessation of all brain function is required for a diagnosis of brain death. In addition, the diagnosis of brain death in children under five years of age must be made with caution.

Cessation of Brain Function
A. Unresponsiveness: The patient must be unresponsive to sensory input, including pain and speech.
B. Absent Brain Stem Reflexes: Pupillary, corneal, and oropharyngeal responses are absent, and attempts to elicit eye movements with the oculocephalic and vestibulo-ocular maneuvers are unsuccessful. Respiratory responses are also absent, with no ventilatory effort after the patient's PCO_2 is permitted to rise to 60 mm Hg, while oxygenation is maintained by giving 100% oxygen by a cannula inserted into the endotracheal tube (**apnea test**).

Irreversibility of Brain Dysfunction
The cause of coma must be known; it must be adequate to explain the clinical picture, and it must be irreversible.

Sedative drug intoxication, hypothermia (32.2 °C [90 °F]), neuromuscular blockade, and shock must be ruled out, since these conditions can produce a clinical picture that resembles brain death but in which neurological recovery may still be possible.

Persistence of Brain Dysfunction
The criteria for brain death described above must persist for an appropriate length of time, as follows:

1. Six hours with a confirmatory isoelectric (flat) EEG, performed according to the technical standards of the American Electroencephalographic Society.

2. Twelve hours without a confirmatory isoelectric EEG.

3. Twenty-four hours for anoxic brain injury without a confirmatory isoelectric EEG.

REFERENCES

General
Buettner UW, Zee DS: Vestibular testing in comatose patients. *Arch Neurol* 1989;46:561–563.
Fisher CM: The neurological examination of the comatose patient. *Acta Neurol Scand* 1969;45(Suppl 36):1–56.
Plum F, Posner JB: *The Diagnosis of Stupor and Coma,* 3rd ed. Vol 19 of: *Contemporary Neurology Series.* Davis, 1980.

Structural Lesions
Chun CH et al: Brain abscess: A study of 45 consecutive cases. *Medicine* 1986;65:415–431.
Dunne JW, Chakera T, Kermode S: Cerebellar hemorrhage— Diagnosis and treatment: A study of 75 consecutive cases. *Quart J Med* 1987; *New Series* 64:739–754.
Ferbert A, Bruckmann H, Drummen R: Clinical features of proven basilar artery occlusion. *Stroke* 1990;21:1135–1142.
Kase CS et al: Lobar intracerebral hematomas: Clinical and CT analysis of 22 cases. *Neurology* 1982;32:1146–1150.
Kushner MJ, Bressman SB: The clinical manifestations of pontine hemorrhage. *Neurology 1985;35:637–643.*

Macdonnell RAL, Kalnins RM, Donnan GA: Cerebellar infarction: Natural history, prognosis, and pathology. *Stroke* 1987;18:849–855.
Poungvarin N et al: Effects of dexamethasone in primary supratentorial intracerebral hemorrhage. *N Engl J Med* 1987;316:1229–1233.
Seelig JM et al: Traumatic acute subdural hematoma: Major mortality reduction in comatose patients treated within four hours. *N Engl J Med* 1981;304:1511–1518.
Wintzen AR: The clinical course of subdural hematoma: A retrospective study of etiological, chronological and pathological features in 212 patients and a proposed classification. *Brain* 1980;103:855–867.

Diffuse Encephalopathies
Caronna JJ: Diagnosis, prognosis, and treatment of hypoxic coma. *Adv Neurol* 1979;26:1–15.
Fischbeck KH, Simon RP: Neurological manifestations of accidental hypothermia. *Ann Neurol* 1981;10:384–387.
Helliwell M et al: Value of emergency toxicological investigations in differential diagnosis of coma. *Br Med J* 1979;2:819–821.

Levy DE et al: Predicting outcome from hypoxic-ischemic coma. *JAMA* 1985;253:1420–1426.

Malouf R, Brust JC: Hypoglycemia: Causes, neurological manifestations, and outcome. *Ann Neurol* 1985; 17:421–430.

Persistent Vegetative State

Executive Board, American Academy of Neurology: Position of the American Academy of Neurology on certain aspects of the care and management of the persistent vegetative state patient. *Neurology* 1989; 39:125–126.

Higashi K et al: Five-year follow-up study of patients with persistent vegetative state. *J Neurol Neurosurg Psychiatry* 1981;44:552–554.

Locked-In Syndrome

McCusker EA et al: Recovery from the "locked-in" syndrome. *Arch Neurol* 1982;39:145–147.

Patterson JR, Grabois M: Locked-in syndrome: A review of 139 cases. *Stroke* 1986;17:758–764.

Brain Death

Lynn J: Guidelines for the determination of death: Report of the Medical Consultants on the Diagnosis of Death to the President's Commission for the Study of Ethical Problems in Medicine and Biomedical and Behavioral Research. *Neurology* 1982;32:395–399.

Neurological Investigations

12

LUMBAR PUNCTURE

Indications

Lumbar puncture is indicated for the following purposes:

1. Diagnosis of meningitis and other infective or inflammatory disorders, subarachnoid hemorrhage, and hepatic encephalopathy.

2. Assessment of the response to therapy in meningitis and other infective or inflammatory disorders.

3. Administration of intrathecal medications or radiological contrast media.

4. Rarely, to reduce CSF pressure.

Contraindications

1. Suspected intracranial mass lesion. In this situation, performing a lumbar puncture can hasten incipient transtentorial herniation.

2. Local infection overlying the site of puncture. Under this circumstance, cervical or cisternal puncture should be performed instead.

3. Coagulopathy. Clotting-factor deficiencies and thrombocytopenia should be corrected before lumbar puncture is undertaken, to reduce the risk of hemorrhage.

4. Suspected spinal cord mass lesion. Lumbar puncture in this case should be performed only in association with myelography, which is used to determine the presence and level of structural spinal pathology.

Preparation

A. Personnel: With a cooperative patient, lumbar puncture can generally be performed by one person. An assistant can be helpful in positioning the patient and handling CSF samples, of course, especially if the patient is uncooperative or frightened.

B. Equipment and Supplies: The following items, which are usually included in preassembled lumbar puncture trays, are required. All must be sterile.

1. Gloves.
2. Iodine-containing solution for sterilizing the skin.
3. Sponges.
4. Drapes.
5. Lidocaine (1%).
6. Syringe (5 mL).
7. Needles (22- and 25-gauge).
8. Spinal needles (20- or 22-gauge) with stylets.
9. Three-way stopcock.
10. Manometer.
11. Collection tubes.
12. Adhesive bandage.

C. Positioning: Lumbar puncture is usually performed with the patient in the lateral decubitus position (Figure 12–1), lying at the edge of the bed and facing away from the person performing the procedure. The patient's lumbar spine should be maximally flexed to open the intervertebral spaces. The spine should be parallel to the surface of the bed and the hips and shoulders aligned in the vertical plane.

Occasionally, it is desirable to perform lumbar puncture with the patient seated. In this case, the patient is seated on the side of the bed, bent over a pillow that rests on a bedside table, while the physician reaches over the bed from the opposite side to perform the procedure.

D. Site of Puncture: The usual practice is to enter the L3–4 or L4–5 interspace, since the spinal cord (conus medullaris) terminates at about the L1–2 level in adults. Thus, the procedure is performed without danger of puncturing the cord. The L3–4 interspace is located at the level of the posterior iliac crests.

Procedure

1. If a comparison between blood and CSF glucose levels is planned, venous blood is drawn for glucose determination. Ideally, blood and CSF glucose levels should be measured in samples obtained simultaneously after the patient has fasted for at least four hours.

2. The necessary equipment and supplies are placed within easy reach.

3. Sterile gloves are worn by the person performing the procedure.

4. A wide area surrounding the interspace to be entered is sterilized, using iodine-containing solution applied to sponges; the solution is then wiped off with clean sponges.

5. The area surrounding the sterile field is draped.

6. The skin overlying the puncture site is anesthetized using lidocaine, a 5-mL syringe, and a 25-gauge needle. A 22-gauge needle is then substituted to anesthetize the underlying tissues.

7. With the stylet in place, the spinal needle is inserted at the midpoint of the chosen interspace. The needle should be parallel to the surface of the bed and angled slightly cephalad, or toward the umbilicus. The bevel of the needle should face upward, toward the face of the person performing the procedure.

8. The needle is advanced slowly until a pop, from penetration of the ligamentum flavum, is felt. The stylet is withdrawn to determine whether the CSF space has been entered, which is indicated by flow of CSF through the needle. If no CSF appears, the stylet is replaced and the needle advanced a short distance; this is continued until CSF is obtained. If at some point the needle cannot be advanced, it is likely that bone has been encountered. The needle is withdrawn partway, maintained parallel to the surface of the bed, and advanced again at a slightly different angle.

9. When CSF is obtained, the stylet is reinserted. The patient is asked to straighten his or her legs, and the stopcock and manometer are attached to the needle. The stopcock is turned to allow CSF to enter the manometer to measure the opening pressure. The pressure should fluctuate with the phases of respiration.

10. The stopcock is turned to allow the CSF to be collected, and the appearance (clarity and color) of the fluid is noted. The amount obtained and the number of tubes required varies, depending on the tests to be performed. Typically, 1–2 mL are collected in each of five tubes for cell count, glucose and protein, VDRL, Gram's stain, and cultures. Additional specimens may be collected for other tests, such as oligoclonal bands and glutamine, and for cytologic study. If the CSF appears to contain blood, additional fluid should be obtained so that the cell count can be repeated on the specimen in the last tube collected. Cytological studies, if desired, require at least 10 mL of CSF.

11. The stopcock and manometer are replaced to record a closing pressure.

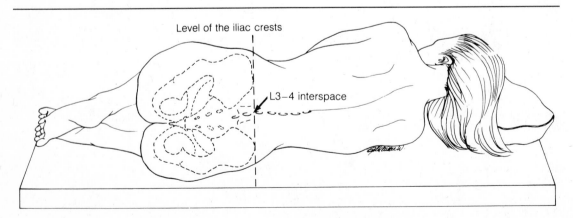

Figure 12–1. Lateral decubitus position for lumbar puncture.

12. The needle is withdrawn and an adhesive bandage applied over the puncture site.

13. It is customary to have the patient lie prone or supine for one or two hours after the procedure to reduce the risk of post-lumbar-puncture headache, but whether this practice is effective is uncertain.

Complications

A. Unsuccessful Tap: A variety of conditions, including marked obesity, degenerative disease of the spine, previous spinal surgery, recent lumbar puncture, and dehydration, can make it difficult to perform lumbar puncture in the conventional manner. When puncture in the lateral decubitus position is impossible, the procedure should be attempted with the patient in a sitting position. If the tap is again unsuccessful, alternative methods include lumbar puncture by an oblique approach or guided by fluoroscopy; lateral cervical puncture; or cisternal puncture. These procedures should be undertaken by a neurologist, neurosurgeon, or neuroradiologist experienced in performing them.

B. Arterial or Venous Puncture: If the needle enters a blood vessel rather than the spinal subarachnoid space, it should be withdrawn and a new needle used to attempt the tap at a different level. Patients who have coagulopathy or are receiving aspirin or anticoagulants should be observed with particular care for signs of spinal cord compression (see Chapter 6) from spinal subdural or epidural hematoma.

C. Post-Lumbar-Puncture Headache: A mild headache, worse in the upright position but relieved by recumbency, is not uncommon following lumbar puncture and will resolve spontaneously over a period of hours to days. It is unclear whether vigorous hydration or keeping the patient in bed for one to two hours after the procedure reduces the likelihood of such headache. The headache usually responds to non-steroidal anti-inflammatory drugs or caffeine (see Chapter 3). Severe and protracted headache can be treated by an autologous blood clot patch, which should be applied by experienced personnel.

Analysis of Results

A. Appearance: The clarity and color of the CSF should be observed as it leaves the spinal needle, and any changes in the appearance of fluid during the course of the procedure should be noted. CSF is normally clear and colorless. It may appear cloudy or turbid with white blood cell counts that exceed about 200/μL, but counts as low as about 50/μL can be detected by holding the tube up to direct sunlight and observing the light-scattering (Tyndall) effect of suspended cells. Color can be imparted to the CSF by hemoglobin (pink), bilirubin (yellow), or, rarely, melanin (black).

B. Pressure: With the patient in the lateral decubitus position, CSF pressure in the lumbar region does not normally exceed 180–200 mm water. When lumbar puncture is performed with patients in the sitting position, they should assume a lateral decubitus posture before CSF pressure is measured. Increased CSF pressure may result from obesity, agitation, or increased intra-abdominal pressure related to position; the latter factor may be eliminated by having the patient extend his or her legs and back once the CSF space has been entered and before the opening pressure is recorded. Pathological conditions associated with increased CSF pressure include intracranial mass lesions, meningoencephalitis, subarachnoid hemorrhage, and pseudotumor cerebri.

C. Microscopic Examination: This may be performed either by the person who performed the lumbar puncture or by a technician at the clinical laboratory; it always includes a cell count and differential. Gram's stain for bacteria, acid-fast stain for mycobacteria, an India ink preparation for *Cryptococcus,* and cytological examination for tumor cells may also be indicated. The CSF normally contains up to five mononuclear leukocytes (lymphocytes or monocytes) per microliter, no polymorphonuclear cells, and no erythrocytes. Erythrocytes may be present, however, if the lumbar puncture is traumatic (see below). Normal CSF is sterile, so that in the absence of CNS infection, no organisms should be observed with the various stains listed above.

D. Bloody CSF: If the lumbar puncture yields bloody CSF, it is crucial to distinguish between CNS hemorrhage and a traumatic tap. The fluid should be watched as it leaves the spinal needle to determine whether the blood clears, which suggests a traumatic tap. This can be established with greater accuracy by comparing cell counts in the first and last tubes of CSF obtained; a marked decrease in the number of red cells supports a traumatic cause. The specimen should be promptly centrifuged and the supernatant examined. With a traumatic lumbar puncture, the supernatant is colorless. In contrast, following CNS hemorrhage, enzymatic degradation of hemoglobin to bilirubin in situ renders the supernatant yellow (xanthochromic). The time course of changes in CSF color following subarachnoid hemorrhage is outlined in Table 12–1.

Blood in the CSF following a traumatic lumbar puncture usually clears within 24 hours; blood is usually present after subarachnoid hemorrhage for at least six days. In addition, blood related to traumatic puncture does not clot, while clotting may occur with subarachnoid hemorrhage. Crenation (shriveling) of red blood cells, however, is of no diagnostic value.

Table 12–1. Pigmentation of the cerebrospinal fluid following subarachnoid hemorrhage.

	Appearance	Maximum	Disappearance
Oxyhemoglobin (pink)	0.5–4 hours	24–35 hours	7–10 days
Bilirubin (yellow)	8–12 hours	2–4 days	2–3 weeks

In addition to breakdown of hemoglobin from red blood cells, other causes of CSF xanthochromia include jaundice with serum bilirubin levels above 4–6 mg/dL, CSF protein concentrations greater than 150 mg/dL, and, rarely, the presence of carotene pigments.

White blood cells seen in the CSF early after subarachnoid hemorrhage or with traumatic lumbar puncture result from leakage of circulating whole blood. If the hematocrit and peripheral white blood cell count are within normal limits, there is approximately one white blood cell for each 1000 red cells. If the peripheral white cell count is elevated, a proportionate increase in this ratio should be expected. In addition, every 1000 red cells present in CSF will increase the CSF protein concentration by about 1 mg/dL.

Procedure Notes

Whenever a lumbar puncture is performed, notes describing the procedure should be recorded in the patient's chart. These notes should provide the following information:

1. Date and time performed.
2. Name of person or persons performing the procedure.
3. Indication.
4. Position of patient.
5. Anesthetic used.
6. Interspace entered.
7. Opening pressure.
8. Appearance of CSF, including changes in appearance during the course of the procedure.
9. Amount of fluid removed.
10. Closing pressure.
11. Tests ordered, eg:
    Tube #1 (1 mL), cell count.
    Tube #2 (1 mL), glucose and protein.
    Tube #3 (1 mL), microbiological stains.
    Tube #4 (1 mL), bacterial, fungal, and mycobacterial cultures.
12. Results of any studies, such as microbiological stains, performed by the operator.
13. Complications, if any.

ELECTROPHYSIOLOGICAL STUDIES

ELECTROENCEPHALOGRAPHY

The electrical activity of the brain can be recorded noninvasively from electrodes placed on the scalp. Electroencephalography (EEG) is easy to perform, is relatively inexpensive, and is helpful in several different clinical contexts.

Evaluation of Suspected Epilepsy

EEG is useful in evaluating patients with suspected epilepsy. The presence of electrographic seizure activity (abnormal, rhythmic electrocerebral activity of abrupt onset and termination) during a behavioral disturbance that could represent a seizure, but about which there is clinical uncertainty, establishes the diagnosis beyond doubt. As seizures occur unpredictably, however, it is not often possible to obtain an EEG during them. Despite that, the EEG findings may be abnormal interictally (at times when the patient is not experiencing clinical attacks) and are therefore still useful for diagnostic purposes. The interictal presence of epileptiform activity (abnormal paroxysmal activity containing some spike discharges) is of particular help in this regard. Such activity is occasionally encountered in patients who have never had a seizure, but its prevalence is greater in epileptics than in normal subjects. Epileptiform activity in the EEG of a patient with an episodic behavioral disturbance that could on clinical grounds be a manifestation of seizures markedly increases the likelihood that the attacks are indeed epileptic, thus providing support for the clinical diagnosis.

Classification of Seizure Disorders

In known epileptics, the EEG findings may help in classifying the seizure disorder and thus in selecting appropriate anticonvulsant medication. For example, in patients with the typical absences of petit mal epilepsy (see Chapter 9) the EEG is characterized both ictally and interictally by episodic generalized spike-and-wave activity (Figure 9–3). In contrast, in patients with episodes of impaired external awareness caused by complex partial seizures, the EEG may be normal or show focal epileptiform discharges interictally. During the seizures there may be abnormal rhythmic activity of variable frequency with a localized or generalized distribution, or, in some instances, there may be no electrographic correlates. The presence of a focal or lateralized epileptogenic source is of particular importance if surgical treatment is under consideration.

Assessment & Prognosis of Seizures

The EEG findings may provide a guide to prognosis and have been used to follow the course of seizure disorders. A normal EEG implies a more favorable prognosis for seizure control, while an abnormal background or profuse epileptiform activity implies a poor prognosis. The EEG findings do not, however, provide a reliable guide to the subsequent development of seizures in patients with head injuries, stroke, or brain tumors. Some physicians have used the electrophysiological findings to determine whether anticonvulsant medication can be discontinued in patients who have been seizure-free for several years. While patients are more likely to be weaned successfully if the EEG is normal, the findings provide only a general guide, and patients can certainly have further seizures, despite a normal EEG, after withdrawal of anticonvulsant medication. Conversely, they may have no further seizures despite a continuing EEG disturbance.

Management of Status Epilepticus

The EEG is of little help in managing tonic-clonic status epilepticus unless patients have received neuromuscular blocking agents and are in pentobarbital-induced coma. In this case, the electrophysiological findings are useful in indicating the level of anesthesia and determining whether the seizures are continuing. The status itself is characterized by repeated electrographic seizures or continuous epileptiform (spike-and-wave) activity. In patients with nonconvulsive status epilepticus, the EEG findings provide the only means of making the diagnosis with confidence and in distinguishing the two main types. In absence status epilepticus, continuous spike-and-wave activity is seen, while repetitive electrographic seizures are found in complex partial status.

Detection of Structural Brain Lesions

Electroencephalography has been used as a noninvasive means of detecting focal structural abnormalities, such as brain tumors. There may be a focal slow-wave disturbance, a localized loss of electrocerebral activity, or a more generalized EEG disturbance that probably relates in part to an altered level of arousal. Noninvasive imaging procedures such as CT and MRI have supplanted the use of EEG in this context.

Diagnosis of Neurological Disorders

Certain neurological disorders produce characteristic but nonspecific abnormalities in the EEG. Their presence is helpful in suggesting, establishing, or supporting the diagnosis. In patients presenting with an acute disturbance of cerebral function, for example, the presence of repetitive slow-wave complexes over one or both temporal lobes suggests a diagnosis of herpes simplex encephalitis. Similarly, the presence of periodic complexes in a patient with an acute dementing disorder suggests a diagnosis of Creutzfeldt-Jakob disease or subacute sclerosing panencephalitis.

Evaluation of Altered Consciousness

The EEG tends to become slower as consciousness is depressed, but the findings depend at least in part upon the etiology of the clinical disorder. The findings, such as the presence of electrographic seizure activity, can suggest diagnostic possibilities that might otherwise be overlooked. Serial records permit the prognosis and course of the disorder to be followed. The electroencephalographic response to external stimulation is an important diagnostic and prognostic guide: electrocerebral responsiveness implies a lighter level of coma. Electrocerebral silence in a technically adequate record implies neocortical death, in the absence of hypothermia or drug overdose. In some patients who appear to be comatose, consciousness is, in fact, preserved. Although there is quadriplegia and a supranuclear paralysis of the facial and bulbar muscles, the EEG is usually normal in such patients with locked-in syndrome (see Chapter 11) and helps in indicating the correct diagnosis.

EVOKED POTENTIALS

The spinal or cerebral potentials evoked by noninvasive stimulation of specific afferent pathways are an important means of monitoring the functional integrity of these pathways. They do not, however, indicate the nature of any lesion that may involve these pathways. The responses are very small compared with the background EEG activity (noise), which has no relationship to the time of stimulation. The responses to a number of stimuli are therefore recorded and averaged (with a computer) to eliminate the random noise.

Types of Evoked Potentials

A. Visual: Monocular visual stimulation with a checkerboard pattern is used to elicit visual evoked potentials, which are recorded from the midoccipital region of the scalp. The most clinically relevant component is the **P100 response,** a positive peak with a latency of approximately 100 msec. The presence and latency of the response are noted. While its amplitude can also be measured, alterations in amplitude are far less helpful in recognizing pathology.

B. Auditory: Monaural stimulation with repetitive clicks is used for eliciting brain stem auditory evoked potentials, which are recorded at the vertex of the scalp. A series of potentials are evoked in the first 10 msec after the auditory stimulus; these represent the sequential activation of various structures in the subcortical auditory pathway. For clinical purposes, attention is directed at the presence, latency, and interpeak intervals of the first five positive potentials recorded at the vertex.

C. Somatosensory: Electrical stimulation of a peripheral nerve is used to elicit the somatosensory evoked potentials, which are recorded over the scalp and spine. The configuration and latency of the responses depend on the nerve that is stimulated.

Indications for Use

Evoked potential studies are useful in several clinical contexts.

A. Detection of Lesions in Multiple Sclerosis: Evoked potentials have been used to detect and localize lesions in the central nervous system. This is particularly important in multiple sclerosis, where the diagnosis depends upon detecting lesions in several regions of the central nervous system. When patients present with clinical evidence of a lesion at only one site, electrophysiological recognition of abnormalities in other locations helps to establish the diagnosis. When patients with suspected multiple sclerosis present with ill-defined complaints, electrophysiological abnormalities in the appropriate afferent pathways are helpful in indicating the organic basis of the symptoms. While noninvasive imaging studies such as MRI are also useful for detecting lesions, they should be used to complement evoked potential studies rather than as a replacement. Evoked potential studies monitor the functional status rather than anatomical integrity of the afferent pathways and can sometimes reveal abnormalities that are not detected by MRI (and the reverse also holds true). Their cost is also considerably lower than MRI. In patients with established multiple sclerosis, the evoked potential findings are sometimes used to follow the course of the disorder or monitor the response to novel forms of treatment, but their value in this regard is unclear.

B. Detection of Lesions in Other Central Nervous System Disorders: Evoked potential abnormalities are encountered in disorders other than multiple sclerosis; multimodal evoked potential abnormalities may be encountered in certain spinocerebellar degenerations, familial spastic paraplegia, and vitamin E or B_{12} deficiency. The diagnostic value of electrophysiological abnormalities therefore depends upon the context in which they are found. While the findings may permit lesions to be localized within broad areas of the central nervous system, precise localization may not be possible because the generators of many of the recorded components are unknown.

C. Assessment and Prognosis Following Central Nervous System Trauma or Hypoxia: Evoked potentials studies can provide information of prognostic relevance. In posttraumatic or postanoxic coma, for example, the bilateral absence of cortically generated components of the somatosensory evoked potential implies that cognition will not be recovered; the prognosis is more optimistic when cortical responses are present on one or both sides. Such studies may be particularly useful in patients with suspected brain death. Somatosensory evoked potentials have also been used to determine the completeness of a traumatic cord lesion; the presence or early return of a response following stimulation of a nerve below the level of the cord injury indicates that the lesion is incomplete and thus suggests a better prognosis.

D. Intraoperative Monitoring: Evoked potentials are also used to monitor the functional integrity of certain neural structures during operative procedures, in an attempt to permit the early recognition of any dysfunction and thereby minimize damage. When the dysfunction relates to a surgical maneuver, it may be possible to prevent or diminish any prominent neurological deficit by reversing the maneuver.

E. Evaluation of Visual or Auditory Acuity: Visual and auditory acuity may be evaluated through evoked potential studies in patients who are unable to cooperate with behavioral testing because of age or abnormal mental state.

ELECTROMYOGRAPHY & NERVE CONDUCTION STUDIES

Electromyography

The electrical activity within a discrete region of an accessible muscle can be recorded by inserting a needle electrode into it. The pattern of electrical activity in muscle (**electromyogram**) both at rest and during activity has been characterized, and abnormalities have been correlated with disorders at different levels of the motor unit.

A. Activity at Rest: Relaxed muscle normally shows no spontaneous electrical activity except in the end-plate region where neuromuscular junctions are located, but various types of abnormal activity occur spontaneously in diseased muscle. **Fibrillation potentials** and **positive sharp waves** (which reflect muscle fiber irritability) are typically found in denervated muscle; they are not invariably present, however. They are sometimes also found in myopathic disorders, especially inflammatory disorders such as polymyositis. Although **fasciculation potentials**—which reflect the spontaneous activation of individual motor units—are occasionally encountered in normal muscle, they are characteristic of neuropathic disorders, especially those with primary involvement of anterior horn cells (eg, amyotrophic lateral sclerosis). Myotonic discharges (high-frequency discharges of potentials from muscle fibers that wax and wane in amplitude and frequency) are found most commonly in such disorders as myotonic dystrophy or myotonia congenita and occasionally in polymyositis or other, rarer disorders. Other types of abnormal spontaneous activity also occur.

B. Activity During Voluntary Muscle Contraction: A slight voluntary contraction of a muscle, activates a small number of motor units. The potentials generated by the muscle fibers of individual units within the detection range of the needle electrode can be recorded. Normal motor-unit potentials have clearly defined limits of duration, amplitude, configuration, and firing rates. These limits depend, in part, on the muscle under study, and the number of units activated for a specified degree of voluntary activity is known within broad limits. In many myopathic disorders, there is an increased incidence of small, short-duration, polyphasic motor units in affected muscles, and an excessive number of units may be activated for a specified degree of voluntary activity. There is a loss of motor units in neuropathic disorders, so that the number of units activated during a maximal contraction will be reduced, and units will fire at a faster rate than normal. In addition, the configuration and dimensions of the potentials may be abnormal, depending on the acuteness of the neuropathic process and on whether reinnervation is occurring. Variations in the configuration and size of individual motor-unit potentials are characteristic of disorders of neuromuscular transmission.

C. Clinical Utility: Lesions can involve the neural or muscle component of the motor unit, or the neuromuscular junction. When the neural component is affected, the pathological process can be either at the level of the anterior horn cells or at some point along the length of the axon as it traverses a nerve root, limb plexus, and peripheral nerve before branching into its terminal arborizations. Electromyography can detect disorders of the motor units and can indicate the site of the underlying lesion. The technique also permits neuromuscular disorders to be recognized when clinical examination is unrewarding because the disease is still at a mild stage—or because poor cooperation on the part of the patient or the presence of other symptoms such as pain makes clinical evaluation difficult. Note that the electromyographic findings do not, of themselves, permit an etiological diagnosis to be reached, and the electrophysiological findings must be correlated with the clinical findings and the results of other laboratory studies.

The electromyographic findings may provide a guide to prognosis. For example, in patients with an acute disorder of a peripheral or cranial nerve (eg, a pressure palsy of the radial nerve or a Bell's palsy) electromyographic evidence of denervation implies a poorer prognosis for recovery than when denervation has not occurred.

Nerve Conduction Studies

A. Motor Nerve Conduction Studies: These studies are performed by recording the electrical response of a muscle to stimulation of its motor nerve at two or more points along its course. This permits conduction velocity to be determined in the fastest-conducting motor fibers between the points of stimulation.

B. Sensory Nerve Conduction Studies: These are performed by analogous means, by determining the conduction velocity and amplitude of action potentials in sensory fibers when these fibers are stimulated at one point and their responses are recorded at another point along the course of the nerve.

C. Indications for Use: Nerve conduction studies provide a means of confirming the presence and extent of peripheral nerve damage. Such studies are particularly helpful when clinical examination is difficult (eg, in children). Nerve conduction studies are particularly helpful in the following contexts.

1. Determining whether sensory symptoms are caused by a lesion proximal or distal to the dorsal root ganglia (in the latter case, sensory conduction studies of the involved fibers will be abnormal) and whether neuromuscular dysfunction relates to peripheral nerve disease.
2. Detecting subclinical involvement of other peripheral nerves in patients who present with a mononeuropathy.
3. Determining the site of a focal lesion and providing a guide to prognosis in patients with a mononeuropathy.
4. Distinguishing between a polyneuropathy and a mononeuropathy multiplex. This distinction may not be possible clinically, but it is important because the causes of these conditions differ.
5. Clarifying the extent to which the disabilities experienced by patients with polyneuropathy relate to superimposed compressive focal neuropathies—which are common complications.
6. Following the progression of peripheral nerve disorders and their response to treatment.
7. Indicating the predominant pathological change in peripheral nerve disorders. In demyelinating neuropathies, conduction velocity is often markedly slowed and conduction block may occur; in axonal neuropathies conduction velocity is usually normal or slowed only mildly, sensory nerve action potentials are small or absent, and electromyography shows evidence of denervation in affected muscles.
8. Detecting hereditary disorders of the peripheral nerves at a subclinical stage in genetic and epidemiological studies.

F-RESPONSE STUDIES

When a stimulus is applied to a motor nerve, impulses travel **antidromically** (toward the spinal cord) as well as **orthodromically** (toward the nerve terminals) and lead to the discharge of a few anterior horn cells. This produces a small motor response that occurs considerably later than the direct muscle response elicited by nerve stimulation. The F wave so elicited is sometimes abnormal in patients with lesions of the proximal portions of the peripheral nervous system, such as the nerve roots. These studies may be helpful in detecting abnormalities when conventional nerve conduction studies are normal.

REPETITIVE NERVE STIMULATION

Description

The size of the electrical response of a muscle to supramaximal electrical stimulation of its motor nerve depends on a number of factors but correlates with the number of activated muscle fibers. Neuromuscular transmission can be tested by recording (with surface electrodes) the response of a muscle to supramaximal stimulation of its motor nerve either repetitively or by single or trains of shocks at selected intervals after a maximal voluntary contraction.

Normal Response

In normal subjects, there is little or no change in the size of the compound muscle action potential following repetitive stimulation of a motor nerve at 10 Hz or less, or with a single stimulus or a train of stimuli delivered at intervals after a voluntary muscle contraction of about ten seconds. This lack of change is the case even though preceding activity in the junctional region influences the amount of acetylcholine released and thus the size of the end-plate potentials elicited by the stimuli. Although the amount of acetylcholine released, is increased briefly after maximal voluntary activity and is then reduced, more acetylcholine is normally released than is required to bring the motor end-plate potentials to the threshold for generating muscle-fiber action potentials.

Response in Disorders of Neuromuscular Transmission

A. Myasthenia Gravis: In myasthenia gravis, depletion of postsynaptic acetylcholine receptors at the neuromuscular junction makes it impossible to compensate for the reduced release of acetylcholine that follows repetitive firing of the motor neuron. Accordingly, repetitive stimulation, particularly between 2 and 5 Hz, may lead to a depression of neuromuscular transmission, with a decrement in the size of the compound muscle action potential recorded from an affected muscle. Similarly, an electrical stimulus of the motor nerve immediately after a ten-second period of maximal voluntary activity may elicit a muscle response that is slightly larger than before, indicating that more muscle fibers are responding. This postactivation facilitation of neuromuscular transmission is followed by a longer-lasting period of depression that is maximal from two to four minutes after the conditioning period and lasts up to ten minutes or so. During this period, the compound muscle action potential is reduced in size.

Decrementing responses to repetitive stimulation at 2–5 Hz can also occur in congenital myasthenic syndromes.

B. Myasthenic Syndrome and Botulism: In Lambert-Eaton myasthenic syndrome, in which there is a defective release of acetylcholine at the neuromuscular junction, the compound muscle action potential elicited by a single stimulus is generally very small. With repetitive stimulation at rates of up to 10 Hz, the first few responses may decline in size, but subsequent responses increase and their amplitude is eventually several times larger than the initial response. Patients with botulism exhibit a similar response to repetitive stimulation, but the findings are somewhat more variable and not all muscles are affected. Incremental responses in Lambert-Eaton syndrome and botulism are more conspicuous with high rates of stimulation and may result from the facilitation of acetylcholine release by the progressive accumulation of calcium in the motor nerve terminal.

CRANIAL IMAGING STUDIES

PLAIN X-RAYS

Abnormalities of bone may be visualized by plain x-rays of the skull. Such abnormalities include metastatic deposits, fractures, and the changes associated with Paget's disease or fibrous dysplasia. In addition, plain films can show areas of abnormal intracranial calcification, alterations in size of the sella turcica, and inflammatory disease of the paranasal sinuses. The advent of CT scanning (which permits visualization of cerebral tissue as well as bone) has led to a decline in the use of plain films.

COMPUTED TOMOGRAPHY

Description

Computed tomographic (CT) scanning is a noninvasive computer-assisted radiological means of examining anatomical structures. It permits the detection of structural intracranial abnormalities with precision, speed, and facility. It is thus of particular use in evaluating patients with progressive neurological disorders or focal neurological deficits in whom a structural lesion is suspected as well as patients with dementia or increased intracranial pressure. Intravenous administration of an iodinated contrast agent improves the ability of CT to detect and define lesions, such as tumors and abscesses, associated with a disturbance of the blood-brain barrier. Because the contrast agents may have an adverse effect on the kidneys, they should be used with discrimination. Contrast-enhanced scans may provide more information than that obtained by unenhanced scans in patients with known or suspected primary or secondary brain tumors, arteriovenous malformations, multiple sclerosis, chronic bilateral isodense subdural hematomas, or hydrocephalus.

Indications for Use

A. Stroke: CT is particularly helpful in evaluating strokes because it can distinguish infarction from intracranial hemorrhage; it is particularly sensitive in detecting intracerebral hematomas, and the location of such lesions may provide a guide to their cause.

B. Tumor: CT scans can indicate the site of a brain tumor, the extent of any surrounding edema, whether the lesion is cystic or solid, and whether it has displaced midline or other normal anatomical structures.

C. Trauma: The CT scan is an important means of evaluating patients following head injury—in particular for detecting traumatic subarachnoid or intracerebral hemorrhage and bony injuries.

D. Dementia: In patients with dementia, CT scan may indicate the presence of a tumor or of hydrocephalus (enlarged ventricles), with or without accompanying cerebral atrophy. The occurrence of hydrocephalus without cerebral atrophy in demented patients suggests normal pressure or communicating hydrocephalus. Cerebral atrophy can occur in demented or normal elderly subjects.

E. Subarachnoid Hemorrhage: In patients with subarachnoid hemorrhage, the CT scan generally indicates the presence of blood in the subarachnoid space and may even suggest the source of the bleeding. If the CT findings are normal despite clinical findings suggestive of subarachnoid hemorrhage, the cerebrospinal fluid should be examined to exclude hemorrhage or meningitis.

MAGNETIC RESONANCE IMAGING

Description

Magnetic resonance imaging (MRI) is an imaging procedure that involves no radiation. The patient lies within a large magnet that aligns some of the protons in the body along the magnet's axis. The protons resonate when stimulated with radio-frequency energy, producing a tiny echo that is strong enough to be detected. The position and intensity of these radio-frequency emissions are recorded and mapped by a computer. The signal intensity depends upon the concentration of mobile hydrogen nuclei (or nuclear-spin density) of the tissues. Spin-lattice (T1) and spin-spin (T2) relaxation times are mainly responsible for the relative differences in signal intensity of the various soft tissues; these parameters are sensitive to the state of water in biological tissues. Pulse sequences with varying dependence on T1 and T2 selectively alter the contrast between soft tissues.

The soft-tissue contrast available with MRI makes it more sensitive than CT scanning in detecting certain structural lesions. MRI provides better contrast than does CT between the grey and white matter of the brain; it is superior for visualizing abnormalities in the posterior fossa and spinal cord and for detecting lesions associated with multiple sclerosis or those that cause seizures. In addition to its greater sensitivity, it is also free of bony artifact and permits multiplane (axial, sagittal, and coronal) imaging with no need to manipulate the position of the patient. Because there are no known hazardous effects, MRI studies can be repeated in a serial manner if necessary.

Gadopentetate dimeglumine is stable, well-tolerated intravenously, and an effective enhancing MRI agent that is useful in identifying small tumors that, because of their similar relaxation times to normal cerebral tissue, may be missed on unenhanced MRI. It also helps to separate tumor from surrounding edema, identify leptomeningeal disease, and provide information about the blood-brain barrier.

Indications for Use & Comparison with CT

A. Stroke: Within a few hours of vascular occlusion, it may be possible to detect and localize cerebral infarcts by MRI; contrast-enhanced CT scans, on the other hand, may be unrevealing for up to 48 hours. After that period, there is little advantage to MRI over CT scanning except for the former's superior imaging ability in the posterior fossa. Nevertheless, CT scanning without contrast is usually the preferred initial study in patients with acute stroke, in order to determine whether hemorrhage has occurred. Intracranial hemorrhage is not easily detected by MRI within the first 48 hours, and CT scan is more reliable for this purpose. Hematomas of more than ten days' duration, however, are better visualized by MRI. While MRI is very effective in detecting and localizing vascular malformations, angiography is still necessary to define their anatomical features and plan effective treatment. In cases of unexplained hematoma, a follow-up MRI obtained three months later may reveal the underlying cause, which is sometimes unmasked as the hematoma resolves.

B. Tumor: Both CT scans and MRI are very useful in detecting brain tumors, but the absence of bone artifacts makes MRI superior for visualizing tumors at the vertex or in the posterior fossa and for detecting acoustic neuromas. Secondary effects of tumors, such as cerebral herniation, can be seen with either MRI or CT scan, but MRI provides more anatomical information. Neither technique, however, permits the nature of the underlying tumor to be determined with any certainty. Pituitary tumors are often visualized more easily by MRI than CT because of the absence of bone or dental metal artifacts.

C. Trauma: Following head injury, CT scan is preferable to MRI because it requires less time, is superior for detecting intracranial hemorrhage, and may reveal bony injuries. Similarly, spinal MRI should not be used in the initial evaluation of patients with spinal injuries because nondisplaced fractures are often not visualized.

D. Dementia: In patients with dementia, while either CT or MRI can help in demonstrating treatable structural causes, MRI appears to be more sensitive.

E. Multiple Sclerosis: In patients with multiple sclerosis, it is often possible to detect lesions in the cerebral white matter or the cervical cord by MRI, even though such lesions may not be visualized on CT scans. The demyelinating lesions detected by MRI may have signal characteristics resembling those of ischemic changes, however, and clinical correlation is therefore always necessary. Gadolinium-enhanced MRI permits lesions of different ages to be distinguished. This ability facilitates the diagnosis of multiple sclerosis: the presence of lesions of different ages suggests a multiphasic disease, whereas lesions of similar age suggest a monophasic disorder, such as acute disseminated encephalomyelitis.

F. Infections: MRI is very sensitive in detecting white-matter edema and probably permits earlier recognition of focal areas of cerebritis and abscess formation than is possible with CT.

Contraindications

Contraindications to MRI include the presence of intracranial clips, metallic foreign bodies in the eye or elsewhere, pacemakers, cochlear implants, and conditions requiring close monitoring of patients. Furthermore, it can be difficult to image patients with claustrophobia, gross obesity, uncontrolled movement disorders, or respiratory disorders that require assisted ventilation or carry any risk of apnea.

POSITRON EMISSION TOMOGRAPHY

Positron emission tomography (PET) is an imaging technique that uses positron-emitting radiopharmaceuticals, such as ^{18}F-fluoro-2-deoxy-D-glucose or ^{18}F-L-dopa, to map brain biochemistry and physiology. PET thus complements other imaging methods that provide primarily anatomical information, such as CT and MRI, and may demonstrate functional brain abnormalities before structural abnormalities are detectable. Although its availability is currently limited, PET has proved useful in several clinical settings. When patients with medically refractory epilepsy are being considered for surgical treatment, PET can help identify focal areas of hypometabolism in the temporal lobe as likely sites of the origin of seizures. PET can also be useful in the differential diagnosis of dementia, since common dementing disorders such as Alzheimer's disease and multi-infarct dementia exhibit different patterns of abnormal cerebral metabolism. PET can help distinguish between clinically similar movement disorders, such as Parkinson's disease and progressive supranuclear palsy, and can provide confirmatory evidence of early Huntington's disease. PET may also be of value in grading gliomas, selecting tumor biopsy sites, and distinguishing recurrent tumors from radiation-induced brain necrosis.

ARTERIOGRAPHY

Description

The intracranial circulation is visualized most satisfactorily by arteriography, a technique in which the major vessels to the head are opacified and radiographed. A catheter is introduced into the femoral or brachial artery and passed into one of the major cervical vessels. A radiopaque contrast material is then injected through the catheter, allowing the vessel (or its origin) to be visualized. The technique, generally performed after noninvasive imaging by CT scanning or MRI, has a definite morbidity and mortality associated with it. It is contraindicated in patients with a stroke in evolution (progressing stroke) and in patients who are allergic to the contrast medium.

Indications for Use

The major indications for arteriography include the following:

1. Diagnosis of **intracranial aneurysms, arteriovenous malformations,** or **fistulas.** Although these lesions can be visualized by CT scan or MRI, their detailed anatomy and the vessels that feed, drain, or are otherwise implicated in them cannot reliably be defined by these other means.
2. Detection and definition of the underlying lesion in patients with **subarachnoid hemorrhage** who are considered good operative candidates (see Table 3–2).
3. Location of vascular lesions in patients with **transient cerebral ischemic attacks** if surgical treatment is being considered.
4. Diagnosis of **cerebral venous sinus thrombosis.**
5. Evaluation of **space-occupying intracranial lesions,** particularly when CT scanning or MRI is unavailable. There may be displacement of the normal vasculature, and in some tumors neovasculature may produce a blush or stain on the angiogram. Meningiomas can be recognized by their blood supply from the external carotid circulation.

DIGITAL SUBTRACTION ANGIOGRAPHY

Digital-subtraction angiography permits images to be obtained with a decreased volume of contrast material. In this technique, angiography is accompanied by computerized subtraction of nonvascular structures. Intravenous (as opposed to intra-arterial) contrast infusions may therefore be adequate to assess the anatomy of such arterial structures as the carotid bifurcation.

MAGNETIC RESONANCE ANGIOGRAPHY

Several imaging techniques that have been used to visualize blood vessels by MRI depend upon certain physical properties of blood to generate contrast. These properties include the rate at which blood is supplied to the imaged area, its velocity and relaxation time, and the absence of turbulent flow. MR angiography has been most useful in visualizing the carotid arteries and proximal portions of the intracranial circulation, where flow is relatively fast. The images are used to screen for stenosis or occlusion of vessels and for large atheromatous lesions. Further research is needed, however, to explore the usefulness of the technique, improve its sensitivity, and define its limitations.

SPINAL IMAGING STUDIES

PLAIN X-RAYS

Plain x-rays of the spine can reveal congenital, traumatic, degenerative or neoplastic bony abnormalities, or narrowing (stenosis) of the spinal canal. Degenerative changes become increasingly common with advancing age, and their clinical relevance depends on the context in which they are found. In patients presenting with neck or low back pain, a plain film is usually the first radiological investigation undertaken.

MYELOGRAPHY

Injecting radiopaque contrast medium into the subarachnoid space permits visualization of part or all of the spinal subarachnoid system. The cord and nerve roots, which are silhouetted by the contrast material in the subarachnoid space, are visualized indirectly. The procedure is invasive and generally requires hospitalization. Until recently, pantopaque was the most commonly used contrast material. Although this is an iodinated compound, patients with allergies to intravenously administered iodinated contrast agents generally tolerate its subarachnoid administration without any problem. Reported complications of myelography with pantopaque include headache, low back pain, confusion, arachnoiditis, inadvertent intravenous injection of contrast material, and vasovagal reactions. Rarely, traumatic herniated intervertebral disks have occurred because of poor technique, as has damage to nerve roots.

Metrizamide, a water-soluble agent, has now become the preferred contrast medium. It is absorbed from the CSF and excreted by the kidneys, with approximately 75% eliminated over the first 24 hours. Unlike pantopaque, it does not produce significant arachnoiditis, but tonic-clonic seizures have been reported in some instances when metrizamide entered the intracranial cavity. Other complications include headaches and nausea and vomiting. Metrizamide myelography may be followed by a CT scan of the spine while the medium is still in place. This shows the soft tissue structures in or about the spinal cord

and provides complementary information to that obtained by the myelogram (see below).

Myelography is indicated in the investigation of patients with suspected spinal cord or nerve root compression or structural anomalies in the foramen magnum region. It is helpful in detecting both extradural and intradural lesions and for providing evidence of an intramedullary abnormality.

COMPUTED TOMOGRAPHY

CT scanning after metrizamide myelography may be helpful when the myelogram either fails to reveal any abnormality or provides poor visualization of the area of interest. The myelogram may be normal, for example, when there is a laterally placed disk protrusion; in such circumstances, a contrast-enhanced CT scan may reveal the lesion. It is also useful in visualizing more fully the area above or below an almost complete block in the subarachnoid space and in providing further information in patients with cord tumors.

MAGNETIC RESONANCE IMAGING

In many instances, the information obtained by myelography can now be obtained more simply by MRI of the spine. Imaging of the spinal canal by MRI is direct and noninvasive, and it permits differentiation of solid from cystic intramedullary lesions. MRI is therefore being used increasingly in place of myelography. In syringomyelia, for example, MRI is the preferred imaging method for visualizing cord cavitation and detecting any associated abnormalities at the craniocervical junction. Congenital abnormalities associated with spinal dysraphism are also easily visualized by MRI. In patients with degenerative disk disease, MRI is probably more accurate than myelography for detecting cord or root compression. When a spinal AVM is suspected, however, the myelogram is the more sensitive screening technique.

ULTRASONOGRAPHY

B-MODE ULTRASONOGRAPHY

In this technique, echoes reflected from anatomical structures are plotted on an oscilloscope screen in two dimensions. The resulting brightness at each point reflects the density of the imaged structure. The technique has been used to image the carotid artery and its bifurcation in the neck, permitting evaluation of the extent of extracranial vascular disease. Blood flowing within an artery does not reflect sound, and the lumen of the vessels therefore appears black. The arterial wall can be seen, however, and atherosclerotic lesions can be detected. Note that with severe stenosis or complete occlusion of the internal carotid artery, it may not be possible to visualize the carotid artery bifurcation.

DOPPLER ULTRASONOGRAPHY

Ultrasound can be used to measure the velocity of blood flow through an artery. Sound waves within a certain frequency range are reflected off red blood cells, and the frequency of the echo provides a guide to the velocity of the flow. Any shift in frequency is proportional to the velocity of the red cells and the angle of the beam of sound waves. When the arterial lumen is narrowed, the velocity of flow increases; increased frequencies are therefore recorded by doppler ultrasonography. Spectral analysis of doppler frequencies is also used to evaluate the anatomical status of the carotid artery.

BIOPSIES

BRAIN BIOPSY

Biopsy of brain tissue can be useful in certain cases when less invasive methods, such as imaging studies, fail to provide a diagnosis. Brain lesions most amenable to biopsy are those that can be localized by imaging studies; are situated in superficial, surgically accessible sites; and do not involve critical brain regions, such as the brain stem or the areas of cerebral cortex involved in language or motor function. Cerebral disorders that can be diagnosed by biopsy include primary and metastatic brain tumors, infectious disorders such as herpes simplex encephalitis or brain abscess, and certain degenerative diseases such as Creutzfeldt-Jakob disease.

MUSCLE BIOPSY

Histopathological examination of a biopsy specimen of a weak muscle can indicate whether the underlying weakness is neurogenic or myopathic in origin. In neurogenic disorders, atrophied fibers occur in groups, with adjacent groups of larger uninvolved fibers. In myopathies, atrophy occurs in a random pattern; the nuclei of muscle cells may be centrally situated, rather than in their normal peripheral location; and fibrosis or fatty infiltration may also be found. Examination of a muscle biopsy specimen may also permit certain inflammatory diseases of muscle, such as polymyositis, to be recognized and treated.

In some patients with a suspected myopathy, although the electromyographic findings are normal, examination of a muscle biopsy specimen reveals the nature of the underlying disorder. Conversely, electromyographic abnormalities suggestive of a myopathy are sometimes found in patients in whom the histological or histochemical studies fail to establish a diagnosis of myopathy. The two approaches are therefore complementary.

NERVE BIOPSY

It is not necessary to undertake nerve biopsy to establish a diagnosis of peripheral neuropathy. The nature of any neuropathological abnormalities can be important, however, in suggesting the underlying disorder of peripheral nerves. In particular, evidence may be found of metabolic storage disease (eg, Fabry's disease, Tangier disease), infection (eg, leprosy), inflammatory change, vasculitis, or neoplastic involvement. The findings are not always of diagnostic relevance, however, and nerve biopsy itself can be performed only on accessible nerves. It is rarely undertaken on more than a single occasion.

ARTERY BIOPSY

In patients with suspected giant cell arteritis, temporal artery biopsy may help to confirming the diagnosis, but the pathological abnormalities are usually patchy in distribution. Therefore, a normal study should not exclude the diagnosis or lead to withdrawal of treatment.

REFERENCES

Lumbar Puncture

Fishman RA: *Cerebrospinal Fluid in Diseases of the Nervous System*, 2nd ed. Saunders, 1992.

Hayward RA, Shapiro MF, Oye RK: Laboratory testing on cerebrospinal fluid: A reappraisal. *Lancet* 1987;1: 1–4.

Marton KI, Gean AD: The spinal tap: A new look at an old test. *Ann Intern Med* 1986;104:840–848.

Electrophysiological Studies

Aminoff MJ (editor): *Electrodiagnosis in Clinical Neurology,* 3rd ed. Churchill Livingstone, 1992.

Aminoff MJ: Evoked potential studies in neurological diagnosis and management. *Ann Neurol* 1990;28:706–710.

Report of the Therapeutics and Technology Assessment Subcommittee of the American Academy of Neurology: Assessment: Intraoperative neurophysiology. *Neurology* 1990;40:1644–1646.

Cranial & Spinal Imaging Studies

Council on Scientific Affairs and American Medical Association: Fundamentals of magnetic resonance imaging. *JAMA* 1098;258:3417–3423.

Miller GM, Forbes GS, Onofrio BM: Magnetic resonance imaging of the spine. *Mayo Clin Proc* 1989;64:986–1004.

Report of the Therapeutics and Technology Assessment Subcommittee of the American Academy of Neurology: Assessment: Positron emission tomography. *Neurology* 1991;41:163–167.

Ross JS et al: Magnetic resonance angiography of the extracranial carotid arteries and intracranial vessels: A review. *Neurology* 1989;39:1369–1376.

Ultrasonography

Lewis BD, James EM, Welch TJ: Current applications of duplex and color Doppler ultrasound imaging: Carotid and peripheral vascular system. *Mayo Clin Proc* 1989;64:1147–1157.

Appendices

APPENDIX A: OUTLINE FOR RECORDING THE NEUROLOGICAL HISTORY & EXAMINATION

Despite recent advances in diagnostic neuroradiology and electrophysiology, an accurate, detailed case history and neurological examination remain the cornerstones of neurological diagnosis. The neurological examination can present a formidable challenge to inexperienced physicians. Conducting and interpreting the examination is facilitated by adopting a standardized, methodical approach that can be used to evaluate a wide variety of neurological complaints and by tailoring the examination of more detailed aspects of neurological function to the particular problem at hand. The following scheme has been found useful in organizing the neurological case history and examination. Even though there is no correct order in which elements of the examination should be performed, an orderly, systematic approach will ensure that no major aspect of the examination is overlooked and that neither the patient nor the examiner emerges exhausted from the ordeal.

HISTORY

Identification
1. Patient's name.
2. Age, sex, and race.
3. Handedness.
4. Reliability.

Chief Complaint
1. Nature.
2. Duration.

History of Present Illness
1. Quality of symptoms.
2. Mode of onset.

3. Course since onset.
4. Frequency of symptoms.
5. Duration of (episodic) symptoms.
6. Severity of symptoms.
7. Precipitating or aggravating factors.
8. Ameliorating factors, including medications.
9. Presence or absence of related symptoms.
10. Previous diagnostic evaluations.

Prior Medical History
1. Perinatal history and developmental milestones, if applicable.
2. Immunizations.
3. Major illnesses.
4. Operations.
5. Trauma.
6. Past and present medications, including dosages and indications.
7. Allergies.

Family History
1. Family tree.
2. Consanguinity.
3. Relatives with problems similar to patient's problem.
4. Age and state of health of living relatives.
5. Age at death and cause of death of deceased relatives.

Social History
1. Education.
2. Employment, including occupational hazards and exposures.
3. Travel.
4. Problems at work or home.

5. Hobbies.
6. Habits, especially alcohol, tobacco, and other drugs.
7. Sexual orientation.

Review of Systems
1. Skin.
2. Eyes, ears, nose, throat.
3. Respiratory.
4. Cardiovascular.
5. Gastrointestinal.
6. Genitourinary.
7. Musculoskeletal.
8. Endocrinological.
9. Immunological.
10. Neurological.
11. Psychiatric.

NEUROLOGICAL EXAMINATION

Higher Cortical Function
(See Chapter 1.)
1. Orientation to person, place, and time.
2. Attention and concentration.
3. Mood and affect.
4. Judgment.
5. Memory.
6. Language and speech.
7. Agnosia.
8. Apraxia.

Gait & Stance
(See p 151.)
1. Normal.
2. Frontal lobe (apraxic) gait.
3. Spastic gait (unilateral or bilateral).
4. Ataxic gait.
5. Parkinsonian gait.
6. Waddling gait.
7. Steppage gait.
8. Romberg's sign.

Cranial Nerves
A. Olfactory (I): Identification by smell of oil of cloves, peppermint, coffee, or tobacco.
B. Optic (II): (See Chapter 5.)
1. Visual acuity in each eye.
2. Visual field in each eye (chart deficits).
3. Ophthalmoscopic examination of cornea, optic disk, retina, macula, and blood vessels in each eye.
C. Oculomotor (III), Trochlear (IV), and Abducens (VI):8 (See Chapter 5.)
1. Pupils
   a. Size.
   b. Shape.
   c. Direct and consensual reaction to light.
   d. Reaction to accommodation.

2. Appearance of eyes
   a. Ptosis.
   b. Exophthalmos.
3. Eye movements
   a. Limitations
      (1) Determine muscles involved by inspection.
      (2) If diplopia is reported, confirm muscles involved by red glass test.
   b. Conjugate movements
   c. Nystagmus
      (1) Precipitating direction of gaze.
      (2) Horizontal, vertical, or rotatory character.
      (3) Direction of fast component.
D. Trigeminal (V):
1. Reflexes
   a. Corneal.
   b. Jaw jerk.
2. Sensory: Touch, pain, and temperature sensation in first (ophthalmic), second (maxillary), and third (mandibular) divisions
3. Motor: Jaw opening and closing
E. Facial (VII):
1. Eye closure.
2. Smile.
3. Wrinkling of forehead.
4. Taste (anterior two-thirds of tongue).
F. Acoustic (VIII):
1. Auditory acuity.
2. Weber test (lateralization).
3. Rinne's test (air versus bone conduction).
4. Oculovestibular (caloric) testing, if applicable.
G. Glossopharyngeal (IX) and Vagus (X):
1. Touch sensation on posterior pharyngeal wall.
2. Gag reflex or swallowing.
3. Elevation of palate (midline or deviated).
H. Accessory (XI):
1. Head turning.
2. Shoulder shrug.
3. Sternocleidomastoid or trapezius atrophy.
I. Hypoglossal (XII):
1. Tongue atrophy or fasciculation.
2. Rapidity and strength of tongue movements.

Motor System
(See Chapter 6.)
A. Muscle Atrophy or Hypertrophy (Indicate location.)
B. Fasciculations: (Indicate location.)
C. Abnormal Movements: (Indicate character, location, precipitating or aggravating factors.)
1. Tremor.
2. Myoclonus.
3. Asterixis.
4. Dystonia.
5. Athetosis.
6. Chorea.
7. Ballismus.

8. Tics.
D. Tone (in all limbs):
1. Normal.
2. Hypotonia.
3. Spasticity.
4. Rigidity (with or without cogwheeling).
5. Paratonia.
E. Power:
1. Strength of individual muscles (a **or** b)
   a. Normal or mild/moderate/severe weakness.
   b. Five-point scale
   0 = No movement.
   1 = Barely discernible movement.
   2 = Movement only with the force of gravity eliminated.
   3 = Movement against gravity only.
   4 = Movement against gravity and resistance.
   5 = Full strength.
2. Pattern of weakness.
   a. Single peripheral nerve.
   b. Single nerve root.
   c. Diffuse, symmetrical, proximal > distal.
   d. Diffuse, symmetrical, distal > proximal.
   e. Pyramidal (extensors > flexors in arms, flexors > extensors in legs).
F. Fine movements:
1. Finger and foot tapping (note rate and regularity).
2. Skilled motor acts (eg, buttoning clothes).
G. Coordination:
1. Finger-to-nose (note intention tremor, past-pointing).
2. Heel-to-shin (note irregularity).
3. Rapid alternating movements (note irregularity).
4. Rebound.
5. Tandem (heel-to-toe) gait.

Sensory System
(See Chapter 7.)
A. Primary Sensory Modalities: (Chart deficits.)
1. Touch.
2. Pain (superficial and deep).
3. Temperature.
4. Vibration.
5. Joint position.
B. Cortical Sensory Modalities:
1. Stereognosis.
2. Graphesthesia.
3. Stimulus localization.
4. Two-point discrimination.
5. Extinction, with double simultaneous stimulation.
C. Sensory Level (if present)
D. Dissociated Sensory Loss (if present)

Reflexes
A. Tendon Reflexes:
1. Grading system
   0 = Absent despite reinforcement.
   1 = Decreased.
   2 = Normal.
   3 = Hyperactive.
   4 = Hyperactive with clonus.
2. Segmental innervation
   a. Jaw jerk (cranial nerve V).
   b. Biceps reflex (C5 and 6).
   c. Brachioradialis reflex (C5 and 6).
   d. Triceps reflex (C7 and 8).
   e. Finger flexor (Hoffmann's) reflex (C8 and T1).
   f. Patellar reflex (L3 and 4).
   g. Hamstring reflex (L5 and S1).
   h. Ankle reflex (S1).
B. Superficial Reflexes:
1. Upper abdominal (T7–10).
2. Lower abdominal (T11 and 12).
3. Cremasteric (L1 and 2).
4. Plantar (S1).
5. Anal (S4 and 5).
C. Primitive Reflexes (frontal release signs):
1. Hand and foot grasps.
2. Suck, snout, rooting, and palmomental reflexes.
3. Glabellar reflex.

Autonomic System
(Note level of deficit, if present)
1. Sweating.
2. Skin temperature.
3. Cyanosis or pallor.
4. Trophic changes of skin or nails.
5. Postural change in blood pressure.

Neurovascular System
1. Brachial pulses and blood pressure in both arms.
2. Carotid pulses at angle of jaw.
3. Carotid or supraclavicular bruits.
4. Temporal artery pulses, tenderness, nodularity.

Skull
1. Size, contour, prominences, deformities.
2. Orbital or cranial bruits.
3. Tenderness to percussion.

Spine
1. Deformity.
2. Tenderness.
3. Bruits.
4. Signs of meningeal irritation (Kernig, Brudzinski).
5. Signs of nerve root irritation (Lasègue).

REFERENCE

Haerer AF (ed): *DeJong's Neurologic Examination,* 5th ed. Lippincott, 1992.

APPENDIX B: A BRIEF EXAMINATION OF THE NERVOUS SYSTEM

Occasionally, a screening neurological examination briefer than that outlined in Appendix A is needed. An approach to such a screening examination follows.

Cognitive Function

The level of consciousness (whether the patient is awake and alert, confused and somnolent or agitated, or comatose) should be noted and orientation to person, place, and time specifically tested. Patients with acute confusional states typically demonstrate impaired orientation to time and place; patients with psychiatric disorders may also be disoriented to person. Language function can be tested rapidly by asking the patient to repeat a phrase such as "no ifs, ands, or buts," since repetition is impaired in most aphasias. The examination of cognitive function is discussed in detail elsewhere (see Chapter 1).

Gait

A singularly helpful test for detecting nervous system dysfunction is observation of the gait (see p 151). Every patient must be observed standing and walking. Standing, starting to walk, stopping, and turning should each be assessed and the associated movements of the limbs noted with each maneuver. These actions require coordination of sensory, motor, cerebellar, visual, and vestibular function and thus provide a sensitive indication of abnormal functioning of these systems.

Cranial Nerves

Cranial nerve abnormalities are the hallmark of brain stem dysfunction and of some neuromuscular disorders. They can also reveal the presence of hemispheric disease or elevated intracranial pressure.

Optic disk swelling (papilledema) is the cardinal sign of increased intracranial pressure; spontaneous venous pulsations upon the disk indicate that intracranial pressure is normal.

Examination of the visual fields surveys the visual pathways of the retina, optic nerves, and chiasm; the lateral geniculate body; the temporal and parietal lobes; and the occipital cortex. A rapid screening technique consists of assessing the patient's ability to detect small movements of the examiner's finger in the temporal fields (or, in obtunded patients, the response to threat).

Unilateral facial weakness that involves especially the lower part of the face is a common sign of contralateral hemispheric lesions. Facial strength should be tested by having patients close their eyes as tightly as possible so that the eyelashes are "buried". Asymmetry of eye closure—or the examiner's ability to open one or both of a patient's eyes against resistance—is a clear sign of motor system dysfunction. Facial grimacing with retraction of the lips when patients are asked to show their teeth may also reveal facial weakness.

Motor System

The most common abnormality affecting the motor system is upper motor neuron, or pyramidal weakness, such as results from hemispheric stroke. Severe hemiparesis or hemiplegia is obvious to even the inexperienced examiner, but even very mild hemiparesis can be detected by observing slowed fine finger movements or minor weakness or increased tone in a pyramidal distribution. Thus, the power of finger abductors, finger and wrist extensors, triceps, dorsiflexors of the foot, and the hamstring muscles should be compared on the two sides.

Sensory System

The distribution of regional or segmental sensory abnormalities can be discerned by asking patients to sketch out on their bodies the limits of the perceived sensory impairment. The peripheral nerve or nerve root to which this pattern of sensory involvement best corresponds can then be determined (see Figure 7–4). Polyneuropathy usually produces distal, symmetrical sensory deficits that are especially prominent in the feet. If present, such deficits should then be differentiated according to whether large nerve fibers (mediating vibratory sense) or small nerve fibers (mediating pain and temperature appreciation) are predominantly affected. The differential diagnosis of these disorders can then be undertaken (see Chapter 7).

Reflexes

The major issue here is whether the deep tendon reflexes are symmetrical, which suggests that no lateralized impairment of upper or lower motor neuron function is present. Reflexes should be elicited by percussing the tendons on both sides with the same force and with the limbs on both sides in similar positions; if no asymmetry is found, the force of percussion should be progressively decreased until the threshold for eliciting the response can be compared from side to side. Impairment of a single reflex is most compatible with nerve root involvement at the level of the reflex (C5–6, biceps and brachioradialis reflex; C7–8, triceps reflex; L3–4, knee jerk; S1, ankle jerk). Bilateral depression or the absence of ankle jerks suggests a polyneuropathy.

In eliciting the plantar reflex, stroking the lateral border of the sole of the foot leads to plantar flexion of the great toe in normal subjects, whereas extension occurs in those with upper motor neuron disturbances (Babinski's sign).

APPENDIX C: CLINICAL EXAMINATION OF COMMON ISOLATED PERIPHERAL NERVE DISORDERS

The accompanying illustrations are a guide for examining sensory and motor function of selected peripheral nerves: radial (Figure 1), median (Figure 2), ulnar (Figure 3), peroneal (Figure 4), and femoral (Figure 5).

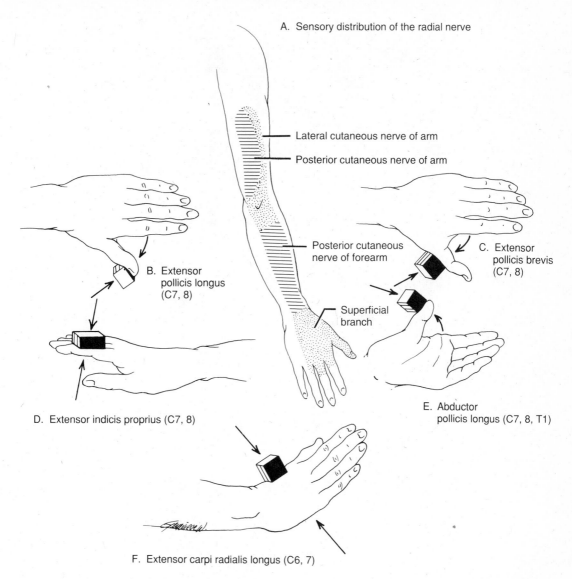

A. Sensory distribution of the radial nerve

Lateral cutaneous nerve of arm

Posterior cutaneous nerve of arm

B. Extensor pollicis longus (C7, 8)

Posterior cutaneous nerve of forearm

C. Extensor pollicis brevis (C7, 8)

Superficial branch

D. Extensor indicis proprius (C7, 8)

E. Abductor pollicis longus (C7, 8, T1)

F. Extensor carpi radialis longus (C6, 7)

Figure 1. Testing the radial nerve. **A:** Sensory distribution. The radial nerve supplies the dorsolateral surface of the upper arm, forearm, wrist, and hand; the dorsal surface of the thumb; the dorsal surface of the index and middle fingers above the distal interphalangeal joints; and the lateral half of the dorsal surface of the ring finger above the distal inter-phalangeal joint. **B:** Extensor pollicis longus. The thumb is extended at the interphalangeal joint against resistance. **C:** Extensor pollicis brevis. The thumb is extended at the metacarpophalangeal joint against resistance. **D:** Extensor indicis proprius. The index finger is extended at the metacarpophalangeal joint against resistance. **E:** Abductor pollicis longus. The thumb is abducted (elevated in a plane at 90 degrees to the palm) at the carpometacarpal joint against resistance. **F:** Extensor carpi radialis longus. The wrist is extended toward the radial (thumb) side against resistance.

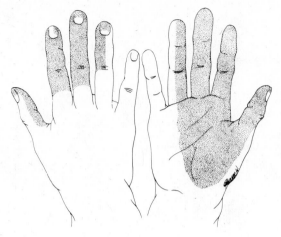

A. Sensory distribution of the median nerve

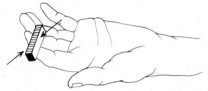

B. Flexor digitorum profundus I and II (C7,**8**, T1)

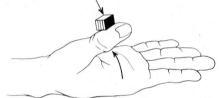

C. Abductor pollicis brevis (C8, **T1**)

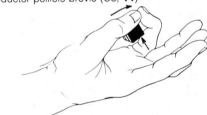

D. Opponens pollicis (C8, **T1**)

Figure 2. Testing the median nerve. **A:** Sensory distribution. The median nerve supplies the dorsal surface of the index and middle fingers; the lateral half of the dorsal surface of the ring finger; the lateral two-thirds of the palm; the palmar surface of the thumb, index finger, middle fingers; and the lateral half of the palmar surface of the ring finger. **B:** Flexor digitorum profundus I and II. The index and middle fingers are flexed at the distal interphalangeal joints against resistance. **C:** Abductor pollicis brevis. The thumb is abducted (elevated at 90 degrees to the plane of the palm) at the metacarpophalangeal joints against resistance. **D:** Opponens pollicis. The thumb is crossed over the palm to touch the little finger against resistance.

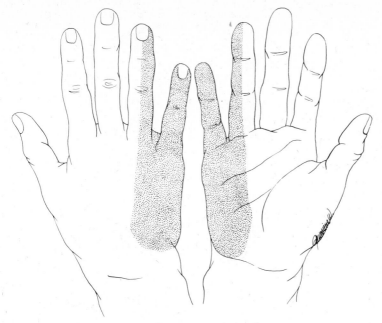

A. Sensory distribution of the ulnar nerve

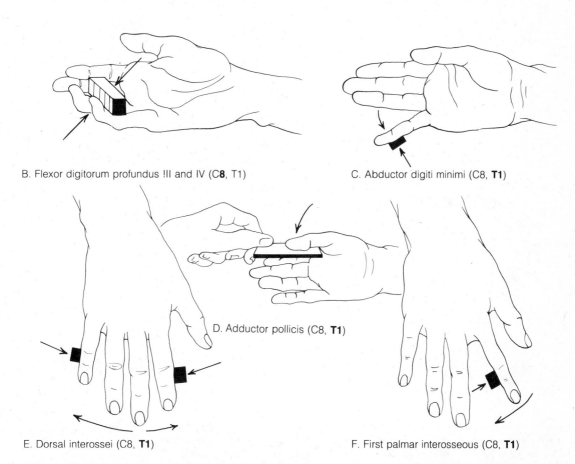

B. Flexor digitorum profundus III and IV (C**8**, T1)

C. Abductor digiti minimi (C8, **T1**)

D. Adductor pollicis (C8, **T1**)

E. Dorsal interossei (C8, **T1**)

F. First palmar interosseous (C8, **T1**)

Figure 3. Testing the ulnar nerve. **A:** Sensory distribution. The ulnar nerve supplies the dorsal and palmar surfaces of the medial one-third of the hand; the dorsal and palmar surfaces of the little finger; and the dorsal and palmar surfaces of the medial half of the ring finger. **B:** Flexor digitorum profundus III and IV. The index and middle fingers are flexed at the distal interphalangeal joints against resistance. **C:** Abductor digiti minimi. The little finger is abducted against resistance. **D:** Adductor pollicis. A piece of paper is grasped between the thumb and the palm with the thumbnail at 90 degrees to the plane of the palm while the examiner tries to pull the paper away. **E:** Dorsal interossei. The fingers are abducted against resistance. **F:** First palmar interosseous. The abducted index finger is adducted against resistance.

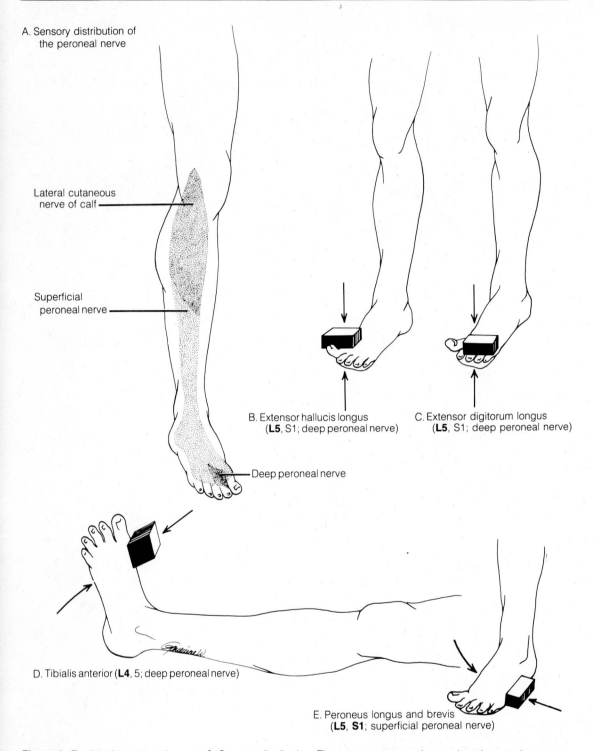

A. Sensory distribution of the peroneal nerve

Lateral cutaneous nerve of calf

Superficial peroneal nerve

B. Extensor hallucis longus (**L5**, S1; deep peroneal nerve)

C. Extensor digitorum longus (**L5**, S1; deep peroneal nerve)

Deep peroneal nerve

D. Tibialis anterior (**L4**, 5; deep peroneal nerve)

E. Peroneus longus and brevis (**L5**, **S1**; superficial peroneal nerve)

Figure 4. Testing the peroneal nerve. **A:** Sensory distribution. The common peroneal nerve has three main sensory branches: The lateral cutaneous nerve of the calf supplies the lateral surface of the calf, the superficial peroneal nerve supplies the lateral surface of the lower leg and the dorsum of the foot, and the deep peroneal nerve supplies a roughly triangular patch of skin on the dorsum of the foot between the first and second toes. **B:** Extensor hallucis longus. The large toe is extended (dorsiflexed) against resistance. **C:** Extensor digitorum longus. The second, third, fourth, and fifth toes are extended against resistance. **D:** Tibialis anterior. The foot is dorsiflexed at the ankle against resistance. **E:** Peroneus longus and brevis. The foot is everted (rotated laterally) at the ankle against resistance.

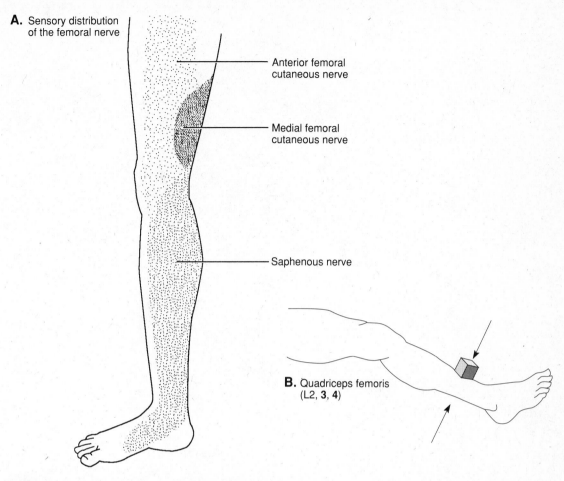

Figure 5. Testing the femoral nerve. **A:** Sensory distribution. The femoral nerve has three main sensory branches. The anterior femoral cutaneous nerve supplies the anterior surface of the thigh, the medial femoral cutaneous nerve supplies the anteromedial surface of the thigh, and the saphenous nerve supplies the medial surface of the lower leg, ankle, and foot. **B:** Quadriceps femoris. The leg is extended at the knee against resistance.

Index

NOTE: Page numbers in boldface type indicate a major discussion. A *t* following a page number indicates tabular material, an *i* following a page number indicates an illustration. All drugs are listed under their generic names.